Current Status and Future Perspective of Neuroblastoma

Current Status and Future Perspective of Neuroblastoma

Edited by **Michael Jones**

hayle medical

New York

Published by Hayle Medical,
30 West, 37th Street, Suite 612,
New York, NY 10018, USA
www.haylemedical.com

Current Status and Future Perspective of Neuroblastoma
Edited by Michael Jones

International Standard Book Number: 978-1-63241-105-1 (Hardback)

Printed in China.

Contents

Preface

Over the recent decade, advancements and applications have progressed exponentially. This has led to the increased interest in this field and projects are being conducted to enhance knowledge. The main objective of this book is to present some of the critical challenges and provide insights into possible solutions. This book will answer the varied questions that arise in the field and also provide an increased scope for furthering studies.

Neuroblastoma is composed of biologically varied tumors. This book provides an extensive analysis into the current prevalence of the disease and its future treatment modalities. Genomic/molecular properties exclusive to the specific tumors firmly link to the clinical results of patients. Formulation of risk stratification models post the analysis of biological characteristics of every case has resulted in huge success in patient management. Nevertheless, the trend of enhancing survival rates in this disease over the past 30 years has begun to level off, and presently available treatment options have nearly reached their maximized intensity. Moreover, aggressive treatment causes serious morbidities to the survivors. The book encompasses valuable data and insights from the world's experts in this field. It will serve as a great source of reference for all the investigators working hard and struggling for the children affected by this disease.

I hope that this book, with its visionary approach, will be a valuable addition and will promote interest among readers. Each of the authors has provided their extraordinary competence in their specific fields by providing different perspectives as they come from diverse nations and regions. I thank them for their contributions.

Editor

Part 1

Neuroblastoma, Clinical Update

1

Recurrent Neuroblastoma

Loretta M.S. Lau[1] and Wendy B. London[2]
[1]The Children's Hospital at Westmead and University of Sydney
[2]Dana-Farber Harvard Cancer Center and Children's Hospital Boston; Children's Oncology Group Statistics and Data Center
[1]Australia
[2]USA

1. Introduction

Advances in neuroblastoma (NB) treatment over the last three decades have resulted in our ability to cure over 70% of children with NB using the current risk-directed therapeutic approach. However, until very recently, improvement in treatment outcome was mainly attributable to the increased survival of low and intermediate-risk patients. The outcome of high-risk NB, especially in children older than 18 months with metastatic disease, remains poor. Despite intensive multimodal therapy, over 50% of patients with high-risk NB relapse with a dismal long-term outcome (Lau et al., 2004; Santana et al., 2008). While immunotherapy has recently increased the post-transplant 2-year event-free survival (EFS) of high-risk NB from 46% to 66% (Yu et al., 2010), longer follow-up is required to monitor for late relapse.

In the last era, children with NB have been offered a wide variety of salvage treatments following disease recurrence. Up to half of these patients achieve some response or stable disease, and survival after relapse is longer in patients who have received salvage therapy (Lau et al., 2004). Chronic NB is also an emerging phenomenon in a subset of patients (Kushner et al., 2002). The longer survival after relapse is also likely due to early detection of disease recurrence as a result of employing more sophisticated surveillance studies in recent years. Furthermore, a proportion of relapsed patients are offered novel agents in phase I/II clinical trials. Unfortunately, response to any form of relapsed therapy is rarely sustained. Future research leading to a better understanding of the factors influencing the clinical course of post-relapse is therefore very important, such that clinicians can select the appropriate salvage therapy: to avoid intensive toxic treatment in patients likely to have short survival following disease recurrence and to test potentially beneficial therapy.

2. Clinical presentation of recurrent NB

Similar to NB at initial diagnosis, the signs and symptoms of relapsed NB reflect the site of local and metastatic disease. However, due to the high frequency of metastatic disease at the presentation of relapse, symptoms and signs related to distant metastases are significantly more common than at diagnosis. Isolated metastatic relapse is found in 60% of patients, followed by combined locoregional and metastatic relapse in 32% of patients (Table 1; (Lau et al., 2004). Isolated local relapse at the primary tumor site is uncommon (6%) and is generally confined to patients with non-metastatic disease at diagnosis. Bone and/or bone marrow disease are present in 75 to 85% of patients with recurrent disease (Kushner et al., 2002; Lau et al., 2004). As a result, bone pain from osteomedullary metastases represents the most common presenting symptom and is reported by 68% of patients with symptomatic relapse (Lau et al., 2004). Other symptoms from distant metastases include lethargy, irritability, soft tissue mass arising from bony involvement of the calvarium, periorbital ecchymosis (raccoon eye), pallor and bruising from bone marrow infiltration and cytopenia, and soft tissue mass from lymph node metastases. Depending on the frequency of follow-up and the type of investigations used to monitor relapse, 30 to 73% of patients are asymptomatic at relapse (Kushner et al., 2009; Lau et al., 2004).

Type of relapse	
Local only	2
Metastatic only	19
Local and metastatic	10
Site of distant relapse	
Bone, bone marrow +/- others	16
Bone and non-bone marrow	6
CNS and bone marrow	1
Bone marrow only	1
CNS only	2
Lung only	2
Lymph node only	1
Symptoms/Signs	
Yes	22
No	9
Time from diagnosis to relapse	median 16.1 months (1.7 – 35.8 months)
Survival post relapse	median 8.4 months (0.2 - 51.1 months)
1-year OS	39%
3-year OS	11%

Table 1. Characteristics of 31 relapsed NB patients from a single institution (Lau et al., 2004)

While central nervous system (CNS) disease is very rare at diagnosis, CNS recurrence has been reported in 1 to 5% of all patients with Stage 4 NB (Kellie et al., 1991; Kramer et al., 2001; Matthay et al., 2003a; Shaw & Eden, 1992). CNS metastases represent 6 to 10% of all disease recurrences and 50 to 70% of these CNS recurrences are isolated CNS relapse. This is thought to be related to prolonged survival of high-risk NB following intensive systemic therapy and the CNS as a sanctuary site for NB. Neuroaxis metastases can be intraparenchymal, leptomeningeal, or both. Patients can present with nausea, vomiting, headaches, seizures, drowsiness, cranial nerve symptoms, motor weakness/paralysis, and back pain (Matthay et al., 2003a).

Fifty percent of relapses present within 18 months from diagnosis and 77% by 24 months (Kushner et al., 2009; Lau et al., 2004; London & Castel et al., 2011; Santana et al., 2008). For CNS recurrence, the median time of relapse was 12 to 20 months (Kellie et al., 1991; Kramer et al., 2001; Matthay et al., 2003a; Shaw & Eden, 1992). Even though late relapse is uncommon, a small number of patients present with first disease recurrence after 5 years and on rare occasions beyond 10 years from diagnosis. Cotterill et al. reported that amongst 406 patients who were in first remission five years from diagnosis, 3% subsequently relapsed and most late relapse patients had Stage 4 disease at diagnosis (Cotterill et al., 2001).

3. Risk of disease recurrence

The 'events' considered for analyses of EFS typically include relapse, progression, secondary malignancy, or death (from any cause prior to the detection of disease relapse or progression). In the majority of NB patients, the first event that patients experience is disease relapse or progression. Therefore, factors that are prognostic of EFS are the same risk factors that are prognostic for NB relapse. Established risk factors for relapse include older age at diagnosis, higher disease stage, *MYCN* amplification, DNA diploidy, and chromosome 1p and 11q aberration.

Since the early 1970's, age at diagnosis has been considered a useful factor in predicting the occurrence of first relapse, disease progression, or death (Evans et al., 1971), and has persisted as highly prognostic despite the discovery of new molecular prognostic factors over the last 30 years. Prior to 2005, an age cut-off of 12 months was used for risk group stratification. Since 2005, a cut-off of 18 months (547 days) has been adopted by the Children's Oncology Group (COG) (London et al., 2005) and was included in the International Neuroblastoma Risk Group (INRG) staging system in 2009 (Monclair et al., 2009). In INRG cohort of 8,800 patients, the 5-year EFS was 42% for patients ≥18 months, compared with 82% for patients <18 months old (Cohn & Pearson et al., 2009) (Table 2). The 5-year EFS for Stage 4 NB was significantly worse than that of non-Stage 4 disease (35% vs. 83%). For tumors with *MYCN* amplification, 11q aberration, 1p aberration, and DNA ploidy ≤ 1, the 5-year EFS were 29%, 35%, 38%, and 55%, respectively. Patients ≥18 months old with Stage 4 *MYCN* amplified NB had the worst outcome (5-year EFS of 19%). In contrast, in spite of Stage 4 disease, the 5-year EFS was 85% for Stage 4 patients younger than 18 months with tumor DNA ploidy >1. In relation to Stage 4S disease, *MYCN* amplification reduced EFS from 82% to 41%, and within the *MYCN* non-amplified group, 11q aberration decreased EFS from 86% to 38% (Ambros et al., 2009).

Moreover, in addition to disease progression on therapy, metastatic response to therapy measured by semi-quantitative metaiodobenzylguanidine (MIBG) score identifies a subgroup of ultra-high-risk patients. In a study of 75 patients, patients with MIBG score >2 after 4 cycles of induction therapy had significantly lower 5-year EFS than those with MIBG score ≤2 (11% vs. 39%) (Matthay et al., 2003b). A recent study of over 250 patients reported a 3-year EFS of 8.3% in patients with a MIBG score >5 post-induction, compared with EFS of 42% in patients with MIBG score ≤ 2 (Yanik et al., 2010). High ferritin levels in Stage 4 patients ≥18 months also reduced 5-year EFS from 48% to 21% for *MYCN* non-amplified tumors and from 28% to 19% for *MYCN* amplified tumors (Cohn & Pearson et al., 2009).

While the majority of disease recurrences occur in high-risk patients, a small percentage of relapsed patients had localized NB at diagnosis and subsequently present with local or metastatic relapse. Factors predictive of relapse in localized NB include the presence of image-defined risk factors (IDRF), tumor histology, *MYCN* amplification, 1q and 11q aberration, and ALK overexpression. In the INRG pretreatment risk classification system, patients with localized NB and IDRF (Stage L2; 5-year EFS of 78%) have significantly worse outcome than those without IDRF (Stage L1; 5-year EFS of 90%) (Monclair et al., 2009). Non-Stage 4 patients with *MYCN* amplified tumors have a 5-year EFS of 46%, compared with *MYCN* non-amplified tumors with a 5-year EFS of 87% (Table 2). Within the *MYCN* non-amplified cohort, the EFS of patients with 11q aberration and/or undifferentiated histology is significantly lower than those without these features (61% vs. 80%)(Cohn & Pearson et al., 2009). Specifically, for patients with stroma-poor localized resectable tumors, the presence of 1q gain and absence of 7p gain may predict relapse (Pezzolo et al., 2009). Furthermore, high ALK protein expression, though uncommon, may be prognostic in Stage 1 and 2 patients. Six of eight Stage 1 and 2 patients with high wild-type ALK expression experience relapse (Parodi et al., 2011).

	5-year EFS ± SE (%)	
	Yes	No
Age ≥18 months	42 ± 1	82 ± 1
Stage 4	35 ± 1	83 ± 1
MYCN amp.		
all stages	29 ± 2	74 ± 1
non-Stage 4	46 ± 4	87 ± 1
Stage 4S	41 ± 9	82 ± 2
Stage 4 & age ≥18 months	19 ± 3	48 ± 5
Stage 4 & ploidy >1		85 ± 3
11q aberration		
all patients	35 ± 5	68 ± 3
non-Stage 4 & MYCN non-amp.	61 ± 11	80 ± 16
Stage 4S & MYCN non-amp.	38 ± 30	87 ± 7
1p	38 ± 3	74 ± 2
DNA ploidy ≤ 1	55 ± 2	76 ± 1

Table 2. EFS by prognostic factors in a cohort of 8,800 patients (Cohn & Pearson et al., 2009)

Furthermore, MYCN amplification, and lumbar puncture at diagnosis were found to be significant risk factors for CNS recurrences in a report of 434 Stage 4 NB patients (Matthay et al., 2003a). In another study of 251 Stage 4 patients, lumbar puncture and elevated serum lactate dehydrogenase (LDH) were reported to be risk factors (Kramer et al., 2001). In these two studies, 28% to 36% of the patients with CNS recurrence had a lumbar puncture during diagnosis. As for late relapse beyond 5 years, a multivariate analysis of 422 patients demonstrated a relative risk of 10.5 for late relapse in patients >12 months with Stage 4 disease at diagnosis, and a relative risk of 4.2 for those with prior relapse (Cotterill et al., 2001). For patients who remained in first remission 5 years from diagnosis, the 10-year progression-free survival (PFS) for patients >12 months with Stage 4 disease at diagnosis was lower for other children (88% vs. 98%).

3.1 Detection of disease recurrence

A multitude of follow-up studies have been used to detect disease recurrence. These include imaging with ultrasonography, computed tomography (CT), magnetic resonance imaging

(MRI), bone scan, MIBG scan and positron emission tomography (PET), as well as bone marrow examination and urine catecholamines. The choice of tests depends on whether the patient presents with symptoms and signs indicative of the location of relapse, and therefore guide the studies to be performed. However, when surveillance studies are undertaken to detect asymptomatic relapse, a number of factors including the risk of relapse, as well as the sensitivity/specificity, invasiveness, and the cost of the studies will need to be taken into consideration.

3.2 Locoregional disease

CT is commonly the test of choice for imaging locoregional recurrence in the thorax (Figure 1), abdomen, and pelvis (Brisse et al., 2011), especially in high risk patients who have received local radiotherapy, and the radiation dose from CT is relatively small compared with that from radiotherapy. For patients with low- and intermediate-risk NB, ultrasound of the abdominal and pelvic region could be considered the first imaging examination to avoid radiation exposure from CT, particularly when there is a low index of suspicion of relapse. MRI provides effective imaging without radiation, but it is limited by availability, cost, and the need for sedation in young children. However, for paraspinal tumors with intraspinal extension, MRI is recommended for better visualization of the spinal cord, nerve roots, and the subarachnoid space (Sofka et al., 1999). MIBG scintigraphy, which is routinely used to detect osteomedullary recurrence, will also demonstrate local recurrence (Figure 1).

3.3 Metastatic disease

Detection of metastases is an integral component of monitoring for NB recurrence, as >95% of relapses are metastatic, and bone and bone marrow are the most common metastatic sites. MIBG scintigraphy is an accurate method for detecting osteomedullary metastases (Figure 1) as there is no physiological uptake of MIBG in bone or bone marrow. MIBG, an analog of norepinephrine and a guanethidine derivative, is taken up and stored in NB cells expressing the norepinephrine transporter and is radio-iodinated for imaging use (Boubaker & Bischof Delaloye, 2008). MIBG scan has a reported sensitivity and specificity of 88% and 83%, respectively (Vik et al., 2009). In comparison, ^{99m}Tc-technetium bone scan is reported to have a sensitivity of 75% and specificity of 50% for the detection of skeletal metastases (Jacobs et al., 1990). As a result, ^{123}I-MIBG imaging has superseded the use of bone scan for demonstrating bone metastases, with the exception of tumors that are not MIBG-avid (Brisse et al., 2011). Approximately 10% of NB tumors do not concentrate MIBG (Carlin et al., 2003). False-negative MIBG scan has been observed when only a small amount of tumor cells are present in the bone marrow (Kushner et al., 2003b). Hence, bilateral bone marrow biopsy is still recommended in order to exclude bone marrow metastases (Matthay et al., 2010). Small hepatic lesions may not be detected by MIBG due to the high physiological uptake in the liver and are better depicted by ultrasound, CT or MRI (Brisse et al., 2011).

^{18}Fluorine-deoxyglucose (FDG) PET scan, which measures the metabolic characteristics of cells, has also been used for detecting NB. Compared with MIBG, FDG-PET was reported to be superior in the evaluation of small soft tissue lesions and Stage 1 and 2 tumors. However, FDG-PET was found to be less sensitive than MIBG in high-risk disease as MIBG was more sensitive than FDG-PET in the detection of bone metastases (Sharp et al., 2009; Taggart et al., 2009). FDG-PET is also limited by the high physiologic uptake of FDG in the brain and can hide skull lesions. Nonetheless, FDG-PET may have a role in monitoring MIBG-negative disease.

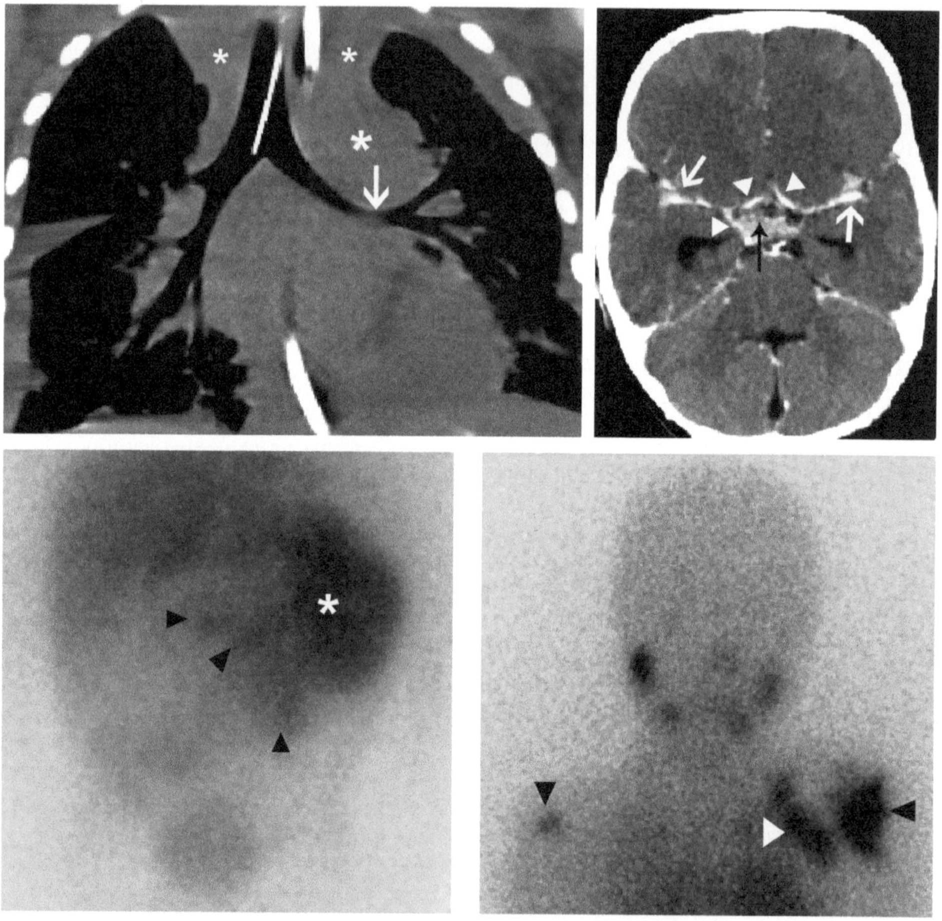

Top left: CT chest shows widespread mediastinal and hilar lymphadenopathy (asterisks) with compression of the left main bronchus (arrow) from distant metastases of recurrent abdominal NB. Patients presented with shortness of breath. Top right: CT brain shows multiple nodular enhancing leptomeningeal deposits in the suprasellar cistern (black arrow) with encasement of the Circle of Willis (Δ) and middle cerebral arteries bilaterally (white arrows) in a NB patient, who presented with increasing drowsiness at the time of isolated CNS relapse. Bottom left: MIBG scan demonstrates a large local recurrence (asterisk) in the left abdomen, with mixed areas of low and intense MIBG uptake. There are also multiple small foci of mild to moderate MIBG uptake in the mesentery and para-aortic locations (▲). Bottom right: MIBG scan shows skeletal metastases in both proximal humeri (▲) and spread to the left axillary lymph nodes (Δ).

Fig. 1. Imaging of NB disease recurrence.

NB patients with symptoms and signs suggestive of CNS metastases are best imaged with CT and/or MRI of the brain and spinal cord for parenchymal brain lesions and leptomeningeal spread (Figure 1). While MIBG can be positive with CNS involvement, the sensitivity of MIBG for CNS metastases is low. Matthay et al. reported that MIBG scans were negative in half of the patients with CNS recurrences (Matthay et al., 2003a). Difficulty in distinguishing cerebral lesions from skull lesions, especially without the help of SPECT images to localize a lesion, and the presence of meningeal disease without bulky lesions make MIBG unsuitable for evaluating CNS metastases.

3.4 Surveillance of asymptomatic relapse

The risk of relapse, the sensitivity and specificity of a specific investigation for detecting relapse, dose of radiation of an imaging study, invasiveness of a test, need of general anesthesia, and the cost of a study are all important factors to be considered when determining a surveillance protocol to detect asymptomatic relapse. For patients with high-risk NB, early detection of recurrence will likely result in better response to salvage therapy than in the setting of bulky metastatic disease. However, it is unclear whether early detection of recurrence prior to the onset of symptoms will lead to increased cure and whether a specific subgroup of NB patients will benefit from surveillance regimens that identify early relapse.

3.4.1 Surveillance of low and intermediate-risk NB

Patients with low probability of relapse should be followed up with tests that are non-invasive, require minimal or no sedation, and involve no or the lowest doses of radiation. Since children are known to have the highest inherent sensitivity to the carcinogenic effects of ionizing radiation (Brody et al., 2007), patients with low- and intermediate-risk NB who have no prior exposure to radiotherapy should be monitored with ultrasound and ^{123}I-MIBG. The radiation dose of ^{123}I-MIBG is 10% of that of ^{131}I-MIBG (Bombardieri et al., 2003). The INRG Task Force recommends post-therapy surveillance MIBG scan at 6-month intervals for 1 year for low-risk Stage 2 patients, and for 2 years for intermediate-risk patients (Matthay et al., 2010). While the measurement of urine catecholamines is a non-invasive test, it is not used as a follow-up investigation due to its poor sensitivity in detecting relapse. The sensitivity of urine catecholamines is only 23% for detecting isolated local recurrence (Simon et al., 2003).

3.4.2 Surveillance of high-risk NB

High-risk NB patients have a significantly higher risk of relapse with a 2-year EFS survival of 46% (Matthay et al., 2009b). Most patients undergo surveillance studies every 3 months until 3 years from diagnosis. CT, MIBG, and bone marrow examination are the most frequently utilized to monitor for disease recurrence. After this critical period, the frequency and type of follow-up studies are generally tailored to the likelihood of relapse of individual patients.

In a recent study of 91 high-risk patients with asymptomatic relapse, ^{123}I-MIBG scan was reported to have the highest sensitivity (82%) of detecting unsuspected relapse, compared with bone scan, bone marrow examination, CT (head), CT (chest/abdomen/pelvis), and urine catecholamines, with sensitivities of 27%, 28%, 22%, 29%, and 18%, respectively (Kushner et al., 2009). ^{123}I-MIBG scan was the sole indicator of unsuspected relapse in 27% of patients, whereas CT chest/abdomen/pelvis was the only positive test in 6% of patients, CT head in 3% of patients, bone marrow histology in 4.5% of patients, bone scan in 3% of patients, and urine catecholamines in none of the patients. However, ^{123}I-MIBG scan failed to reveal unsuspected relapse in the bone marrow in 25% of patients, in extracranial soft tissue in 21% of patients, and in head/orbits in 13% of patients. This study confirms the limitations of MIBG to detect low levels of bone marrow infiltration, small liver lesions, and

CNS metastases. In addition, urine catecholamine levels have limited use in diagnosing early recurrence with small tumor burden.

3.4.3 Surveillance of minimal residual disease

Minimal residual disease (MRD) in NB refers to the small number of circulating tumor cells present in the bone marrow, peripheral blood, or peripheral blood stem cells. Although histological examination of bone marrow is considered the gold standard for assessing bone marrow metastases, this conventional tool has a detection level of only 1% tumor cells (N.K. Cheung et al., 1997) and does not have sufficient sensitivity to detect MRD. Significant effort has therefore been directed towards the development of MRD detection methods in the last two decades. The ability to measure occult tumor cells is important for increasing the sensitivity of detecting metastases at diagnosis, evaluating response during treatment, and detecting early relapse post therapy.

The three main MRD detection techniques are immunocytology (IC), quantitative reverse transcriptase polymerase chain reaction (QRT-PCR), and flow cytometry (FC) (Beiske et al., 2005). For IC, both the SIOPEN Bone Marrow Committee and the INRG Task Force have recommended disialoganglioside (G_{D2}) as a target cell surface antigen and have developed standardized protocol for IC (Beiske et al., 2009; Swerts et al., 2005). Similarly, standard operating procedures have been developed by the SIOPEN Research Network and INRG Task Force for QRT-PCR, using tyrosine hydroxylase as target mRNA (Beiske et al., 2009; Viprey et al., 2007). The use of multiple molecular markers in QRT-PCR to increase the sensitivity and specificity of MRD detection has also been investigated (I.Y. Cheung et al., 1998; I.Y. Cheung et al., 2008; Stutterheim et al., 2009). FC has the advantage of measuring several antigens on single cells and can screen a large number of cells in a short time. CD9, CD56, CD45, CD81, anti-G_{D2} are the commonly used markers (Beiske et al., 2005). However, FC is considered to be less sensitive than IC for MRD detection in NB.

Despite all the technological advances made in MRD detection, the clinical relevance of MRD remains unclear. While the majority of studies demonstrated the prognostic value of MRD in bone marrow and blood, the level of clinically significant MRD and the timing of MRD were not consistent in these studies (Burchill et al., 2001; Cai et al., 2007; I.Y. Cheung et al., 2003; Moss et al., 1991; Seeger et al., 2000; Stutterheim et al., 2011). The clinical utility of MRD in NB at various stages of therapy requires validation in large prospective multi-center clinical trials using standardized protocols. Which marker(s) should be exploited? What level of MRD is indicative of relapse? Does very early intervention based on MRD improve survival post relapse? Answers to these questions will no doubt influence future surveillance program to monitor early relapse.

4. Survival following disease recurrence

Long-term cure after NB relapse is considered rare. For patients treated in the 1990's, the 5-year post-recurrence survival is 11% (Santana et al., 2008) and the median survival is 8 months (Lau et al., 2004). Patients who relapse within 12 to 16 months from diagnosis did even worse and median survival was only 2.5 months (Lau et al., 2004; Santana et al., 2008). Prognostic factors at diagnosis continue to have a significant impact on survival post relapse (London & Castel et al., 2011). In addition, a small number of patients are reported to have a protracted clinical course after relapse. Chronic NB may become more apparent in the next decade when prolonged survival with multiple recurrences is encountered with increasing frequency with novel therapeutics.

4.1 Factors predictive of survival after relapse

Many of the factors at diagnosis that are prognostic of EFS and overall survival (OS) also influence OS after disease progression or relapse. As stated above, the COG uses age (<18 months, ≥18 months), INSS stage, *MYCN* status, histopathology, and ploidy to assign patients to the appropriate level of treatment intensity at the time of diagnosis. In an INRG analysis of 2,266 patients who experienced first progression/relapse, the median time to relapse was 13 months, and 5-year OS from the time of first relapse was 20% (London & Castel et al., 2011). After disease progression or relapse, factors identified as most highly prognostic of poor OS were age ≥18 months, use of intensive multi-modality treatment at diagnosis, stage 4, elevated serum ferritin, elevated LDH, unfavorable histology, high MKI, and *MYCN* amplification, whereby the presence of any one of these adverse features doubled the risk for death post-relapse. Furthermore, time from diagnosis to first relapse/progression had a significant impact on survival after relapse. However, time-to-first-relapse (TTFR) was associated with OS time in a complex non-linear relationship; patients with TTFR of 36 months or longer had the lowest risk of death, followed by patients who relapsed in the period of 0 to less than 6 months or 18 to 36 months. Patients who relapsed between 6 and 18 months after diagnosis had the highest risk of death. TTFR, older age, higher INSS stage, and *MYCN* amplification were independently prognostic of worse post relapse OS in multivariable analysis. Within the subgroup of patients with *MYCN* amplified tumors and stage 3 and 4 disease, TTFR was the most highly predictive of OS post relapse (London & Castel et al., 2011).

In a retrospective study describing 781 children with NB experiencing tumor recurrence, the 10-year OS was 6.8% after progression and 14.4% after relapse (Garaventa et al., 2009). Similar to the findings of London & Castel et al. (2011), the factors worsening outcome in univariate analysis were age >18 months, advanced stage, high LDH, *MYCN* amplification, and abdominal primary (no multivariable analysis). Most relapses occurred early (median 7.8 months), but 86 (24%) occurred late (median 28 months). Early relapses had a more rapid, unfavorable course, with ~80% of deaths occurring within 2 years, whereas survival time was longer for late relapses. From the German protocols NB90, NB97, and NB2004 (451 high-risk patients), Simon et al. presented data on 232 patients with NB who relapsed after autologous stem cell transplantation (ASCT) as part of initial treatment (Simon et al., 2011). *MYCN* amplification, early recurrence within 18 or 24 months after diagnosis, as well as bone marrow and lung/pleura metastasis at relapse were independently predictive of poor survival in multivariate analysis. Of the patients who received second-line chemotherapy, the 23 patients who underwent a second ASCT had better outcome than the 135 patients who did not have a second ASCT (3 year OS of 43.5% vs. 9.6%).

Two previous single-institution studies in NB also showed that shorter time to first relapse was a significant adverse factor for survival. Lau et al. reviewed 31 patients with NB with relapsed disease and found that patients who relapsed less than 12 months from diagnosis, patients who did not receive salvage therapy, and patients with tumor *MYCN* amplification had significantly shorter survival time (Lau et al., 2004). Santana et al. addressed the study of disease-control intervals in 91 high-risk patients with NB (Santana et al., 2008). The estimated median times to disease recurrence were 18.3, 8.7, and 3.8 months for the first, second, and third recurrences, respectively. Patients with longer initial disease control had a significant post-recurrence survival advantage. This study emphasized the importance of knowing the intervals of disease progression as end points for the design of protocols with new agents.

Ultimately, understanding the genetic differences in early versus late relapsing patients will facilitate selection of appropriate targeted therapy. Meanwhile, it is appropriate to perform stratification of relapsed patients according to the timing of first relapse, as well as stage, age, and *MYCN* status; this is critical in certain types of study designs, such as randomized phase II trials, to maintain a balance of less favorable patients between treatment arms.

4.2 Outcome of CNS recurrence

If patients recur with neuraxis involvement, the outcome has always been considered ominous, either with or without treatment. The median survival from CNS recurrence ranged from 2 to 14 months and survival beyond 18 months was very rare (Kellie et al., 1991; Kramer et al., 2001; Matthay et al., 2003a; Shaw & Eden, 1992). It was also suggested that patients with meningeal recurrence had the shortest survival (0.9 months) (Matthay et al., 2003a). However, CNS-directed radioimmunotherapy may improve the outcome of these patients (Croog et al., 2010; Kramer et al., 2010) (refer to Section 5.2 for details).

4.3 Chronic neuroblastoma and late relapse

Chronic or indolent NB generally refers to active NB beyond four to five years from diagnosis. This can arise from persistent stable disease, first recurrence followed by a protracted disease course with multiple recurrences or from late relapse with or without prolonged survival.

4.3.1 Chronic neuroblastoma in adolescents and adults

Indolent NB is a more common phenomenon in adolescents and adults than in children, but the actual number of adolescents and adults with NB is very small, since over 90% of NB patients are diagnosed before the of age 10 years. Despite an indolent course and the absence of *MYCN* amplification, the outcome of these patients is very poor. Of the 1,950 NB patients registered with the Children's Cancer Group from 1973 to 1993, 2% of patients were aged between 13 and 18 years, and survival was 7% at 5 years compared with 30% survival in patients aged 1 to 13 years (Franks et al., 1997). Only one tumor from the older age group had *MYCN* amplification. In a report of 1116 children and 53 adolescence (age 10 -18 years), adolescence were also found to have worse outcome than children (10-year OS 20% vs. 39%) and had an indolent course post-recurrence (Conte et al., 2006). Franks et al. described 15 of the 16 NB patients aged between 13 and 33 years subsequently relapsed and 13 died. The median OS was 3.5 years, which is significantly longer than the post-relapse median survival of eight months in children. Moreover, in adolescents and adults, non-Stage 4 patients have an even more protracted course following relapse than Stage 4 patients (median survival 7.8 vs. 2.8 years).

4.3.2 Chronic neuroblastoma in children

Childhood NB may follow a chronic course and has partly been attributed to improved salvage regimens that have become available in the last decade. Children with chronic NB can be separated according to the timing of relapse. In a study by Kushner et al. describing NB patients who were younger than 10 years old at diagnosis and had metastatic disease five years or more from diagnosis, 21 Stage 4 patients had first relapse <4 years from diagnosis (Kushner et al., 2002). All 21 patients had a second recurrence and 13 had a third recurrence. Seventeen (81%) died of NB between 5 and 9.8 years from diagnosis, and four were alive with disease 5.6 to 7.8 years from diagnosis. The study also included Stage 4 patients who presented with late first relapse (4.3 to 13 years from diagnosis). This group of late relapse patients appears to have an even more chronic course. Three of the nine patients died of NB at 7.3 to 10.4 years from diagnosis, three were alive with disease 6.7 to 14.1 years, and three were in second remission 6.8 to 19.5 years. Multiple recurrences were also described by Santana et al. (Santana et al., 2008). In a cohort of 66 relapsed NB patients, 12% had one recurrence (median 15.7 months from diagnosis), 21% had two recurrences (median 7.2 months from last relapse), and 67% had at least three recurrences (median 3.5 months). The interval between each successive recurrence decreased.

4.3.3 Late relapse

First relapse occurring more than five years from initial diagnosis is uncommon and is observed in 3% of NB patients who remain in remission for the first five years. In a study where 406 remission patients were followed up >5 years from diagnosis, 18 patients relapsed and 14 of these were late first recurrences (Cotterill et al., 2001). Only two patients were alive at the time of report. A literature review described 30 cases of late NB recurrences (published between 1950 and 1990) (Cervera et al., 1990). In 29 patients, relapse occurred between 5 and 16 years from diagnosis. The outcome was only known in 24 patients, of whom 17 died of NB at 6.5 to 24.7 years from diagnosis. One case was exceptional in that a man, who was 29 years old at diagnosis, relapsed 52 years later (Mir et al., 1987). Kushner et al. also reported a man, who relapsed 38 years after he was diagnosed at age 8 years (Kushner et al., 2002).

5. Therapeutic strategies for relapsed NB

Extensive effort has been put into the development of drugs to treat high-risk NB. The most recent advance is the use of anti-G_{D2} immunotherapy to eradicate MRD (Yu et al., 2010). However, at this point of time, 50% of high-risk NB patients will relapse after receiving conventional treatment without immunotherapy. Current salvage regimens can induce response or arrest disease progression in 60% of relapsed patients (Lau et al., 2004), but to date no salvage treatment regimens are known to be curative. A number of novel agents with anti-NB activities are currently under investigation and are mostly available to relapsed patients who are eligible for specific phase I/II clinical trials.

5.1 Conventional chemotherapeutics

Intensive regimens using conventional chemotherapeutic agents were used in relapsed NB patients in the 1990's, and they include various combinations of high doses of carboplatin, cisplatin, cyclophosphamide, ifosfamide, doxorubicin, and etoposide (Alvarado et al., 1997; Campbell et al., 1993; Kreissman et al., 1997). Although these treatments achieved responses in 35 to 50% of patients, they were accompanied by unacceptably high toxicities with no improvement in long-term outcome and are rarely indicated in current settings. Myeloablative therapy is also rarely indicated for the same reason, with the exception of metastatic relapse in patients with low and intermediate-risk NB, who may be salvaged with frontline myeloablative regimen used for high-risk disease. However, the use of moderate dose of conventional chemotherapy in combination with new agents is an important means of assessing new agents in phase I/II studies.

5.2 Palliative radiotherapy

While radiotherapy (RT) cannot cure relapse, it provides rapid and effective symptom control and palliation for skeletal, soft tissue, and CNS metastases. NB often remains radiosensitive at relapse. Palliative RT is given for bone pain, obstructive symptoms from soft tissue mass and neurological symptoms from CNS disease. 200 to 300cGy is delivered for each fraction and the number of fractions given depends on response (Caussa et al., 2011; Paulino, 2003). The median total RT dose is around 2000cGy. RT can achieve a response rate of 63 to 79% in skeletal metastases, 67 to 84% in soft tissue sites, and 44 to 80% in CNS metastases (Caussa et al., 2011; Halperin & Cox, 1986; Paulino, 2003).

5.3 Second-line chemotherapy

Further dose intensification with conventional chemotherapeutics is not a practical option with disease recurrence. Second line chemotherapies with mild to modest toxicities that have not been included in frontline treatment are often considered for salvage. Topotecan, irinotecan, temozolomide are commercially available drugs. Other agents such as fenretinide and vorinostat are still undergoing clinical trials for NB treatment.

5.3.1 Topoisomerase I inhibitors

Over the past decade, topotecan and irinotecan, both topoisomerase I inhibitors with proven anti-NB activity, have been frequently used in relapsed NB. Targeting the DNA-relaxing enzyme topoisomerase I results in failure of DNA re-ligation during DNA replication and repair. In a phase II trial, partial responses (PR) or better were observed in 32% of the 57 relapsed patients receiving topotecan and cyclophosphamide and in 19% of the 62 patients in the topotecan alone group. While the topotecan/cyclophosphamide group had a significantly better 3-year PFS (10% vs. 0%), there was no difference in 3-year OS (17% vs. 14%) (London et al., 2010). The combination of topotecan and cyclophosphamide has been the most extensively utilized salvage regimen, and 60% of relapsed patients are expected to experience grade 3 or 4 hematological toxicity. Vincristine or etoposide have also been added as a third drug to topotecan/cyclophosphamide, and PR or better were obtained in 52% and 61% of relapsed patients, respectively (Kushner et al., 2010; Simon et al., 2007).

In many cases, irinotecan is combined with temozolomide. A phase II study of irinotecan/ oral temozolomide demonstrated a response rate of 19% and stable disease (SD) of 56% in relapsed patients (Bagatell et al., 2011). Diarrhoea is a common side effect of irinotecan, and Grade 3 or 4 diarrhoea was reported in 6% of patients. Oral irinotecan/temozolomide, which has the benefit of home administration and reduced costs, has also been tested, with 50% of patients achieving response or stable disease (Wagner et al., 2009). High dose carboplatin/irinotecan/temozolomide had a response rate of 68% (Kushner et al., 2011).

5.3.2 Fenretinide

Fenretinide (N-4-hydroxyphenyl retinamide, [4-HPR]) is a synthetic retinoid with cytotoxic and growth inhibitory effects on NB cell lines. Unlike 13-cis- and all-trans-retinoic acids, fenretinide does not induce cellular differentiation, but induces apoptosis (Di Vinci et al., 1994). The mechanisms of action include de novo ceramide synthesis, generation of reactive oxygen species (Maurer et al., 1999), anti-angiogenesis (Ribatti et al., 2003), and increased natural-killer cell activity (Villa et al., 1993). Phase I trials of oral fenretinide in relapsed NB patients demonstrated SD in 43% to 77% of patients (Garaventa et al., 2003; Villablanca et al., 2006). One NB patient had a complete response (CR). However, capsule formulation of fenretinide has poor bioavailability and wide interpatient variation, and the large capsules present a major challenge for children to ingest. LYM-X-SORB, a novel organized lipid matrix, can increase the oral bioavailability of fenretinide (Maurer et al., 2007). A phase I study of fenretinide/LYM-X-SORB oral powder formulation in NB patients is underway.

5.3.3 Vorinostat

Vorinostat (suberoylanilide hydroxamic acid, [SAHA]) is an oral histone deacetylase (HDAC) inhibitor. HDAC inhibition leads to histone acetylation, opening of chromatin structure, and reactivation of previously silenced genes (Johnstone, 2002). In NB, HDAC inhibitors have been shown to induce apoptosis and impair VEGF production (Muhlethaler-Mottet et al., 2008), restore the p53 pathway (Condorelli et al., 2008), synergize with retinoic acid to inhibit growth (Coffey et al., 2001), and enhance RT (S. Mueller et al., 2011). In a phase I trial of vorinostat, one CR was observed in a NB patient receiving vorinostat in combination with 13-cis-retinoic acid (Fouladi et al., 2010).

5.4 Immunotherapy

G_{D2}, disialoganglioside, is the most common tumor-associated antigen targeted in NB immunotherapy. G_{D2} is an ideal target as it is a ubiquitous and abundant surface glycolipid that is present on NB cells but in normal tissue except for neurons. The three main anti-G_{D2} monoclonal antibodies (MoAb) are 3F8, ch14.18, and hu14.18-IL-2. Tumor cells are killed via complement activation and antibody-dependent cell-mediated cytotoxicity (ADCC) that can be augmented by cytokines, e.g. interleukin-2 (IL-2) and GM-CSF (Hank et al., 1990; Imai et al., 2005; B.M. Mueller et al., 1990). Chimeric antibody Ch14.18/IL-2/GM-CSF immunotherapy is effective against MRD in the post-consolidation setting, as shown in a recent phase III randomized trial in primary NB (Yu et al., 2010). In recurrent NB, unsustained response to immunotherapy is restricted to non-bulky disease in the bone marrow and small MIBG-avid lesions. Common side effects include pain, capillary leak syndrome, hypotension, and allergic reaction.

3F8 is a murine MoAb and is the first MoAb to be studied in NB patients (N.K. Cheung et al., 1987). In a phase II study of 3F8/GMCSF, CR in five of 10 patients was restricted to the bone marrow and all developed progressive disease at other sites (Kushner et al., 2001). Similar results were seen in a phase II study of humanized 14.18-IL-2, a fusion protein of humanized 14.18 anti-G_{D2} MoAb linked to IL-2 (Shusterman et al., 2010). Of the 20 patients with small disease burden, CR was achieved in five patients, three of whom had bone marrow disease only by histology at relapse, one had a single MIBG-avid lesion, and one had both bone marrow and bone disease.

Unlike high-risk patients, patients who have locoregional NB and relapse with metastatic disease may be salvaged with immunotherapy. Kushner et al. reported three of five patients, who were initially treated with surgery alone for low-risk NB and subsequently relapsed with metastatic disease, were in CR at four to seven years (Kushner et al., 2003a). These patients received an intensive salvage regimen containing intensive chemotherapy, 3F8 MoAb, ^{131}I-3F8, local RT, and 13-cis-retinoic acid.

5.5 Radionuclide therapy

MIBG is taken up by 90% of NB tumors. MIBG labeled with therapeutic isotope ^{131}I is used to deliver target specific RT in NB for >20 years. ^{131}I-MIBG therapy is generally well tolerated, except for myelosuppression that may require stem cell support in heavily pretreated patients (DuBois et al., 2004). MIBG monotherapy achieved responses in up to a third of relapsed patients at doses ≥12 mCi/kg, but with no long-term cure (DuBois & Matthay, 2008). In a large phase II trial of 164 patients receiving 12 to 18 mCi/kg of ^{131}I-MIBG, the overall response rate was 36% and SD rate was 36%, and the 2-year OS was 29% (Matthay et al., 2007). The additional benefits of dose intensification with tandem ^{131}I-MIBG

infusions (Matthay et al., 2009a) and of including ^{131}I-MIBG with myeloablative therapy requires further studies (Matthay et al., 2006).
^{131}I-MIBG therapy may be enhanced with radiosensitizers such as cisplatin (Mastrangelo et al., 1997) and topotecan (Gaze et al., 2005) or with non-carrier added radiolabeled MIBG. Conventional preparation of ^{131}I-MIBG has large quantities of unlabeled or cold (non-radioactive) MIBG in the final formulation. Saturation of the norepinephrine transporter by unlabeled MIBG reduces the efficacy while increasing the side-effects. This can be circumvented by using the Ultratrace solid-phase preparation technique to synthesize non-carrier added radiolabeled MIBG (Ultratrace ^{131}I-MIBG). This novel formulation resulted in greater tumor uptake and efficacy in NB xenografts (Barrett et al., 2010). The increased uptake and retention of Ultratrace ^{131}I-MIBG may have therapeutic benefit by allowing further intensification of MIBG therapy.

5.6 Targeted therapies

Targeted therapies with potential anti-NB activities include small molecule inhibitors against ALK (anaplastic lymphoma kinase), aurora A kinase, trk tyrosine kinase, Akt/PI3-kinase, and EGFR, and monoclonal antibodies against VEGF, IGF-1, and TRAIL receptor.

5.6.1 ALK inhibition

Anaplastic lymphoma kinase (ALK) is a receptor tyrosine kinase and was identified as a NB predisposition gene (Mosse et al., 2008). *ALK* somatic mutations and amplification are found in 8% of primary NB. Of interest, a subset of tumors expressing high mRNA levels of wild-type *ALK* have similar genotype and poor clinical outcome to tumors with *ALK* mutations/amplification (Schulte et al., 2011). Preclinical data show that ALK inhibition diminishes growth in cells with *ALK* mutations, as well as in cells overexpressing wild-type *ALK* (Janoueix-Lerosey et al., 2008). Hence, ALK inhibitors may potentially be effective in NB tumors expressing high levels of ALK. A phase I/II trial of a small molecule inhibitor of ALK is in progress.

5.6.2 Anti-angiogenesis

NB is a highly vascular tumor and tumor angiogenesis is associated with metastatic disease and poor outcome (Meitar et al., 1996). Bevacizumab (MoAb against vascular endothelial growth factor (VEGF)), did not lead to any objective responses when used as a single agent in children with refractory solid tumors (Glade Bender et al., 2008). The efficacy of bevacizumab in combination with irinotecan/temozolomide and with the radiolabeled ^{131}I-3F8 antibody in relapsed NB is currently being investigated.

5.6.3 TRK inhibition

TrkB, a member of the Trk (NTRK) neurotrophin tyrosine kinase receptors, is highly expressed in unfavorable NB (Brodeur et al., 2009; Nakagawara et al., 1994). TrkB overexpression results in increased chemoresistance in NB cells (Ho et al., 2002). Lestaurtinib (CEP-701), a selective Trk tyrosine kinase inhibitor, has anti-tumor activity in NB xenograft models, both as a single agent and in combination with topotecan/cyclophosphamide and with irinotecan/temozolomide (Iyer et al., 2010). In a phase I trial of lestaurtinib, two PR and nine SD were reported in 46 patients with refractory NB (Minturn et al., 2011).

5.7 Treatment of CNS relapse

The outcome of CNS recurrence is dismal with conventional chemotherapeutic agents. The use of CNS-directed radioimmunotherapy (RIT) may improve the prognosis of this group of patients. RIT enables the targeted delivery of RT to tumor cells (Kramer et al., 2007). In a retrospective analysis of 14 patients who received craniospinal irradiation together with irinotecan as a radiosensitizer, followed by intra-Ommaya (IO) RIT (^{131}I-8H9 or ^{131}I-3F8), 10 were alive with no CNS disease at 15.2 to 62.7 months from CNS relapse, three were alive with disease at 24.6 to 30.2 months, and one died from other cause but without disease at 21.9 months (Croog et al., 2010). This is in contrast with the 12 patients, who only received whole/partial brain or partial spine radiotherapy and all succumbed 4.2 to 23.9 months later. In addition, the same group treated 21 patients with CNS recurrences with an intensive regimen containing IO RIT (^{131}I-8H9 or ^{131}I-3F8) with promising results (Kramer et al., 2010). Seventeen patients were alive without CNS disease at 7 to 74 months post CNS relapse. In addition to IO RIT, patients also received CSI with irinotecan, irinotecan/temozolomide/carboplatin, systemic immunotherapy (anti-3F8 with GMCSF), and maintenance treatment with 13-cis-retinoic acid and oral temozolomide. The long-term treatment consequences of CNS directed RIT are yet to be evaluated.

The use of IO topotecan has also been described in a NB case report of isolated CNS metastases. This patient, who received both IO and IV topotecan, had a CR of both parenchymal and leptomeningeal disease and was progression-free for 18 weeks (Sirachainan et al., 2008).

6. Conclusion

Although long-term disease-free survival after recurrent NB remains extremely poor, salvage regimens in the recent era have altered the natural disease course and prolong post-relapse survival, with a small subset of chronic patients experiencing multiple recurrences or non-remitting disease. However, it is difficult to predict response to salvage therapy and survival time post relapse. Knowledge in this area is limited. Which patients should be offered multi-modality treatment and which patients should receive oral agents with minimal toxicity? How can we ensure quality of life is not jeopardized by unrealistic expectations? These are difficult questions clinicians must face whenever a child with NB relapses.

Furthermore, surveillance for disease recurrence can cause significant emotional and financial burden. Can detection of early asymptomatic relapse improve quality of life or change long-term survival? Can the detection of early molecular relapse by monitoring MRD improve response to salvage therapy and increase survival? What is a clinical significant MRD level? Further research is needed to provide answers to these questions to facilitate development of effective surveillance protocols.

7. Acknowledgement

LMS Lau is supported in part by National Health and Medical Research Council (Australia) and Cure Cancer Australia Foundation. WBL is supported in part by NIH/NCI grant U10 CA98413-06 to the Children's Oncology Group Statistics and Data Center, and support for her INRG research is provided by the Little Heroes Pediatric Cancer Research Foundation. We thank Dr Peter J Shaw for his comments.

8. References

Alvarado, C.S., Kretschmar, C., Joshi, V.V., Toledano, S., Cantor, A., Strother, D., Nitschke, R. & Castleberry, R.P. (1997). Chemotherapy for patients with recurrent or refractory neuroblastoma: a POG Phase II study. *J Pediatr Hematol Oncol*, Vol.19, No.1, pp. 62-67.

Ambros, P.F., Ambros, I.M., Brodeur, G.M., Haber, M., Khan, J., Nakagawara, A., Schleiermacher, G., Speleman, F., Spitz, R., London, W.B., Cohn, S.L., Pearson, A.D. & Maris, J.M. (2009). International consensus for neuroblastoma molecular diagnostics: report from the International Neuroblastoma Risk Group (INRG) Biology Committee. *Br J Cancer*, Vol.100, No.9, pp. 1471-1482.

Bagatell, R., London, W.B., Wagner, L.M., Voss, S.D., Stewart, C.F., Maris, J.M., Kretschmar, C. & Cohn, S.L. (2011). Phase II study of irinotecan and temozolomide in children with relapsed or refractory neuroblastoma: a Children's Oncology Group study. *J Clin Oncol*, Vol.29, No.2, pp. 208-213.

Barrett, J.A., Joyal, J.L., Hillier, S.M., Maresca, K.P., Femia, F.J., Kronauge, J.F., Boyd, M., Mairs, R.J. & Babich, J.W. (2010). Comparison of high-specific-activity ultratrace 123/131I-MIBG and carrier-added 123/131I-MIBG on efficacy, pharmacokinetics, and tissue distribution. *Cancer Biother Radiopharm*, Vol.25, No.3, pp. 299-308.

Beiske, K., Ambros, P.F., Burchill, S.A., Cheung, I.Y. & Swerts, K. (2005). Detecting minimal residual disease in neuroblastoma patients-the present state of the art. *Cancer Lett*, Vol.228, No.1-2, pp. 229-240.

Beiske, K., Burchill, S.A., Cheung, I.Y., Hiyama, E., Seeger, R.C., Cohn, S.L., Pearson, A.D. & Matthay, K.K. (2009). Consensus criteria for sensitive detection of minimal neuroblastoma cells in bone marrow, blood and stem cell preparations by immunocytology and QRT-PCR: recommendations by the International Neuroblastoma Risk Group Task Force. *Br J Cancer*, Vol.100, No.10, pp. 1627-1637.

Bombardieri, E., Aktolun, C., Baum, R.P., Bishof-Delaloye, A., Buscombe, J., Chatal, J.F., Maffioli, L., Moncayo, R., Mortelmans, L. & Reske, S.N. (2003). 131I/123I-metaiodobenzylguanidine (MIBG) scintigraphy: procedure guidelines for tumour imaging. *Eur J Nucl Med Mol Imaging*, Vol.30, No.12, pp. BP132-139.

Boubaker, A. & Bischof Delaloye, A. (2008). MIBG scintigraphy for the diagnosis and follow-up of children with neuroblastoma. *Q J Nucl Med Mol Imaging*, Vol.52, No.4, pp. 388-402.

Brisse, H.J., McCarville, M.B., Granata, C., Krug, K.B., Wootton-Gorges, S.L., Kanegawa, K., Giammarile, F., Schmidt, M., Shulkin, B.L., Matthay, K.K., Lewington, V.J., Sarnacki, S., Hero, B., Kaneko, M., London, W.B., Pearson, A.D., Cohn, S.L. & Monclair, T. (2011). Guidelines for Imaging and Staging of Neuroblastic Tumors: Consensus Report from the International Neuroblastoma Risk Group Project. *Radiology*.

Brodeur, G.M., Minturn, J.E., Ho, R., Simpson, A.M., Iyer, R., Varela, C.R., Light, J.E., Kolla, V. & Evans, A.E. (2009). Trk receptor expression and inhibition in neuroblastomas. *Clin Cancer Res*, Vol.15, No.10, pp. 3244-3250.

Brody, A.S., Frush, D.P., Huda, W. & Brent, R.L. (2007). Radiation risk to children from computed tomography. *Pediatrics*, Vol.120, No.3, pp. 677-682.

Burchill, S.A., Lewis, I.J., Abrams, K.R., Riley, R., Imeson, J., Pearson, A.D., Pinkerton, R. & Selby, P. (2001). Circulating neuroblastoma cells detected by reverse transcriptase polymerase chain reaction for tyrosine hydroxylase mRNA are an independent poor prognostic indicator in stage 4 neuroblastoma in children over 1 year. *J Clin Oncol*, Vol.19, No.6, pp. 1795-1801.

Cai, J.Y., Tang, Y.J., Jiang, L.M., Pan, C., Chen, J. & Tang, J.Y. (2007). Prognostic influence of minimal residual disease detected by flow cytometry and peripheral blood stem cell transplantation by CD34+ selection in childhood advanced neuroblastoma. *Pediatr Blood Cancer*, Vol.49, No.7, pp. 952-957.

Campbell, L.A., Seeger, R.C., Harris, R.E., Villablanca, J.G. & Matthay, K.K. (1993). Escalating dose of continuous infusion combination chemotherapy for refractory neuroblastoma. *J Clin Oncol*, Vol.11, No.4, pp. 623-629.

Carlin, S., Mairs, R.J., McCluskey, A.G., Tweddle, D.A., Sprigg, A., Estlin, C., Board, J., George, R.E., Ellershaw, C., Pearson, A.D., Lunec, J., Montaldo, P.G., Ponzoni, M., van Eck-Smit, B.L., Hoefnagel, C.A., van den Brug, M.D., Tytgat, G.A. & Caron, H.N. (2003). Development of a real-time polymerase chain reaction assay for prediction of the uptake of meta-[(131)I]iodobenzylguanidine by neuroblastoma tumors. *Clin Cancer Res*, Vol.9, No.9, pp. 3338-3344.

Caussa, L., Hijal, T., Michon, J. & Helfre, S. (2011). Role of palliative radiotherapy in the management of metastatic pediatric neuroblastoma: a retrospective single-institution study. *Int J Radiat Oncol Biol Phys*, Vol.79, No.1, pp. 214-219.

Cervera, A., Kingston, J.E. & Malpas, J.S. (1990). Late recurrence of neuroblastoma: a report of five cases and review of the literature. *Pediatr Hematol Oncol*, Vol.7, No.4, pp. 311-322.

Cheung, I.Y., Barber, D. & Cheung, N.K. (1998). Detection of microscopic neuroblastoma in marrow by histology, immunocytology, and reverse transcription-PCR of multiple molecular markers. *Clin Cancer Res*, Vol.4, No.11, pp. 2801-2805.

Cheung, I.Y., Feng, Y., Gerald, W. & Cheung, N.K. (2008). Exploiting gene expression profiling to identify novel minimal residual disease markers of neuroblastoma. *Clin Cancer Res*, Vol.14, No.21, pp. 7020-7027.

Cheung, I.Y., Lo Piccolo, M.S., Kushner, B.H. & Cheung, N.K. (2003). Early molecular response of marrow disease to biologic therapy is highly prognostic in neuroblastoma. *J Clin Oncol*, Vol.21, No.20, pp. 3853-3858.

Cheung, N.K., Heller, G., Kushner, B.H., Liu, C. & Cheung, I.Y. (1997). Detection of metastatic neuroblastoma in bone marrow: when is routine marrow histology insensitive? *J Clin Oncol*, Vol.15, No.8, pp. 2807-2817.

Cheung, N.K., Lazarus, H., Miraldi, F.D., Abramowsky, C.R., Kallick, S., Saarinen, U.M., Spitzer, T., Strandjord, S.E., Coccia, P.F. & Berger, N.A. (1987). Ganglioside GD2 specific monoclonal antibody 3F8: a phase I study in patients with neuroblastoma and malignant melanoma. *J Clin Oncol*, Vol.5, No.9, pp. 1430-1440.

Coffey, D.C., Kutko, M.C., Glick, R.D., Butler, L.M., Heller, G., Rifkind, R.A., Marks, P.A., Richon, V.M. & La Quaglia, M.P. (2001). The histone deacetylase inhibitor, CBHA, inhibits growth of human neuroblastoma xenografts in vivo, alone and synergistically with all-trans retinoic acid. *Cancer Res*, Vol.61, No.9, pp. 3591-3594.

Cohn, S.L., Pearson, A.D., London, W.B., Monclair, T., Ambros, P.F., Brodeur, G.M., Faldum, A., Hero, B., Iehara, T., Machin, D., Mosseri, V., Simon, T., Garaventa, A., Castel, V. & Matthay, K.K. (2009). The International Neuroblastoma Risk Group (INRG) classification system: an INRG Task Force report. *J Clin Oncol*, Vol.27, No.2, pp. 289-297.

Condorelli, F., Gnemmi, I., Vallario, A., Genazzani, A.A. & Canonico, P.L. (2008). Inhibitors of histone deacetylase (HDAC) restore the p53 pathway in neuroblastoma cells. *Br J Pharmacol*, Vol.153, No.4, pp. 657-668.

Conte, M., Parodi, S., De Bernardi, B., Milanaccio, C., Mazzocco, K., Angelini, P., Viscardi, E., Di Cataldo, A., Luksch, R. & Haupt, R. (2006). Neuroblastoma in adolescents: the Italian experience. *Cancer*, Vol.106, No.6, pp. 1409-1417.

Cotterill, S.J., Pearson, A.D., Pritchard, J., Kohler, J.A. & Foot, A.B. (2001). Late relapse and prognosis for neuroblastoma patients surviving 5 years or more: a report from the European Neuroblastoma Study Group "Survey". *Med Pediatr Oncol*, Vol.36, No.1, pp. 235-238.

Croog, V.J., Kramer, K., Cheung, N.K., Kushner, B.H., Modak, S., Souweidane, M.M. & Wolden, S.L. (2010). Whole neuraxis irradiation to address central nervous system relapse in high-risk neuroblastoma. *Int J Radiat Oncol Biol Phys*, Vol.78, No.3, pp. 849-854.

Di Vinci, A., Geido, E., Infusini, E. & Giaretti, W. (1994). Neuroblastoma cell apoptosis induced by the synthetic retinoid N-(4-hydroxyphenyl)retinamide. *Int J Cancer*, Vol.59, No.3, pp. 422-426.

DuBois, S.G. & Matthay, K.K. (2008). Radiolabeled metaiodobenzylguanidine for the treatment of neuroblastoma. *Nucl Med Biol*, Vol.35 Suppl 1, pp. S35-48.

DuBois, S.G., Messina, J., Maris, J.M., Huberty, J., Glidden, D.V., Veatch, J., Charron, M., Hawkins, R. & Matthay, K.K. (2004). Hematologic toxicity of high-dose iodine-131-metaiodobenzylguanidine therapy for advanced neuroblastoma. *J Clin Oncol*, Vol.22, No.12, pp. 2452-2460.

Evans, A.E., D'Angio, G.J. & Randolph, J. (1971). A proposed staging for children with neuroblastoma. Children's cancer study group A. *Cancer*, Vol.27, No.2, pp. 374-378.

Fouladi, M., Park, J.R., Stewart, C.F., Gilbertson, R.J., Schaiquevich, P., Sun, J., Reid, J.M., Ames, M.M., Speights, R., Ingle, A.M., Zwiebel, J., Blaney, S.M. & Adamson, P.C. (2010). Pediatric phase I trial and pharmacokinetic study of vorinostat: a Children's Oncology Group phase I consortium report. *J Clin Oncol*, Vol.28, No.22, pp. 3623-3629.

Franks, L.M., Bollen, A., Seeger, R.C., Stram, D.O. & Matthay, K.K. (1997). Neuroblastoma in adults and adolescents: an indolent course with poor survival. *Cancer*, Vol.79, No.10, pp. 2028-2035.

Garaventa, A., Luksch, R., Lo Piccolo, M.S., Cavadini, E., Montaldo, P.G., Pizzitola, M.R., Boni, L., Ponzoni, M., Decensi, A., De Bernardi, B., Bellani, F.F. & Formelli, F. (2003). Phase I trial and pharmacokinetics of fenretinide in children with neuroblastoma. *Clin Cancer Res*, Vol.9, No.6, pp. 2032-2039.

Garaventa, A., Parodi, S., De Bernardi, B., Dau, D., Manzitti, C., Conte, M., Casale, F., Viscardi, E., Bianchi, M., D'Angelo, P., Zanazzo, G.A., Luksch, R., Favre, C., Tamburini, A. & Haupt, R. (2009). Outcome of children with neuroblastoma after progression or relapse. A retrospective study of the Italian neuroblastoma registry. *Eur J Cancer*, Vol.45, No.16, pp. 2835-2842.

Gaze, M.N., Chang, Y.C., Flux, G.D., Mairs, R.J., Saran, F.H. & Meller, S.T. (2005). Feasibility of dosimetry-based high-dose 131I-meta-iodobenzylguanidine with topotecan as a radiosensitizer in children with metastatic neuroblastoma. *Cancer Biother Radiopharm*, Vol.20, No.2, pp. 195-199.

Glade Bender, J.L., Adamson, P.C., Reid, J.M., Xu, L., Baruchel, S., Shaked, Y., Kerbel, R.S., Cooney-Qualter, E.M., Stempak, D., Chen, H.X., Nelson, M.D., Krailo, M.D., Ingle, A.M., Blaney, S.M., Kandel, J.J. & Yamashiro, D.J. (2008). Phase I trial and pharmacokinetic study of bevacizumab in pediatric patients with refractory solid tumors: a Children's Oncology Group Study. *J Clin Oncol*, Vol.26, No.3, pp. 399-405.

Halperin, E.C. & Cox, E.B. (1986). Radiation therapy in the management of neuroblastoma: the Duke University Medical Center experience 1967-1984. *Int J Radiat Oncol Biol Phys*, Vol.12, No.10, pp. 1829-1837.

Hank, J.A., Robinson, R.R., Surfus, J., Mueller, B.M., Reisfeld, R.A., Cheung, N.K. & Sondel, P.M. (1990). Augmentation of antibody dependent cell mediated cytotoxicity following in vivo therapy with recombinant interleukin 2. *Cancer Res*, Vol.50, No.17, pp. 5234-5239.

Ho, R., Eggert, A., Hishiki, T., Minturn, J.E., Ikegaki, N., Foster, P., Camoratto, A.M., Evans, A.E. & Brodeur, G.M. (2002). Resistance to chemotherapy mediated by TrkB in neuroblastomas. *Cancer Res*, Vol.62, No.22, pp. 6462-6466.

Imai, M., Landen, C., Ohta, R., Cheung, N.K. & Tomlinson, S. (2005). Complement-mediated mechanisms in anti-GD2 monoclonal antibody therapy of murine metastatic cancer. *Cancer Res*, Vol.65, No.22, pp. 10562-10568.

Iyer, R., Evans, A.E., Qi, X., Ho, R., Minturn, J.E., Zhao, H., Balamuth, N., Maris, J.M. & Brodeur, G.M. (2010). Lestaurtinib enhances the antitumor efficacy of chemotherapy in murine xenograft models of neuroblastoma. *Clin Cancer Res*, Vol.16, No.5, pp. 1478-1485.

Jacobs, A., Delree, M., Desprechins, B., Otten, J., Ferster, A., Jonckheer, M.H., Mertens, J., Ham, H.R. & Piepsz, A. (1990). Consolidating the role of *I-MIBG-scintigraphy in childhood neuroblastoma: five years of clinical experience. *Pediatr Radiol*, Vol.20, No.3, pp. 157-159.

Janoueix-Lerosey, I., Lequin, D., Brugieres, L., Ribeiro, A., de Pontual, L., Combaret, V., Raynal, V., Puisieux, A., Schleiermacher, G., Pierron, G., Valteau-Couanet, D., Frebourg, T., Michon, J., Lyonnet, S., Amiel, J. & Delattre, O. (2008). Somatic and germline activating mutations of the ALK kinase receptor in neuroblastoma. *Nature*, Vol.455, No.7215, pp. 967-970.

Johnstone, R.W. (2002). Histone-deacetylase inhibitors: novel drugs for the treatment of cancer. *Nat Rev Drug Discov*, Vol.1, No.4, pp. 287-299.

Kellie, S.J., Hayes, F.A., Bowman, L., Kovnar, E.H., Langston, J., Jenkins, J.J., 3rd, Pao, W.J., Ducos, R. & Green, A.A. (1991). Primary extracranial neuroblastoma with central nervous system metastases characterization by clinicopathologic findings and neuroimaging. *Cancer*, Vol.68, No.9, pp. 1999-2006.

Kramer, K., Humm, J.L., Souweidane, M.M., Zanzonico, P.B., Dunkel, I.J., Gerald, W.L., Khakoo, Y., Yeh, S.D., Yeung, H.W., Finn, R.D., Wolden, S.L., Larson, S.M. & Cheung, N.K. (2007). Phase I study of targeted radioimmunotherapy for leptomeningeal cancers using intra-Ommaya 131-I-3F8. *J Clin Oncol*, Vol.25, No.34, pp. 5465-5470.

Kramer, K., Kushner, B., Heller, G. & Cheung, N.K. (2001). Neuroblastoma metastatic to the central nervous system. The Memorial Sloan-kettering Cancer Center Experience and A Literature Review. *Cancer*, Vol.91, No.8, pp. 1510-1519.

Kramer, K., Kushner, B.H., Modak, S., Pandit-Taskar, N., Smith-Jones, P., Zanzonico, P., Humm, J.L., Xu, H., Wolden, S.L., Souweidane, M.M., Larson, S.M. & Cheung, N.K.

(2010). Compartmental intrathecal radioimmunotherapy: results for treatment for metastatic CNS neuroblastoma. *J Neurooncol*, Vol.97, No.3, pp. 409-418.

Kreissman, S.G., Rackoff, W., Lee, M. & Breitfeld, P.P. (1997). High dose cyclophosphamide with carboplatin: a tolerable regimen suitable for dose intensification in children with solid tumors. *J Pediatr Hematol Oncol*, Vol.19, No.4, pp. 309-312.

Kushner, B.H., Kramer, K. & Cheung, N.K. (2001). Phase II trial of the anti-G(D2) monoclonal antibody 3F8 and granulocyte-macrophage colony-stimulating factor for neuroblastoma. *J Clin Oncol*, Vol.19, No.22, pp. 4189-4194.

Kushner, B.H., Kramer, K. & Cheung, N.K. (2002). Chronic neuroblastoma. *Cancer*, Vol.95, No.6, pp. 1366-1375.

Kushner, B.H., Kramer, K., LaQuaglia, M.P. & Cheung, N.K. (2003a). Curability of recurrent disseminated disease after surgery alone for local-regional neuroblastoma using intensive chemotherapy and anti-G(D2) immunotherapy. *J Pediatr Hematol Oncol*, Vol.25, No.7, pp. 515-519.

Kushner, B.H., Kramer, K., Modak, S. & Cheung, N.K. (2009). Sensitivity of surveillance studies for detecting asymptomatic and unsuspected relapse of high-risk neuroblastoma. *J Clin Oncol*, Vol.27, No.7, pp. 1041-1046.

Kushner, B.H., Kramer, K., Modak, S. & Cheung, N.K. (2011). High-dose carboplatin-irinotecan-temozolomide: treatment option for neuroblastoma resistant to topotecan. *Pediatr Blood Cancer*, Vol.56, No.3, pp. 403-408.

Kushner, B.H., Kramer, K., Modak, S., Qin, L.X. & Cheung, N.K. (2010). Differential impact of high-dose cyclophosphamide, topotecan, and vincristine in clinical subsets of patients with chemoresistant neuroblastoma. *Cancer*, Vol.116, No.12, pp. 3054-3060.

Kushner, B.H., Yeh, S.D., Kramer, K., Larson, S.M. & Cheung, N.K. (2003b). Impact of metaiodobenzylguanidine scintigraphy on assessing response of high-risk neuroblastoma to dose-intensive induction chemotherapy. *J Clin Oncol*, Vol.21, No.6, pp. 1082-1086.

Lau, L., Tai, D., Weitzman, S., Grant, R., Baruchel, S. & Malkin, D. (2004). Factors influencing survival in children with recurrent neuroblastoma. *J Pediatr Hematol Oncol*, Vol.26, No.4, pp. 227-232.

London, W.B., Castel, V., Monclair, T., Ambros, P.F., Pearson, A.D.J., Cohn, S.L., Berthold, F., Nakagawara, A., Ladenstein, R.L., Iehara, T. & Matthay, K.K. (2011). Clinical and biologic features predictive of survival after relapse of neuroblastoma: A report from the International Neuroblastoma Risk Group (INRG) Project. *J Clin Oncol (Jul 18, Epub ahead of print)*.

London, W.B., Castleberry, R.P., Matthay, K.K., Look, A.T., Seeger, R.C., Shimada, H., Thorner, P., Brodeur, G., Maris, J.M., Reynolds, C.P. & Cohn, S.L. (2005). Evidence for an age cutoff greater than 365 days for neuroblastoma risk group stratification in the Children's Oncology Group. *J Clin Oncol*, Vol.23, No.27, pp. 6459-6465.

London, W.B., Frantz, C.N., Campbell, L.A., Seeger, R.C., Brumback, B.A., Cohn, S.L., Matthay, K.K., Castleberry, R.P. & Diller, L. (2010). Phase II randomized comparison of topotecan plus cyclophosphamide versus topotecan alone in children with recurrent or refractory neuroblastoma: a Children's Oncology Group study. *J Clin Oncol*, Vol.28, No.24, pp. 3808-3815.

Mastrangelo, R., Tornesello, A., Lasorella, A., Iavarone, A., Mastrangelo, S., Riccardi, R., Diociaiuti, L., Rufini, V., Pession, A. & Troncone, L. (1997). Optimal use of the 131-I-metaiodobenzylguanidine and cisplatin combination in advanced neuroblastoma. *J Neurooncol*, Vol.31, No.1-2, pp. 153-158.

Matthay, K.K., Brisse, H., Couanet, D., Couturier, J., Benard, J., Mosseri, V., Edeline, V., Lumbroso, J., Valteau-Couanet, D. & Michon, J. (2003a). Central nervous system metastases in neuroblastoma: radiologic, clinical, and biologic features in 23 patients. *Cancer*, Vol.98, No.1, pp. 155-165.

Matthay, K.K., Edeline, V., Lumbroso, J., Tanguy, M.L., Asselain, B., Zucker, J.M., Valteau-Couanet, D., Hartmann, O. & Michon, J. (2003b). Correlation of early metastatic response by 123I-metaiodobenzylguanidine scintigraphy with overall response and event-free survival in stage IV neuroblastoma. *J Clin Oncol*, Vol.21, No.13, pp. 2486-2491.

Matthay, K.K., Quach, A., Huberty, J., Franc, B.L., Hawkins, R.A., Jackson, H., Groshen, S., Shusterman, S., Yanik, G., Veatch, J., Brophy, P., Villablanca, J.G. & Maris, J.M. (2009a). Iodine-131--metaiodobenzylguanidine double infusion with autologous stem-cell rescue for neuroblastoma: a new approaches to neuroblastoma therapy phase I study. *J Clin Oncol*, Vol.27, No.7, pp. 1020-1025.

Matthay, K.K., Reynolds, C.P., Seeger, R.C., Shimada, H., Adkins, E.S., Haas-Kogan, D., Gerbing, R.B., London, W.B. & Villablanca, J.G. (2009b). Long-term results for children with high-risk neuroblastoma treated on a randomized trial of myeloablative therapy followed by 13-cis-retinoic acid: a children's oncology group study. *J Clin Oncol*, Vol.27, No.7, pp. 1007-1013.

Matthay, K.K., Shulkin, B., Ladenstein, R., Michon, J., Giammarile, F., Lewington, V., Pearson, A.D. & Cohn, S.L. (2010). Criteria for evaluation of disease extent by (123)I-metaiodobenzylguanidine scans in neuroblastoma: a report for the International Neuroblastoma Risk Group (INRG) Task Force. *Br J Cancer*, Vol.102, No.9, pp. 1319-1326.

Matthay, K.K., Tan, J.C., Villablanca, J.G., Yanik, G.A., Veatch, J., Franc, B., Twomey, E., Horn, B., Reynolds, C.P., Groshen, S., Seeger, R.C. & Maris, J.M. (2006). Phase I dose escalation of iodine-131-metaiodobenzylguanidine with myeloablative chemotherapy and autologous stem-cell transplantation in refractory neuroblastoma: a new approaches to Neuroblastoma Therapy Consortium Study. *J Clin Oncol*, Vol.24, No.3, pp. 500-506.

Matthay, K.K., Yanik, G., Messina, J., Quach, A., Huberty, J., Cheng, S.C., Veatch, J., Goldsby, R., Brophy, P., Kersun, L.S., Hawkins, R.A. & Maris, J.M. (2007). Phase II study on the effect of disease sites, age, and prior therapy on response to iodine-131-metaiodobenzylguanidine therapy in refractory neuroblastoma. *J Clin Oncol*, Vol.25, No.9, pp. 1054-1060.

Maurer, B.J., Kalous, O., Yesair, D.W., Wu, X., Janeba, J., Maldonado, V., Khankaldyyan, V., Frgala, T., Sun, B.C., McKee, R.T., Burgess, S.W., Shaw, W.A. & Reynolds, C.P. (2007). Improved oral delivery of N-(4-hydroxyphenyl)retinamide with a novel LYM-X-SORB organized lipid complex. *Clin Cancer Res*, Vol.13, No.10, pp. 3079-3086.

Maurer, B.J., Metelitsa, L.S., Seeger, R.C., Cabot, M.C. & Reynolds, C.P. (1999). Increase of ceramide and induction of mixed apoptosis/necrosis by N-(4-hydroxyphenyl)-retinamide in neuroblastoma cell lines. *J Natl Cancer Inst*, Vol.91, No.13, pp. 1138-1146.

Meitar, D., Crawford, S.E., Rademaker, A.W. & Cohn, S.L. (1996). Tumor angiogenesis correlates with metastatic disease, N-myc amplification, and poor outcome in human neuroblastoma. *J Clin Oncol*, Vol.14, No.2, pp. 405-414.

Minturn, J.E., Evans, A.E., Villablanca, J.G., Yanik, G.A., Park, J.R., Shusterman, S., Groshen, S., Hellriegel, E.T., Bensen-Kennedy, D., Matthay, K.K., Brodeur, G.M. & Maris, J.M. (2011). Phase I trial of lestaurtinib for children with refractory neuroblastoma: a new approaches to neuroblastoma therapy consortium study. *Cancer Chemother Pharmacol.*

Mir, R., Phillips, S.L., Schwartz, G., Mathur, R., Khan, A. & Kahn, L.B. (1987). Metastatic neuroblastoma after 52 years of dormancy. *Cancer*, Vol.60, No.10, pp. 2510-2514.

Monclair, T., Brodeur, G.M., Ambros, P.F., Brisse, H.J., Cecchetto, G., Holmes, K., Kaneko, M., London, W.B., Matthay, K.K., Nuchtern, J.G., von Schweinitz, D., Simon, T., Cohn, S.L. & Pearson, A.D. (2009). The International Neuroblastoma Risk Group (INRG) staging system: an INRG Task Force report. *J Clin Oncol*, Vol.27, No.2, pp. 298-303.

Moss, T.J., Reynolds, C.P., Sather, H.N., Romansky, S.G., Hammond, G.D. & Seeger, R.C. (1991). Prognostic value of immunocytologic detection of bone marrow metastases in neuroblastoma. *N Engl J Med*, Vol.324, No.4, pp. 219-226.

Mosse, Y.P., Laudenslager, M., Longo, L., Cole, K.A., Wood, A., Attiyeh, E.F., Laquaglia, M.J., Sennett, R., Lynch, J.E., Perri, P., Laureys, G., Speleman, F., Kim, C., Hou, C., Hakonarson, H., Torkamani, A., Schork, N.J., Brodeur, G.M., Tonini, G.P., Rappaport, E., Devoto, M. & Maris, J.M. (2008). Identification of ALK as a major familial neuroblastoma predisposition gene. *Nature*, Vol.455, No.7215, pp. 930-935.

Mueller, B.M., Romerdahl, C.A., Gillies, S.D. & Reisfeld, R.A. (1990). Enhancement of antibody-dependent cytotoxicity with a chimeric anti-GD2 antibody. *J Immunol*, Vol.144, No.4, pp. 1382-1386.

Mueller, S., Yang, X., Sottero, T.L., Gragg, A., Prasad, G., Polley, M.Y., Weiss, W.A., Matthay, K.K., Davidoff, A.M., DuBois, S.G. & Haas-Kogan, D.A. (2011). Cooperation of the HDAC inhibitor vorinostat and radiation in metastatic neuroblastoma: efficacy and underlying mechanisms. *Cancer Lett*, Vol.306, No.2, pp. 223-229.

Muhlethaler-Mottet, A., Meier, R., Flahaut, M., Bourloud, K.B., Nardou, K., Joseph, J.M. & Gross, N. (2008). Complex molecular mechanisms cooperate to mediate histone deacetylase inhibitors anti-tumour activity in neuroblastoma cells. *Mol Cancer*, Vol.7, pp. 55.

Nakagawara, A., Azar, C.G., Scavarda, N.J. & Brodeur, G.M. (1994). Expression and function of TRK-B and BDNF in human neuroblastomas. *Mol Cell Biol*, Vol.14, No.1, pp. 759-767.

Parodi, F., Passoni, L., Massimo, L., Luksch, R., Gambini, C., Rossi, E., Zuffardi, O., Pistoia, V. & Pezzolo, A. (2011). Identification of novel prognostic markers in relapsing localized resectable neuroblastoma. *OMICS*, Vol.15, No.3, pp. 113-121.

Paulino, A.C. (2003). Palliative radiotherapy in children with neuroblastoma. *Pediatr Hematol Oncol*, Vol.20, No.2, pp. 111-117.

Pezzolo, A., Rossi, E., Gimelli, S., Parodi, F., Negri, F., Conte, M., Pistorio, A., Sementa, A., Pistoia, V., Zuffardi, O. & Gambini, C. (2009). Presence of 1q gain and absence of 7p gain are new predictors of local or metastatic relapse in localized resectable neuroblastoma. *Neuro Oncol*, Vol.11, No.2, pp. 192-200.

Ribatti, D., Raffaghello, L., Marimpietri, D., Cosimo, E., Montaldo, P.G., Nico, B., Vacca, A. & Ponzoni, M. (2003). Fenretinide as an anti-angiogenic agent in neuroblastoma. *Cancer Lett*, Vol.197, No.1-2, pp. 181-184.

Santana, V.M., Furman, W.L., McGregor, L.M. & Billups, C.A. (2008). Disease control intervals in high-risk neuroblastoma. *Cancer*, Vol.112, No.12, pp. 2796-2801.

Schulte, J.H., Bachmann, H.S., Brockmeyer, B., De Preter, K., Oberthuer, A., Ackermann, S., Kahlert, Y., Pajtler, K., Theissen, J., Westermann, F., Vandesompele, J., Speleman, F., Berthold, F., Eggert, A., Brors, B., Hero, B., Schramm, A. & Fischer, M. (2011). High ALK receptor tyrosine kinase expression supersedes ALK mutation as a determining factor of an unfavorable phenotype in primary neuroblastoma. *Clin Cancer Res*.

Seeger, R.C., Reynolds, C.P., Gallego, R., Stram, D.O., Gerbing, R.B. & Matthay, K.K. (2000). Quantitative tumor cell content of bone marrow and blood as a predictor of outcome in stage IV neuroblastoma: a Children's Cancer Group Study. *J Clin Oncol*, Vol.18, No.24, pp. 4067-4076.

Sharp, S.E., Shulkin, B.L., Gelfand, M.J., Salisbury, S. & Furman, W.L. (2009). 123I-MIBG scintigraphy and 18F-FDG PET in neuroblastoma. *J Nucl Med*, Vol.50, No.8, pp. 1237-1243.

Shaw, P.J. & Eden, T. (1992). Neuroblastoma with intracranial involvement: an ENSG Study. *Med Pediatr Oncol*, Vol.20, No.2, pp. 149-155.

Shusterman, S., London, W.B., Gillies, S.D., Hank, J.A., Voss, S.D., Seeger, R.C., Reynolds, C.P., Kimball, J., Albertini, M.R., Wagner, B., Gan, J., Eickhoff, J., DeSantes, K.B., Cohn, S.L., Hecht, T., Gadbaw, B., Reisfeld, R.A., Maris, J.M. & Sondel, P.M. (2010). Antitumor activity of hu14.18-IL2 in patients with relapsed/refractory neuroblastoma: a Children's Oncology Group (COG) phase II study. *J Clin Oncol*, Vol.28, No.33, pp. 4969-4975.

Simon, T., Berthold, F., Borkhardt, A., Kremens, B., De Carolis, B. & Hero, B. (2011). Treatment and outcomes of patients with relapsed, high-risk neuroblastoma: results of German trials. *Pediatr Blood Cancer*, Vol.56, No.4, pp. 578-583.

Simon, T., Hero, B., Hunneman, D.H. & Berthold, F. (2003). Tumour markers are poor predictors for relapse or progression in neuroblastoma. *Eur J Cancer*, Vol.39, No.13, pp. 1899-1903.

Simon, T., Langler, A., Harnischmacher, U., Fruhwald, M.C., Jorch, N., Claviez, A., Berthold, F. & Hero, B. (2007). Topotecan, cyclophosphamide, and etoposide (TCE) in the treatment of high-risk neuroblastoma. Results of a phase-II trial. *J Cancer Res Clin Oncol*, Vol.133, No.9, pp. 653-661.

Sirachainan, N., Visudtibhan, A., Tuntiyatorn, L., Pakakasama, S., Chuansumrit, A. & Hongeng, S. (2008). Favorable response of intraommaya topotecan for leptomeningeal metastasis of neuroblastoma after intravenous route failure. *Pediatr Blood Cancer*, Vol.50, No.1, pp. 169-172.

Sofka, C.M., Semelka, R.C., Kelekis, N.L., Worawattanakul, S., Chung, C.J., Gold, S. & Fordham, L.A. (1999). Magnetic resonance imaging of neuroblastoma using current techniques. *Magn Reson Imaging*, Vol.17, No.2, pp. 193-198.

Stutterheim, J., Gerritsen, A., Zappeij-Kannegieter, L., Yalcin, B., Dee, R., van Noesel, M.M., Berthold, F., Versteeg, R., Caron, H.N., van der Schoot, C.E. & Tytgat, G.A. (2009). Detecting minimal residual disease in neuroblastoma: the superiority of a panel of real-time quantitative PCR markers. *Clin Chem*, Vol.55, No.7, pp. 1316-1326.

Stutterheim, J., Zappeij-Kannegieter, L., Versteeg, R., Caron, H.N., van der Schoot, C.E. & Tytgat, G.A. (2011). The prognostic value of fast molecular response of marrow disease in patients aged over 1 year with stage 4 neuroblastoma. *Eur J Cancer*, Vol.47, No.8, pp. 1193-1202.

Swerts, K., Ambros, P.F., Brouzes, C., Navarro, J.M., Gross, N., Rampling, D., Schumacher-Kuckelkorn, R., Sementa, A.R., Ladenstein, R. & Beiske, K. (2005). Standardization of the immunocytochemical detection of neuroblastoma cells in bone marrow. *J Histochem Cytochem*, Vol.53, No.12, pp. 1433-1440.

Taggart, D.R., Han, M.M., Quach, A., Groshen, S., Ye, W., Villablanca, J.G., Jackson, H.A., Mari Aparici, C., Carlson, D., Maris, J., Hawkins, R. & Matthay, K.K. (2009). Comparison of iodine-123 metaiodobenzylguanidine (MIBG) scan and [18F]fluorodeoxyglucose positron emission tomography to evaluate response after iodine-131 MIBG therapy for relapsed neuroblastoma. *J Clin Oncol*, Vol.27, No.32, pp. 5343-5349.

Vik, T.A., Pfluger, T., Kadota, R., Castel, V., Tulchinsky, M., Farto, J.C., Heiba, S., Serafini, A., Tumeh, S., Khutoryansky, N. & Jacobson, A.F. (2009). (123)I-mIBG scintigraphy in patients with known or suspected neuroblastoma: Results from a prospective multicenter trial. *Pediatr Blood Cancer*, Vol.52, No.7, pp. 784-790.

Villa, M.L., Ferrario, E., Trabattoni, D., Formelli, F., De Palo, G., Magni, A., Veronesi, U. & Clerici, E. (1993). Retinoids, breast cancer and NK cells. *Br J Cancer*, Vol.68, No.5, pp. 845-850.

Villablanca, J.G., Krailo, M.D., Ames, M.M., Reid, J.M., Reaman, G.H. & Reynolds, C.P. (2006). Phase I trial of oral fenretinide in children with high-risk solid tumors: a report from the Children's Oncology Group (CCG 09709). *J Clin Oncol*, Vol.24, No.21, pp. 3423-3430.

Viprey, V.F., Corrias, M.V., Kagedal, B., Oltra, S., Swerts, K., Vicha, A., Ladenstein, R. & Burchill, S.A. (2007). Standardisation of operating procedures for the detection of minimal disease by QRT-PCR in children with neuroblastoma: quality assurance on behalf of SIOPEN-R-NET. *Eur J Cancer*, Vol.43, No.2, pp. 341-350.

Wagner, L.M., Villablanca, J.G., Stewart, C.F., Crews, K.R., Groshen, S., Reynolds, C.P., Park, J.R., Maris, J.M., Hawkins, R.A., Daldrup-Link, H.E., Jackson, H.A. & Matthay, K.K. (2009). Phase I trial of oral irinotecan and temozolomide for children with relapsed high-risk neuroblastoma: a new approach to neuroblastoma therapy consortium study. *J Clin Oncol*, Vol.27, No.8, pp. 1290-1296.

Yanik, G.A., Parisi, M.T., Naranjo, A., Matthay, K.K., London, W.B., McGrady, P.W., Kreissman, S.G. & Shulkin, B.L. (2010). MIBG scoring as a prognostic indicator in patients with stage IV neuroblastoma: A COG study. *Journal of Clinical Oncology*, Vol.28, No.15s (abstract 9516).

Yu, A.L., Gilman, A.L., Ozkaynak, M.F., London, W.B., Kreissman, S.G., Chen, H.X., Smith, M., Anderson, B., Villablanca, J.G., Matthay, K.K., Shimada, H., Grupp, S.A., Seeger, R., Reynolds, C.P., Buxton, A., Reisfeld, R.A., Gillies, S.D., Cohn, S.L., Maris, J.M. & Sondel, P.M. (2010). Anti-GD2 antibody with GM-CSF, interleukin-2, and isotretinoin for neuroblastoma. *N Engl J Med*, Vol.363, No.14, pp. 1324-1334.

2

Genetic Factors Influencing the Risk and Clinical Outcome of Neuroblastoma

Diana T. Lau and Lesley J. Ashton
Children's Cancer Institute Australia for Medical Research,
Lowy Cancer Research Centre, UNSW,
Australia

1. Introduction

Neuroblastoma is an embryonal malignancy of the sympathetic nervous system arising from neuroblasts. It is the most common solid tumor in children under the age of 5 and accounts for 8-10% of all childhood cancers (Brodeur & Maris, 2006). The disease occurs almost exclusively in infants and children below the age of 4, with median age of diagnosis approximately 17 months (Ries et al., 1999; London et al., 2005). Prognostic factors such as age at diagnosis, clinical stage, Shimada histology, amplification of *MYCN*, DNA ploidy, and molecular defects such as allelic loss of chromosome 1p and 11q in tumor cells are used for risk stratification and treatment assignment. The amplification of *MYCN* oncogene occurs in 20% to 25% of primary neuroblastomas and is consistently associated with poor outcome in neuroblastoma (Brodeur & Seeger, 1986). Although the overall 5-year survival of patients with neuroblastoma have improved considerably over the past decade, survival rates among children with high-risk neuroblastoma remains below 50%, despite marked intensification of chemotherapy (Baade et al., 2010).

A particular hallmark of neuroblastoma is its clinical heterogeneity, where some patients experience spontaneous regression or differentiation of the tumor into benign ganglioneuroma, while others are affected by rapid and fatal tumor progression (Schwab et al., 2003). Although the disease is often diagnosed in the perinatal period, environmental or parental risk factors have not been identified consistently and the molecular basis of neuroblastoma development and progression is still poorly understood (Hamrick et al., 2001; Urayama et al., 2007; Munzer et al., 2008). Recent advances in genome-wide studies have proven to be a useful prognostic tool for identifying genetic alleles or regions that may be used as risk markers for neuroblastoma development. In recent years, a number of genetic and genomic changes have been identified in neuroblastoma tumors that are relevant to clinical progression, allowing tumors to be classified into subsets with distinct clinical behavior. Genome-wide association studies (GWAS) have described genetic factors influencing the risk and clinical outcome of neuroblastoma such as rare mutations in the *ALK* gene for familial neuroblastoma, common single nucleotide polymorphisms (SNPs) at 6p22 in *FLJ22536* and *FLJ44180*, 2q35 in *BARD1*, 11p15.4 in *LMO1*, and copy number variation at 1q21.1 in *NBPF23*. Moreover, several regions with chromosomal alterations have been identified and many of these regions are speculated to harbor tumor suppressor genes.

However, no single genetic change has been found to be common to all neuroblastoma tumors suggesting a complex underlying genetics of neuroblastoma and that aberrant expression or regulation of multiple genes may work together to initiate the malignant transformation of undifferentiated neuroblasts.

More recently, it has become apparent that the biology of neuroblastoma is determined not only by the tumor's genetic profile but also the tumor epigenetic profile. Distinct CpG island methylation patterns have been suggested to characterize different clinical groups of neuroblastoma (Alaminos et al., 2004; Yang et al., 2004; Banelli et al., 2005b; Abe et al., 2007) . Indeed, several potential tumor suppressor genes such as *CASP8* and *RASSF1* have been identified to be frequently hypermethylated and silenced in neuroblastoma. Therefore, epigenetic biomarkers may be considered as a potential prognostic marker for predicting risk groups and response to therapy.

This chapter reviews the genetic changes that are associated with the risk and outcome in neuroblastoma with particular focus on recently identified SNPs, copy number variations, genomic changes and epigenetic alterations that have been linked to the tumorigenesis and progression of neuroblastoma. Knowledge of the genetics of neuroblastoma offers opportunities to understand the underlying mechanisms for the heterogeneity of neuroblastoma and will facilitate the discovery of new therapeutic targets.

2. Genetic alterations in neuroblastoma

2.1 PHOX2B and *ALK* mutations in familial neuroblastoma

Familial neuroblastoma accounts for approximately 1% of all cases and the disease appears to inherit in an autosomal dominant mode with incomplete penetrance (Maris et al., 2007). Some patients with neuroblastoma have been described with other congenital disorders of neural crest-derived cells, such as central congenital hypoventilation syndrome (CCHS) or Hirschsprung disease (Maris et al., 1997; Amiel et al., 2003). Hence, the co-existence of these disorders and neuroblastoma suggests a common underlying genetic cause. In CCHS, mutations in the paired-like homeobox 2B (*PHOX2B*) gene at chromosome 4p12 is commonly detected, which prompted researchers to examine mutations of *PHOX2B* in neuroblastoma (Weese-Mayer et al., 2005). *PHOX2B* encodes a transcription factor that regulates the development of the autonomic nervous system. Linkage studies of neuroblastoma cases have revealed several germline *PHOX2B* mutations found exclusively in patients with congenital abnormalities of the neural crest (Table 1) (Mosse et al., 2004; Trochet et al., 2004). Although only 6.4% of familial neuroblastoma cases have shown to harbor these mutations, *PHOX2B* was the first gene to be considered as a candidate gene for predisposition to familial neuroblastoma (Raabe et al., 2007). Analysis of *PHOX2B* mutations in sporadic neuroblastoma has also revealed several frameshift mutations (Table 1) (Limpt et al., 2004) and although these mutations occur in less than 3% in sporadic neuroblastomas, they suggest a role for *PHOX2B* in the oncogenesis of neuroblastoma.

For cases that were not associated with other congenital disorders of neural crest development, several groups have independently discovered mutations of the anaplastic lymphoma kinase (*ALK*) gene in familial neuroblastoma as well as sporadic neuroblastoma (Caren et al., 2008; Chen et al., 2008; George et al., 2008; Janoueix-Lerosey et al., 2008; Mosse et al., 2008). Findings from these studies have shown that the frequency of somatic *ALK* mutations ranged from 4-8% in primary neuroblastoma tumors (Janoueix-Lerosey et al., 2008; Mosse et al., 2008).

Gene	Chromosome location	Gene function	Genetic variations^	References
PHOX2B	4p12	Regulator of autonomic nervous system development	R110L, R141G, G299T, G216fs*88, A241fs*64, G239fs*82	(Limpt et al., 2004; Mosse et al., 2004; Trochet et al., 2004)
ALK	2q23	Encodes for tyrosine kinase	R1275Q, F1275L, F1174L, F1174I, F1174C, F1174V, F1245C, F1245L, F1245V, F1245I, D1091N, A1234T, G1128A, I1171N, I1250T, K1062M, M1166R, R1192P, T1087I, T1151M, Y1278S	(Chen et al., 2008; George et al., 2008; Janoueix-Lerosey et al., 2008; Mosse et al., 2008)
FLJ22536 *FLJ44180*	6p22	Unknown	rs693940, rs4712653, rs9295536	(Maris et al., 2008)
BARD1	2q35	Interacts with *BRCA1*	rs6435862, rs3768716, rs17487792, rs6712055, rs7587476, rs6715570	(Capasso et al., 2009)
LMO1	11q15.4	Transcriptional regulator	rs110419, rs4758051, rs10840002, rs204938	(Wang et al., 2011)
DUSP12	1q23.3	Encodes for Ser/Thr and Tyr protein phosphatases	rs1027702$^{\phi}$	(Nguyễn et al., 2011)
DDX4	5q11.2	Putative RNA helicases	rs2619046$^{\phi}$	(Nguyễn et al., 2011)
IL31RA	5q11.2	Encodes for type I cytokine receptor family protein	rs10055201$^{\phi}$	(Nguyễn et al., 2011)
HSD17B12	11q11.2		rs11037575$^{\phi}$	(Nguyễn et al., 2011)
NBF23	1q21.1	Unknown	CNV	(Diskin et al., 2009)

^Only missense mutations are listed. $^{\phi}$Most significant SNP identified.

Table 1. A summary of significant SNPs and CNV at each described predisposition locus identified by GWAS.

The *ALK* gene maps to chromosome 2p23, which also contains *MYCN*, the well-known oncogene in neuroblastoma. The protein product of *ALK* is a tyrosine kinase, an enzyme that regulates the activity of other proteins through phosphorylation. *ALK* plays a critical role in controlling cell proliferation, differentiation and survival in normal cells, especially in the development of the brain and the autonomic nervous system (Wellmann et al., 1997; *The NCBI handbook*, 2002). In many human cancers, *ALK* functions as an oncogene by the activation of *ALK* signaling to form oncogenic fusion proteins through chromosomal translocation events (Mosse et al., 2009). More than 20 *ALK* mutations have been identified in neuroblastoma patients and cell lines (Table 1), including F1174L, F1174S, F1245C and R1275Q which are located in the conserved regions of the kinase domain and have been shown to activate *ALK* signaling, suggesting their functional importance for the regulation of kinase activity (Chen et al., 2008; Janoueix-Lerosey et al., 2008; Mosse et al., 2008; Martinsson et al., 2011). *ALK* mutations tend to be associated with advanced stage neuroblastoma. In particular, F1174L mutations have been observed to occur at a higher frequency in *MYCN*-amplified tumors, and be associated with poorer outcome, suggesting an interactive role between both aberrations (De Brouwer et al., 2010). Other genetic defects such as amplification and overexpression of the *ALK* gene have been found to correlate with unfavorable features, such as metastatic tumors and poor outcome in neuroblastoma (Caren et al., 2008; Janoueix-Lerosey et al., 2008; Passoni et al., 2009). In addition, the expression levels of *ALK* and *PHOX2B* were directly correlated in neuroblastoma cell lines (Bachetti et al., 2010). Hence, *ALK* has been identified as a novel target gene of *PHOX2B*, indicating that these two genes are jointly involved in the tumorigenesis of neuroblastoma (Bachetti et al., 2010). Since mutations of *ALK* and *PHOX2B* account for the majority of familial neuroblastoma cases, patients with a family history of neuroblastoma are routinely offered genetic counseling and testing for *ALK* and *PHOX2B* mutations (www.ncbi.nlm.nih.gov/sites/GeneTests).

2.2 Genetic variations in sporadic neuroblastoma

The vast majority of neuroblastoma tumors develop sporadically without family history of the disease (Capasso & Diskin, 2010). Genetic variation appears to play a central role in determining neuroblastoma susceptibility with most cases likely to arise from the interaction between multiple genetic variants (Maris et al., 2007). The use of high-density SNP genotyping arrays in GWAS has proven to be a powerful tool in identifying genetic determinants of complex disease. The first report that identified common genetic variants predisposing to neuroblastoma came from a GWAS using blood samples from nearly 2000 neuroblastoma patients and more than 4000 healthy control subjects of European descent (Maris et al., 2008). In this study, over half a million SNPs were genotyped and 3 common SNPs within the *FLJ22536* and *FLJ44180* genes at chromosome 6p22.3 were identified to be associated with the predisposition of sporadic neuroblastoma (Table 1). Investigations also showed that patients that were homozygous for these high-risk alleles were more likely to develop a clinically aggressive form of neuroblastoma, including metastatic neuroblastoma, *MYCN* amplification, and subsequently relapse. Although the function of *FLJ22536* and *FLJ44180* in the tumorigenesis of neuroblastoma is not yet known, these findings suggest that common variants of these two genes may have a distinctive role in the etiology of more aggressive forms of neuroblastoma; a hypothesis examined in subsequent GWAS limited to patients with high-risk neuroblastoma (Capasso et al., 2009). These investigators not only replicated the findings of candidate SNPs at 6p22, a further 6 SNPs within the *BRCA1*-associated RING domain 1 (*BARD1*) gene at 2q35 were found to be associated with aggressive neuroblastoma (Table 1). *BARD1* has been previously implicated to have a role in several types of cancers, including breast cancer. The BARD1 protein heterodimerizes with BRCA1 protein and the formation of a stable complex between these proteins is thought to be important for the tumor suppressor function of *BRCA1* (Capasso et al., 2009). However, further studies are required to characterize the biological consequences of genetic variations in the *BARD1* gene which may lead to the identification of potential therapeutic target for high-risk neuroblastoma.

A further GWAS examining over 2000 patients with neuroblastoma and 6000 control subjects of European ancestry reported that common genetic variants within the *LMO1* gene at 11p15.4 were significantly associated with the risk of neuroblastoma (Table 1) (Wang et al., 2011). *LMO1* encodes a cysteine-rich transcriptional regulator, and its paralogs (*LMO2, LMO3* and *LMO4*) have each been implicated in other cancers (Curtis & McCormack, 2010; Wang et al., 2011). Similar to those observed for the 6p22 and *BARD1* loci, the risk alleles of *LMO1* were also found to be associated with high-risk neuroblastoma and decreased survival. In particular, the *LMO1* SNP, rs110419, displayed the strongest association with the aggressive form of the disease. Moreover, presence of the rs110419 variant allele and copy number gains of *LMO1* were associated with increased expression of *LMO1* in neuroblastoma cell lines and primary tumors, suggesting a gain-of-function role of these genetic defects in the tumorigenesis of neuroblastoma (Wang et al., 2011).

More recently, a novel gene-centric approach examined the combined effect of all SNPs within 10 kilobases of 15,885 target genes (Nguyễn et al., 2011). This method correctly identified three genes previously reported to be associated with high-risk neuroblastoma (*FLJ22536, BARD1* and *LMO1*). When the analyses were enriched for low-risk neuroblastoma cases, SNPs within four novel genes, dual specificity phosphatase 12 (*DUSP12*), DEAD box polypeptide 4 isoform (*DDX4*), interleukin 31 receptor A precursor (*IL31RA*) and hydroxysteroid (17-beta) dehydrogenase 12 (*HSD17B12*) were identified as being associated with the less aggressive form of neuroblastoma. These susceptibility loci were successfully replicated in two independent cohorts highlighting the importance of robust phenotypic data and the use of alternative methods that focus on individual genes, instead of individual SNPs in GWAS.

Copy number variation (CNV) is another form of genetic variation that has been linked to cancer susceptibility. CNVs are structural variants that comprise of copy number change involving a DNA fragment that is at least one kilobases long (Freeman et al., 2006). Previous investigations identified a deletion CNV at chromosome 1q21.1 that was highly associated with neuroblastoma (Diskin et al., 2009). Sequencing of this region found a previously unknown transcript with high sequence similarity to several neuroblastoma breakpoint family (*NBPF*) genes and this novel transcript was termed *NBPF23* (Diskin et al., 2009). The expression level of *NBPF23* was directly correlated with CNV and NBPF23 was shown to preferentially express in normal fetal brain and fetal sympathetic tissues, implicating its role in early tumorigenesis of neuroblastoma (Diskin et al., 2009).

2.3 Genomic changes in neuroblastoma

Over the last two decades, many chromosomal and molecular anomalies have been identified in patients with neuroblastoma and the biological and clinical relevance of these genetic changes have been reported. In order to establish reliable genetic markers, several reported molecular defects have been evaluated by the International Neuroblastoma Risk Group (INRG) in a cohort of 8800 neuroblastoma patients to determine their value as a prognostic marker, and some of these markers have been incorporated into risk assessment strategies (Ambros et al., 2009; Cohn et al., 2009).

2.3.1 *MYCN* amplification and chromosome alterations

The most important of these biologic markers is *MYCN*, an oncogene that is amplified in approximately 20-25% of all neuroblastoma cases and is more common in patients with advanced-stage disease (Brodeur & Seeger, 1986). The process of amplification usually results in 50 to 400 copies of the gene per cell, with correspondingly high levels of MYCN protein expression (Seeger et al., 1988). Patients with amplification of *MYCN* tend to have rapid tumor progression and poor prognosis, even in the presence of other favorable factors such as low-stage neuroblastoma. Amplification of *MYCN* is often associated with other chromosomal aberrations such as the deletion of chromosome 1p, which was identified in 25-35% of all neuroblastoma cases (Attiyeh et al., 2005; White et al., 2005). Studies have shown that the addition of an intact human chromosome 1p to a 1p-deleted neuroblastoma cell line can induce cellular differentiation and/or death (Bader et al., 1991), suggesting that the 1p chromosome region harbors tumor suppressor genes (TSGs) or genes that are likely to control neuroblast differentiation. While only a few candidate TSGs have been identified in this region (Okawa et al., 2008), deletion of the 1p region has been associated with unfavorable clinical outcome, independent of age and stage (Caron et al., 1996b) and most 1p-deletions have been found in the 1p36 area of the chromosome; a region showing loss of heterozygosity (LOH) in 20-40% of neuroblastoma tumors (Caren et al., 2007).

Another common chromosomal aberration is the deletion of 11q identified in more than half of all neuroblastoma cases, has found to be highly associated with chromosome 3p LOH (George et al., 2007). As 11q deletions were inversely correlated to *MYCN* amplification, this aberration represents a powerful biomarker of poor outcome in cases without *MYCN* amplification (Attiyeh et al., 2005). Hence, 11q status has recently been included as a criterion in the INRG classification system (Cohn et al., 2009). To a lesser extent, other allelic losses of chromosome segments 3p, 4p, 9p, and 14q have been shown to have varying degrees of prognostic importance (Fong et al., 1992; Caron et al., 1996a; Ejeskar et al., 1998; Vandesompele et al., 1998).

The partial gain of chromosome 17q has been observed in more than 70% of primary neuroblastoma tumors, indicating that a 17q gain is one of the most frequent genetic abnormalities observed in neuroblastoma (Plantaz et al., 1997; George et al., 2007). Unbalanced 17q gain is associated with *MYCN* amplification, loss of 1p, and adverse outcome (Bown et al., 1999). Although this feature may be useful for treatment stratification, the underlying molecular mechanisms conferring the adverse phenotype of neuroblastoma are still unclear.

While recent genome-wide approaches have provided a comprehensive overview of genetic alterations present in neuroblastoma, segmental chromosomal aberrations have also been reported to be associated with clinically aggressive disease and high-risk of relapse (Janoueix-Lerosey et al., 2009; Schleiermacher et al., 2010). In contrast, neuroblastoma patients with whole chromosomal gains or losses have shown better survival and association with favorable clinical disease stage (Lastowska et al., 2001). These findings place a greater emphasis on overall genomic pattern rather than individual conventional markers for inclusion in future treatment stratification system for neuroblastoma.

2.3.2 DNA content

DNA content or ploidy and structural abnormalities, such as chromosomal deletions or gains, have been extensively studied in neuroblastoma. A strong correlation has been found between increased chromosome number in neuroblastoma cells (diploid versus hyperdiploid) and response to therapy, especially in children less than 1 year of age (Look et al., 1991). While patients with favorable neuroblastoma tend to have a hyperdiploid or near-triploid DNA content (Kaneko et al., 1987), the majority of neuroblastoma cell lines and advanced primary tumors from older patients have either a near-diploid or near-tetraploid DNA content (Maris & Matthay, 1999). Diploid or tetraploid tumors in older patients usually have several structural rearrangements, including amplification, deletion, and unbalanced translocations, while hyperdiploid and triploid tumors in infants generally have whole chromosome gains without structural rearrangements (Kaneko et al., 1987; Maris & Matthay, 1999). These observations are consistent with the findings mentioned earlier that segmental chromosome defects confer a more aggressive phenotype than those with whole chromosome gains or losses.

3. DNA methylation and cancer

Cancer development is an intricate multistep process that involves the malfunction of proto-oncogenes, tumor suppressor genes (TSGs), and other key cellular genes essential for cell differentiation, progression and genome integrity. Malfunction or inactivation of these genes is thought to be predominantly caused by genetic events such as DNA mutations and chromosomal deletions. Until recently, epigenetic alterations were recognized as an alternative mechanism associated with inappropriate gene silencing. Epigenetic changes are heritable alterations in the expression of genes that occur without changing the nucleotide gene sequence of DNA (Das & Singal, 2004). The most well characterized epigenetic event in the mammalian genome is DNA methylation; an essential process that regulates gene transcription and normal cell development. DNA methylation silences gene expression through the addition of methyl groups to cytosine residues within CpG-rich dinucleotides present in the promoter region of genes, where transcription is initiated. Although CpG sites are relatively uncommon in most of the human genome, CpG-rich sequences occurs at a much higher frequency proximal to gene promoter regions and are known as CpG islands (CGIs) and these islands are mostly free of methylation in normal cells (Jones & Baylin, 2002).

In recent years, a growing number of cancer-related genes have been identified to harbor dense methylation in normally unmethylated promoter CGI (Jones & Baylin, 2002). Hypermethylation of the promoter region is often associated with transcriptional silencing of downstream genes such as tumor suppressor genes (Esteller & Herman, 2002). Indeed, many genes implicated in pathways controlling growth, genomic stability and cell survival have been reported to be silenced by promoter hypermethylation. In cancer, gene silencing through methylation occurs at least as frequently as mutations or deletions (Baylin, 2005), while a global decrease in methylated CpG content or hypomethylation is rather uncommon (Kulis & Esteller, 2010). Nevertheless, changes in methylation patterns may lead to chromosomal instability, activation of endogenous parasitic sequences, loss of imprinting, inappropriate expression, aneuploidy, and mutations (Esteller & Herman, 2002). Thus, aberrant methylation is recognized as an important component of tumorigenesis and methylation changes in multiple genes may represent the characteristics of different tumors or tumor subtypes with unique biological and clinical features. Hence, methylation is considered a promising biomarker for diagnostic and prognostic stratification of cancer patients.

3.1 DNA methylation in neuroblastoma

Although *MYCN* amplification is a strong prognostic marker that identifies a subgroup of patients at high risk of tumor progression and intensive therapy, the majority of metastatic neuroblastomas do not show amplification of this oncogene and these patients can also present with aggressive forms of neuroblastoma (Ambros et al., 2009). Therefore, identification of additional predictive biomarkers is needed for better stratification of patient risk groups and therapeutic regimens.

In the past decade, a growing list of aberrantly methylated genes including those involved in apoptosis, cell-cycle regulation, differentiation and development has been described in neuroblastoma (Table 2). This list is likely to expand as large scale methods for the detection of methylation continue to improve. Despite the current lack of evidence supporting the role of global hypomethylation in neuroblastoma, methylation studies have provided clues for the molecular basis of neuroblastoma and the search for epigenetic signatures that could be associated with defined clinical and biological parameters in neuroblastoma continues. A list of methylation studies and their findings are presented in Table 3. Several studies have found distinct promoter methylation patterns that were able to characterize different clinical groups in neuroblastoma (Abe et al., 2005; Banelli et al., 2005b). The latest findings describing the role of methylation in uncultured or primary neuroblastoma tumors are discussed below.

3.1.1 Tumor suppressor genes

Inactivation of TSGs is a critical step in cancer development. Functional loss of TSGs is usually mediated by oncogenic mutations or chromosomal deletions. In recent years, CGI hypermethylation has been recognized as an alternative mechanism for TSG inactivation and several potential TSGs has been described to be frequently hypermethylated and down-regulated in neuroblastoma.

Allelic losses of chromosome 3p21.3 are frequently detected in many cancers. Several candidate tumor-suppressor genes have been identified in this region, including *RASSF1* (Ras-association domain family 1). This gene encodes for an anaphase inhibitor that prevents cell proliferation by negatively regulating cell-cycle progression through the inhibition of cyclin D1 protein (Nguyễn et al., 2011). Loss or altered expression of *RASSF1* has been associated with the tumorigenesis of other cancers, suggesting the tumor suppressor function of this gene (Burbee et al., 2001). *RASSF1* is consistently methylated in primary neuroblastoma tumors and is frequently inactivated by promoter hypermethylation resulting in loss of expression (Harada et al., 2002; Michalowski et al., 2008). Silencing of *RASSF1* has been postulated to contribute to aberrations of *RAS* signal pathways observed in neuroblastomas (Tanaka et al., 1998). Furthermore, several investigators have reported methylation of *RASSF1* to be associated with unfavorable features. For example, neuroblastoma patients with older age (>1 year) have been shown to have higher levels of *RASSF1* methylation (Harada et al., 2002; Yang et al., 2004), while complete methylation of *RASSF1* has been found to be more prevalent in patients with *MYCN* amplification than

Gene	Gene function	Methylation frequency (%), (no. of samples)	References
APAF1	Proapoptotic gene	28% (23/82)	(Grau et al., 2010)
CASP8	Apoptotic gene, potential TSG	56% (24/42) 60% (21/35) 38% (17/45)	(Hoebeeck et al., 2009) (Lazcoz et al., 2006) (Michalowski et al., 2008)
HOXA9	Development regulator	39% (57/145)‡	(Alaminos et al., 2004)
PYCARD	Induces apoptosis	31% (45/145)‡	(Alaminos et al., 2004)
RASSF1	Anaphase inhibitor	71% (30/42) 52% (14/27) 70% (39/56) 83% (34/41) 93% (42/45) 84% (26/31) 55% (37/67) 94% (64/68)	(Hoebeeck et al., 2009) (Harada et al., 2002) (Yang et al., 2004) (Lazcoz et al., 2006) (Michalowski et al., 2008) (Banelli et al., 2005b) (Astuti et al., 2001) (Misawa et al., 2009)
SFN	Inhibits cell-cycle progression	100% (31/31)	(Banelli et al., 2005b)
TIMP3	Inhibitor of tissue metallo-proteases, matrix remodeling, tissue invasion	51% (23/45)	(Michalowski et al., 2008)
THBS1	Angiogenesis inhibitor	55% (31/56) 64% (24/38)	(Yang et al., 2004) (Gonzalez-Gomez et al., 2003)
TNRSF10C	Anti-apoptotic decoy receptors	11% (5/45) 21% (6/28)	(Michalowski et al., 2008) (van Noesel et al., 2002)
TNRSF10D	Anti-apoptotic decoy receptors	25% (11/45) 25% (7/28) 42% (13/31)	(Michalowski et al., 2008) (van Noesel et al., 2002) (Banelli et al., 2005b)
ZMYND10	Cell-cycle regulation, potential TSG	15% (6/42) 8% (3/41) 34% (15/45) 41% (20/49)	(Hoebeeck et al., 2009) (Lazcoz et al., 2006) (Michalowski et al., 2008) (Agathanggelou et al., 2003)

‡Included 27 relapse samples corresponding to the same patients from whom primary tumors were also available.

Table 2. Genes commonly silenced by promoter methylation in primary neuroblastoma tumors.

Gene(s) examined	Detection method	Sample size	Findings	Reference
PTEN, MGMT, PRDM2, hMLH1, CD44, THBS1, GSTP1, CFTR, TNFRSF10A, ZMYND10, RASSF5, RARβ, CASP8, PYCARD, APAF1, RB1, EMP3, CCND2, RASSF1, SYK	MSP	82	Hypermethylation of *CASP8, PYCARD* and *THBS1* were associated with *MYCN* amplification and poor EFS and OS. Combined analysis of hypermethylation of apoptotic genes (*CASP8, PYCARD* and *APAF1*) was suggested as a good prognostic indicator of NB progression.	(Grau et al., 2010)
SFN	Pyro-sequencing & MSP	122	A methylation threshold of 85% for the *SFN* gene distinguished NB patients with progressive disease from those with favorable outcome.	(Banelli et al., 2010)
ROBO1, PRMD2, TP73, DCC, CDH1, ZMYND10, PTEN, CASP8, RASSF1, CD44	MSP	42	Hypermethylation of *CASP8* and *CDH1* was associated with poor EFS. Meta-analysis of 115 NB tumors demonstrated that *CASP8* methylation and *MYCN* amplification are correlated.	(Hoebeeck et al., 2009)
RASSF1	MSP	68	Hypermethylation of *RASSF1* was found in 94% of NB tumors and 25% in matched serum samples. Serum methylation of *RASSF1* was associated with age at diagnosis (≥1 year), stage 4 NB and *MYCN* amplification.	(Misawa et al., 2009)
TIMP3, CASP8, ZMYND10, TNFRSF10C, TNFRSF10D, CDKN2B, RARβ, DAPK1, FHIT, NF2, CDKN2A, CDKN2A, APC, RB1, SMARCB1, NF2, CFLAR, CDH1, MGMT	MSP	45 & 17 relapse	Methylation of *RASSF1, TIMP3, CASP8, ZMYND10* was detected at diagnosis as well as relapse and were associated with unfavorable stage.	(Michalowski et al., 2008)
HIC1, PYCARD, TNFRSF10D, ZMYND10, TNFRSF10A, CDH1, SCGB3A1, RARRES1, IRF7, CDH13, EDNRB, MGMT, BRCA1, RB1, P27, DKK3, VHL, SLC16A1, PTEN	MSP	70	*TNFRSF10D, CASP8* and *SCGB3A1* were associated with high-risk NB and poor outcome.	(Yang et al., 2007)
RASSF1, RASSF5, ZMYND10, CASP8	MSP	41	A correlation was found between the methylation levels of *RASSF1* and *CASP8*. No association was detected between methylation and known prognostic factors.	(Lazcoz et al., 2006)
PCDHB gene family, *PCDHA* gene family, *MST1, MST1P9, DKFZp451I127, FBLN7, ZBTB22, CYP26C1*	MS-RDA & MSP	145	Multiple CGIs were simultaneously methylated in patients with poor prognosis, conforming to the concept of CpG island methylator phenotype (CIMP). Almost all cases with *MYCN* amplification exhibited CIMP.	(Abe et al., 2005)

Gene(s) examined	Detection method	Sample size	Findings	Reference
SFN, RASSF1, CDKN2A, CDH1, CASP8, TNFRSF10D, RARβ, TNFRSF10A, MGMT, TAp73, ΔNp73	MSP, COBRA & direct sequencing	31	Methylation of *SFN, RASSF1* and intragenic segment of *CASP8* was different between *MYCN* amplified and non-amplified NB tumors. Hypermethylation of *TNRSF10D* was associated with reduced overall survival.	(Banelli et al., 2005b)
TNFRSF10A, PYCARD, RARβ, SYK, PRDM2, FOLH1, CDKN2A, CCND2, LMX1A, HOXA9	MSP	118 & 27 relapse	Hypermethylation of *HOXA9* was associated with poor survival in patients <1 year of age and with no amplification of *MYCN*.	(Alaminos et al., 2004)
SPARC, TIMP3, THBS1, DAPK1, TP73, FAS, CDKN2A, CDKN1A RASSF1, RARβ2, CASP8	MSP	56	Hypermethylation of *RASSF1* was associated with age >1 year, high-risk NB and poor survival. No association between *THBS1* methylation and prognostic factors or survival was observed.	(Yang et al., 2004)
ZMYND10, RASSF1	MSP & COBRA	49	Methylation of *ZMYND10* was detected in 41% of primary NB tumors. No correlation was found between methylation of *RASSF1* and *ZMYND10*.	(Agathanggelou et al., 2003)
MGMT, DAPK1, CDKN2A, THBS1, TIMP3, TP73, CDKN2A, RB1, CASP8, TP53, GSTP1	MSP	38	A high frequency of methylation (64%) was detected in *THBS1*, while all other genes have intermediate or low methylation frequency (0-30%).	(Gonzalez-Gomez et al., 2003)
TNFRSF10A, TNFRSF10B, TNFRSF10C, TNFRSF10D	MSP	28	Hypermethylation was observed for *TNFRSF10C* and *TNFRSF10D*, while *TNFRSF10A* and *TNFRSF10B* were frequently expressed in NB tumors with no methylation was observed.	(van Noesel et al., 2002)
CDKN2A, MGMT, GSTP1, RASSF1, APC, DAPK1, RARβ2, CDH1, CDH13	MSP	27	Methylation of *RASSF1* had the highest frequency (52%) when compared to other genes (<6%). Hypermethylation of *RASSF1* was associated with age >1 year.	(Harada et al., 2002)
RASSF1, CASP8	MSP & COBRA	67	*RASSF1* was methylated in the majority of primary NB tumors and *RASSF1* promoter methylation is was associated with transcriptional silencing of *RASSF1* in NB cell lines. Methylation of *RASSF1* and *CASP8* was found to be correlated.	(Astuti et al., 2001)

Abbreviation: MSP = methylation specific PCR; COBRA = combined bisulfite restriction analysis; MS-RDA = methylation-sensitive representational difference analysis; EFS = event-free survival; OS = overall survival; CGI = CpG island; NB=neuroblastoma.

Table 3. A summary of findings from methylation studies in primary neuroblastoma tumors.

those without (Banelli et al., 2005b). However, associations between *RASSF1* methylation and clinical outcome of neuroblastoma have been variable. One study found significant association between *RASSF1* methylation and high-risk neuroblastoma as well as poor survival (Yang et al., 2004), while other studies were unable to detect any associations (Harada et al., 2002; Wong et al., 2004; Lazcoz et al., 2006). Nevertheless, when the combined methylation levels of both *RASSF1* and *TNFRSF10D* are considered, their clinical association with reduced overall survival and progressive tumors becomes more apparent (Banelli et al., 2005b). Similarly, methylation patterns in *RASSF1* and *CASP8* have been reported to be correlated, although the clinical significance of this association is yet to be established (Astuti et al., 2001; Lazcoz et al., 2006). More recently, a study examining the level of promoter hypermethylation of *RASSF1* in serum DNA samples of patients with neuroblastoma found increased levels of *RASSF1* hypermethylation associated with older age, stage 4 disease, and *MYCN* amplification (Misawa et al., 2009). These promising findings indicate that screening for methylation status of *RASSF1* and other genes in patient serum at diagnosis may be further developed for use as a non-surgical prognostic predictor of neuroblastoma outcome.

ZMYND10 (zinc finger, MYND-type containing 10, also known as *BLU*) is another candidate tumor suppressor gene residing in the 3q21 region, and is thought to regulate entry into the cell cycle. Overexpression of *ZMYND10* has been shown to inhibit cell growth in neuroblastoma, while methylation of the *ZMYND10* promoter has been correlated with reduce *ZMYND10* gene expression in neuroblastoma cell lines (Agathanggelou et al., 2003) and hypermethylation of *ZMYND10* has been reported in a broad spectrum of tumors including neuroblastoma (Agathanggelou et al., 2003; Qiu et al., 2004). Methylation of *ZMYND10* has been shown to be associated with clinical stage, with stages 1, 2, and 4S showing significantly less methylation than stages 3 and 4 (Michalowski et al., 2008). An association between *ZMYND10* methylation and *MYCN* amplification has also been reported but the underlying mechanism for this is yet to be determined (Hoebeeck et al., 2009). Although *ZMYND10* is located immediately upstream of *RASSF1*, no correlation has been found between the methylation levels of these two genes in neuroblastoma, suggesting that methylation or inactivation of *ZMYND10* is an independent event and does not result from a common deleted region (Agathanggelou et al., 2003).

3.1.2 Apoptosis-related genes

Neuroblastoma has the highest rate of spontaneous regression among other malignant tumors (Hero et al., 2008). The molecular basis of spontaneous regression is often explained by the ability of neuroblastoma cells to differentiate into ganglion cells or to delay activation of apoptosis (Oue et al., 1996). Apoptosis is a process of programmed cell death dependent on the coordinated control of multiple highly conserved genes that leads to cell disruption. Alterations in the apoptosis pathway have been implicated in several aspects of tumor cell growth. Indeed, the level of expression in molecules involved in apoptosis has been shown to be a prognostic factor in patients with neuroblastoma (Islam et al., 2000; Casciano et al., 2004; Takita et al., 2004).

Methylation of the pro-apoptotic gene *PYCARD* (PYD and CARD domain-containing protein, also known as *TMS1*), has been reported in patients with advanced stage neuroblastoma, while no evidence of hypermethylation of *PYCARD* was found in patients with spontaneous regression (Alaminos et al., 2004; Grau et al., 2010). *PYCARD* induces apoptosis, and inhibits tumor cell survival. Hence its silencing via methylation could confer a growth advantage for tumor cells allowing escape from the apoptotic process (Banelli et al., 2005a). The absence of *PYCARD* expression driven by methylation has been demonstrated in other cancers (Martinez et al., 2007; Zhang et al., 2007).

Similar to the *PYCARD* gene, hypermethylation of the *APAF1* (apoptotic peptidase activating factor 1) gene has been reported to be associated with poorer prognosis in neuroblastoma patients (Grau et al., 2010). This gene has been described as a pro-apoptotic gene and a putative TSG in *MYCN* amplified neuroblastoma (Teitz et al., 2002). *APAF1* is a cytoplasmic protein that initiates apoptosis through activation of caspase-9 (Hausmann et al., 2000). Hence, silenced expression of *APAF1* through hypermethylation could dampen the initiation of the caspase cascade, thereby reducing the apoptotic activity of the gene.

The *CASP8* (caspase-8) gene is located at chromosome band 2q33, a region associated with LOH in neuroblastomas and several other tumor types (van Noesel & Versteeg, 2004). This gene encodes for cysteine protease, a key enzyme at the top of the apoptotic cascade and is activated in programmed cell death. Down-regulation of *CASP8* is one of the most well-known apoptotic defects in neuroblastoma. Indeed, it has been shown that the loss of *CASP8* expression was highly correlated with the amplification of *MYCN* (Teitz et al., 2000). Hypermethylation of *CASP8* has frequently been reported in neuroblastoma and the aberrant methylation of this gene is often associated with *MYCN* amplification (Teitz et al., 2000; Casciano et al., 2004; Hoebeeck et al., 2009). However, structural analysis of *CASP8* has revealed that the region showing differential methylation patterns between *MYCN*-amplified and non-amplified tumors was an intragenic sequence between exons 2 and 3 in the *CASP8* gene which lacked promoter activity (Banelli et al., 2002). Although subsequent studies have identified a *CASP8* promoter, the effect of DNA methylation in the promoter region of *CASP8* has not been shown to have a direct impact on gene expression (Banelli et al., 2002; Banelli et al., 2005a). Nonetheless, neuroblastoma cell lines treated with demethylation agent 5-aza-2′ deoxcytidine (5-AZA) activates *CASP8* expression, suggesting that demethylation of a trans-acting factor or gene controls the activity of *CASP8* (van Noesel, 2004).

TRAIL (tumor necrosis factor-related apoptosis-inducing ligand) is a member of the tumor necrosis factor (TNF) family of ligands capable of initiating apoptosis in a variety of cancer cells but not in most normal cells (van Noesel et al., 2002). Apoptotic signaling of TRAIL is induced by interacting with its death receptors (DRs) encoded by *TNFRSF10A* and *TNFRSF10B* genes. However, two anti-apoptotic decoy receptors (DcRs) encoded by *TNFRSF10C* and *TNFRSF10D* genes, compete with death receptors for binding to TRAIL and prevent normal cells from TRAIL-mediated apoptosis (van Noesel et al., 2002). Hence, the balanced expression of all four receptors is required to prevent TRAIL-induced apoptosis in normal cells.

Methylation of the death receptors, *TNFRSF10A* and *B*, has not been detected in primary neuroblastoma tissue and these receptors are frequently expressed (van Noesel et al., 2002). However, DcR proteins encoded by the *TNFRSF10C* and *D* genes are silenced by promoter methylation in a variety of tumors including neuroblastoma (van Noesel et al., 2002; Banelli et al., 2005b). Methylation of *TNFRSF10D* has been shown to be associated with reduced overall survival in neuroblastoma patients independent of *MYCN* amplification, suggesting that aberrant methylation of *TNFRSF10D* may be a potential prognostic biomarker for unfavorable outcome (Banelli et al., 2005b; Yagyu et al., 2008). In addition, the strong correlation between methylation of *TNFRSF10D* in sera and in neuroblastoma tumors, further supports the possibility of using serum measures of gene methylation as prognostic markers for clinical outcome in neuroblastoma (Yagyu et al., 2008). However, the biological significance of *TNFRSF10D* in carcinogenesis remains unclear.

3.1.3 Cell cycle, signal transduction and other genes

THBS1 (thrombospondin-1, also known as *TSP-1*), is a well-known inhibitor of angiogenesis and altered expression of *THBS1* is thought to contribute to neo-vascularization and metastasis in human cancer (Roberts, 1996). Studies have shown that *THBS1* promoter is frequently methylated and silenced in neuroblastoma (Gonzalez-Gomez et al., 2003; Yang et al., 2003). However, there has been an absence of any association detected between methylation of *THBS1* and clinical features such as *MYCN* amplification, deletion of 1p in neuroblastoma, and tumor type (Yang et al., 2003)

The *SFN* (stratifin, also known as 14.3.3δ) gene is directly regulated by p53 and is thought to function as a G2/M phase cell-cycle regulator by inhibiting cell-cycle progression, causing cells to leave the stem-cell compartment and undergo differentiation (Hermeking, 2003). Inactivation of *SFN* has been shown to be involved in tumor development in a variety of malignant tumors (Hermeking, 2003) with demethylation of the *SFN* promoter significantly increasing the expression of this gene in neuroblastoma (Banelli et al., 2010). *SFN* has been found to be fully methylated in *MYCN*-amplified neuroblastoma and partially methylated in non-amplified tumors (Banelli et al., 2005b). More recently, quantitative pyrosequencing analysis has identified that a methylation threshold level of 85% for the *SFN* gene distinguishes neuroblastoma patients presenting with progressive disease from those with a more favorable outcome, independent of other prognostic markers (Banelli et al., 2010).

The *HOXA9* (homeobox A9) gene encodes a sequence-specific transcription factor which is part of a developmental regulatory system that provides cells with specific positional identities on the anterior-posterior axis of an organism (*The NCBI handbook*, 2002). Dysregulated expression of *HOXA9* has been described in several malignancies including non-small-cell lung cancer (Calvo et al., 2000) and breast cancer (Gilbert et al., 2010). Neuroblastoma cell lines treated with demethylating agents have been reported to display increased levels of *HOXA9* gene expression (Margetts et al., 2008). Comprehensive methylation profiling of a large series of neuroblastoma tumors has shown that promoter hypermethylation of *HOXA9* is associated with poorer survival of patients aged ≥1 year and patients without *MYCN*-amplification (Alaminos et al., 2004). Currently, no clinical or pathologic prognostic markers have been identified for these two groups of patients. Hence, *HOXA9* methylation may be a useful biomarker that can predict the clinical outcome of these subgroups.

3.1.4 *MYCN* and methylation

As mentioned earlier, numerous reports have demonstrated that hypermethylation of certain tumor-related genes such as *CASP8, RASSF1,* and *ZMYND10* is most evident in *MYCN*-amplified neuroblastomas. Although these observations may have occurred by chance, there may be additional mechanisms driving the methylation of certain genes in tumors with *MYCN*-amplification. *MYCN* encodes for a transcription factor that binds to recognition sites such as E-box promoter sequence of target genes to activate the transcriptional activity of the associated genes. *c-MYC*, a functional homolog of *MYCN*, does not appear to bind to recognition sequences that include a methylated CpG, resulting in transcriptional repression and *MYCN* could interact in a similar manner (Prendergast & Ziff, 1991). Another possible explanation is that epigenetic alterations may have a specific role in more aggressive subtypes of neuroblastoma. This hypothesis is supported by observations from a genome-wide screen of neuroblastoma tumor samples where the methylation of multiple CGIs of particular genes were dependent upon each other and this phenotype was significantly associated with poor survival and *MYCN* amplification (Abe et al., 2005). These findings indicate that some genes may become methylated in a coordinated manner, suggesting a "CpG islands methylator phenotype" (CIMP) which was originally recognized in colorectal cancer (Abe et al., 2005). Recent evidence supporting the presence of CIMP in neuroblastoma comes from a genome-wide DNA methylation analysis of neuroblastoma tumors identifying large-scale blocks of contiguously hypermethylated CGIs, with a highly biased distribution towards the telomeric or terminal regions of the chromosome (Buckley et al., 2011). The aberrant methylation of multiple genes giving rise to distinctive neuroblastoma tumors or tumor subtypes may explain the biologically and clinically variable features observed in neuroblastoma. Furthermore, clustering of methylation data from neuroblastoma cell lines distinguished those with *MYCN* amplification from others (Alaminos et al., 2004). Therefore, it is possible that both *MYCN* amplification and CIMP contribute to a more aggressive type of neuroblastoma and the detection of methylation of certain genes in the aggressive type of neuroblastoma coincided with *MYCN* amplification. Taken together, the molecular mechanism for *MYCN* and methylation is still unclear and warrants further studies.

3.2 Considerations for future methylation analysis

While there have been many reports demonstrating gene inactivation driven by DNA methylation in neuroblastoma, the frequency of methylation varies considerably between different studies. The observed variation is likely to reflect the genetic heterogeneity of neuroblastoma, where primary tumors are comprised of multiple cell types such as the S-type (substrate adherent), N-type (neuroblastic), and I-type (stem) cells; with each type of cell having a distinct methylation and gene expression profile (Alaminos et al., 2004). Hence, inherent variability may not reflect the real differences in hypermethylation profiles of primary tumors but distinct cell types. Moreover, neuroblastoma is a cancer of the developing neural crest in which several of the cell types are pluripotent and have the capacity to differentiate into other neurolastoma cell types. Thus, differences that are seen in hypermethylation profiles in a particular neuroblastoma cell may reflect changes in methylation of a normal differentiating cell rather than development of a cancer phenotype (Ross & Spengler, 2004). Future studies may benefit from incorporating immunocytochemical studies to identify the proportion of each cell type and evaluate the level of methylation to the particular cell type accordingly. The use of different techniques for detecting DNA methylation presents another source of variation. Hence, standardized methods and scoring systems should be established for more comparable results between laboratories.

Over the past decade, an increasing number of genes are discovered to be epigenetically silenced in tumors. Methylation analysis is rapidly progressing from the study of a single or few genes into that of the high-throughput determination of the methylation status of thousands of CGIs by microarray analysis. Similar limitations of GWAS also apply to the genome-wide search for epigenetic markers. The large number of comparisons performed increases the error. Therefore, adjustment for multiple-testing should be considered such as the use of false discovery rate for the identification of as many true associations as possible while minimizing the overall proportion of false-positive tests (Foley et al., 2009).

Whether a candidate gene or genomic approach is used, studies should aim to identify genes with promoter CGI hypermethylation that results in subsequent gene silencing. Although demethylating agents are commonly used in studies to identify genes that are reactivated, using demethylating agents alone is not a definite proof that the gene has methylation-associated silencing since gene expression can be indirectly induced through other transcriptional factors that are epigenetically controlled. A more effective plan of investigation might be to first identify genes with CGI hypermethylation, then test for the functionality of methylation using demethylating agents. When treating cell lines with demethylating agents, it is important to include a control cell line with low or no methylation and assess the level of candidate gene expression pre- and post- treatment. Change in expression in the control cell line indicates that other transcriptional activators were methylated and that expression is not due to methylation-induced silencing of the gene. In addition, it is also possible that candidate TSGs that are unmethylated but upregulated by demethylating agents may be indirect markers for downstream epigenetically inactivated TSGs.

Although methylated promoter CGIs generally disable the transcription of the correlated gene, other concomitant epigenetic events such as changes in histone proteins may affect DNA organization and gene expression. Changes in chromatin structure also influence gene expression as genes are inactivated when the chromatin is condensed and expressed when the chromatin is in an open configuration (Rodenhiser & Mann, 2006). These dynamic chromatin states are controlled by histone modifications, involving the histone deacetylase (HDACs) family of enzymes in this reversible epigenetic process. Active promoter regions normally have unmethylated DNA and high levels of acetylated histones, while inactive regions of chromatin contain methylated DNA and deacetylated histones. Therefore, a full evaluation of promoter DNA hypermethylation, histone modification and quantitative gene expression will help to decipher the entire epigenome. The International Human Epigenome Project (IHEP), is an international collaboration that aims to identify, catalogue and interpret genome-wide DNA methylation patterns of all human genes in all major tissues. This project will provide high-resolution reference epigenome maps to the research community (The American Association for Cancer Research Human Epigenome Task Force; The European Union Network of Excellence Scientific Advisory Board, 2008). These maps will integrate the various epigenetic layers of detailed DNA methylation, histone modification, nucleosome occupancy and expression patterns of coding and non-coding RNA in different normal and disease cell types which will be a rich source of information for the study of tumorigenesis and for the identification of cancer-specific methylation biomarkers.

4. Future directions: Clinical implications of DNA methylation in neuroblastoma

In the next few years, an increasing number of novel biomarkers for neuroblastoma will continue to be identified through epigenomic profiling. This approach will not only help further understand the molecular mechanisms governing neuroblastoma, the clinical relevance of these novel biomarkers will also serve to stratify tumor types, identify prognostic groups, predict therapeutic response and assess the risk of relapse. As DNA methylation patterns are relatively easy to detect and specific to tumor types, specific methylation patterns may be useful in the clinical setting. In addition, studies have accurately detected aberrant methylation of particular genes in biological fluids such as serum, sputum, or urine which will allow early diagnosis of cancer without the need for invasive surgery. However, the sensitivity and specificity of DNA methylation markers in cancer diagnosis depends on tumor type, the gene studied, the type of body fluid used, and the technique involved. Therefore, DNA methylation detection methods need to become more standardized to facilitate sensitive, accurate and reproducible results in the clinical setting. To date, studies examining the relationship between DNA methylation and individual treatment response in neuroblastoma are limited. Moreover, the DNA methylation profiling may also be useful in the continued assessment of patients throughout treatment.

Unlike genetic alterations, DNA methylation can be reversed to restore the function of key control pathways in malignant and premalignant cells by treatment with demethylating agents. DNA methylation inhibitors such as azacitidine and decitabine can induce functional re-expression of aberrantly silenced genes in cancer, causing growth arrest and apoptosis in tumor cells (Jones & Baylin, 2002). More recently, several inhibitors of chromatin-modifying enzymes, including histone deacetylase (HDAC) inhibitors and DNA methyltransferase (DNMT) inhibitors have now been approved by US Food and Drug Association (FDA) and are being used in clinical practice with good prognosis for tumor regression. For example, DNMT inhibitors such as 5-azacytidine (Vidaza®) and decitabine (Dacogen™) have been approved for the treatment of myelodysplastic syndrome and leukemia (Mack, 2006). However, the treatment of solid tumors with DNMT inhibitors showed response rates of less than 10% and is considerably less successful than the treatment of leukemias (Goffin & Eisenhauer, 2002). Recently, decitabine was used in a phase I clinical trial as an anticancer drug for children with solid tumor and neuroblastoma (George et al., 2010). Although patients had tolerable toxicity to low-dose decitabine in combination with doxorubicin/cyclophosphamide, doses of decitabine capable of producing clinically relevant biologic effects were not well tolerated with this combination. Therefore, further studies are required to examine the efficacy of HDAC and DNMT inhibitors in combination with current treatment protocols to identify best treatment options for neuroblastoma.

5. Conclusion

It is clear that both genetic and epigenetic changes play a crucial role in the tumorigenesis of neuroblastoma. The genetic heterogeneity of neuroblastoma suggests that the initiation and progression of this disease requires multiple interacting genetic factors including genetic variants in susceptibility loci, copy number variations, amplification of oncogenes, deletion of tumor suppressor genes, and other genetic mechanisms such as DNA methylation. These genetic events may act alternatively or synergistically in the multistep process of carcinogenesis. With recent technological advances in whole-genome microarrays, both genetic and epigenetic screens should be undertaken to enumerate the full spectrum of alterations in the human cancer genome to facilitate the identification of novel biomarkers for the most efficient grouping of neuroblastoma. More importantly, it will direct future efforts towards new therapeutic approaches that will target specific molecular alterations in the tumor cell.

6. References

Abe, M., Ohira, M., Kaneda, A., Yagi, Y., Yamamoto, S., Kitano, Y., Takato, T., Nakagawara, A. & Ushijima, T. (2005). CpG island methylator phenotype is a strong determinant of poor prognosis in neuroblastomas. *Cancer Res* 65(3): 828-34.

Abe, M., Westermann, F., Nakagawara, A., Takato, T., Schwab, M. & Ushijima, T. (2007). Marked and independent prognostic significance of the CpG island methylator phenotype in neuroblastomas. *Cancer Lett* 247(2): 253-8.

Agathanggelou, A., Dallol, A., Zochbauer-Muller, S., Morrissey, C., Honorio, S., Hesson, L., Martinsson, T., Fong, K. M., Kuo, M. J., Yuen, P. W., Maher, E. R., Minna, J. D. & Latif, F. (2003). Epigenetic inactivation of the candidate 3p21.3 suppressor gene BLU in human cancers. *Oncogene* 22(10): 1580-8.

Alaminos, M., Davalos, V., Cheung, N. K., Gerald, W. L. & Esteller, M. (2004). Clustering of gene hypermethylation associated with clinical risk groups in neuroblastoma. *J Natl Cancer Inst* 96(16): 1208-19.

Ambros, P. F., Ambros, I. M., Brodeur, G. M., Haber, M., Khan, J., Nakagawara, A., Schleiermacher, G., Speleman, F., Spitz, R., London, W. B., Cohn, S. L., Pearson, A. D. & Maris, J. M. (2009). International consensus for neuroblastoma molecular diagnostics: report from the International Neuroblastoma Risk Group (INRG) Biology Committee. *Br J Cancer* 100(9): 1471-82.

Amiel, J., Laudier, B., Attie-Bitach, T., Trang, H., de Pontual, L., Gener, B., Trochet, D., Etchevers, H., Ray, P., Simonneau, M., Vekemans, M., Munnich, A., Gaultier, C. & Lyonnet, S. (2003). Polyalanine expansion and frameshift mutations of the paired-like homeobox gene PHOX2B in congenital central hypoventilation syndrome. *Nat Genet* 33(4): 459-461.

Astuti, D., Agathanggelou, A., Honorio, S., Dallol, A., Martinsson, T., Kogner, P., Cummins, C., Neumann, H. P., Voutilainen, R., Dahia, P., Eng, C., Maher, E. R. & Latif, F. (2001). RASSF1A promoter region CpG island hypermethylation in phaeochromocytomas and neuroblastoma tumours. *Oncogene* 20(51): 7573-7.

Attiyeh, E. F., London, W. B., Mosse, Y. P., Wang, Q., Winter, C., Khazi, D., McGrady, P. W., Seeger, R. C., Look, A. T., Shimada, H., Brodeur, G. M., Cohn, S. L., Matthay, K. K. & Maris, J. M. (2005). Chromosome 1p and 11q deletions and outcome in neuroblastoma. *N Engl J Med* 353(21): 2243-53.

Baade, P. D., Youlden, D. R., Valery, P. C., Hassall, T., Ward, L., Green, A. C. & Aitken, J. F. (2010). Population-based survival estimates for childhood cancer in Australia during the period 1997-2006. *Br J Cancer* 103(11): 1663-70.

Bachetti, T., Di Paolo, D., Di Lascio, S., Mirisola, V., Brignole, C., Bellotti, M., Caffa, I., Ferraris, C., Fiore, M., Fornasari, D., Chiarle, R., Borghini, S., Pfeffer, U., Ponzoni, M., Ceccherini, I. & Perri, P. (2010). PHOX2B-mediated regulation of ALK expression: in vitro identification of a functional relationship between two genes involved in neuroblastoma. *PLoS One* 5(10).

Bader, S. A., Fasching, C., Brodeur, G. M. & Stanbridge, E. J. (1991). Dissociation of suppression of tumorigenicity and differentiation in vitro effected by transfer of single human chromosomes into human neuroblastoma cells. *Cell Growth Differ* 2(5): 245-55.

Banelli, B., Bonassi, S., Casciano, I., Mazzocco, K., Di Vinci, A., Scaruffi, P., Brigati, C., Allemanni, G., Borzi, L., Tonini, G. P. & Romani, M. (2010). Outcome prediction and risk assessment by quantitative pyrosequencing methylation analysis of the SFN gene in advanced stage, high-risk, neuroblastic tumor patients. *Int J Cancer* 126(3): 656-68.

Banelli, B., Casciano, I., Croce, M., Di Vinci, A., Gelvi, I., Pagnan, G., Brignole, C., Allemanni, G., Ferrini, S., Ponzoni, M. & Romani, M. (2002). Expression and methylation of CASP8 in neuroblastoma: identification of a promoter region. *Nat Med* 8(12): 1333-5; author reply 1335.

Banelli, B., Di Vinci, A., Gelvi, I., Casciano, I., Allemanni, G., Bonassi, S. & Romani, M. (2005a). DNA methylation in neuroblastic tumors. *Cancer Lett* 228(1-2): 37-41.

Banelli, B., Gelvi, I., Di Vinci, A., Scaruffi, P., Casciano, I., Allemanni, G., Bonassi, S., Tonini, G. P. & Romani, M. (2005b). Distinct CpG methylation profiles characterize different clinical groups of neuroblastic tumors. *Oncogene* 24(36): 5619-28.

Baylin, S. B. (2005). DNA methylation and gene silencing in cancer. *Nat Clin Pract Oncol* 2 Suppl 1: S4-11.

Bown, N., Cotterill, S., Lastowska, M., O'Neill, S., Pearson, A. D., Plantaz, D., Meddeb, M., Danglot, G., Brinkschmidt, C., Christiansen, H., Laureys, G., Speleman, F., Nicholson, J., Bernheim, A., Betts, D. R., Vandesompele, J. & Van Roy, N. (1999). Gain of chromosome arm 17q and adverse outcome in patients with neuroblastoma. *N Engl J Med* 340(25): 1954-61.

Brodeur, G. M. & Maris, J. M. (2006). Neuroblastoma. *Principles and Practice of Pediatric Oncology*. P. A. Pizzo & D. G. Poplack, Lippincott Williams & Wilkins: 933-970.

Brodeur, G. M. & Seeger, R. C. (1986). Gene amplification in human neuroblastomas: basic mechanisms and clinical implications. *Cancer Genet Cytogenet* 19(1-2): 101-11.

Buckley, P. G., Das, S., Bryan, K., Watters, K. M., Alcock, L., Koster, J., Versteeg, R. & Stallings, R. L. (2011). Genome-wide DNA methylation analysis of neuroblastic tumors reveals clinically relevant epigenetic events and large-scale epigenomic alterations localized to telomeric regions. *Int J Cancer* 128(10): 2296-305.

Burbee, D. G., Forgacs, E., Zöchbauer-Müller, S., Shivakumar, L., Fong, K., Gao, B., Randle, D., Kondo, M., Virmani, A., Bader, S., Sekido, Y., Latif, F., Milchgrub, S., Toyooka, S., Gazdar, A. F., Lerman, M. I., Zabarovsky, E., White, M. & Minna, J. D. (2001). Epigenetic Inactivation of RASSF1A in Lung and Breast Cancers and Malignant Phenotype Suppression. *Journal of the National Cancer Institute* 93(9): 691-699.

Calvo, R., West, J., Franklin, W., Erickson, P., Bemis, L., Li, E., Helfrich, B., Bunn, P., Roche, J., Brambilla, E., Rosell, R., Gemmill, R. M. & Drabkin, H. A. (2000). Altered HOX and WNT7A expression in human lung cancer. *Proc Natl Acad Sci U S A* 97(23): 12776-81.

Capasso, M., Devoto, M., Hou, C., Asgharzadeh, S., Glessner, J. T., Attiyeh, E. F., Mosse, Y. P., Kim, C., Diskin, S. J., Cole, K. A., Bosse, K., Diamond, M., Laudenslager, M., Winter, C., Bradfield, J. P., Scott, R. H., Jagannathan, J., Garris, M., McConville, C., London, W. B., Seeger, R. C., Grant, S. F., Li, H., Rahman, N., Rappaport, E., Hakonarson, H. & Maris, J. M. (2009). Common variations in BARD1 influence susceptibility to high-risk neuroblastoma. *Nat Genet* 41(6): 718-723.

Capasso, M. & Diskin, S. J. (2010). Genetics and genomics of neuroblastoma. *Cancer Treat Res* 155: 65-84.

Caren, H., Abel, F., Kogner, P. & Martinsson, T. (2008). High incidence of DNA mutations and gene amplifications of the ALK gene in advanced sporadic neuroblastoma tumours. *Biochem J* 416(2): 153-9.

Caren, H., Fransson, S., Ejeskar, K., Kogner, P. & Martinsson, T. (2007). Genetic and epigenetic changes in the common 1p36 deletion in neuroblastoma tumours. *Br J Cancer* 97(10): 1416-24.

Caron, H., van Sluis, P., Buschman, R., Pereira do Tanque, R., Maes, P., Beks, L., de Kraker, J., Voute, P. A., Vergnaud, G., Westerveld, A., Slater, R. & Versteeg, R. (1996a). Allelic loss of the short arm of chromosome 4 in neuroblastoma suggests a novel tumour suppressor gene locus. *Hum Genet* 97(6): 834-7.

Caron, H., van Sluis, P., de Kraker, J., Bökkerink, J., Egeler, M., Laureys, G., Slater, R., Westerveld, A., Voûte, P. A. & Versteeg, R. (1996b). Allelic Loss of Chromosome 1p as a Predictor of Unfavorable Outcome in Patients with Neuroblastoma. *New England Journal of Medicine* 334(4): 225-230.

Casciano, I., Banelli, B., Croce, M., De Ambrosis, A., di Vinci, A., Gelvi, I., Pagnan, G., Brignole, C., Allemanni, G., Ferrini, S., Ponzoni, M. & Romani, M. (2004). Caspase-8 gene expression in neuroblastoma. *Ann N Y Acad Sci* 1028: 157-67.

Chen, Y., Takita, J., Choi, Y. L., Kato, M., Ohira, M., Sanada, M., Wang, L., Soda, M., Kikuchi, A., Igarashi, T., Nakagawara, A., Hayashi, Y., Mano, H. & Ogawa, S. (2008). Oncogenic mutations of ALK kinase in neuroblastoma. *Nature* 455(7215): 971-4.

Cohn, S. L., Pearson, A. D., London, W. B., Monclair, T., Ambros, P. F., Brodeur, G. M., Faldum, A., Hero, B., Iehara, T., Machin, D., Mosseri, V., Simon, T., Garaventa, A., Castel, V. & Matthay, K. K. (2009). The International Neuroblastoma Risk Group (INRG) classification system: an INRG Task Force report. *J Clin Oncol* 27(2): 289-97.

Curtis, D. J. & McCormack, M. P. (2010). The Molecular Basis of Lmo2-Induced T-Cell Acute Lymphoblastic Leukemia. *Clinical Cancer Research* 16(23): 5618-5623.

Das, P. M. & Singal, R. (2004). DNA methylation and cancer. *J Clin Oncol* 22(22): 4632-42.

De Brouwer, S., De Preter, K., Kumps, C., Zabrocki, P., Porcu, M., Westerhout, E. M., Lakeman, A., Vandesompele, J., Hoebeeck, J., Van Maerken, T., De Paepe, A., Laureys, G., Schulte, J. H., Schramm, A., Van Den Broecke, C., Vermeulen, J., Van Roy, N., Beiske, K., Renard, M., Noguera, R., Delattre, O., Janoueix-Lerosey, I., Kogner, P., Martinsson, T., Nakagawara, A., Ohira, M., Caron, H., Eggert, A., Cools, J., Versteeg, R. & Speleman, F. (2010). Meta-analysis of neuroblastomas reveals a skewed ALK mutation spectrum in tumors with MYCN amplification. *Clin Cancer Res* 16(17): 4353-62.

Diskin, S. J., Hou, C., Glessner, J. T., Attiyeh, E. F., Laudenslager, M., Bosse, K., Cole, K., Mosse, Y. P., Wood, A., Lynch, J. E., Pecor, K., Diamond, M., Winter, C., Wang, K., Kim, C., Geiger, E. A., McGrady, P. W., Blakemore, A. I., London, W. B., Shaikh, T. H., Bradfield, J., Grant, S. F., Li, H., Devoto, M., Rappaport, E. R., Hakonarson, H. & Maris, J. M. (2009). Copy number variation at 1q21.1 associated with neuroblastoma. *Nature* 459(7249): 987-91.

Ejeskar, K., Aburatani, H., Abrahamsson, J., Kogner, P. & Martinsson, T. (1998). Loss of heterozygosity of 3p markers in neuroblastoma tumours implicate a tumour-suppressor locus distal to the FHIT gene. *Br J Cancer* 77(11): 1787-91.

Esteller, M. & Herman, J. G. (2002). Cancer as an epigenetic disease: DNA methylation and chromatin alterations in human tumours. *J Pathol* 196(1): 1-7.

Foley, D. L., Craig, J. M., Morley, R., Olsson, C. A., Dwyer, T., Smith, K. & Saffery, R. (2009). Prospects for epigenetic epidemiology. *Am J Epidemiol* 169(4): 389-400.

Fong, C. T., White, P. S., Peterson, K., Sapienza, C., Cavenee, W. K., Kern, S. E., Vogelstein, B., Cantor, A. B., Look, A. T. & Brodeur, G. M. (1992). Loss of heterozygosity for chromosomes 1 or 14 defines subsets of advanced neuroblastomas. *Cancer Res* 52(7): 1780-5.

Freeman, J. L., Perry, G. H., Feuk, L., Redon, R., McCarroll, S. A., Altshuler, D. M., Aburatani, H., Jones, K. W., Tyler-Smith, C., Hurles, M. E., Carter, N. P., Scherer, S. W. & Lee, C. (2006). Copy number variation: new insights in genome diversity. *Genome Res* 16(8): 949-61.

George, R. E., Attiyeh, E. F., Li, S., Moreau, L. A., Neuberg, D., Li, C., Fox, E. A., Meyerson, M., Diller, L., Fortina, P., Look, A. T. & Maris, J. M. (2007). Genome-wide analysis of neuroblastomas using high-density single nucleotide polymorphism arrays. *PLoS One* 2(2): e255.

George, R. E., Lahti, J. M., Adamson, P. C., Zhu, K., Finkelstein, D., Ingle, A. M., Reid, J. M., Krailo, M., Neuberg, D., Blaney, S. M. & Diller, L. (2010). Phase I study of decitabine with doxorubicin and cyclophosphamide in children with neuroblastoma and other solid tumors: a Children's Oncology Group study. *Pediatr Blood Cancer* 55(4): 629-38.

George, R. E., Sanda, T., Hanna, M., Frohling, S., Luther, W., 2nd, Zhang, J., Ahn, Y., Zhou, W., London, W. B., McGrady, P., Xue, L., Zozulya, S., Gregor, V. E., Webb, T. R., Gray, N. S., Gilliland, D. G., Diller, L., Greulich, H., Morris, S. W., Meyerson, M. & Look, A. T. (2008). Activating mutations in ALK provide a therapeutic target in neuroblastoma. *Nature* 455(7215): 975-8.

Gilbert, P. M., Mouw, J. K., Unger, M. A., Lakins, J. N., Gbegnon, M. K., Clemmer, V. B., Benezra, M., Licht, J. D., Boudreau, N. J., Tsai, K. K., Welm, A. L., Feldman, M. D., Weber, B. L. & Weaver, V. M. (2010). HOXA9 regulates BRCA1 expression to modulate human breast tumor phenotype. *J Clin Invest* 120(5): 1535-50.

Goffin, J. & Eisenhauer, E. (2002). DNA methyltransferase inhibitors-state of the art. *Ann Oncol* 13(11): 1699-716.

Gonzalez-Gomez, P., Bello, M. J., Lomas, J., Arjona, D., Alonso, M. E., Aminoso, C., Lopez-Marin, I., Anselmo, N. P., Sarasa, J. L., Gutierrez, M., Casartelli, C. & Rey, J. A. (2003). Aberrant methylation of multiple genes in neuroblastic tumours. relationship with MYCN amplification and allelic status at 1p. *Eur J Cancer* 39(10): 1478-85.

Grau, E., Martinez, F., Orellana, C., Canete, A., Yanez, Y., Oltra, S., Noguera, R., Hernandez, M., Bermudez, J. D. & Castel, V. (2010). Hypermethylation of apoptotic genes as independent prognostic factor in neuroblastoma disease. *Mol Carcinog* 50(3): 153-62.

Hamrick, S. E., Olshan, A. F., Neglia, J. P. & Pollock, B. H. (2001). Association of pregnancy history and birth characteristics with neuroblastoma: a report from the Children's Cancer Group and the Pediatric Oncology Group. *Paediatr Perinat Epidemiol* 15(4): 328-37.

Harada, K., Toyooka, S., Maitra, A., Maruyama, R., Toyooka, K. O., Timmons, C. F., Tomlinson, G. E., Mastrangelo, D., Hay, R. J., Minna, J. D. & Gazdar, A. F. (2002).

Aberrant promoter methylation and silencing of the RASSF1A gene in pediatric tumors and cell lines. *Oncogene* 21(27): 4345-9.

Hausmann, G., O'Reilly, L. A., van Driel, R., Beaumont, J. G., Strasser, A., Adams, J. M. & Huang, D. C. (2000). Pro-apoptotic apoptosis protease-activating factor 1 (Apaf-1) has a cytoplasmic localization distinct from Bcl-2 or Bcl-x(L). *J Cell Biol* 149(3): 623-34.

Hermeking, H. (2003). The 14-3-3 cancer connection. *Nat Rev Cancer* 3(12): 931-943.

Hero, B., Simon, T., Spitz, R., Ernestus, K., Gnekow, A. K., Scheel-Walter, H. G., Schwabe, D., Schilling, F. H., Benz-Bohm, G. & Berthold, F. (2008). Localized infant neuroblastomas often show spontaneous regression: results of the prospective trials NB95-S and NB97. *J Clin Oncol* 26(9): 1504-10.

Hoebeeck, J., Michels, E., Pattyn, F., Combaret, V., Vermeulen, J., Yigit, N., Hoyoux, C., Laureys, G., De Paepe, A., Speleman, F. & Vandesompele, J. (2009). Aberrant methylation of candidate tumor suppressor genes in neuroblastoma. *Cancer Lett* 273(2): 336-46.

Islam, A., Kageyama, H., Takada, N., Kawamoto, T., Takayasu, H., Isogai, E., Ohira, M., Hashizume, K., Kobayashi, H., Kaneko, Y. & Nakagawara, A. (2000). High expression of Survivin, mapped to 17q25, is significantly associated with poor prognostic factors and promotes cell survival in human neuroblastoma. *Oncogene* 19(5): 617-23.

Janoueix-Lerosey, I., Lequin, D., Brugieres, L., Ribeiro, A., de Pontual, L., Combaret, V., Raynal, V., Puisieux, A., Schleiermacher, G., Pierron, G., Valteau-Couanet, D., Frebourg, T., Michon, J., Lyonnet, S., Amiel, J. & Delattre, O. (2008). Somatic and germline activating mutations of the ALK kinase receptor in neuroblastoma. *Nature* 455(7215): 967-70.

Janoueix-Lerosey, I., Schleiermacher, G., Michels, E., Mosseri, V., Ribeiro, A., Lequin, D., Vermeulen, J., Couturier, J., Peuchmaur, M., Valent, A., Plantaz, D., Rubie, H., Valteau-Couanet, D., Thomas, C., Combaret, V., Rousseau, R., Eggert, A., Michon, J., Speleman, F. & Delattre, O. (2009). Overall genomic pattern is a predictor of outcome in neuroblastoma. *J Clin Oncol* 27(7): 1026-33.

Jones, P. A. & Baylin, S. B. (2002). The fundamental role of epigenetic events in cancer. *Nat Rev Genet* 3(6): 415-28.

Kaneko, Y., Kanda, N., Maseki, N., Sakurai, M., Tsuchida, Y., Takeda, T., Okabe, I. & Sakurai, M. (1987). Different Karyotypic Patterns in Early and Advanced Stage Neuroblastomas. *Cancer Research* 47(1): 311-318.

Kulis, M. & Esteller, M. (2010). DNA methylation and cancer. *Adv Genet* 70: 27-56.

Lastowska, M., Cullinane, C., Variend, S., Cotterill, S., Bown, N., O'Neill, S., Mazzocco, K., Roberts, P., Nicholson, J., Ellershaw, C., Pearson, A. D. & Jackson, M. S. (2001). Comprehensive genetic and histopathologic study reveals three types of neuroblastoma tumors. *J Clin Oncol* 19(12): 3080-90.

Lazcoz, P., Munoz, J., Nistal, M., Pestana, A., Encio, I. & Castresana, J. S. (2006). Frequent promoter hypermethylation of RASSF1A and CASP8 in neuroblastoma. *BMC Cancer* 6: 254.

Limpt, V. v., Schramm, A., Lakeman, A., Sluis, P. v., Chan, A., Noesel, M. v., Baas, F., Caron, H., Eggert, A. & Versteeg, R. (2004). The Phox2B homeobox gene is mutated in sporadic neuroblastomas. *Oncogene* 23(57): 9280-9288.

London, W. B., Castleberry, R. P., Matthay, K. K., Look, A. T., Seeger, R. C., Shimada, H., Thorner, P., Brodeur, G., Maris, J. M., Reynolds, C. P. & Cohn, S. L. (2005). Evidence for an age cutoff greater than 365 days for neuroblastoma risk group stratification in the Children's Oncology Group. *J Clin Oncol* 23(27): 6459-65.

Look, A. T., Hayes, F. A., Shuster, J. J., Douglass, E. C., Castleberry, R. P., Bowman, L. C., Smith, E. I. & Brodeur, G. M. (1991). Clinical relevance of tumor cell ploidy and N-myc gene amplification in childhood neuroblastoma: a Pediatric Oncology Group study. *J Clin Oncol* 9(4): 581-91.

Mack, G. S. (2006). Epigenetic cancer therapy makes headway. *J Natl Cancer Inst* 98(20): 1443-4.

Margetts, C. D. E., Morris, M., Astuti, D., Gentle, D. C., Cascon, A., McRonald, F. E., Catchpoole, D., Robledo, M., Neumann, H. P. H., Latif, F. & Maher, E. R. (2008). Evaluation of a functional epigenetic approach to identify promoter region methylation in phaeochromocytoma and neuroblastoma. *Endocrine-Related Cancer* 15(3): 777-786.

Maris, J. M., Chatten, J., Meadows, A. T., Biegel, J. A. & Brodeur, G. M. (1997). Familial neuroblastoma: a three-generation pedigree and a further association with Hirschsprung disease. *Med Pediatr Oncol* 28(1): 1-5.

Maris, J. M., Hogarty, M. D., Bagatell, R. & Cohn, S. L. (2007). Neuroblastoma. *Lancet* 369(9579): 2106-20.

Maris, J. M. & Matthay, K. K. (1999). Molecular biology of neuroblastoma. *J Clin Oncol* 17(7): 2264-79.

Maris, J. M., Mosse, Y. P., Bradfield, J. P., Hou, C., Monni, S., Scott, R. H., Asgharzadeh, S., Attiyeh, E. F., Diskin, S. J., Laudenslager, M., Winter, C., Cole, K. A., Glessner, J. T., Kim, C., Frackelton, E. C., Casalunovo, T., Eckert, A. W., Capasso, M., Rappaport, E. F., McConville, C., London, W. B., Seeger, R. C., Rahman, N., Devoto, M., Grant, S. F., Li, H. & Hakonarson, H. (2008). Chromosome 6p22 locus associated with clinically aggressive neuroblastoma. *N Engl J Med* 358(24): 2585-93.

Martinez, R., Schackert, G. & Esteller, M. (2007). Hypermethylation of the proapoptotic gene TMS1/ASC: prognostic importance in glioblastoma multiforme. *J Neurooncol* 82(2): 133-9.

Martinsson, T., Eriksson, T., Abrahamsson, J., Caren, H., Hansson, M., Kogner, P., Kamaraj, S., Schonherr, C., Weinmar, J., Ruuth, K., Palmer, R. H. & Hallberg, B. (2011). Appearance of the novel activating F1174S ALK mutation in neuroblastoma correlates with aggressive tumor progression and unresponsiveness to therapy. *Cancer Res* 71(1): 98-105.

Michalowski, M. B., de Fraipont, F., Plantaz, D., Michelland, S., Combaret, V. & Favrot, M. C. (2008). Methylation of tumor-suppressor genes in neuroblastoma: The RASSF1A gene is almost always methylated in primary tumors. *Pediatr Blood Cancer* 50(1): 29-32.

Misawa, A., Tanaka, S., Yagyu, S., Tsuchiya, K., Iehara, T., Sugimoto, T. & Hosoi, H. (2009). RASSF1A hypermethylation in pretreatment serum DNA of neuroblastoma patients: a prognostic marker. *Br J Cancer* 100(2): 399-404.

Mosse, Y. P., Laudenslager, M., Khazi, D., Carlisle, A. J., Winter, C. L., Rappaport, E. & Maris, J. M. (2004). Germline PHOX2B mutation in hereditary neuroblastoma. *Am J Hum Genet* 75(4): 727-30.

Mosse, Y. P., Laudenslager, M., Longo, L., Cole, K. A., Wood, A., Attiyeh, E. F., Laquaglia, M. J., Sennett, R., Lynch, J. E., Perri, P., Laureys, G., Speleman, F., Kim, C., Hou, C., Hakonarson, H., Torkamani, A., Schork, N. J., Brodeur, G. M., Tonini, G. P., Rappaport, E., Devoto, M. & Maris, J. M. (2008). Identification of ALK as a major familial neuroblastoma predisposition gene. *Nature* 455(7215): 930-5.

Mosse, Y. P., Wood, A. & Maris, J. M. (2009). Inhibition of ALK signaling for cancer therapy. *Clin Cancer Res* 15(18): 5609-14.

Munzer, C., Menegaux, F., Lacour, B., Valteau-Couanet, D., Michon, J., Coze, C., Bergeron, C., Auvrignon, A., Bernard, F., Thomas, C., Vannier, J. P., Kanold, J., Rubie, H., Hemon, D. & Clavel, J. (2008). Birth-related characteristics, congenital malformation, maternal reproductive history and neuroblastoma: the ESCALE study (SFCE). *Int J Cancer* 122(10): 2315-21.

The NCBI handbook (2002). [Internet] Bethesda (MD): National Library of Medicine (US), National Center for Biotechnology Information.

Nguyễn, L. B., Diskin, S. J., Capasso, M., Wang, K., Diamond, M. A., Glessner, J., Kim, C., Attiyeh, E. F., Mosse, Y. P., Cole, K., Iolascon, A., Devoto, M., Hakonarson, H., Li, H. K. & Maris, J. M. (2011). Phenotype Restricted Genome-Wide Association Study Using a Gene-Centric Approach Identifies Three Low-Risk Neuroblastoma Susceptibility Loci. *PLoS genetics* 7(3): e1002026.

Okawa, E. R., Gotoh, T., Manne, J., Igarashi, J., Fujita, T., Silverman, K. A., Xhao, H., Mosse, Y. P., White, P. S. & Brodeur, G. M. (2008). Expression and sequence analysis of candidates for the 1p36.31 tumor suppressor gene deleted in neuroblastomas. *Oncogene* 27(6): 803-10.

Oue, T., Fukuzawa, M., Kusafuka, T., Kohmoto, Y., Imura, K., Nagahara, S. & Okada, A. (1996). In situ detection of DNA fragmentation and expression of bcl-2 in human neuroblastoma: relation to apoptosis and spontaneous regression. *J Pediatr Surg* 31(2): 251-7.

Passoni, L., Longo, L., Collini, P., Coluccia, A. M., Bozzi, F., Podda, M., Gregorio, A., Gambini, C., Garaventa, A., Pistoia, V., Del Grosso, F., Tonini, G. P., Cheng, M., Gambacorti-Passerini, C., Anichini, A., Fossati-Bellani, F., Di Nicola, M. & Luksch, R. (2009). Mutation-independent anaplastic lymphoma kinase overexpression in poor prognosis neuroblastoma patients. *Cancer Res* 69(18): 7338-46.

Plantaz, D., Mohapatra, G., Matthay, K. K., Pellarin, M., Seeger, R. C. & Feuerstein, B. G. (1997). Gain of chromosome 17 is the most frequent abnormality detected in neuroblastoma by comparative genomic hybridization. *Am J Pathol* 150(1): 81-9.

Prendergast, G. & Ziff, E. (1991). Methylation-sensitive sequence-specific DNA binding by the c-Myc basic region. *Science* 251(4990): 186-189.

Qiu, G.-H., Tan, L. K. S., Loh, K. S., Lim, C. Y., Srivastava, G., Tsai, S.-T., Tsao, S. W. & Tao, Q. (2004). The candidate tumor suppressor gene BLU, located at the commonly deleted region 3p21.3, is an E2F-regulated, stress-responsive gene and inactivated by both epigenetic and genetic mechanisms in nasopharyngeal carcinoma. *Oncogene* 23(27): 4793-4806.

Raabe, E. H., Laudenslager, M., Winter, C., Wasserman, N., Cole, K., LaQuaglia, M., Maris, D. J., Mosse, Y. P. & Maris, J. M. (2008). Prevalence and functional consequence of PHOX2B mutations in neuroblastoma. *Oncogene* 27(4): 469-476.

Ries, L.A.G., Smith, M.A., Gurney, J.G., Linet, M., Tamra, T., Young, J. L. & Bunin, G. R. (1999). Cancer Incidence and Survival among Children and Adolescents: United

States SEER Program 1975-1995. National Cancer Institute, SEER Program. Bethesda, MD. NIH Pub. No. 99-4649: 17-34.

Roberts, D. D. (1996). Regulation of tumor growth and metastasis by thrombospondin-1. *FASEB J* 10(10): 1183-91.

Rodenhiser, D. & Mann, M. (2006). Epigenetics and human disease: translating basic biology into clinical applications. *CMAJ* 174(3): 341-8.

Ross, R. A. & Spengler, B. A. (2004). The conundrum posed by cellular heterogeneity in analysis of human neuroblastoma. *J Natl Cancer Inst* 96(16): 1192-3.

Schleiermacher, G., Janoueix-Lerosey, I., Ribeiro, A., Klijanienko, J., Couturier, J., Pierron, G., Mosseri, V., Valent, A., Auger, N., Plantaz, D., Rubie, H., Valteau-Couanet, D., Bourdeaut, F., Combaret, V., Bergeron, C., Michon, J. & Delattre, O. (2010). Accumulation of segmental alterations determines progression in neuroblastoma. *J Clin Oncol* 28(19): 3122-30.

Schwab, M., Westermann, F., Hero, B. & Berthold, F. (2003). Neuroblastoma: biology and molecular and chromosomal pathology. *Lancet Oncol* 4(8): 472-80.

Seeger, R. C., Wada, R., Brodeur, G. M., Moss, T. J., Bjork, R. L., Sousa, L. & Slamon, D. J. (1988). Expression of N-myc by neuroblastomas with one or multiple copies of the oncogene. *Prog Clin Biol Res* 271: 41-9.

Takita, J., Ishii, M., Tsutsumi, S., Tanaka, Y., Kato, K., Toyoda, Y., Hanada, R., Yamamoto, K., Hayashi, Y. & Aburatani, H. (2004). Gene expression profiling and identification of novel prognostic marker genes in neuroblastoma. *Genes Chromosomes Cancer* 40(2): 120-32.

Tanaka, T., Sugimoto, T. & Sawada, T. (1998). Prognostic discrimination among neuroblastomas according to Ha-ras/trk A gene expression: a comparison of the profiles of neuroblastomas detected clinically and those detected through mass screening. *Cancer* 83(8): 1626-33.

Teitz, T., Wei, T., Liu, D., Valentine, V., Valentine, M., Grenet, J., Lahti, J. M. & Kidd, V. J. (2002). Caspase-9 and Apaf-1 are expressed and functionally active in human neuroblastoma tumor cell lines with 1p36 LOH and amplified MYCN. *Oncogene* 21(12): 1848-58.

Teitz, T., Wei, T., Valentine, M. B., Vanin, E. F., Grenet, J., Valentine, V. a., Behm, F. G., Look, A. T., Lahti, J. M. & Kidd, V. J. (2000). Caspase 8 is deleted or silenced preferentially in childhood neuroblastomas with amplification of MYCN. *Nat Med* 6: 529-535.

The American Association for Cancer Research Human Epigenome Task Force; The European Union Network of Excellence Scientific Advisory Board (2008). Moving AEAD with an international human epigenome project. *Nature* 454: 711-715.

Trochet, D., Bourdeaut, F., Janoueix-Lerosey, I., Deville, A., de Pontual, L., Schleiermacher, G., Coze, C., Philip, N., Frebourg, T., Munnich, A., Lyonnet, S., Delattre, O. & Amiel, J. (2004). Germline mutations of the paired-like homeobox 2B (PHOX2B) gene in neuroblastoma. *Am J Hum Genet* 74(4): 761-4.

Urayama, K. Y., Von Behren, J. & Reynolds, P. (2007). Birth characteristics and risk of neuroblastoma in young children. *Am J Epidemiol* 165(5): 486-95.

van Noesel, M. M., van Bezouw, S., Salomons, G. S., Voute, P. A., Pieters, R., Baylin, S. B., Herman, J. G. & Versteeg, R. (2002). Tumor-specific down-regulation of the tumor necrosis factor-related apoptosis-inducing ligand decoy receptors DcR1 and DcR2 is associated with dense promoter hypermethylation. *Cancer Res* 62(7): 2157-61.

van Noesel, M. M. & Versteeg, R. (2004). Pediatric neuroblastomas: genetic and epigenetic 'danse macabre'. *Gene* 325: 1-15.

Vandesompele, J., Van Roy, N., Van Gele, M., Laureys, G., Ambros, P., Heimann, P., Devalck, C., Schuuring, E., Brock, P., Otten, J., Gyselinck, J., De Paepe, A. & Speleman, F. (1998). Genetic heterogeneity of neuroblastoma studied by comparative genomic hybridization. *Genes Chromosomes Cancer* 23(2): 141-52.

Wang, K., Diskin, S. J., Zhang, H., Attiyeh, E. F., Winter, C., Hou, C., Schnepp, R. W., Diamond, M., Bosse, K., Mayes, P. A., Glessner, J., Kim, C., Frackelton, E., Garris, M., Wang, Q., Glaberson, W., Chiavacci, R., Nguyen, L., Jagannathan, J., Saeki, N., Sasaki, H., Grant, S. F., Iolascon, A., Mosse, Y. P., Cole, K. A., Li, H., Devoto, M., McGrady, P. W., London, W. B., Capasso, M., Rahman, N., Hakonarson, H. & Maris, J. M. (2011). Integrative genomics identifies LMO1 as a neuroblastoma oncogene. *Nature* 469(7329): 216-20.

Weese-Mayer, D. E., Berry-Kravis, E. M. & Marazita, M. L. (2005). In pursuit (and discovery) of a genetic basis for congenital central hypoventilation syndrome. *Respir Physiol Neurobiol* 149(1-3): 73-82.

Wellmann, A., Doseeva, V., Butscher, W., Raffeld, M., Fukushima, P., Stetler-Stevenson, M. & Gardner, K. (1997). The activated anaplastic lymphoma kinase increases cellular proliferation and oncogene up-regulation in rat 1a fibroblasts. *FASEB J* 11(12): 965-72.

White, P. S., Thompson, P. M., Gotoh, T., Okawa, E. R., Igarashi, J., Kok, M., Winter, C., Gregory, S. G., Hogarty, M. D., Maris, J. M. & Brodeur, G. M. (2005). Definition and characterization of a region of 1p36.3 consistently deleted in neuroblastoma. *Oncogene* 24(16): 2684-94.

Wong, I. H., Chan, J., Wong, J. & Tam, P. K. (2004). Ubiquitous aberrant RASSF1A promoter methylation in childhood neoplasia. *Clin Cancer Res* 10(3): 994-1002.

Yagyu, S., Gotoh, T., Iehara, T., Miyachi, M., Katsumi, Y., Tsubai-Shimizu, S., Kikuchi, K., Tamura, S., Tsuchiya, K., Imamura, T., Misawa-Furihata, A., Sugimoto, T., Sawada, T. & Hosoi, H. (2008). Circulating methylated-DCR2 gene in serum as an indicator of prognosis and therapeutic efficacy in patients with MYCN nonamplified neuroblastoma. *Clin Cancer Res* 14(21): 7011-9.

Yang, Q., Kiernan, C. M., Tian, Y., Salwen, H. R., Chlenski, A., Brumback, B. A., London, W. B. & Cohn, S. L. (2007). Methylation of CASP8, DCR2, and HIN-1 in neuroblastoma is associated with poor outcome. *Clin Cancer Res* 13(11): 3191-7.

Yang, Q., Zage, P., Kagan, D., Tian, Y., Seshadri, R., Salwen, H. R., Liu, S., Chlenski, A. & Cohn, S. L. (2004). Association of epigenetic inactivation of RASSF1A with poor outcome in human neuroblastoma. *Clin Cancer Res* 10(24): 8493-500.

Yang, Q. W., Liu, S., Tian, Y., Salwen, H. R., Chlenski, A., Weinstein, J. & Cohn, S. L. (2003). Methylation-associated silencing of the thrombospondin-1 gene in human neuroblastoma. *Cancer Res* 63(19): 6299-310.

Zhang, C., Li, H., Zhou, G., Zhang, Q., Zhang, T., Li, J., Zhang, J., Hou, J., Liew, C. T. & Yin, D. (2007). Transcriptional silencing of the TMS1/ASC tumour suppressor gene by an epigenetic mechanism in hepatocellular carcinoma cells. *J Pathol* 212(2): 134-42.

Part 2

Neuroblastoma, Biology Update

3

The Cell Biology of Neuroblastoma

John B. Denny
Department of Ophthalmology
University of Texas Health Science Center, San Antonio
Texas
USA

1. Introduction

Neuroblastoma is the third most common solid tumor in children and is the most common extracranial solid tumor in children (Maris, 2010; Coulter et al., 2008; Wickstrom et al., 2007). It is highly malignant and has a poor outcome despite aggressive treatment, even with autologous stem cell transplantation (Sartelet et al., 2008). It is a disease of the neural crest and the sympathetic nervous system, and most often originates from the adrenal gland. Neuroblastoma occurs as low risk, medium risk, and high risk forms, with the high risk form being difficult to treat even with the most advanced protocols. The prognosis for neuroblastoma is poor in advanced stages of the disease. Low risk forms may regress spontaneously, and may require no surgery and only observation (Kitanaka et al., 2002). Spontaneous remission occurs more commonly in neuroblastoma than in other cancers (Carlsen, 1990; Hero et al., 2008). The reasons for this are not at present understood. The overall cure rate is 40%, which indicates that new therapeutic strategies are needed (Sartelet et al., 2008). This chapter will focus on the cell and molecular biology of neuroblastoma, and the development of therapeutic strategies for its treatment. It will emphasize biologically unfavorable and clinically aggressive neuroblastomas rather than biologically favorable neuroblastomas.

2. Cancer cell growth

Tumor cells require the action of growth factors to proliferate. The initial step is the interaction of growth factors and cytokines with various receptors, followed by the subsequent activation of other signaling molecules. Neuroblastic (N-type) cells are the predominant cell type in neuroblastoma, as oppoed to stromal (S-type) cells (Armstrong et al., 2006).

2.1 Growth factors binding to Receptor Tyrosine Kinases (RTKs)

Receptor tyrosine kinases (RTKs) are transmembrane proteins that contain tyrosine kinase activity and include the receptor for insulin, the receptor for IGF-1 (insulin-like growth factor-1), called IGF1R, the TrkA high affinity receptor for nerve growth factor (NGF), the eph receptors for the neuronal guidance factors known as ephrins, the TrkB receptor for brain-derived neurotrophic factor (BDNF), and the receptors for the acidic and basic forms of fibroblast growth factor (FGF), GDNF (glial cell line-derived neurotrophic factor), VEGF (vascular endothelial growth factor), PDGF (platelet-derived growth factor), and EGF (epidermal growth factor) (Sartelet et al., 2008). NGF binding to TrkA causes the neuronal growth-associated protein GAP-43 to become phosphorylated by protein kinase C in isolated growth cones (Denny, 2006). NGF causes an increase in the production of GAP-43 by PC12 cells (Denny, 2006). RTKs activate PI3K (phosphatidylinositol 3-kinase), which leads to activation of the protein kinase Akt. The IGF1R has been implicated in the pathogenesis of neuroblastoma (Coulter et al., 2008). IGF1R signals through the Ras/Raf/MEK(mitogen-activated protein kinase)/ERK(extracellular signal-regulated kinase) pathway to induce proliferative growth and through the PI3K/Akt pathway for anti-apoptosis (Coulter et al., 2008). BDNF/TrkB are expressed in cases of neuroblastoma that have a poor prognosis (Jaboin et al., 2002; Li and Thiele, 2007). BDNF/TrkB protects neuroblastoma cells from chemotherapy-induced apoptosis (Jaboin et al., 2002). This is mediated by the PI3K/Akt pathway, making Akt a target to improve the prognosis (Li and Thiele, 2007). BDNF/TrkB also prevents axotomized retinal ganglion cell death, by acting through the MAPK and PI3K pathways (Nakazawa et al., 2002). The specific inhibitors LY294002 (PI3K) and U0126 (MAPK) were used (Nakazawa et al., 2002). The gene for the transcription factor MYCN is amplified in approximately 20% of human neuroblastomas and gives a poor prognosis (Petroni et al., 2011). MYCN overexpression sensitizes neuroblastoma cells to apoptosis, which requires the phosphorylation of p53 at Ser-46 by the protein kinase HIPK2 (Petroni et al., 2011). MYCN expression is disrupted when the IGF1R is blocked by a specific antibody, αIR3 (Coulter et al., 2008). N1E-115 neuroblastoma cells produce GAP-43 when they are differentiated by low serum and dimethylsulfoxide (DMSO) (Ollom and Denny, 2008).. It has been proposed that when NCAM on a growth cone encounters a suitable substrate, FGF receptors are clustered and GAP-43 is phosphorylated at Ser-41 by protein kinase C, leading to cytoskeletal changes and growth cone advance. (Denny, 2006).. The expression of GAP-43 in neuroblastoma cells suggests that the cells are attempting to function as neurons by extending growth cones and neurites.The expression of GAP-43 by differentiated N1E-115 cells is particularly intense (Ollom and Denny, 2008; Baker and Storm, 1997), whereas its expression in the retinal ganglion cell line RGC-5 is much weaker (Ollom and Denny, unpublished results). Differentiation of N1E-115 cells also causes the up-regulation of angiotensin II receptors (Reagan et al., 1990). The N1E-115 cells were differentiated by the presence of 0.5% serum and 1.5% DMSO (Reagan et al., 1990). These cells incorporated radioactive palmitate into GAP-43, but the palmitoylated protein was only immunoprecipitated by an antibody directed toward the C-terminal 10 amino acids of GAP-43 (Ollom and Denny, unpublished results). The presence of the palmitate chains may block the binding of antibodies at other sites in the protein. Protein palmitoylation in N1E-115 cells was not affected by norepinephrine, Sema3A, or netrin-1. GAP-43 was crosslinked to calmodulin but not to actin following analysis by two-dimensional electrophoresis (Ollom and Denny, 2008). Full-length GAP-43 phosphorylated at Ser-41 was immunoprecipitated from differentiated N1E-115 cells with an antibody specific for that phosphorylated residue, and a 34 kDa fragment containing that epitope was detected on Western blot. Nogo-A is a transmembrane protein that was initially thought to block nerve regeneration through its expression on oligodendrocytes, but it has been shown to be expressed on N1E-115 cells and SH-SY5Y cells (Liu et al.,

2002) as well as on normal hippocampal neurons (Zagrebelsky et al., 2010). Melatonin protected neuroblastoma cells, acting as cultured neurons, from the effects of Alzheimer amyloid peptide (Pappolla et al., 1997)

2.2 Cytokines

Cytokines include tumor necrosis factor-α (TNF-α), TNF-β, interleukins, and interferons (IFNs). They bind to receptors other than RTKs. TNF-α causes inflammation and kills tumor cells *in vitro.* It can be administered to patients as an anti-cancer agent, but has not been successful due to its toxicity and the development of resistance. The binding of IL-3 (interleukin-3) to its receptor activates Raf/MEK/ERK, PI3K/Akt, and JAK/STAT (Janus kinase/ Signal Transducer and Activator of Transcription), which results in cell proliferation and prevention of apoptosis (Steelman et al., 2004). Bacterial products cause macrophages to release TNF-α and IL-12, which cause NK (natural killer) cells to release interferon-γ (IFN-γ). This interferon in turn causes macrophages to secrete more TNF-α and IL-12. IFN-γ is the only type II interferon. It is produced by NK cells, NKT (natural killer T) cells, and by CD4 (cluster of differentiation 4) T helper cells and CD8 cytotoxic T cells. IFN-γ is the main factor that causes macrophage activation. It also activates cytotoxic T cells and NK cells. T helper cells secrete many interleukins which include IL-2, -3, -4, -5, and -6. Activated macrophages can kill both parasites and cancer cells. The secretion of IL-12 and TNF-α by macrophages is inhibited by IL-10. Human type I interferons include IFN-α and IFN-β, which inhibit neuroblastoma angiogenesis and growth (Streck et al., 2004) and are secreted by NK cells, B-cells, T-cells, fibroblasts, endothelial cells, macrophages, and osteoblasts. They stimulate an anti-viral response in both NK cells and macrophages. Alpha IFNs slow the rate of tumor cell division until the cells can no longer survive, and can also increase the level of IL-6. The commercially available alpha IFN Intron-A (interferon alfa-2b) is currently used to treat hairy cell leukemia, bladder cancer, chronic myelogenous leukemia (CML), ovarian cancer, multiple myeloma, malignant melanoma, non-Hodgkins lymphoma (NHL), and Kaposi's sarcoma, but not, as yet, neuroblastoma. Both type I and type II interferons contain approximately 166 amino acids and bind to the type II cytokine receptor. The IFNs can increase Class I and Class II major histocompatability complex (MHC) antigen expression. IFN-γ increases the expression of Class I MHC antigens on neuroblastoma cells, increasing the likelihood of infiltration of T cells into the tumor *in vivo* (Reid et al., 2009). One of the most common means by which solid tumor cells evade the immune response is by downregulation of Class I MHC antigen expression (Garcia-Lora, et al., 2003) IL-6 promotes the survival of neuroblastoma cells in bone marrow (Ara al., 2009). It has been suggested by Robert Seeger and Yves DeClerck that inflammation may promote neuroblastoma. Consistent with this is the finding that TNF functions as a growth factor for neurob;astoma (Goillot et al., 1992). C1300 neuroblastoma cells retrovirally transduced with the IL-4 gene had reduced tumorigenicity in syngeneic A/J and nude mice when compared with wild type cells (Yoshida et al., 1998).

2.3 G-Protein coupled receptors

G-protein coupled receptors (GPCRs) are proteins that cross the plasma membrane seven times and act through heterotrimeric G-proteins, which are active in the GTP-bound state and inactive in the GDP-bound state. The rate of cell division can be increased by G-protein stimulation of PI3K and Ras, and also by activation of phospholipase C (PLC), which leads to the formation of diacylglycerol (DAG) and the activation of protein kinase C (PKC). PKC is also stimulated by calcium and phosphatidylserine. Another source of DAG is phosphatidylcholine, utilizing the enzyme phospholipase D (PLD) (Denny, 2006). PKC then activates Raf and the Raf/MEK/ERK pathway, leading to cell division. PKC also activates the transcription factor NF-KB (nuclear factor-KB), which affects transcription in the nucleus. There are six catecholamine receptors and include D1, D2, β1,β2, α1, and α2. All six receptors are GPCRs. Adenylate cyclase (AC) is stimulated by D_1 dopamine receptors and inhibited by D_2 receptors. The β receptors both activate AC. α1 receptors constrict arterioles and raise blood pressure, and α2 receptors are located presynaptically on neurons in the vasomotor center of the brainstem. Clonidine, acting as an agonist at these α2 receptors, lowers the concentration of norepinephrine in the plasma, thereby lowering blood pressure. When epinephrine or norepinephrine bind to the β-adrenergic receptor (either β_1 or β_2), the stimulatory G-protein Gs is activated, which then activates adenylate cyclase, leading to the formation of cAMP and the activation of protein kinase A (PKA). This leads to the activation of the transcription factor CREB (cAMP response element-binding), which alters gene expression in the nucleus. A different G-protein activates guanylate cyclase, leading to the formation of cGMP. The binding of acetylcholine to the muscarinic acetylcholine receptor activates PLC and PKC. The muscarinic receptor can also interact with the inhibitory G-protein Gi, leading to an inhibition of adenylate cyclase. The metabotropic glutamate receptor and the receptors for many peptides in the brain, including angiotensin II, are GPCRs (Denny et al., 1991) . GPCR activation of PI3K does not always lead to cell division but can cause an increase in neurite outgrowth instead. Angiotensin II, binding to the angiotensin type I receptor and stimulating the PI3K/Akt pathway, caused an increase in the expression of the growth-associated protein GAP-43 and neurite outgrowth rather than an increase in the rate of cell division (Yang et al., 2002). Both GAP-43 and the G-protein Go are found in high concentrations in neuronal growth cones (Denny, 2006).

A cyclic nucleotide phosphodiesterase (PDE) breaks down the cyclic nucleotides cAMP and cGMP. The PDE inhibitors Zaprinast and DC-TA-46 inhibit SK-N-MC neuroblastoma growth, both *in vitro* and in a xenograft model of nude mice (Giorgi et al., 2001). The concentrations for 50% inhibition (IC50 values) in clonal density experiments were 3.3 μM and 1.9 μM, respectively.

2.4 Integrins

Integrins are heterodimeric transmembrane proteins that activate focal adhesion kinase (FAK) and the tyrosine kinase Src. Src phosphorylates FAK, and FAK then activates Ras. Like Src, FAK is a tyrosine protein kinase. Integrins also activate the Rho GTPase Cdc42. Integrins bind extracellular matrix molecules such as laminin. Cancer cells become invasive and lose their ability to be guided by the extracellular matrix. GAP-43 is phosphorylated at Ser-41 by protein kinase C when laminin binds to its integrin (Lalli and Hall, 2005), which shows the activating effect of the extracellular matrix on neurons in culture. GAP-43 is expressed in neurons as a result of prostate cancer, and causes axon sprouting (Jimenez-Andrade et al., 2010). Other proteins present intracellularly at the integrin site include talin, vinculin, paxillin, F-actin, and microtubules.

2.5 Ras

The Ras superfamily contains 21 kDa monomeric GTPases that are important in many aspects of normal cell function. The Ras superfamily contains a subfamily also called Ras, which is involed in cell proliferation. Subfamily Rho is important in neuronal development (Denny, 2006). This subfamily controls the dynamics of the cytoskeleton and includes the GTPases RhoA, RhoB, RhoC, RhoD, RhoF, RhoG, Cdc42 and Rac-1. Rac-1 promotes the formation of the actin-rich lamellipodium that surrounds the central core of the growth cone in growing neurons. From the lamellipodium are formed actin-containing filopodia. The formation of filopodia is promoted by Cdc42 (Denny, 2006). Other subfamilies include Rab (involved in membrane trafficking), Ran (a single member involved in nuclear transport), Arf (involved in vesicular transport), and Rheb (Ras homolog enriched in brain). Rheb functions in cell proliferation as described below. The Ras subfamily contains H-Ras, K-Ras, N-Ras, R-Ras, TC21 (R-Ras2), Rap1A, Rap1B, Rap2A, Rap2B, RalA, RalB, and M-Ras (R-Ras3) (Denny, 2006, 2008; Kimmelman et al., 2002). Ral GTPases have been shown to regulate neurite branching *via* GAP-43 and in this way contribute to cell growth (Lalli and Hall, 2005). Point mutations in the genes H-*ras*, K-*ras*, or N-*ras* can give rise to protein products which can transform NIH-3T3 cells to a fully malignant phenotype (Gutierrez and Magee, 1991). These cells exhibit transformed characteristics in culture but are inhibited by tumor suppressor mechanisms when injected into wild-type mice. This suppression is overcome when the cells are injected into athymic (nude) mice, and tumors develop (Chambers et al., 1990). The activated form of Ras proteins binds GTP and the unactivated form binds GDP. A mutation can diminish the GTPase activity and cause Ras to remain in the GTP-bound form. Such a mutation in Ras will lock the Raf/MEK/ERK pathway in the "on" position and contribute to the cell becoming cancerous.

2.6 Lipid modifications of proteins

Palmitoylation refers to the addition of the 16 carbon fatty acid palmitate to proteins, primarily in reversible thioester linkage to cysteine (Denny, 2008). Many proteins involved in cell growth and division are palmitoylated, including GPCRs, heterotrimeric G-protein α-subunits, monomeric GTPases, GAP-43, integrins, and NCAM (neural cell adhesion molecule)-140 and NCAM-180 (Denny, 2008). The Src family of protein tyrosine kinases include Src, Lyn, Yes, Lck, and Fyn. Lyn is palmitoylated while c-Src (cellular Src) is not (Kasahara et al., 2007). Src was found not to be palmitoylated while Yes, Lck, and Fyn were palmitoylated and myristoylated (Koegl et al., 1994). Myristoylation refers to the addition of the 14 carbon fatty acid myristate to the N-terminus of a protein in permanent amide linkage. Heterotrimeric G-protein α-subunits are palmitoylated and myristoylated (Denny, 2008). Ras proteins are modified by both palmitoylation and prenylation, the latter involving the addition of either the 15 carbon farnesyl group or the 20 carbon geranylgeranyl group (Denny, 2008). These modifications are required for the activity of Ras (Denny, 2008). Blockade of the farnesylation of Ras is a therapeutic approach in cancer (Margaritora, et al., 2005; Omer et al., 1997), as is the blockade of geranylgeranyltransferase I (Philips and Cox, 2007).

2.7 PI3K/PTEN/Akt/mTOR pathway

The serine/threonine protein kinase Akt (also called protein kinase B) lies at the center of a pathway that promotes cancer cell survival and protects cells from apoptosis (Sartelet et al., 2008). Pathological activation of Akt frequently occurs in neuroblastoma and correlates with a poor prognosis (Fulda, 2009). Phosphatidylinositol 3-kinase (PI3K) converts the phospholipid phosphatidylinositol 4,5 bisphosphate (PI (4,5) P2 or PIP2) to phosphatidylinositol 3,4,5 triphosphate (PI (3,4,5) P3 or PIP3). PIP3 causes the protein kinase PDK1 to bind to the plasma membrane and phosphorylate Akt at Thr-308. PI3K is heterodimeric with an 85 kDa regulatory subunit and a 110 kDa catalytic subunit. Full activation of Akt occurs following a second phosphorylation at Ser-473, which is carried out by mTORC2 (Martelli et al., 2010), as described below. PI3K is the initial molecule to be activated by RTKs, GPCRs, and Ras. The oncogenic version of Ras requires an interaction with PI3K to produce its transforming effect (Carnero et al., 2008). Inhibition of Akt by the inhibition of PI3K has been studied, as well as drugs, such as geldanamycin and rapamycin, that modify the expression of Akt (Sartelet et al., 2008). The blockade of Akt signaling has been shown to result in apoptosis and growth inhibition of tumor cells (Tokunaga et al., 2008). Phosphorylated Akt phosphorylates and thereby inhibits TSC2, which is a GAP (GTPase activating protein) that together with TSC1 inactivates the small GTPase Rheb. When TSC2 is inhibited, Rheb accumulates in the GTP-bound form. This form activates the protein kinase activity of mTORC1, leading to activation of the protein kinase p70S6K and phosphorylation of ribosomal protein S6. This pathway leads to decreased apoptosis, and increased cell metabolism, proliferation, ribosome biogenesis, and translation (Martelli et al., 2010). Phosphorylated Akt activates MDM2, which inhibits p53. Since p53 promotes the apoptosis of tumor cells, this constitutes another mechanism whereby activated Akt inhibits apoptosis and promotes cancer growth (Martelli et al., 2010). The inhibition of Akt appears to be an excellent future course for the treatment of neuroblastoma (Sartelet et al., 2008).

The mammalian target of rapamycin (mTOR) is a 289 kDa serine/threonine protein kinase that regulates cell-cycle progression, autophagy, and cell survival, and was discovered as the binding site for rapamycin (Sarbassov et al., 2005). It is a single chain of 2,549 amino acids. Rapamycin binds to the 12 kDa protein FKBP12, and this complex binds to and inhibits mTOR (Marelli et al., 2010). The kinase domain of mTOR is located toward the C-terminus, between residues 2181 and 2431 (Martelli et al., 2010). Two complexes exist that contain mTOR, called mTORC1 and mTORC2 (Martelli et al., 2010). Both complexes contain the protein deptor (Peterson et al., 2009; Martelli et al., 2010). In normal cells, deptor holds mTORC1 and mTORC2 in check, helping to prevent transformation to the cancerous phenotype. In most cancers the expression of deptor is low, which allows mTORC1 and mTORC2 kinase activities to promote cell growth and survival and convert the cell to the cancerous phenotype. A major mechanism in this regard is the direct activation of Akt by mTORC2. By contrast, mTORC1 inhibits the activating pathways upstream of Akt. Treating cells with rapamycin, which binds to mTORC1, therefore leads to Akt activation, and may limit the usefulness of rapamycin and its analogs as anti-cancer drugs (Peterson et al., 2009). Nevertheless, the inhibition of the IGFR combined with rapamycin or temsirolimus inhibited the growth of the neuroblastoma cell lines BE-2 (c) and IMR-32 (Coulter et al., 2008). In contrast to most cancers, a subset of multiple myelomas that contain translocations in cyclinD1/D3 or c-MAF/MAFB contain highly overexpressed deptor, and its inhibition of mTORC1 unexpectedly leads to the activation of the PI3K/mTORC2/Akt pathway (Peterson et al., 2009). A decrease in deptor levels in these cells leads to apoptosis (Peterson et al., 2009). Inhibitors of mTOR are being used to treat advanced renal cell carcinoma (Kapoor and Figlin, 2009).

2.8 Raf/MEK/ERK pathway

Raf is a serine/threonine protein kinase that is coded for by the *c-raf* proto-oncogene. The Raf/MEK/ERK pathway is located downstream of Ras. Mutations in Ras can cause the

Raf/MEK/ERK pathway to be permanently activated, leading to the formation of cancer cells (Steelman et al., 2008). The activation of this pathway leads to the activation of the transcription factor Fos. It also leads to the activation of *c-jun* N-terminal kinases (JNKs) which activate the transcription factor Jun. The combination of Fos and Jun is called AP-1.

2.9 JAK/STAT pathway

This pathway can also be activated by mutated Ras (Steelman et al., 2008). The binding of cytokines to their receptors activates a JAK (Janus Kinase), which undergoes autophosphorylation by tyrosine kinase activity. The phosphorylated form of JAK binds seven different STATs (Signal Transducer and Activator of Transcription), which are transcription factors which enter the nucleus, bind to seven different promoters, and alter gene expression. In the cytosol, a STAT can stimulate Bcl-xL. This is anti-apoptotic, since Bcl-xL blocks the activating effect of mitochondrial cytochrome c on caspase-9. Interferon-β induces apoptosis in the SH-SY5Y cell line through activation of JAK/STAT signaling and down-regulation of the PI3K/Akt pathway (Dedoni et al., 2010). Apoptosis was accompanied by the cleavage of caspases -9, -7, and -3, cytochrome c release, and the phosphorylation of STAT1 (Dedoni et al., 2010). IL-6 promotes the survival of neuroblastoma cells in bone marrow (Ara al., 2009). IL-6 and IL-10 contribute to neuroblastoma progression, with IL-6 acting through STAT3 (Song et al., 2007).

2.10 Anaplastic Lymphoma Kinase (ALK)

The gene for anaplastic lymphoma kinase (ALK) is the major gene that predisposes an individual to familial neuroblastoma (Maris, 2010; Mosse et al., 2008). Although ALK is important in the normal development of the brain, the mutation of its gene is associated with 10-15% of neuroblastomas (Mosse et al., 2008). ALK, also known as CD246, is a novel receptor tyrosine kinase and its inhibition is an approach in cancer therapy (Mosse et al., 2009).

2.11 Cytogenetic alterations in neuroblastoma

The outlook in neuroblastoma, as it is in other cancers, is better if the patient possesses a normal karyotype. The above pathways may become activated as a result of cytogenetic alterations, in which parts of chromosomes are deleted and added or translocated to other chromosomes. This places promoters near genes that they would normally not affect, and this increases the likelihood of converting a proto-oncogene to an oncogene. In the highest risk form of neuroblastoma the cells contain cytogenetic alterations such as MYCN amplification or 1p deletion (Wickstrom et al., 2007). The 6p22 locus is associated with clinically aggressive neuroblastoma (Maris et al., 2008). By contrast, the gain of whole chromosomes occurs most commonly in biologically favorable neuroblastomas, as the gain of chromosome 17 is the most frequent abnormality detected in neuroblastoma (Plantaz et al., 1997).

How chromosomal translocations result in cancer has been studied in B-cells. Translocation of the *c-myc* gene close to the enhancer for antibody heavy chains yields cancerous B-cells in Burkitt's lymphoma (Adams and Cory, 1998). Myc is a transcription factor and its major effect is on B- cell proliferation. MYCN codes for a member of the Myc family that is specifically associated with neuroblastoma. In cancerous B-cells, the part of chromosome 18 containing the *bcl-2* locus undergoes a reciprocal translocation with the part of chromosome

14 that contains the antibody heavy chain locus. This is a t(14:18) translocation, which places the *bcl-2* gene close to the heavy chain gene enhancer. All of the resulting leukemias are called chronic lymphocytic leukemia (CLL). Because Bcl-2 is pro-survival and is now expressed at a high level, it prevents apoptosis, which should normally occur in the B-cell once an infection has passed. This causes the B-cell to continue to divide and to become cancerous. More than just the translocation is necessary, however, since 50% of the population contains the above B-cell translocation but the individuals do not have cancer. This shows that it is possible for an individual to have cancer cells but not have cancer.

2.12 NBPF10

NBPF10 (neuroblastoma breakpoint family member 10) has its gene in humans located at 1q21.1. It is highly conserved and contains DUF1220 repeats. It is thought to be related to the 1q21.1 deletion syndrome and the 1q21.1 duplication syndrome.

2.13 Angiogenesis and neuroblastoma

Angiogenesis in neuroblastoma has been reviewed (Ribatti et al., 2004). Imatinib has been used on neuroblastoma tumorigenesis and vascular endothelial growth factor (VEGF) expression (Beppo et al., 2009).Tumors increase vascularization to provide a greater blood supply. Lenalidomide (Revlimid) is related to thalidomide and possesses immunomodulatory and antiangiogenic properties. It inhibits the secretion of pro-inflammatory cytokines and promotes the release of anti-inflammatory cytokines from peripheral blood mononuclear cells. It decreases the activity of TNF-α. Lenalidomide blocks the proliferation of some cancer cell lines but not others. Lenalidomide blocks growth factor-induced angiogenesis and growth factor-induced endothelial cell migration, which may be due to an inhibition of Akt phosphorylation (Dredge et al., 2005). It also blocks the basic fibroblast growth factor (bFGF)-induced increase in the phosphorylation of Akt *in vitro* (Dredge et al., 2005). It is currently used in the treatment of multiple myeloma but could have use in neuroblastoma.

2.14 Neuroblastoma-derived cell lines

The cell line N1E-115 is one of many clones that were derived from the spontaneous mouse neuroblastoma C-1300 (Amano et al., 1972). The growth of cell lines in serum-free medium containing the growth factors insulin, transferrin, progesterone, putrescine, and sodium selenite was pioneered using the rat neuroblastoma cell line B104 (Bottenstein and Sato, 1979). When N1E-115 cells are placed in serum-free medium and are thereby deprived of growth factors, they stop dividing and develop neuronal characteristics, rather than undergo apoptosis (Baker and Storm, 1997). A marked increase in the level of GAP-43 is seen following the differentiation of N1E-115 cells (Denny, 2006; Ollom and Denny, 2008). By contrast, most cancer cells undergo apoptosis when deprived of growth factors (Kilic et al., 2002). The main executioner caspase was caspase-3 in apoptosis induced by serum starvation in AKR-2B fibroblasts (Kilic et al., 2002). An apoptosome of molecular weight 600 kDa was formed and free activated caspase-12 was detected in the cytosol (Kilic et al., 2002). No cleavage of caspase-9 was detected (Kilic et al., 2002).

SH-SY5Y cells were derived from a human neuroblastoma, show neuronal characteristics, and respond to the application of norepinephrine (Laifenfeld et al., 2002). Norepinephrine-treated SH-SY5Y cells showed alterations in the expression of 44 genes, as determined in a

neurobiology cDNA microarray (Laifenfeld et al., 2002). The expression of the genes for GAP-43, the cell adhesion molecule L1, and laminin were increased (Laifenfeld et al., 2002).
Neurons grow, using Akt, but in the sense of extending axons instead of creating daughter cells. Axonal growth is channeled through tissues during development without disrupting them, while invasion of tissue by cancer cells is disruptive and may result in the death of the host. The semaphorin Sema3A inhibits neurite outgrowth by inhibiting the phosphorylation of Akt (Chadborn et al., 2006).
We have found that the protein kinase inhibitor staurosporine is lethal for N1E-115 cells when applied to undifferentiated cells (C.M. Ollom and J.B. Denny, unpublished results). By contrast, it causes the retinal ganglion cell line RGC-5 to differentiate into neuronal-like cells (Lieven et al., 2007). In addition, staurosporine causes the differentiation of SH-SY5Y cells (Prince and Oreland, 1997). One explanation for these results is that N1E-115 cells lack sufficient Bcl-2 to prevent the apoptosis that is induced by staurosporine. Bcl-2 has been shown to be protective against the cytotoxic effects of staurosporine (Takeda et al., 1997). By contrast, either low serum (Baker and Storm, 1997) or low serum and dimethylsulfoxide (Ollom and Denny, 2008) cause N1E-115 cells to stop dividing and to undergo neurite extension. Growth has been switched in these cases from abnormal cell division to a more normal neurite extension. How does this switch occur? Why do these cancer cells not undergo apoptosis when deprived of growth factors in low serum? N1E-115 cells appear to have retained many genes, especially those involved in cytoskeletal dynamics, that allow neurite extension to occur (Oh, et al., 2006). N1E-115 cells were differentiated by the addition of dimethylsulfoxide, and most of the pathways described above were involved in the differentiation process, including protein kinases A and C, TrkA, B. and C, MAP kinases, raf kinases, ERK, and c-jun N-terminal kinases (Oh et al., 2005, 2006).

3. Tumor suppression

3.1 PTEN (Phosphatase and Tensin Homolog)

A point mutation in an oncogene may not result in cancer, because a second event may be required, such as the inhibition of NK cell function or the mutation of the gene for PTEN, which will raise the level of PIP3 in the cell and allow the activation of Akt. If normal PTEN is present, it may nullify the mutation in Ras by decreasing the level of PIP3 to the point that Akt cannot be continuously activated. PTEN (phosphatase and tensin homolog) carries out the reverse reaction of PI3K and thereby decreases the level of PIP3 in the cell. This decreases the amount of activated Akt and reduces the ability of the cell to divide. Mutations in the PTEN gene are associated with many human cancers. A small fraction of neuroblastomas were found to harbor PTEN alterations when 45 primary neuroblastoma tumors and 12 neuroblastoma cell lines were screened (Munoz et al., 2004). The level of activated Akt is therefore determined by the level of PI3K, which promotes its formation, and by the level of PTEN, which decreases its formation.

3.2 p53

p53 is encoded by the *TP53* gene located on the short arm of chromosome 17 in humans. Human p53 contains 393 amino acids. The protein can activate DNA repair mechanisms and arrest cells prior to the entrance into S phase of the cell cycle to allow this repair to occur. If the DNA damage is not repairable, p53 initiates apoptosis of the cell. If p53 is altered by mutation, the block for cells entering S phase will not occur, and cells will divide uncontrollably, leading to cancer. Tumor suppression is therefore greatly reduced if the *TP53* gene is altered. Mutations in p53 were reported to be infrequent in neuroblastoma (Tweddle et al., 2003). The protein p73 has been shown to cause the differentiation of a neuroblastoma cell line (De Laurenzi et al., 2000). P73 and p63 are related to p53.

3.3 Selenium and vitamin E as anti-oxidants

Selenium is a cofactor for glutathione peroxidase, which uses glutathione to decrease the levels of hydrogen peroxide and organic hydroperoxides in the cell. Vitamin E has a similar anti-oxidant role. Epidemiological studies suggest that selenium may protect against cancer. Anti-oxidants were neuroprotective in SH-SY5Y cells overexpressing the familial Parkinson's disease alpha-synuclein A53T mutation (Ma et al., 2010). DHA (docosahexaenoic acid) is the most abundant polyunsaturated fatty acid in the retina and has neuroprotective effects against oxidative stress in retinal ganglion cells.

3.4 DNA repair and tumor suppression

NF1 is a tumor suppressor in neuroblastoma that controls the response to retinoic acid and the disease outcome (Holzel et al., 2010). NF1 codes for the protein neurofibromin, which is an enzyme controlling Ras. Loss of NF1 activates Ras-MEK signaling, and neuroblastomas with low levels of NF1 and ZNF423 have an extremely poor outcome (Holzel et al., 2010). NF1 regulates TSC2 and mTOR. A repressible DNA repair system exists in mouse neuroblastoma cells (McCombe and Kidson, 1975). MicroRNA-542-5p has been shown to be a novel tumor suppressor in neuroblastoma (Bray et al., 2011). DNA repair can contribute to tumor suppression by repairing mutated sites in the genome that can lead to cancer. A common example is the removal of thymine dimers that are formed each day in skin cells as a result of exposure to the UV-B wavelength band of UV light from the sun. The presence of these dimers can result in a mutation that may lead to skin cancer if not removed. The enzyme carrying out DNA repair in the nuclear genome in humans is DNA polymerase β, while that acting on the mitochondrial genome is DNA polymerase γ. The repair activity in mitochondria is much less efficient than that occurring in the nucleus, leading to a much greater rate of mutation in the mitochondrial genome compared to the nuclear genome. The loss of this thymine dimer excision is clearly a loss of tumor suppression.

3.5 The immune response

There is ample evidence that cancer cells cause an immune response in the host. Immunodeficiency leads to an increased likelihood of cancer, as in the development of Kaposi's sarcoma in patients infected with the human immunodeficiency virus (HIV). In addition, there is an increase in Epstein-Barr virus (EBV)-induced lymphoma in transplant patients. Finally, the fact that neuroblastoma can regress spontaneously suggests that immunological mechanisms can come into play (Carlsen, 1990). If the tumor cell load is reduced by chemotherapeutic agents, it is possible that the immune system can control the residual tumor. Without immune system attack, those tumor cells that escape chemotherapeutic agents can regrow and kill the host. It may be necessary for the tumor cell load to be low for the immune system to control or destroy the cells that evaded attack by chemotherapeutic agents. The immune response to neuroblastoma has been increased by increasing the immunogenicity of neuroblastoma cells using IL-2 (Bowman et al., 1998).

3.6 Natural Killer (NK) cells

Natural killer (NK) cells are lymphocytes that kill certain neuroblastoma cells lines in culture (Ogbomo et al., 2006). The cell lines were UKF-NB-2 and UKF-NB-4 obtained from bone marrow metastases of neuroblastoma patients with stage IV disease (Ogbomo et al., 2006). NK cells are inhibited by alcohol (Boyadjieva et al., 2004), which could be a factor in the onset of neuroblastoma in children born to mothers who consumed alcohol during pregnancy. The inhibition of NK cells could alone account for the carcinogenic properties of alcohol. NK cells are tumoricidal without the need for Class I MHC antigen participation.

3.7 Tumor Specific Transplantation Antigens (TSTAs) and Tumor Associated Transplantation Antigens (TATAs)

Tumor cell antigens that can induce this immune response include tumor specific transplantation antigens (TSTAs), which are unique to the tumor cell, are not expressed on normal cells, and are responsible for tumor rejection. Tumor associated transplantation antigens (TATAs) are expressed by both tumor cells and normal cells. Although antibodies may develop against TSTAs, cell-mediated immunity appears to be most important in tumor rejection. Activated macrophages can, in addition, be tumoricidal.

This response has been called immune surveillance. Does immune surveillance prevent the formation of many cancers and why does it sometimes fail? It is possible that the TSTAs may not be sufficiently immunogenic to elicit the required immune response, or the cells may not express sufficient Class I MHC antigens, or they may secrete antigens that block antibody and cell-mediated responses. Tumor cells can escape immune detection by downregulating Class I MHC molecules, which decreases the detection of TSTAs. Antibodies may bind to NK cells, B-lymphocytes, macrophages, and granulocytes without binding to the tumor cells. All of this constitutes an escape from immune surveillance, which allows the tumor cells to proliferate. Neuroblastoma cells are of neuroectodermal origin and express a number of cancer germline (CG) antigens (Wolfl et al., 2005). Screening of 68 tumor specimens for CG antigens revealed expression of MAGE-A1 in 44%, MAGE-A3/A6 in 21%, and NY-ESO-1 in 28% of cases (Wolfl et al., 2005). None of the selected tumors showed expression of MHC class I or class II antigens, which would limit the immunogenicity of the tumors in the host.

3.8 Antibody treatment of neuroblastoma

Antibodies directed toward the disialoganglioside GD-2, located on the cell surface, have been used in the treatment of neuroblastoma (Navid, et. al., 2010; Cheung et al., 1998). This ganglioside is not widely expressed on normal cells, making it an attractive target for antibody therapy in neuroblastoma and other cancers. Treatment of high risk neuroblastoma with antibody to GD-2 and the cytokines GM-CSF (granulocyte-macrophage colony-stimulating factor) and IL-2 gave superior outcomes when compared to treatment with six cycles of isotretinoin (Yu et al., 2010).

4. Cancer cell apoptosis

An important approach in cancer treatment is to modulate the apoptosis of cancer cells. Programmed cell death (PCD) can be either caspase-dependent (apoptosis) or caspase-independent (Kang et al., 2004). Neuronal PCD occurs normally in brain development but also occurs in pathological states. The PCD of cancer cells is a desirable end point in terms of either curing a patient's cancer or decreasing the cancer cell load. Although NGF is a growth factor when it binds to TrkA, it can cause apoptosis when it binds to the low affinity receptor $p75^{NTR}$ (Wang et al., 2001).

4.1 Caspases

The caspases are cysteine-dependent, aspartate-directed proteases, and make up a family of 14 enzymes, termed caspases 1-14 (Kang et al., 2004). Only seven of these participate in apoptosis. These include the initiator caspases -2, -8, -9, and -10 and the effector or executioner caspases -3, -6, and -7. Caspase-8 expression is thought to be silenced in most high stage neuroblastomas (Hopkins-Donaldson et al., 2002). Interestingly, caspase-3 participates in long-term depression (LTD) and AMPA receptor internalization, giving the enzyme a broader role in the nervous system than simply being an executioner caspase involved in apoptosis (Zheng et al., 2010).

4.2 Death receptors

The binding of the ligands TNF-α, FasL, and TRAIL (TNF-related apoptosis-inducing ligand) to their receptors TNFR (TNF receptor), Fas, and DR4 or DR5, respectively, termed death receptors of the TNFR superfamily, induces apoptosis (Kang et al., 2004). The binding of TRAIL to DR4 or DR5 induces rapid apoptosis. Caspases-2, -3, and -7 have been shown to be involved in thapsigargin-induced apoptosis of SH-SY5Y cells (Dahmer, 2005). Fas is also known as Cluster of Differentiation 95 or CD95. FasL is therefore also called CD95L.

4.3 Bcl-2

The Bcl-2 family of cytoplasmic proteins contains three subfamilies (Adams and Cory, 1998). Proteins most like Bcl-2 itself promote cell survival, while those more distantly related promote apoptosis. The fate of the cell is thus a result of the balance between these two types of proteins. Bcl stands for B-cell leukemia or B-cell lymphoma. The first subfamily is also called Bcl-2. It is pro-survival and anti-apoptotic, and includes the proteins Bcl-2, Bcl-xL, Bcl-w, Mcl-1, and A1. By contrast, the Bax subfamily is pro-apoptotic and includes the proteins Bax, Bak, and Bok. Bax is stimulated by p53, which promotes apoptosis. The BH3 subfamily is also pro-apoptotic and includes the proteins Bad, Bid, Bik, Blk, Hrk, BNIP3, and BimL. Akt inhibits Bad and thereby inhibits apoptosis and promotes growth. Bcl-2 is a 25 kDa protein with a C-terminal hydrophobic section of 21 amino acids that is important for docking to the cytoplasmic face of the mitochondrial membrane. Its gene *bcl-2* is also a proto-oncogene. The Fas (CD95/APO-1/TNFRSF6) receptor-ligand system is one of the key regulators of apoptosis. Fas is triggered by binding to its ligand FasL, either as membrane-bound FasL on FasL-expressing cells or through the crosslinking of soluble FasL. Fas then recruits Fas-associated death domain protein (FADD) and procaspase-8 to form the death-inducing signaling complex (DISC), which activates the caspase cascade, causing cell death (Kischkel et al., 1995). It has been shown that palmitoylation is required for efficient Fas cell death signaling (Chakrabandhu et al., 2007). The binding of norepinephrine and other α-agonists to α-1 adrenergic receptors blocks neuronal cell death associated with glutamate-induced excitotoxicity, and does so in the retinal ganglion cell line RGC-5 by regulating calcium and Bax levels and the activation of caspase-3 (Tchedre and Yorio, 2008). Bcl-2 is a regulator for retinoic-acid induced apoptotic cell death in neuroblastoma (Niizuma et al.,

2006). Cell lines that downregulated Bcl-2 (CHP134 and NB-39-nu cells) underwent apoptosis in the presence of all-*trans*-retinoic acid (ATRA), whereas those cell lines highly expressing Bcl-2 (LA-N-5 cells and RTBM1 cells) underwent differentiation instead of apoptosis (Niizuma et al., 2006).

4.4 Nitric Oxide

Nitric oxide (NO) is produced from L-arginine and molecular oxygen by nitric oxide synthase (NOS) isotypes that include neuronal NOS (nNOS), inducible NOS (iNOS), and endothelial NOS (eNOS) (Kang et al., 2004). Neuronal NOS mRNA was detected in four of nine human neuroblastoma cell lines (Fujisawa et al., 1994). A shorter mRNA was also detected (Fujisawa et al., 1994). Nitric oxide binds to the heme moiety of soluble guanylate cyclase, activating the enzyme and thereby stimulating the conversion of GMP to cGMP. At low levels, NO protects cells from apoptosis that is induced by growth factor deprivation, whereas stimulation of NMDA receptors by glutamate yields high levels of NO by activating nNOS via calcium/calmodulin, which leads to neuronal apoptosis (Kang et al., 2004; Denny, 2006). NO prevents the serum deprivation-induced apoptosis of SH-SY5Y cells by increasing the expression of cytoprotective genes such as thioredoxin (Andoh et al., 2002) and thioredoxin peroxidase, and cGMP may play a role in this increase in gene expression (Kang et al., 2004).

By contrast, nitric oxide induced apoptosis in SH-SY5Y cells (Moriya, et al., 2000). NO caused the cleavage of the short peptides DEVD-AFC, VDVAD-AFC, and LEHD-AFC, which are substrates for caspases -3, and -7, caspase-2, and caspase-9, respectively (Moriya et al., 2000). Each substrate contains one or two aspartic acid residues. The pro forms of caspases -2, -3, -6, and -7 decreased during apoptosis (Moriya et al., 2000). There was a subsequent loss of mitochondrial membrane potential (Moriya et al., 2000). Paclitaxel also induced the apoptosis of SH-SY5Y cells, an effect that was inhibited by *trans*-resveratrol (Nicolini et al., 2001).

5. Chemotherapy

The previous information presented in this chapter will now be applied to chemotherapeutic agents that have been used in the treatment of neuroblastoma. Twelve drugs are currently indicated for the treatment of neuroblastoma: carboplatin, cisplatin, cyclophosphamide, dacarbazine, doxorubicin, etoposide, fenretinide, iobenguane, isotretinoin, melphalan, teniposide, and vincristine. Only three of these, cyclophosphamide, doxorubicin, and vincristine, are FDA-approved for this use at present. The remaining nine drugs are being used experimentally in neuroblastoma therapy, as are bleomycin, bortezomib, and dexamethosone. Iobenguane is currently FDA-approved only for imaging purposes.

5.1 Alkylating agents

The alkylating agents cyclophosphamide (Cytoxan), melphalan (Alkeran), and BCNU (bis-chloroethylnitrosourea), also called Carmustine, have two alkyl chloride groups capable of reacting with the nucleophilic nitrogen atom at position seven of guanine, yielding crosslinking of adjacent DNA strands. Dacarbazine is also thought to act as an alkylating agent. These reactions cause DNA strand scission, which blocks replication and transcription and results in cell death. All of these agents have shown activity against neuroblastoma. Chlorambucil is an alkylating agent with a structure similar to melphalan but is mainly used to treat CLL. BCNU inhibited the growth of the SK-N-MC neuroblastoma (Giorgi et al., 2001). Melphalan is used for stem cell transplant preparation in neuroblastoma. High dose melphalan, with stem cell support, has been used in the treatment of advanced neuroblastoma (Pritchard et al., 2005). It consolidates the response to induction chemotherapy (Pritchard et al., 2005). The melphalan prodrug J1 (L-melphalanyl-p-L-fluorophenylalanine ethyl ester) displayed high cytotoxic activity *in vitro* against seven neuroblastoma cell lines, with IC50 values in the submicromolar range (Wickstrom et al., 2007). J1 induced caspase-3 cleavage and apoptotic morphology, had additive effects with doxorubicin, cyclophosphamide, carboplatin, and vincristine, and killed otherwise drug-resistant cells when combined with etoposide (Wickstrom et al., 2007). Also susceptible to J1 were athymic rats and mice carrying neuroblastoma xenografts containing SH-SY5Y and SK-N-BE(2) cells (Wickstrom et al., 2007).

Of all the alkylating agents, cyclophosphamide stands at the forefront of therapy in neuroblastoma. The most commonly used induction chemotherapy regimen includes dose-intensive cycles of cisplatin and etoposide alternating with vincristine, doxorubicin, and cyclophosphamide (Kushner, et al., 1994).

5.2 Doxorubicin

Doxorubicin is also called Adriamycin, and the liposomal form is called Doxil. Doxorubicin, but not Doxil, is FDA-approved for the treatment of neuroblastoma. Doxorubicin intercalates between the bases of DNA, changing its geometry and causing a cytotoxic effect. Doxorubicin also produces cytotoxicity by interacting with topoisomerase II. Doxorubicin-induced death in stromal or S-type cells in neuroblastoma does not involve death receptors such as Fas and is caspase-independent in N-type cells (Hopkins-Donaldson et al., 2002). Doxorubicin was applied to the caspase-8 silenced N-type invasive neuroblastoma cells lines LAN-1 and IMR-32 and to the S-type noninvasive SH-EP neuroblastoma cells expressing caspase-8 (Hopkins-Donaldson et al., 2002). Doxorubicin induced caspase-3, -7, -8, and –9 and Bid cleavage in S-type cells and death was blocked by caspase inhibitors. Doxorubicin-treated S-type cells showed apoptotic nuclei while N-type cells did not (Hopkins-Donaldson et al., 2002). Both doxorubicin and cisplatin were found to activate caspase-9 and caspase-3 but not caspase-8 in S-type cells (Bian et al., 2004). The central effect of caspase-9 was augmented by the expression of CD95/Fas (Bian et al., 2004).

5.3 Fenretinide

Fenretinide (4-hydroxy(phenyl)retinamide) is a synthetic retinoid that is used in the treatment of neuroblastoma. It may cause the accumulation of a ceramide and reactive oxygen species in tumor cells, causing cell death *via* apoptosis (Wu et al., 2001).

5.4 Isotretinoin

Isotretinoin is a retinoid, which resembles vitamin A and is a mediator of cell proliferation and apoptosis. The retinoid receptors are part of the steroid-thyroid superfamily of nuclear receptors called retinoid X receptors (RXRs) and retinoic acid receptors (RARs) (Denny, 2006). Isotretinoin acts mainly on RARs. Isotretinoin is part of the standard therapy during the first remission in patients with high-risk neuroblastoma (Maris, 2010).

5.5 Iobenguane

Iobenguane (metaiodobenzylguanidine, MIBG) containing radioactive iodine (^{131}I) is currently being used experimentally to destroy tumor cells in relapsed or high-risk neuroblastoma (Howard et al., 2005). K. Matthay has used this compound along with vorinostat to incrase its effectiveness in neuroblastoma. Vorinostat is a histone deacetylase inhibitor that sensitizes neuroblastoma to radiation. ^{131}I is primarily a beta emitter but about 10% of its radiation output is gamma radiation. Iobenguane iodinated with ^{123}I or ^{131}I has been used in imaging. ^{123}I is a gamma emitter, but at the energy primarily used for imaging, rather than for the destruction of cells. Iobenguane resembles norepinephrine and is therefore concentrated in adrenergic tissue. This allows for the diagnosis and therapy of both neuroblastoma and pheochromocytoma.

5.6 Carboplatin, Cisplatin, Bleomycin, Etoposide, and Vincristine

Cisplatin (CDDP; *cis*-diamminedichloroplatinum (II)) interacts electrostatically with the same nucleophilic nitrogen atom in guanine that reacts with the alkylating agents. As with alkylating agents, this generates DNA crosslinks. Cisplatin also binds to nitrogen at the seven position in adenine. Increased DNA repair overcomes the effect of cisplatin, generating resistance. The chlorine atoms are replaced by the 1,1-cyclobutanedicarboxylato ligand in carboplatin. Bleomycin acts by forming a complex with DNA. If this cytotoxic action is repaired, the anti-cancer effect of the drug is blocked and resistance occurs. Etoposide binds to a complex of DNA and topoisomerase II, which is cytotoxic. Teniposide functions similarly to etoposide Bleomycin was used in conjunction with etoposide and cisplatin in the treatment of adult neuroblastoma arising from the broad ligament of the uterus (Milam et al., 2007). The patient died 20 months after diagnosis (Milam et al., 2007). Cisplatin, vinblastine, and bleomycin (CVB) have been used in the treatment of relapsed, disseminated neuroblastoma (Bostrom et al., 1984).

5.7 Bortezomib

Bortezomib (Velcade) is an effective inhibitor of neuroblastoma cell growth and angiogenesis (Combaret et al., 2008). The drug is used in the treatment of multiple myeloma (Combaret et al., 2008). Bortezomib inhibits the action of the 26S proteasome, which is a large protease complex located in the cytosol and nucleus. The action of the 20S proteasome on GAP-43 was studied *in vitro* (Denny, 2004). If the proteasome degradation of the proteins p21cip, p27kip, and cyclins is inhibited, the cells are sensitized to apoptosis (Martelli et al., 2010). An advantage for bortezomib is that cancer cells are much more sensitive to proteasome inhibition than are normal cells. This is in contrast to alkylating agents, which have considerable cytotoxic effects on both normal and cancer cells, causing hair loss due to the action of the drugs on normal cells in the hair follicles. Carfilzomib is a second generation proteasome inhibitor for the treatment of multiple myeloma.

Bortezomib inhibits the activation of NF-KB by stabilizing its inhibitor protein IKB. Activation of NF-KB results in the production of VEGF, which promotes angiogenesis, interleukin-6, VCAM-1 (vascular cell adhesion molecule-1), and anti-apoptotic factors such as Bcl-2. VCAM-1 is also called CD106. It causes the adherence of malignant plasma cells to bone marrow stromal tissue in multiple myeloma. Bortezomib links the death receptor to the mitochondrial pathway in neuroblastoma cells, which leads to TRAIL-induced apoptosis (Naumann et al., 2011). Bortezomib enhances the TRAIL-induced cleavage of Bid into tBid, accumulation of tBid in the cytosol, and insertion of tBid into the mitochondrial membrane (Naumann et al., 2011). Bortezomib stabilizes tBid, promoting apoptosis (Naumann et al.,

2011). Our results with staurosporine and N1E-115 cells are consistent with the proposed mechanism of action of bortezomib. If the proteasomal degradation of IKB is blocked by bortezomib, IKB is present to block NF-KB and less Bcl-2 is produced, leading to an increased susceptibility of the cancer cells to apoptosis.

5.8 PI-103

PI3K is inhibited by Wortmannin and LY294002, and mTOR is inhibited by rapamycin, but it has been found that inhibiting PI3K and mTOR at the same time with the drug PI-103 is more effective in the treatment of T-cell acute lymphoblastic leukemia (T-ALL) than is the inhibition of PI3K and mTOR separately (Chiarini et al., 2009). PI-103 induced the apoptosis of T-ALL cells that was characterized by the activation of caspase-3 and caspase-9 (Chiarini et al., 2009). A similar approach may be fruitful in neuroblastoma.

5.9 Treatment with glucocorticoids

Although the glucocorticoids betamethasone, dexamethasone, prednisolone, and prednisone inhibit tumor cell growth and are used in the treatment of many cancers, they are presently not indicated in the treatment of neuroblastoma. However, consistent with its anti-cancer effect, dexamethasone has been found to block the migration of the human neuroblastoma cell line SK-N-SH (Casulari et al., 2006). A study sponsored by the Children's Oncology Group and the National Cancer Institute (NCI), with ClinicalTrials.gov identifier NCT00033293 and entitled "Cyclophosphamide and prednisone with or without immunoglobulin in treating abnormal muscle movement in children with neuroblastoma", is recruiting participants in 2011.

6. Concluding remarks

New treatment modalities are needed for neuroblastoma, which continues to have an overall cure rate of only 40%. Promising approaches include those involving immunotherapy, with antibodies directed toward the GD-2 antigen. The use of interferons, used currently in other cancers, also shows promise, with their inherent stimulation of the tumoricidal effects of NK cells and activated macrophages. The combination of immunotherapy and conventional chemotherapy and radiotherapy utilizing iobenguane and radioactive iodine appear to be useful approaches. The use of isotretinoin and fenretinide, as well as bortezomib and lenalidomide, may be helpful in this disease. The inhibition of the protein kinases Akt, mTOR, and ALK, which lie at the center of the abnormalities of the neuroblastoma cell, may prove very fruitful. Promotion of the effect of PTEN, which counters the effect of Akt, is also a useful approach. It is clearly important to initiate the apoptosis of neuroblastoma cells. The use of existing neuroblastoma cell lines and the cloning of new cell lines will continue to be a very useful research technique for the development of new therapies. Many new treatment options now exist and will be forthcoming for a very serious disease that affects such a young population.

7. Acknowledgments

This work was supported by a grant from the San Antonio Area Foundation and by an unrestricted grant to the Department of Ophthalmology from Research to Prevent Blindness (RPB), New York, NY.

8. References

Adams, J.M., and Cory, S. (1998) The Bcl-2 protein family: Arbiters of cell survival. *Science* 281(5381):1322-1326.

Amano, T., Richelson, E., and Nirenberg, M. (1972) Neurotransmitter synthesis by neuroblastoma clones. *Proc. Natl. Acad. Sci. USA* 69(1):258-263.

Andoh, T., Chock, O.B., and Chiueh, C.C. (2002) The roles of thioredoxin in protection against oxidative stress-induced apoptosis in SH-SY5Y cells. *J. Biol. Chem.* 277(12): 9655-9660.

Ara, T., Song, L., Shimada, H., Keshelava, N., Russell, H.V., Metelitsa, L.S., Groshen, S.G.Seeger, R., and DeClerck, Y.A. (2009) Interleukin-6 in the bone marrow microenvironment promotes the growth and survival of neuroblastoma cells. *Cancer Res.* 69:329-337.

Armstrong, M.B., Bian, X., Liu, Y., Subramanian, C., Ratanaproeska, A.B., Shao, F., Yu, V.C., Kwok, R.P.S., Opipare, Jr., A.W., Castle, V.P. (2006) Signaling from p53 to NF-kB determines the chemotherapy responsiveness of neuroblastoma. *Neoplasia* 8(1): 967-977.

Baker, L.P., and Storm, D.R. (1997) Dynamic palmitoylation of neuromodulin (GAP-43) in cultured rat cerebellar neurons and mouse N1E-115 cells. *Neurosci. Lett.* 234(2-3): 156-160.

Beppu, K., Jaboine, J., Marchant, M.S., Marshal, C.S., and Thiele, C.S. (2003) Effect of imatinib mesylate on neuroblastoma tumorigenesis and vascular endothelial growth factor expression. J. Natl. *Cancer Insti.*86(1):46-55.

Bian, X., Giordano, T.D., Lin, H.J., Solomon, G., Castle, V.P., and Opipari, A.W., Jr. (2004) Chemotherapy-induced apoptosis of S-type neuroblastoma cells requires caspase-9 and is augmented by CD95/Fas stimulation. *J. Biol. Chem.* 279(6): 4663-4669.

Bostrom, B., Woods, W.G., Ramsay, N.K., Krivit, W., Levine, P., and Nesbit, M.E., Jr. (1984) Cisplatin, vinblastine, and bleomycin (CVB) therapy for relapsed disseminated neuroblastoma. *Cancer Treat. Rep.* 68(9):1157-1158.

Bottenstein, J.E., and Sato, G.H. (1979) Growth of a rat neuroblastoma cell line in serum-free supplemented medium. *Proc. Natl. Acad. Sci. USA* 76(1):514-517.

Bowman, L., Grossmann, M., Rill, D., Brown, M., Zhong, W.Y., Alexander, B., Leimig, T., Coustan-Smith, E., Campana, D., Jenkins, J., Woods, D., Kitchingman, G., Vanin, E., and Brenner, M. (1998) IL-2 adenovector-transduced autologous tumor cells induce antitumor immune responses in patients with neuroblastoma. *Blood* 92(6):1941-1949.

Boyadjieva, N.I., Chaturvedi, K., Poplawski, M.M., and Sarkar, D.K. (2004) Opioid antagonist naltrexone disrupts feedback interaction between μ and δ opioid receptors in splenocytes to prevent alcohol inhibition of NK cell function. *J. Immunol.* 173: 42-49.

Bray, I., Tivnan, A., Bryan, K., Foley, N.H., Watters, K.M., Tracey, L., Davidoff, A.M., and Stallings, R.L. (2011) MicroRNA-542-5p as a novel tumor suppressor in neuroblastoma. *Cancer Lett.* 303(1): 56-64.

Carlsen, N.L. (1990) How frequent is spontaneous remission of neuroblastoma? Implications for screening. *Br. J. Cancer* 61:441-446.

Carnero, A., Blanco-Aparicio, C., Renner, O., Link, W., and Leal, J.F. (2008) The PTEN/PI3K/AKT signalling pathway in cancer therapeutic implications. *Curr. Cancer Drug Targets* 8: 187-198.

Casulari, L.A., Dondi, D., Maggi, R., Demissie, M., Piccolella, M., and Piva, F. (2006) Dexamethasone blocks the migration of the human neuroblastoma cell line SK-N-SH. *Braz. J. Med. Biol. Res.* 39(9): 1233-1240.

Chadborn, N.H., Ahmed, A.I., Holt, M.R., Prinjha, R., Dunn, G.A., Jones, G.E., and Eickholt, B.J. (2006) PTEN couples Sema3A signalling to growth cone collapse. *J. Cell Sci.* 119: 951-957.

Chakrabandhu, K., Herincs,, Z., Huault, S., Dost, B., Peng, L., Conchonaud, F., Marguet, D., He, H.-T., and Hueber, A.-O. (2007) Palmitoylation is required for efficient Fas cell death signaling. *EMBO J.* 26: 209-220.

Chambers, A.F., Denhardt, G.H., and Wilson, S.M. (1990) Ras-transformed NIH 3T3 cell lines, selected for metastatic ability in chick embryos, have increased proportions of p21-expressing cells and are metastatic in nude mice. *Invasion Metastasis* 10(4): 225-240.

Cheung, N.K., Kushner, B.H., Yeh, S.D., and Larson, S.M. (1998) 3F8 monoclonal antibody treatment of patients with stage 4 neuroblastoma: a phase II study. *Int. J. Oncol.* 12(6):1299-1306.

Chiarini, F., Fala, F., Tazzari, P.L., Ricci, F., Astolfi, A., Pession, A., Pagliaro, P., McCubrey, J.A., and Martelli, A.M. (2009) Dual inhibition of class IA phosphatidylinositol 3-kinase and mammalian target of rapamycin as a new therapeutic option for T-cell acute lymphoblastic leukemia. *Cancer Res.* 69(8): 3520-3528.

Combaret, V., Boyault, S., Iacono, I., Brejon, S., Rousseau, R., and Puisieux, A. (2008) Effect of bortezomib on human neuroblastoma: analysis of molecular mechanisms involved in cytotoxicity. *Mol. Cancer* 7: 50-61.

Coulter, D.W., Blatt, J., D'Ercole, A.J., and Moats-Staats, B.M. (2008) IGF-1 receptor inhibition combined with rapamycin or temsirolimus inhibits neuroblastoma cell growth. *Anticancer Res.* 28: 1509-1516.

Dahmer, M.K. (2005) Caspases-2, -3, and –7 are involved in thapsigargin-induced apoptosis of SH-SY5Y neuroblastoma cells. *J. Neurosci. Res.* 80: 576-583.

De LaurenziV., Raschella, G., Barcaroli, D., Annicchiarico-Petrazzelli, M., Ranalli, M., Catani, M.V.Tanno, B., Constanzo, A., Levrero, M., and Melino, G. (2000) Induction of neuronal differentiation by p73 in a neuroblastoma cell line. *J Biol. Chem.* 275(20): 15226-15231.

Dedoni, S., Olianas, M.C., and Onali, P. (2010) Interferon-β induces apoptosis in human SH-SY5Y neuroblastoma cells through activation of JAK-STAT signaling and down-regulation of PI3K/Akt pathway. *J. Neurochem.* 115(6): 1421-1433.

Denny, J.B. (2004) Growth-associated protein of 43 kDa (GAP-43) is cleaved nonprocessively by the 20S proteasome. *Eur. J. Biochem.* 271: 2480-2493.

Denny, J.B. (2006) Molecular mechanisms, biological actions, and neuropharmacology of the growth-associated protein GAP-43. *Curr. Neuropharm.* 4: 293-304.

Denny, J.B. (2008) Protein palmitoylation in neuronal growth and plasticity. *Curr. Top. Peptide & Protein Res.* 9: 57-69.

Denny, J.B., Polan-Curtain, J., Wayner, M.J., and Armstrong, D.L. (1991) Angiotensin II blocks hippocampal long-term potentiation. *Brain Res.* 567: 321-324.

Dredge, K., Horsfall, R., Robinson, S.P., Zhang, L.H., Lu, L., Tang, Y., Shirley, M.A., Muller, G., Schafer, P., Stirling, D., Dalgleish, A.G., and Bartlett, J.B. (2005) Orally administered lenalidomide (CC-5013) is anti-angiogenic in vivo and inhibits endothelial cell migration and Akt phosphorylation in vitro. *Microvasc. Res.* 69: 56-63.

Fujisawa, H., Ogura, T., Kurashima, Y., Yokoyama, T., Yamashita, J., and Esumi, H. (1994) Expression of two types of nitric oxide synthase mRNA in human neuroblastoma cell lines. *J. Neurochem.* 63(1):140-145.

Fulda, S. (2009) The PI3K/Akt/mTOR pathway as therapeutic target in neuroblastoma. *Curr Cancer Drug Targets* 9: 729-737.

Garcia-Lora, A., Algarra, I., Collado, A., and Garrido, F. (2003) Tumor immunology, vaccination and escape strategies. *Eur. J. Immunogenet.* 30:177-183.

Giorgi, M., Leonetti, C., Citro, G., and Augusti-Tocco, G. (2001) In vitro and in vivo inhibition of SK-N-MC neuroblastoma growth using cyclic nucleotide phosphodiesterase inhibitors. *J. Neuro-Oncol.* 51(1):25-31.

Goillot, E., Combaret, V., Landenstein, R., Baubet, D., Blay, J-Y., Thierry, P. and Favrot, M.C. (1992) Tumor necrosis factor functions as an autocrine growth factor for neuroblastomas. *Cancer Res.* 52:3194-3200.

Gutierrez, L., and Magee, A.I. (1991) Characterization of an acyltransferase acting on $p21^{N\text{-}ras}$ protein in a cell-free system. *Biochim. Biophys. Acta* 1078: 147-154.

Hero, B., Simon, T., Spitz, R., Ernestus, K., Gnekow, A.K., Scheel-Walter, H.-G., Schwabe, D., Schilling, F.H., Benz-Bohm, G., and Berthold, F. (2008) Localized infant neuroblastomas often show spontaneous regression: results of the prospective trials NB95-S and NB97. *J. Clin. Oncol.* 26(9): 1504-1510.

Holzel, M., Huang, S., Koster, J., Ora, I., Lakeman, A., Caron, H., Nijkamp, W., Xie, J., Callens, T., Asgharzadeh, S., Seeger, R.C., Messiaen, L., Versteeg, R., and Bernards, R. (2010) NF1 is a tumor suppressor in neuroblastoma that determines retinoic acid response and disease outcome. *Cell* 142(2): 218-229.

Hopkins-Donaldson, S., Yan, P., Bourloud, K.B., Muhlethaler, A., Bodmer, J.L., and Gross, N. (2002) Doxorubicin-induced death in neuroblastoma does not involve death receptors in S-type cells and is caspase-independent in N-type cells. *Oncogene* 21(39): 6132-6137.

Howard, J.P., Maris, J.M., Kersun, L.S., Huberty, J.P., Cheng, S-C., Hawkins, R.A., and Matthay, K.K. (2005) Tumor response and toxicity with multiple infusions of high dose ^{131}I-MIBG in refractory neuroblastoma. *Ped. Blood & Cancer 44(3):232-239.*

Jaboin, J., Kim, C.J., Kaplan, D.R., and Thiele, C.J. (2002) Brain-derived neurotrophic factor activation of TrkB protects neuroblastoma cells from chemotherapy-induced apoptosis via phosphatidylinositol 3'-kinase pathway. *Cancer Res.* 62: 6756-6763.

Jimenez-Andrade, J.M., Bloom, A.P., Stake, J.I., Mantyh, W. G., Taylor, R.N., Greeman, K.T., Ghilardi, J.R., Kuskowski, M.A., and Mantyh, P.W. (2010) Pathological sprouting of adult nociceptors in chronic prostate cancer-induced bone pain. *J. Neurosci* 30(44):14649-14656.

Kang. Y.-C., Kim, P.K., Choi, B.-M., Chung, H.-T., Ha, K.-S., Kwon, Y.-G., and Kim, Y.-M. (2004) Regulation of programmed cell death in neuronal cells by nitric oxide. *In Vivo* 18: 367-376.

Kapoor, A., and Figlin, R.A. (2009) Targeted inhibition of mammalian target of rapamycin for the treatment of advanced renal cell carcinoma. *Cancer* 115(16): 3618-3630.

Kasahara, K., Nakayama, Y., Kihara, A., Matsuda, D., Ikeda, K., Kuga, T., Fukumoto, Y., Igarashi, Y., and Yamaguchi, N. (2007) Rapid trafficking of c-Src, a non-palmitoylated Src-family kinase, between the plasma membrane and late endosomes/lysosomes. *Exp. Cell Res.* 313(12): 2651-2666.

Kilic, M., Schafer, R., Hoppe, J., and Kagerhuber, U. (2002) Formation of noncanonical high molecular weight caspase-3 and -6 complexes and activation of caspase-12 during serum starvation induced apoptosis in AKR-2B mouse fibroblasts. *Cell Death & Diff.* 9(2):125-137.

Kimmelman, A.C., Nunez Rodriguez, N., and Chan, A.M. (2002) R-Ras3/M-Ras induces neuronal differentiation of PC12 cells through cell-type-specific activation of the mitogen-activated protein kinase cascade. *Mol. Cell Biol.* 22(16):5946-5961.

Kischkel, F.C., Hellbardt, S., Behrmann, I., Germer, M., Pawlita, M., Krammer, P.H., and Peter, M.E. (1995) Cytotoxicity-dependent APO-1 (Fas/CD95)-associated proteins form a death-inducing signaling complex (DISC) with the receptor. *EMBO J.* 14: 5579-5588.

Kitanaka, C., Kato, K., Ijiri, R., Sakurada, K., Tomiyama, A., Noguchi, K., Nagashima, Y., Nakagawara, A., Momoi, T., Toyoda, Y., Kigasawa, H., Nishi, T., Shirouzu, M., Yokoyama, S., Tanaka, Y., and Kuchino, Y. (2002) Increased Ras expression and caspase-independent neuroblastoma cell death: possible mechanism of spontaneous neuroblastoma regression. *J. Natl. Cancer Inst.* 94(5): 358-368.

Koegl, M., Zlatkine, P., Ley, S.C., Courtneidge, S.A., and Magee, A.I. (1994) Palmitoylation of multiple Src-family kinases at a homologous N-terminal motif. *Biochem. J.* 303: 749-753.

Kushner, B.H., LaQuaglia, M.P., Bonilla, M.A., Lindsley, K., Rosenfield, N., Yeh, S., Eddy, J., Gerald, W.L., Heller, G., and Cheung, N.-K.V. (1994) Highly effective induction therapy for stage 4 neuroblastoma in children over 1 year of age. *J. Clin. Oncol.* 12(12):2607-2613.

Laifenfeld, D., Klein, E., and Ben-Shachar, D. (2002) Norepinephrine alters the expression of genes involved in neuronal sprouting and differentiation: relevance for major depression and antidepressant mechanisms. *J. Neurochem.* 83: 1054-1064.

Lalli, G., and Hall, A. (2005) Ral GTPases regulate neurite branching through GAP-43 and the exocyst complex. *J. Cell Biol.* 171(5):857-869.

Li, Z., and Thiele, C.J. (2007) Targeting Akt to increase the sensitivity of neuroblastoma to chemotherapy: lessons learned from the brain-derived neurotrophic factor/TrkB signal transduction pathway. *Expert Opin. Ther. Targets* 11: 1611-1621.

Lieven, C.J., Millet, L.E., Hoegger, M.J., and Levin, L.A. (2007) Induction of axon and dendrite formation during early RGC-5 cell differentiation. *Exp. Eye Res.* 85(5):678-683.

Liu, H., Ng, C.E.L., and Tang, B.L. (2002) Nogo-A expression in mouse central nervous system neurons. *Neurosci. Lett.* 328(3):257-260.

Ma, L., Cao, T.T., Kandpal, G., Warren, L., Fred Hess, J., Seabrook, G.R. and Ray, W.J. (2010) Genome-wide microarray analysis of the differential neuroprotective effects of antioxidants in neuroblastoma cells overexpressing the familial Parkinson's disease alpha-synuclein A53T mutation. *Neurochem Res.* 35(1): 130-142.

Margaritora, S., Cesario, A., Porziella, V., Granone, P., Catassi, A., and Russo, P. (2005) Farnesyltransferase inhibitors: overview of their action and role in solid malignancy therapy. *Lett. Drug Design & Discov.* 2:26-35.

Maris, J.M. (2010) Recent advances in neuroblastoma. *N. Engl. J. Med.* 362 (23): 2202-2211.

Maris, J.M., Mosse, Y.P., Bradfield, J.P., Hou, C., Monni, S., Scott, R.H., Asgharzadeh, S., Attiyeh, E.F., Diskin, S.J., Laudenslager, M., Winter, C., Cole, K.A., Glessner, J.T., Kim, C., Frackelton, E.C., Casalunovo, T., Eckert, A.W., Capasso, M., Rappaport, E.F., McConville, C., London, W.B., Seeger, R.C., Rahman, N., Devoto, M., Grant, S.F.A., Li, H. and Hakonarson, H.(2008) Chromosome 6p22 locus associated with clinically aggressive neuroblastoma. *N. Engl. J. Med.* 358: 2585-2593.

Martelli, A.M., Evangelisti, C., Chiarini, F., and McCubrey, J.A. (2010) The phosphatidylinositol 3-kinase/Akt/mTOR signaling network as a therapeutic target in acute myelogenous leukemia patients. *Oncotarget.* 1(2):89-103.

McCombe, P. and Kidson, C. (1975) A repressible DNA-repair system in mouse neuroblastoma cells. *Basic Life Sci.* 5B: 813-815.

Milam, M.R., Gabel, S.F., Milam, R.A., Liu, J., and Ramirez, P.T. (2007) Neoadjuvant bleomycin, etoposide, and cisplatin in adult neuroblastoma arising from the broad ligament of the uterus. *Gynecol. Oncol.* 107(2): 350-354.

Moriya, R., Uehara, T., and Nomura, Y. (2000) Mechanism of nitric oxide-induced apoptosis in human neuroblastoma SH-SY5Y cells. *FEBS Lett.* 484(3): 253-260.

Mosse, Y.P., Laudenslager, M., Longo, L., Cole, K.A., Wood, A., Attiyeh, E.F., Laquaglia, M.J., Sennett, R., Lynch, J.E., Perri, P., Laureys, G., Speleman, F., Kim, C., Hou, C., Hakonarson, H., Torkamani, A., Schork, N.J., Brodeur, G.M., Tonini, G.P., Rappaport, E., Devoto, M., and Maris, J.M. (2008) Identification of ALK as a major familial neuroblastoma predisposition gene. *Nature* 455 (7215):930-935.

Mosse, Y.P., Wood, A., and Maris, J.M. (2009) Inhibition of ALK signaling for cancer therapy. *Clin. Cancer Res.* 15 (18): 5609-5614.

Munoz, J., Lazcoz, P., Inda, M.M., Nistal., M., Pestana, A., Encio, I.J., and Castresana, J.S. (2004) Homozygous deletion and expression of PTEN and DMBT1 in human primary neuroblastoma and cell lines. *Int. J. Cancer* 109:673-679.

Nakazawa, T., Tamai, M., and Mori, N. (2002) Brain-derived neurotrophic factor prevents axotomized retinal ganglion cell death through MAPK and PI3K pathways. *Invest Ophthalmol. Vis. Sci.*43(10):3319-3326.

Naumann, I., Kappler, R., von Schweinitz, D., Debatin, K.-M., and Fulda, S. (2011) Bortezomib primes neuroblastoma cells for TRAIL-induced apoptosis by linking the death receptor to the mitochondrial pathway. *Clin. Cancer Res.* 17(10): 3204-3218.

Navid, F., Santana, V.M., and Barfield, R.C. (2010) Anti-GD2 antibody therapy for GD2-expressing tumors. *Curr. Cancer Drug Targets* 10(2):200-209.

Nicolini, G., Rigolio, R., Miloso, M., Bertelli, A.A.E., and Tredici, G. (2001) Anti-apoptotic effect of *trans*-resveratrol on paclitaxel-induced apoptosis in the human neuroblastoma SH-SY5Y cell line. *Neurosci. Lett.* 302 (1): 41-44.

Niizuma, H., Nakamura, Y., Ozaki, T., Nakanishi, H., Ohira, M., Isogai, E., Kageyama, H., Imaizumi, M., and Nakagawara, A. (2006) Bcl-2 is a key regulator for the retinoic acid-induced apoptotic cell death in neuroblastoma. *Oncogene* 25: 5046-5055.

Ogbomo, H., Hahn, A., Geiler, J., Michaelis, M., Doerr, H.W., and Cinatl, J.Jr. (2006) NK sensitivity of neuroblastoma cells determined by a highly sensitive coupled luminescent method. *Biochem. Biophys. Res. Commun.* 339: 375-379.

Oh, J.-E., Karlmark, K.R., Shin, J.-H., Pollak, A., Freilinger, A., Hengstschlager, M., and Lubec, G. (2005) Differentiation of neuroblastoma cell line N1E-115 involves several signaling cascades. *Neurochem. Res.* 30(3):333-348.

Oh, J.-E., Karlmark, K.R., Shin, J.-H., Pollak, A., Hengstschlager, M., and Lubec, G. (2006) Cytoskeleton changes following differentiation of N1E-115 neuroblastoma cell line. *Amino Acids* 31(3):289-293.

Ollom, C.M., and Denny. J.B. (2008) A crosslinking analysis of GAP-43 interactions with other proteins in differentiated N1E-115 cells. *Int. J. Mol. Sci.* 9: 1753-1771.

Omer, C.A., Anthony, N.J., Buser-Doepner, C.A., Burkhardt, A.L., deSolms, S.J., Dinsmore, C.J., Gibbs, J.B., Hartman, G.D., Koblan, K.S., Lobell, R.B., Oliff, A., Williams, T.M., and Kohl, N.E. (1997) Farnesyl:proteintransferase inhibitors as agents to inhibit tumor growth. *Biofactors* 6(3):359-366.

Pappolla, M.A., Sos, M., Omar, R.A., Bick, R.J., Hickson-Bick, D.L.M., Reiter, R.J., Efthimiopoulos, and Robakis, N.K. (1997) Melatonin prevents death of neuroblastoma cells exposed to the Alzheimer amyloid peptide. *J. Neurosci.* 17(5): 1683-1690.

Peterson, T.R., Laplante, M., Thoreen, C.C., Sancak, Y., Kang, S.A., Kuehl, W.M., Gray, N.S., and Sabatini, D.M. (2009) DEPTOR is an mTOR inhibitor frequently overexpressed in multiple myeloma cells and required for their survival. *Cell* 137: 873-886.

Petroni, M., Veschi, V., Prodosmo, A., Rinaldo, C., Massimi, I., Carbonari, M., Dominici, C., McDowell, H.P., Rinaldi, C., Screpanti, I., Frati, L., Bartolazzi, A., Gulino, A., Soddu, S., and Giannini, G. (2011) MYCN sensitizes human neuroblastoma to apoptosis by HIPK2 activation through a DNA damage response. *Mol. Cancer Res.* 9(1): 67-77.

Philips, M.R., and Cox, A.D. (2007) Geranylgeranyltransferase I as a target for anti-cancer drugs. *J. Clin. Invest.* 117(5):1223-1225.

Plantaz, D., Mohapatra, G., Matthay, K.K., Pellarin, M., Seeger, R.C., and Feurerstein, B.G. (1997) Gain of chromosome 17 is the most common abnormality detected in neuroblastoma by comparative genomic hybridization. *Am. J. Pathol.*150(1):81-89.

Prince, J.A., and Oreland, L. (1997) Staurosporine differentiated human SH-SY5Y neuroblastoma cultures exhibit transient apoptosis and trophic factor independence. *Brain Res. Bull.* 43(6):515-523.

Pritchard, J., Cotterill, S.J., Germond, S.M., Imeson, J., de Kraker, J., and Jones, D.R. (2005) High dose melphalan in the treatment of advanced neuroblastoma: results of a randomised trial (ENSG-1) by the European Neuroblastoma Study Group. *Pediatr. Blood Cancer* 44(4):348-357.

Reagan, L.P., Ye, X.R., Mir, R., DePalo, L.R., and Fluharty, S.J. (1990) Up-regulation of angiotensin II receptors by in vitro differentiation of murine N1E-115 neuroblastoma cells. *Mol. Pharmacol.* 38(6): 878-886.

Reid, G.S.D., Shan, X., Coughlin, C.M., Lassoued, W., Pawel, B.R., Wexler, L.H., Thiele, C.J., Tsokos, M., Pinkus, J.L., Pinkus, G.S., Grupp, S.A., and Vonderheide, R.H. (2009) Interferon-γ-dependent infiltration of human T cells into neuroblastoma tumors *in vivo*. *Clin. Cancer Res.* 15(21):6602-6608.

Ribatti, D., Marimpietri, D., Pastorino, F., Brignole, C., Nico, B., Vacca, A., and Ponzoni, M. (2004) Angiogenesis in neuroblastoma. *Ann. N.Y. Acad. Sci.* 1028:133-142.

Sarbassov, D.D., Ali, S.M., and Sabatini, D.M. (2005) Growing roles for the mTOR pathway. *Curr. Opin. Cell Biol.* 17: 596-603.

Sartelet, H., Oligny, L.L., and Vassal, G. (2008) AKT pathway in neuroblastoma and its therapeutic implication. *Expert Rev. Anticancer Ther.* 8(5): 757-769.

Song,, L., Ara, T., Saio, J., Deng, Z-b., Asgharzdeh, S., Ji, L., Sposto, R., DeClerck, Y.A., Seeger, R.C. and Metelitsa, L.S. (2007) The role of paracrine IL-6 and IL-10 in neuroblastoma progression. *J. Immunol.* 178:49.9.

Steelman, L.S., Abrams, S.L., Whelan, J., Bertrand, F.E., Ludwig, D.E., Basecke, J., Libra, M., Stivala, F., Milella, M., Tafuri, A., Lunghi, P., Bonati, A., Martelli, A.M., and McCubrey, J.A. (2008) Contributions of the Raf/MEK/ERK, PI3K/PTEN/Akt/mTOR and Jak/STAT pathways to leukemia. *Leukemia* 22:686-707.

Steelman, L.S., Pohnert, S.C., Shelton, J.G., Franklin, R.A., Bertrand, F.E., and McCubrey, A. (2004) JAK/STAT, Raf/MEK/ERK, PI3K/Akt and BCR-ABL in cell cycle progression and leukemogenesis. *Leukemia* 18:189-218.

Streck, C.J., Zhang, Y., Miyamoto, R., Zhou, J., Ng, C.Y., Nathwani, A.C., and Davidoff, A.M. (2004) Restriction of neuroblastoma angiogenesis and growth by interferon-alpha/beta. *Surgery* 136(2):183-189.

Takeda, M., Kobayashi, M., Osaki, T., Shirato, I., and Endou, H. (1997) Staurosporine-induced apoptosis of immortalized mouse proximal tubule cells is modulated by *bcl-2* expression level. *Int. Union of Biochem. Mol. Biol. Life* 42: 649-656.

Tchedre, K.T., and Yorio, T. (2008) α-1 receptors protect RGC-5 cells from apoptosis by regulating intracellular calcium, bax levels, and caspase-3 activation. *Invest. Ophthal. Vis. Sci.* 49:2577-2588.

Tokunaga, E., Oki, E., Egashira, A., Sadanaga, N., Morita, M., Kakeji, Y., and Maehara, Y. (2008) Deregulation of the Akt pathway in human cancer. *Curr. Cancer Drug Targets* 8(1):27-36.

Tweddle, D.A., Pearson, A.D.J., Haber, M., Norris, M.D., Xue, C., Flemming, C., and Lunec. J. (2003) The p53 pathway and its inactivation in neuroblastoma. *Cancer Lett.* 197(1): 93-98.

Wang, X., Bauer, J.H., Li, Y., Shao, Z., Zetoune, F.S., Cattaneo, E., and Vincenz, C. (2001) Characterization of a p75 (NTR) apoptotic signaling pathway using a novel cellular model. *J. Biol. Chem.* 276(36): 33812-33820.

Wickstrom, M., Johnsen, J.I., Ponthan, F., Segerstrom, L., Sveinbjomsson, B., Lindskog, M., Lovborg, H., Viktorsson, K., Lewensohn, R., Kogner, P., Larsson, R., and Gullbo, J. (2007) The novel melphalan prodrug J1 inhibits neuroblastoma growth *in vitro* and *in vivo*. *Mol. Cancer Ther.* 6: 2409-2417.

Wolfl, M., Jungbluth, A.A., Garrido, F., Cabrera, T., Meyen-Southard, S., Spitz, R., Ernestus, K., and Berthold, F. (2005) Expression of MHC class I, MHC class II, and cancer germline antigens in neuroblastoma. *Cancer Immunol. Immunother.* 54:400-406.

Wu, J., DiPietrantonio, A., and Hsieh, T. (2001) Mechanism of fenretinide (4-HPR)-induced cell death. *Apoptosis* 6(5):377-388.

Yang, H., Shaw, G., and Raizada, M.K. (2002) ANG II stimulation of neuritogenesis involves protein kinase B in brain neurons. *Am. J. Physiol. Regul. Integr. Comp. Physiol.* 283:R107-R114.

Yoshida, H., Enomoto, H., Miyauchi, M., Takanaga, K., Ohnuma, N., Sakiyama, S., and Tagawa, M. (1998) Impaired tumorigenicity of IL-4 produciing murine neuroblastoma cells in immunodeficient nude mice. *Int. J. Oncol.* 12(5);1067-1071.

Yu, A.L., Gilman, A., Ozkaynak, F., London, W.B., Kreissman, S., Chen, H.X., Smith, M., Anderson, B., Villablanca, J., Matthay, K.K., Shimada, H., Grupp, S.A., Seeger, R., Reynolds, P., Buxton, A., Reisfeld, R.A., Gillies, S.D., Cohn, S.L., Maris, J.M., and Sondel, P.M. (2010) Anti-GD2 antibody with GM-CSF, interleukin-2, and isotretinoin for neuroblastoma. *N. Engl. J. Med.* 363: 1324-1334.

Zagrebelsky, M., Schweigreiter, R., Bandtlow, C.E., Schwab, M.E. and Korte, M. (2010) Nogo-A stabilizes the architecture of hippocampal neurons. *J. Neurosci.* 30(40): 13220-13234.

Zechel, C. (2005) Requirement of retinoic acid receptor isotypes α, β, and γ during the initial steps of neural differentiation of PCC7 cells. *Mol. Endocrinol.* 19(6): 1629-1645.

Zheng, L., Jo, J., Jia, J.-M., Lo, S.-C., Whitcomb, D.J., Jiao, S., Cho, K., and Sheng, M. (2010) Caspase-3 activation via mitochondria is required for long-term depression and AMPA receptor internalization. *Cell* 141(5): 859-871

4

Neuroblastoma: A Malignancy Due to Cell Differentiation Block

Andrew Tee, Pei Y. Liu, Glenn M. Marshall and Tao Liu
Children's Cancer Institute Australia for Medical Research
Australia

1. Introduction

Neuroblastoma originates from precursor neuroblasts of the sympathetic nervous system. Unlike most other cancer types, neuroblastoma is characterized by a unique capacity for spontaneous complete regression, at least partly through neuronal differentiation, in a proportion of patients, and is therefore regarded as a cancer due to cell differentiation block. The first demonstration of *in vitro* differentiation of human neuroblastoma cells was published 30 years ago, when human SK-N-SH and SH-SY5Y neuroblastoma cells were shown to differentiate morphologically (neurite outgrowth) and biochemically in response to 12-O-tetradecanoyl-phorbol-13-acetate (TPA) treatment (Påhlman et al., 1981). The differentiated cells showed an increased expression of noradrenaline, adrenaline and neuron-specific enolase (NSE), differentiation markers which are employed for the diagnosis of neuroblastoma in patients. In 1982, retinoic acid (RA) was shown to induce concentration-dependent morphologic differentiation and growth inhibition in the LA-N-1 human neuroblastoma cell line (Sidell, 1982). The RA-induced morphologic differentiation and growth inhibition persisted despite removal of the drug. These observations demonstrate that RA promotes the differentiation of LA-N-1 neuroblastoma cells and results in a reduced expression of the malignant phenotype, and suggest that patients with advanced neuroblastoma may be successfully treated by RA to induce their tumour cells to differentiate and to undergo growth inhibition. In the last three decades, a number of factors, such as up-regulation of the expression of retinoic acid receptors, have been identified as crucial for the induction or blockage of neuroblastoma cell differentiation. Importantly, naturally occurring and synthetic retinoids have shown great promise in the clinic when used as differentiation agents in neuroblastoma patients with minimal residual disease, while the mechanism of retinoid anticancer signalling in neuroblastoma is still not fully understood (Liu et al., 2005; Reynolds et al., 2003).

2. Neurotrophin and neurotrophin receptor-induced neuroblastoma cell differentiation

Among the best characterized factors involved in pre-cancerous neuroblast and neuroblastoma cell differentiation are the tyrosine kinase receptor (TRK), its ligands nerve growth factor (NGF), brain-derived neurotrophic factor (BDNF), neurotrophin-3 (NT-3) and neurotrophin-4/5 (NT-5). Neuroblastoma cell lines generally lack functional neurotrophin receptors of the TRK gene family and therefore do not differentiate when stimulated with neurotrophins including NGF, BDNF, NTF3 or NTF5, and absence of TRKA and TRKC gene expression in neuroblastoma tissues correlates with poor prognosis in neuroblastoma patients (Kogner et al., 1993; Suzuki et al., 1993; Yamashiro et al., 1996). When transfected with either TRKA or TRKC, neuroblastoma cell lines can differentiate into sympathetic neurons in response to treatment with their cognate ligands NGF and NT-3 (Edsjo et al., 2001; Lavenius et al., 1995). Moreover, treatment with growth inhibition agents such as aphidicolin and all-trans RA (atRA) results in NGF responsiveness through induction of TRKA gene expression, demonstrating that TRK-negative cells retain a capacity to respond to TRK-mediated cell differentiation (Hishiki et al., 1998; Poluha, Poluha, and Ross, 1995). Taken together, these data show that many neuroblastoma cell lines have the capacity to respond to physiological differentiation stimuli, although they have lost this capacity with regard to stimulation with NGF or with other neurotrophins unless the neuroblastoma cells are triggered to express the cognate receptors [reviewed in (Edsjö, Holmquist, and Påhlman, 2007)].

While TRKA- and TRKC-mediated signalling decreases neuroblastoma cell proliferation and aggressiveness, BDNF/TRKB signalling corresponds with poor outcome in neuroblastoma patients [reviewed in (Edsjö, Holmquist, and Påhlman, 2007)]. BDNF treatment of neuroblastoma cells transfected with a TRKB over-expressing construct does not induce differentiation (Ho et al., 2011), and BDNF stimulation of neuroblastoma cell lines expressing TRKB as a result of RA treatment does not affect proliferation, but increases survival and invasiveness (Matsumoto et al., 1995). In addition to these effects of TRKA and TRKB signalling, recent data also suggest a difference with respect to therapy resistance, invasiveness, angiogenesis, and possibly also genomic stability (Schramm et al., 2005).

atRA treatment of neuroblastoma cells can also induce the expression of the proto-oncogene RET, which codes for a tyrosine kinase growth factor receptor specifically binding glial cell line-derived neurotrophic factor (GDNF) (Airaksinen and Saarma, 2002). GDNF is required for the proper development of enteric and parasympathetic neuroblasts (Airaksinen and Saarma, 2002), and atRA-treated neuroblastoma cells differentiate further in response to GDNF (Hishiki et al., 1998). Additionally, activation of RET by GDNF leads to differentiation of neuroblasts and neuroblastoma cells into ganglia cells (D'Alessio et al., 1995), and GDNF synergizes with ciliary neurotrophic factor (CNTF) to enhance TRKA receptor expression, thereby strengthening NGF-mediated cell differentiation signal (Peterson and Bogenmann, 2004).

3. Fyn and Fyn kinase induce neuroblastoma cell differentiation

Other factors involved in neuroblastoma cell differentiation include the Fyn nonreceptor kinase. Expression of active Fyn induces differentiation and growth arrest in neuroblastoma cells (Berwanger et al., 2002). High expression of Fyn and high Fyn kinase activity are restricted to low-stage human neuroblastoma tissues, and expression of Fyn predicts long-term survival independently of MYCN gene amplification (Berwanger et al., 2002).

4. N-Myc blocks neuroblastoma cell differentiation

The most powerful endogenous blocker of neuroblastoma cell differentiation is the *MYCN* oncogene. N-Myc is well-known to repress neuroblastoma cell differentiation partly through repressing TRKA gene expression. A recent study demonstrates that N-Myc blocks TRKA gene expression by recruiting histone deacetylase 1 (HDAC1) to TRKA gene promoter and repressing its transcription (Iraci et al., 2011). Additionally, N-Myc represses the expression of growth arrest specific1 (GAS1), leading to increased RET tyrosine 1062 phosphorylation and decreased GDNF signaling (Lopez-Ramirez et al., 2008).

5. Histone deacetylase 1 and tissue transglutaminase in neuroblastoma cell differentiation

The transamidation activity of tissue transglutaminase (TG2) has been shown to be essential for the neuroblastoma and leukemia cell differentiation response to retinoid therapy (Balajthy et al., 2006; Tucholski, Lesort, and Johnson, 2001), and TG2 overexpression alone induces neuronal differentiation in neuroblastoma cells (Tucholski, Lesort, and Johnson, 2001). We have recently shown that repression of TG2 gene expression and reduction in transamidation activity are essential for N-Myc-induced neuroblastoma cell differentiation block (Liu et al., 2007). Importantly, dual step cross-linking chromatin immunoprecipitation and protein coimmunoprecipitation assays show that N-Myc acts as a transrepressor by recruiting HDAC1 protein to an Sp1-binding site in the TG2 gene core promoter in a manner distinct from it's action as a transactivator at E-Box binding sites (Liu et al., 2007). Histone deacetylase inhibitor treatment blocks the N-Myc-mediated HDAC1 recruitment and TG2 repression *in vitro*. In neuroblastoma-bearing N-Myc transgenic mice, histone deacetylase inhibitor treatment induces TG2 expression and demonstrates marked antitumor activity *in vivo*. Taken together, these data indicate the critical roles of HDAC1 and TG2 in N-Myc-induced oncogenesis and have significant implications for the use of histone deacetylase inhibitor therapy in N-Myc-driven neuroblastoma.

6. Opposing effects of two tissue transglutaminase protein isoforms in neuroblastoma cell differentiation

Uniquely, two isoforms of TG2 mRNA and protein, a short form (TG2-S) and a full length form (TG2-L), have been characterized (Begg et al., 2006). We have shown that TG2-L and TG2-S exert opposing effects on cell differentiation (Tee et al., 2010). Repression of TG2-L with small interfering RNA, which does not affect TG2-S expression, induces dramatic neuronal differentiation in neuroblastoma cells. In contrast, overexpression of TG2-S or a GTP-binding-deficient mutant of TG2-L (R580A), both of which lack the GTP-binding Arg-580 residue, induces neuroblastoma cell differentiation, which is blocked by an inhibitor of transamidase activity. Whereas N-Myc represses and retinoid activates both TG2 isoforms, repression of TG2-L, but not simultaneous repression of TG2-L and TG2-S, enhances neuroblastoma cell differentiation due to N-Myc small interfering RNA or retinoid. Moreover, suppression of vasoactive intestinal peptide (VIP) expression alone induces neuroblastoma cell differentiation, and VIP can be up-regulated by TG2-L, but not TG2-S. Taken together, these data indicate that TG2-L and TG2-S exert opposite effects on cell differentiation due to differences in GTP binding and modulation of VIP gene transcription (Tee et al., 2010).

7. Retinoid differentiation therapy

Conventional therapy of neuroblastoma patients now includes the differentiation agent retinoid. Unlike chemo-radiotherapy, retinoid differentiation therapy shows minimal side effects on normal cells, because normal non-malignant cells are already differentiated. The effects of retinoids are mediated by two classes of non-steroid nuclear hormone receptors, the retinoic acid (RAR α, β, γ) and the retinoic X (RXR α, β, γ) receptors (Reynolds et al., 2003). The naturally occurring all-trans-retinoic acid (atRA), 9-cis-retinoic acid and the synthetic 13-cis-retinoic acid (13-cis-RA) are examples of retinoids studied in neuroblastoma. It has long been established that atRA stimulation of neuroblastoma cells results in growth inhibition and neuronal differentiation as indicated by neurite outgrowth, increased NSE activity and accumulation of norepinephrine (Pahlman et al., 1984; Sidell, 1982) . Even though atRA induces neuronal differentiation, the outcome differs depending on the neuroblastoma cell line studied. While some cell lines develop a sympathetic noradrenergic phenotype, a cholinergic switch has been suggested in other cell lines (Handler et al., 2000; Hill and Robertson, 1997). Mechanism studies have revealed that the down-regulation of the proto-oncogenes N-Myc, MYB and HRAS precedes the morphological differentiation, with changes in the expression of other proto-oncogenes following thereafter (Thiele, Deutsch, and Israel, 1988; Thiele, Reynolds, and Israel, 1985). As discussed in the previous sections, atRA treatment can also result in neuroblastoma cell differentiation by up-regulating the expression of the neurotrophin receptors TRKA, TRKB and RET, leading to responsiveness to their ligands NGF, BDNF and GDNF (Cerchia et al., 2006; Hishiki et al., 1998).

Phase I clinical trials show that higher and more sustained drug levels can be obtained with 13-cis-RA relative to atRA, and a phase III randomized clinical trial shows that high-dose, pulse therapy with 13-cis-RA given after completion of intensive chemoradiotherapy (with or without autologous bone marrow transplantation) significantly improved event-free survival in high-risk neuroblastoma patients (Reynolds et al., 2003) (Matthay et al., 1999). Moreove, *In vitro* as well as clinical data indicate that synthetic retinoids such as Fenretinide might be effective against neuroblastoma cells resistant to 13-cis-RA therapy. This effect seems to be independent of retinoid receptors, does not involve differentiation but is involved in the induction of programmed cell death (Reynolds et al., 2003).

8. Combination differentiation therapy with retinoids and histone deacetylase inhibitors

Although 13-cis-RA significantly improves event-free survival in high-risk neuroblastoma patients (Matthay et al., 1999), resistance to retinoid therapy eventually develops in more than 50% of neuroblastoma patients. Combination therapies with retinoids and other anti-cancer agents have therefore been studied extensively. Interestingly, during screening a small-molecule library for compounds enhancing histone deacetylase inhibitor-induced neuroblastoma cell differentiation, retinoids were found to be the top hit compounds (Hahn et al., 2008). Secondary assays confirmed greater neuroblastoma differentiation with the combination therapy of histone deacetylase inhibitors and retinoids. In a xenograft model of neuroblastoma, animals treated with the combination therapy with the histone deacetylase inhibitor SAHA and atRA had the longest survival. This work suggests that combination therapy with histone deacetylase inhibitors and retinoids could be a promising new strategy for differentiation therapy of children with neuroblastoma (Hahn et al., 2008).

9. References

Airaksinen, M. S., and Saarma, M. (2002). The GDNF family: Signalling, biological functions and therapeutic value. *Nat Rev Neurosci* 3(5), 383-394.

Balajthy, Z., Csomos, K., Vamosi, G., Szanto, A., Lanotte, M., and Fesus, L. (2006). Tissue-transglutaminase contributes to neutrophil granulocyte differentiation and functions. *Blood* 108(6), 2045-54.

Begg, G. E., Carrington, L., Stokes, P. H., Matthews, J. M., Wouters, M. A., Husain, A., Lorand, L., Iismaa, S. E., and Graham, R. M. (2006). Mechanism of allosteric regulation of transglutaminase 2 by GTP. *Proc Natl Acad Sci U S A* 103(52), 19683-8.

Berwanger, B., Hartmann, O., Bergmann, E., Bernard, S., Nielsen, D., Krause, M., Kartal, A., Flynn, D., Wiedemeyer, R., Schwab, M., Schafer, H., Christiansen, H., and Eilers, M.

(2002). Loss of a FYN-regulated differentiation and growth arrest pathway in advanced stage neuroblastoma. *Cancer Cell* 2(5), 377-86.

Cerchia, L., D'Alessio, A., Amabile, G., Duconge, F., Pestourie, C., Tavitian, B., Libri, D., and de Franciscis, V. (2006). An autocrine loop involving ret and glial cell-derived neurotrophic factor mediates retinoic acid-induced neuroblastoma cell differentiation. *Mol Cancer Res* 4(7), 481-8.

D'Alessio, A., De Vita, G., Cali, G., Nitsch, L., Fusco, A., Vecchio, G., Santelli, G., Santoro, M., and de Franciscis, V. (1995). Expression of the RET oncogene induces differentiation of SK-N-BE neuroblastoma cells. *Cell Growth Differ* 6(11), 1387-94.

Edsjo, A., Hallberg, B., Fagerstrom, S., Larsson, C., Axelson, H., and Pahlman, S. (2001). Differences in Early and Late Responses between Neurotrophin-stimulated trkA- and trkC-transfected SH-SY5Y Neuroblastoma Cells. *Cell Growth Differ* 12(1), 39-50.

Edsjö, A., Holmquist, L., and Påhlman, S. (2007). Neuroblastoma as an experimental model for neuronal differentiation and hypoxia-induced tumor cell dedifferentiation. *Semin Cancer Biol.* 17(3), 248-56.

Hahn, C. K., Ross, K. N., Warrington, I. M., Mazitschek, R., Kanegai, C. M., Wright, R. D., Kung, A. L., Golub, T. R., and Stegmaier, K. (2008). Expression-based screening identifies the combination of histone deacetylase inhibitors and retinoids for neuroblastoma differentiation. *Proc Natl Acad Sci U S A* 105(28), 9751-6.

Handler, A., Lobo, M. D., Alonso, F. J., Paino, C. L., and Mena, M. A. (2000). Functional implications of the noradrenergic-cholinergic switch induced by retinoic acid in NB69 neuroblastoma cells. *J Neurosci Res* 60(3), 311-20.

Hill, D. P., and Robertson, K. A. (1997). Characterization of the cholinergic neuronal differentiation of the human neuroblastoma cell line LA-N-5 after treatment with retinoic acid. *Brain Res Dev Brain Res* 102(1), 53-67.

Hishiki, T., Nimura, Y., Isogai, E., Kondo, K., Ichimiya, S., Nakamura, Y., Ozaki, T., Sakiyama, S., Hirose, M., Seki, N., Takahashi, H., Ohnuma, N., Tanabe, M., and Nakagawara, A. (1998). Glial cell line-derived neurotrophic factor/neurturin-induced differentiation and its enhancement by retinoic acid in primary human neuroblastomas expressing c-Ret, GFR alpha-1, and GFR alpha-2. *Cancer Res* 58(10), 2158-65.

Ho., R., Minturn, J. E., Simpson, A. M., Iyer, R., Light, J. E., Evans, A. E., and Brodeur, G. M. (2011). The effect of P75 on Trk receptors in neuroblastomas. *Cancer Lett* 305(1):76-85.

Iraci, N., Diolaiti, D., Papa, A., Porro, A., Valli, E., Gherardi, S., Herold, S., Eilers, M., Bernardoni, R., Della Valle, G., and Perini, G. (2011). A SP1/MIZ1/MYCN repression complex recruits HDAC1 at the TRKA and p75NTR promoters and affects neuroblastoma malignancy by inhibiting the cell response to NGF. *Cancer Res* 71(2), 404-12.

Kogner, P., Barbany, G., Dominici, C., Castello, M. A., Raschella, G., and Persson, H. (1993). Coexpression of messenger RNA for TRK protooncogene and low affinity nerve growth factor receptor in neuroblastoma with favorable prognosis. *Cancer Res* 53(9), 2044-50.

Lavenius, E., Gestblom, C., Johansson, I., N°anberg, E., and P°ahlman, S. (1995). Transfection of TRK-A into human neuroblastoma cells restores their ability to differentiate in response to nerve growth factor. . *Cell Growth Differ* 6, 727-36.

Liu, T., Bohlken, A., Kuljaca, S., Lee, M., Nguyen, T., Smith, S., Cheung, B., Norris, M. D., Haber, M., Holloway, A. J., Bowtell, D. D., and Marshall, G. M. (2005). The retinoid anticancer signal: mechanisms of target gene regulation. *Br J Cancer* 93(3), 310-8.

Liu, T., Tee, A. E., Porro, A., Smith, S. A., Dwarte, T., Liu, P. Y., Iraci, N., Sekyere, E., Haber, M., Norris, M. D., Diolaiti, D., Della Valle, G., Perini, G., and Marshall, G. M. (2007). Activation of tissue transglutaminase transcription by histone deacetylase inhibition as a therapeutic approach for Myc oncogenesis. *Proc Natl Acad Sci U S A* 104(47), 18682-7.

Lopez-Ramirez, M. A., Dominguez-Monzon, G., Vergara, P., and Segovia, J. (2008). Gas1 reduces Ret tyrosine 1062 phosphorylation and alters GDNF-mediated intracellular signaling. *Int J Dev Neurosci* 26(5), 497-503.

Matsumoto, K., Wada, R., Yamashiro, J., Kaplan, D., and Thiele, C. (1995). Expression of brain-derived neurotrophic factor and p145TrkB affects survival, differentiation, and invasiveness of human neuroblastoma cells. *Cancer Res* 55, 1798-806.

Matthay, K. K., Villablanca, J. G., Seeger, R. C., Stram, D. O., Harris, R. E., Ramsay, N. K., Swift, P., Shimada, H., Black, C. T., Brodeur, G. M., Gerbing, R. B., and Reynolds, C. P. (1999). Treatment of high-risk neuroblastoma with intensive chemotherapy, radiotherapy, autologous bone marrow transplantation, and 13-cis-retinoic acid. Children's Cancer Group. *N Engl J Med* 341(16), 1165-73.

Påhlman, S., Odelstad, L., Larsson, E., Grotte, G., and Nilsson, K. (1981). Phenotypic changes of human neuroblastoma cells in culture induced by 12-Otetradecanoyl-phorbol-13-acetate. *Int J Cancer* 28, 583-9.

Pahlman, S., Ruusala, A. I., Abrahamsson, L., Mattsson, M. E., and Esscher, T. (1984). Retinoic acid-induced differentiation of cultured human neuroblastoma cells: a comparison with phorbolester-induced differentiation. *Cell Differ* 14(2), 135-44.

Peterson, S., and Bogenmann, E. (2004). The RET and TRKA pathways collaborate to regulate neuroblastoma differentiation. *Oncogene* 23(1), 213-25.

Poluha, W., Poluha, D. K., and Ross, A. H. (1995). TrkA neurogenic receptor regulates differentiation of neuroblastoma cells. *Oncogene* 10(1), 185-9.

Reynolds, C. P., Matthay, K. K., Villablanca, J. G., and Maurer, B. J. (2003). Retinoid therapy of high-risk neuroblastoma. *Cancer Lett* 197(1-2), 185-92.

Schramm, A., Schulte, J., Astrahantseff, K., Apostolov, O., Limpt, V., and Sieverts, H. (2005). Biological effects of TrkA and TrkB receptor signaling in neuroblastoma. *Cancer Lett* 228, 143-53.

Sidell, N. (1982). Retinoic acid-induced growth inhibition and morphologic differentiation of human neuroblastoma cells in vitro. *J Natl Cancer Inst* 68(4), 589-96.

Suzuki, T., Bogenmann, E., Shimada, H., Stram, D., and Seeger, R. C. (1993). Lack of high-affinity nerve growth factor receptors in aggressive neuroblastomas. *J Natl Cancer Inst* 85(5), 377-84.

Tee, A. E., Marshall, G. M., Liu, P. Y., Xu, N., Haber, M., Norris, M. D., Iismaa, S. E., and Liu, T. (2010). Opposing effects of two tissue transglutaminase protein isoforms in neuroblastoma cell differentiation. *J Biol Chem* 285(6), 3561-7.

Thiele, C. J., Deutsch, L. A., and Israel, M. A. (1988). The expression of multiple proto-oncogenes is differentially regulated during retinoic acid induced maturation of human neuroblastoma cell lines. *Oncogene* 3(3), 281-8.

Thiele, C. J., Reynolds, C. P., and Israel, M. A. (1985). Decreased expression of N-myc precedes retinoic acid-induced morphological differentiation of human neuroblastoma. *Nature* 313(6001), 404-6.

Tucholski, J., Lesort, M., and Johnson, G. V. (2001). Tissue transglutaminase is essential for neurite outgrowth in human neuroblastoma SH-SY5Y cells. *Neuroscience* 102(2), 481-91.

Yamashiro, D. J., Nakagawara, A., Ikegaki, N., Liu, X. G., and Brodeur, G. M. (1996). Expression of TrkC in favorable human neuroblastomas. *Oncogene* 12(1), 37-41.

5

Alternative TrkA Splicing and Neuroblastoma

Antonietta R. Farina et al.*
Department of Experimental Medicine, University of L'Aquila
L'Aquila
Italy

1. Introduction

Neuroblastoma is one of the most frequent solid paediatric tumours of the nervous system, accounting for up to 10% of all paediatric tumours. The majority of NBs originate from a sympathoadrenal cell lineage of neural crest origin during sympathetic nervous system development, and represent a heterogeneous group of tumours that exhibit a high degree of genetic and biological variability, including not infrequent spontaneous regression or differentiation to ganglioneuroma (Evans, 2004; Nakagawara, 2004). A large percentage of NB patients present with stage 4 disease characterised by dissemination primarily to bone; bone marrow; lymph node; liver and skin sites, with metastatic bone disease carrying automatic stage 4 diagnosis and the poorest prognosis. A subset of stage 4 NBs that disseminate primarily to liver skin and bone marrow sites exhibit frequent spontaneous regression and are classified as stage 4S. Genetic alterations that associated with aggressive NB include: amplification of the proto-oncogenic transcription factor N-myc in up to 20% of all NBs and up to 40% of aggressive NB; gain of chromosome 17 and loss of distal material from the chromosomes 1p32-pter (minimal common region 1p36.2); 14p23-qter; 11q23 and 18, regions likely to contain oncosuppressors (Evans, 2004; Nakagawara, 2004; Jiang et al., 2011; Takita et al., 2000). Despite general improvements in therapy, the age of onset plus high frequency of post-therapeutic relapse have meant that survival rates in patients with NB remain poor, highlighting the need for a greater understanding of the molecular mechanisms involved in this tumor type and the translation of this information into novel therapies.

Receptor tyrosine kinases (RTKs) regulate cellular growth, differentiation and survival during development. In general, RTK function depends upon appropriate ligand binding, with inappropriate activation and temporary duration of activation regulated by molecular domain, glycosylation status; protein chaperones; phosphorylation status and associated protein tyrosine phosphatases. The deregulation of RTK function is involved in tumour pathology, with over 30 RTKs associated with different malignancies, and is associated with

*Lucia Cappabianca[1], Pierdomenico Ruggeri[1], Natalia Di Ianni[1], Marzia Ragone[1], Stefania Merolle[1], Alberto Gulino[2] and Andrew R. Mackay[1]
[1]*Department of Experimental Medicine, University of L'Aquila, Aquila, Italy*
[2]*Department of Experimental Medicine and Pathology, University of Rome "La Sapienza",Rome, Italy*

a change in any one or combination of RTK regulatory mechanisms. Direct oncogenic activation of RTKs has been shown to result from gene amplification; novel chimera formation; deletion and point-mutation; and also by alternative and/or aberrant splicing (Bennasruone et al., 2004).

Alternative splicing is a fundamental physiological mechanism for differential protein expression from a single gene through alternative exon usage, is largely responsible for the proteomic complexity of higher organisms (Modek & Lee, 2002) and is also involved in cancer at the level of both oncogene activation and oncosuppressor inactivation. RTK oncogenes reported to be activated by alternative or aberrant splicing include the EGF receptor, FGF receptor-1; insulin receptor and nerve growth factor (NGF) receptor tropomyosin related tyrosine kinase (Trk) A (Kalnina et al., 2005; Tacconelli et al., 2004).

TrkA is the preferred receptor for NGF, plays a critical role in sympathetic nervous system development and is essential for the formation, differentiation and survival of normal sympathetic neurons that originate from cells of neural crest origin (Bibel & Barde, 2000). Not surprisingly, since the majority of NBs arise from a sympathoadrenal cell lineage of neural crest origin they also exhibit varying degrees of TrkA gene expression (Nakagawara et al., 1992; Nakagawara & Koger, 2000; Nakagawara, 2001). Mutation-activated TrkA oncogenes, however, have not been reported in NB and a possible NB tumour-suppressor function for TrkA has been suggested by an inverse relationship between expression and NB stage. Indeed, TrkA expression is considered to be a marker of better prognosis, potentially involved in both spontaneous and therapy-induced NB regression (Nakagawara et al., 1992; Nakagawara & Koger, 2000; Nakagawara, 2001). This hypothesis is supported by reports of TrkA tumour-suppressing activity in NB models, characterised by growth inhibition; differentiation, apoptosis and the inhibition of angiogenesis (Tacconelli et al., 2004; Nakagawara, 2001; Matsushima & Bogenmann, 2000; Lavenius et al., 1995; Lucarelli et al., 1997; Eggert et al., 2002).

Recently, however, the concept that TrkA plays an exclusively tumour suppressing role in NB has been challenged by discovery of a novel stress-regulated alternative TrkAIII splice variant, expressed by advanced stage primary human NBs, which exhibits tumour promoting activity in NB models and oncogenic activity in NIH-3T3 fibroblasts (Tacconelli et al., 2004).

In this chapter, therefore, we review current concepts concerning alternative TrkA splicing in NB, through comparative analysis of alternative TrkA splice variant structure, spontaneous versus ligand-mediated activation, post receptor signalling, regulation of expression, and tumour suppressing versus oncogenic activity. We also discuss the potential prognostic value of assessing alternative TrkAIII splicing and therapeutic ways to reduce TrkAIII involvement in NB.

2. The TrkA proto-oncogene

Trk-A is a member of the tyrosine kinase neurotrophin receptor family that includes TrkB and TrkC and is the preferred receptor for NGF but also binds the neurotrophin NT-3 (Klein et al., 1991; Patapoutian & Reichardt, 2001). The 25kb human TrkA gene is organised into 17 exons and maps to chromosome 1q21-q22 (Greco et al., 1996; Weier et al., 1995). Identification of the TrkA proto-oncogene was preceded by the discovery of the first tumour-associated TrkA oncogene (Klein et al., 1991; Martin-Zanca et al., 1986, 1989).

TrkA expression is absolutely required for the development, maturation and maintenance of the central and peripheral nervous systems. Within the peripheral nervous system TrkA regulates the formation, differentiation and survival of sympathetic neurones that originate from progenitors of neural crest origin (Bibel & Barde, 2000; Kaplan & Miller, 2000; Oppenheim, 1991; Ernsberger, 2009). TrkA is also critical for the development and function of the immune system (Vega et al., 2003; Fiore et al., 2009).

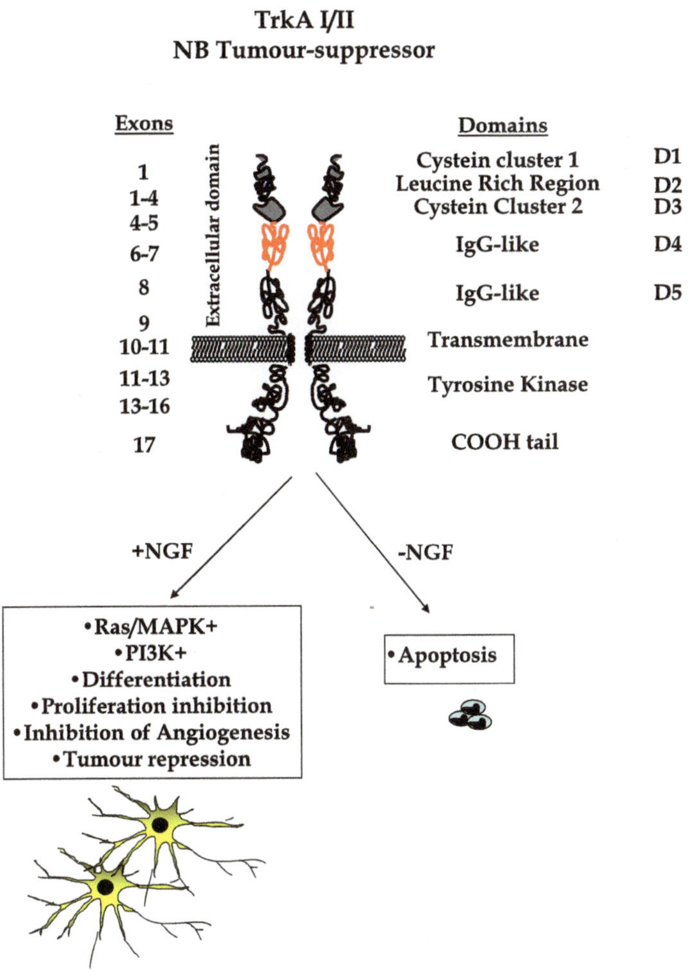

Representation of the exon and domain structure of TrkAI/II receptors and the biological effects of TrkA upon NB cell behaviour.

Fig. 1. The TrkAI/II NB tumour suppressor

The TrkA protein is expressed as a predominant 140kDa cell surface transmembrane tyrosine kinase receptor, comprised of an extracellular domain containing two cysteine-rich clusters (D1 and D3) interrupted by a leucine rich domain (D2) and 2 immunoglobulin (Ig)-

like domains (D4 and D5) involved in ligand-binding. Receptor transmembrane and juxta-membrane regions are critical for signal internalisation and transduction, whereas the intracellular tyrosine-rich carboxyl-terminal cytoplasmic domain exhibits tyrosine kinase activity upon ligand-mediated activation and is responsible for propagating post-receptor signal transduction (Windisch et al., 1995; Arevalo et al., 2000; Peng et al., 1995; Monshipouri et al., 2000; Kaplan et al., 1991; Holden et al., 1997; Wiesman et al., 2000) (Figure 1).

In the absence of ligand, cell surface TrkA receptors are maintained as inactive oligomers (Mischel et al., 2002) that concentrate within caveolin-1 and cholesterol-containing cell membrane caveolae invaginations, which also contain components of the Ras signalling pathway (Paratcha & Ibanez, 2002). In the absence of ligand, receptor oligomers are maintained in an inactive state by a mature extracellular domain N-glycosylation status, the presence of intact D4 and D5 domains and by receptor-associated protein tyrosine phosphatases (PTPases) (Arevalo et al., 2000; Marsh et al., 2003; Watson et al., 1999; Ostman & Bohmer, 2001; Sastry & Elferink, 2011). Upon ligand binding, oligomeric TrkA receptors alter conformation and acquire tyrosine kinase activity, which is facilitated by temporary inactivation of receptor-associated PTPases. This results in auto- and trans-phosphorylation of receptor tyrosine residues Y490, Y674/675, Y751 and Y785, which act as phosphorylation-dependent binding sites for a variety of signalling proteins. The adapters Shc and FRS-2 bind to phosphorylated Y490; Grb-2 and SOS bind to phosphorylated Y674 and Y675; the IP3K p85α subunit binds phosphorylated Y751 and PLCγ binds phosphorylated Y785. These interactions provide avenues for signal transduction through the Ras/MAPK, PI3K/Akt/NF-κB and PKC pathways, which mediate the effects of NGF upon cell differentiation, proliferation, survival and apoptosis (Kaplan & Stevens, 1994; Green & Kaplan, 1995; Hallberg et al., 1998; Meakin et al., 1999; Cunningham et al., 1997; Obermeier et al., 1993, 1994; Segal et al., 1996; Yao & Cooper, 1995). Neurotrophin activity is further modulated by interaction between TrkA and the low affinity $p75^{NTR}$ receptor (Peng et al., 1995; Hempstead et al., 1991; Majdan et al., 2001; Zaccaro et al., 2002; Nykjaer et al., 2005).

An additional feature of NGF/TrkA receptors is retrograde transport signalling within the cell. This depends upon receptor/ligand interaction, internalisation and retrograde transport of NGF-activated TrkA receptors, resulting in signal transduction within the cell body. Sympathetic neurons most dramatically illustrate this activity, with retrograde transport of NGF-activated TrkA along the axonal length to the neuronal cell body. This phenomenon appears to involve ubiquitin-mediated receptor internalisation through interaction with $p75^{NTR}$ and TRAF6, receptor endocytosis within clatherin coated vesicles and receptor endocytosis facilitated by the endocytosis inducing protein EHD4/Pincher (Moises et al., 2007; Howe et al., 2004; Valdez et al., 2005).

In addition to a cell surface localisation, immature forms of the TrkA receptor also localise to intracellular membranes of the Golgi Network (GN), where they can be trans-activated by agonists of the G-protein linked A_{2A} adenosine receptor, providing evidence for intracellular neurotrophin-independent TrkA activation. Furthermore, post-receptor signal transduction from GN-associated TrkA differs from that of NGF-activated cell surface TrkA by signalling through PI3K/Akt but not Ras/MAPK, inducing NF-κB transcription factor activity and a more stress-resistant phenotype. TrkA localisation to the GN may not only reflect the transient passage of de-novo synthesised receptors but also alterations in receptor extracellular domain N-glycosylation and/or folding (Watson et al., 1999; Rajagopal et al., 2004).

2.1 TrkA oncogenes

The first TrkA oncogene was identified in colon cancer as a novel constitutively active cytoplasmic chimera bearing tropomyosin substitution of the TrkA extracellular domain (Martin-Zanca et al., 1986, 1989). Subsequently, Trk-T1, Trk-T2 and Trk-T3 oncogenes were identified in papillary thyroid and colon tumours and characterised as constitutively active non-cell surface chimeric oncogenes. Trk-T1 and Trk-T2 oncogenes bear different extracellular domain substitutions with tropomyosin and Trk-T3 bears an extracellular substitution with Trk-fused gene, located on chromosome 3q11-12 (Coulier et al., 1990; Greco et al., 2010). Non-chimeric TrkA oncogenes include a constitutively active extracellular domain point mutated TrkA oncogene identified in prostate cancer (George et al., 1998) and a TrkA oncogene bearing an extracellular deletion of the D5 Ig-like domain identified in acute myeloid leukaemia (Reuther et al., 2000). Under experimental conditions TrkA oncogenes have been generated by: C345S and P203A point mutations within the receptor extracellular domain; by in-frame deletion of extracellular domain sequences encoding the Ig-like domains D4 and D5; and by duplication of the TrkA tyrosine kinase domain (Arevalo et al., 2000; Coulier et al., 1990).

In general, activated TrkA oncogenes are expressed as constitutively phosphorylated receptors, which exhibit spontaneous ligand-independent tyrosine kinase activity and signal chronically through PI3K/Akt/NF-κB, PKC and/or Ras/MAPK pathways, resulting in cellular transformation associated with alterations in proliferation and survival (Nakagawara, 2001; Martin-Zanca et al, 1989; Arevalo et al., 2000, 2001; Watson et al., 1999; Meakin et al., 1999; Coulier et al., 1990; Greco et al., 2010). Therefore in non-mutated TrkA, an intact fully N-glycosylated extracellular domain is critical for preventing ligand-independent receptor oligomerisation and spontaneous oncogenic activation, with essential roles played by extracellular domain P203 and C345 residues and by the extracellular D4 and D5 Ig-like domains (Arevalo et al., 2000, 2001; Watson et al., 1999; Coulier et al., 1990).

2.2 TrkA as an NB tumour-suppressor

NB arises from cells of neural crest origin during sympathetic nervous system development (Evans, 2004; Nakagawara, 2004; Jiang et al., 2011) and as a consequence exhibit varying degrees of TrkA expression (Tacconelli et al., 2004; Nakagawara et al., 1992; Nakagawara & Koger, 2000; Nakagawara, 2001). However, despite the absolute requirement for TrkA in the formation, differentiation and maintenance of the sympathetic nervous system; variable TrkA expression and the presence of non-coding TrkA gene polymorphisms and mutations in NBs (Scaruffi et al., 1999), there are no reports that associate mutation-activated TrkA oncogenes with this tumour type. On the contrary, TrkA is considered to be a potential NB tumour-suppressor. This concept is derived from the association between high level TrkA expression and low stage NB and has led to TrkA expression being considered a marker of better prognosis, and to the suggestion that TrkA expression may be required for both spontaneous and therapy-induced NB regression (Nakagawara et al., 1992; Nakagawara & Koger, 2000; Nakagawara, 2001; Brodeur et al., 2009; Tanaka et al., 1998; Suzuki et al., 1993). This hypothesis is supported by evidence that NB cells exhibit multiple defects in NGF receptor signalling (Azar et al., 1990); reports that NB differentiating agents such as retinoic acid and γ-interferon augment TrkA expression (Sugimoto et al., 2001), and reports that

TrkA gene transduction restores NGF-responsiveness to NB cells, inducing ligand-dependent signalling through PI3K, Ras/MAPK and PKC pathways, resulting in growth arrest, differentiation and the inhibition of angiogenesis and NB tumour xenograft growth (Tacconelli et al., 2004; Matsushima et al., 1990; Lavenius et al., 1995; Lucarelli et al., 1997; Eggert et al., 2002). A potential NB tumour-suppressor function for TrkA suggests that reduced TrkA expression would facilitate tumour progression. This is supported by the inverse relationship exhibited by TrkA expression and NB stage (Nakagawara et al., 1992; Nakagawara & Koger, 2000; Nakagawara, 2001) and suggests that the reintroduction of adequate TrkA expression levels and/or the activation of post cell surface TrkA receptor signalling represents an important potential therapeutic goal in NB.
Recently, however, a darker side to TrkA involvement in NB has been revealed by the discovery of an alternative TrkA splice variant "TrkAIII" expressed by advanced stage primary human NBs that exhibits oncogenic activity in NB models (Tacconelli et al., 2004; Farina et al., 2009a, 2009b).

3. Alternative TrkA splice variants

The human 25kb TrkA gene localises to chromosome 1p21-22, is organised into 17 exons (Greco et al., 1996; Weier et al., 1995) and exhibits alternative splicing. Alternative TrkA splice variants include: TrkA L0 and L1, which exhibit differential exons 2-4 usage (Dubus et al., 2000); TrkAI and TrkAII, which exhibit differential exon 9 use (Barker et al., 1993); and TrkAIII, which exhibits inframe skipping of exons 6 and 7, combined with exon 9 omission (Tacconelli et al., 2004).

3.1 TrkA L0 and L1

Alternative use of TrkA exons 2, 3 and 4 leads to the expression of alternative TrkA L0 (exons 2, 3 and 4 alternatively spliced) and L1 (exons 2 and 3 alternatively spliced) splice variants, originally described during rat development (Dubus et al., 2000). These variants would be expected to yield truncated receptors bearing inframe deletions of leucine-rich sequences encoded within exons 2-4 (Greco et al., 1996). Since, TrkA leucine rich motifs modulate ligand-binding to TrkA Ig-like domains (Windisch et al., 1995), L1 and L0 variants may exhibit altered ligand-binding activity, similar to that described for analogous alternative TrkB splice variants (Ninkina et al., 1997). Within the developing rat, the TrkA L1 variant is expressed within the thymus, testis, lung and kidney (Dubus et al., 2000). There are no reports that directly link TrkAL0 and L1 splice variants to tumour pathology. However, an uncharacterised 80kDa truncated TrkA isoform has been reported in human thymomas but it remains to be elucidated whether this represents an alternative splice variant, deletion mutant or degradation product (Parrens et al., 1998).

3.2 TrkAI and TrkAII

The differential use of exon 9, which encodes the amino acid sequence VSFSPV, results in the expression of alternative TrkAI (exon 9 exclusion) and TrkAII (exon 9 inclusion) splice variants (Barker et al., 1993). Both TrkAI and TrkAII variants are expressed as approximately 140kDa cell surface transmembrane receptors and the omission of exon 9 sequence does not result in ligand-independent receptor activation. Both variants bind NGF and NT3 neurotrophins (Barker et al., 1993; Clary et al., 1994) and exhibit a degree of tissue-specific expression, with TrkAII expressed predominantly by nervous system tissues and TrkAI expressed predominantly in thymic tissues (Barker et al., 1993). At the functional level, TrkAII exhibits a higher level of NT3-mediated activation when co-expressed with the low affinity neurotrophin receptor $p75^{NTR}$ (Clary et al., 1994), which promotes apoptosis in the absence of TrkA signalling and regulates both ligand-dependent and independent TrkA activation to augment cell survival (Peng et al., 1995; Hempstead et al., 1991; Majdan et al., 2001; Zaccaro et al., 2002; Nykjaer et al., 2005). There are no other reported functional differences between the alternative TrkAI and TrkAII splice variants, suggesting that both isoforms are likely to be involved in nervous and immunological system development, maturation and maintenance through the regulation of proliferation, differentiation, apoptosis and survival, with potential for tissue-specific functional differences. There are no reports linking alternative TrkAI and TrkAII splicing to NB, suggesting that combined expression may represent a marker of better prognosis, inversely correlated with malignant NB behaviour (Tacconelli et al., 2004; Nakagawara et al., 1992; Nakagawara & Koger, 2000; Nakagawara, 2001, Brodeur et al., 2009; Tanaka et al., 1998; Suzuki et al., 1993; Cao et al., 2010).

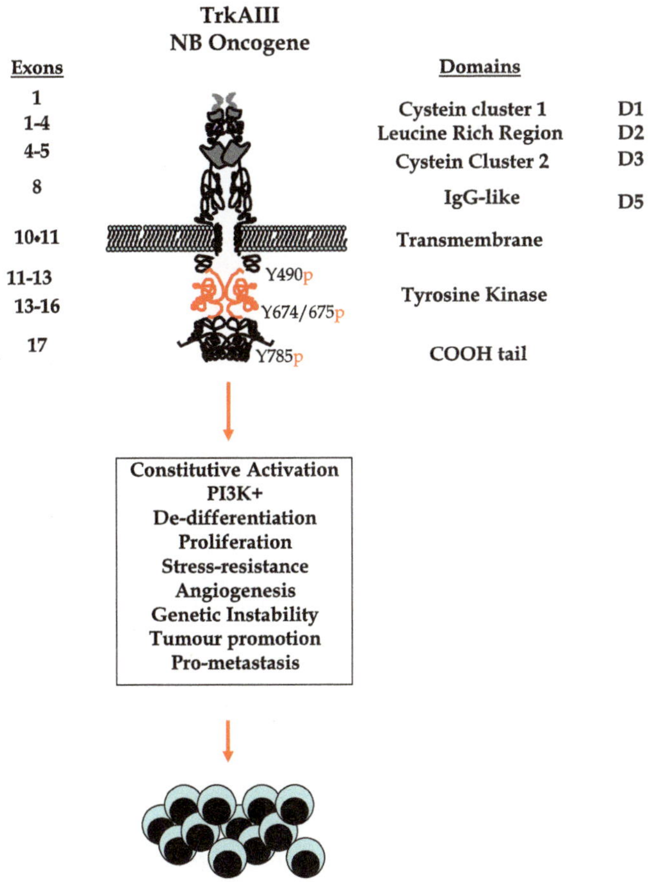

Representation of the exons and domain-structure of the TrkAIII receptor and its biological effects upon NB cells.

Fig. 2. The TrkAIII oncogene

3.3 The alternative TrkAIII splice variant

TrkAIII was originally identified as an unexpected RT-PCR product in mRNAs purified from primary human NBs and was subsequently cloned from the human SH-SY5Y NB cell line. TrkAIII was characterised as a novel alternative splice variant, exhibiting inframe skipping of exons 6 and 7, in addition to exon 9 omission (Figure 2) (Tacconelli et al., 2004).
The skipping of exon 6 and 7 results in an in-frame deletion of amino acids 192-284, which encode the entire extracellular D4 Ig-like domain; introduces a valine substitution at the novel exon 5/8 splice junction; and causes the loss of several functional N-glycosylation sites (Tacconelli et al., 2004).

3.3.1 TrkAIII expression by primary NBs and NB cell lines

Originally identified in an advanced stage 4 primary human NB, preliminary data in 24 primary human NBs indicated predominant TrkAIII expression with respect to TrkAI/II in advanced stage 3 and 4 disease (Tacconelli et al., 2004). This has been recently confirmed in an independent study of 39 primary human NBs, in which a significant relationship between high TrkAIII expression and high stage was reported (Cao et al., 2010).
TrkAIII is expressed by human SK-N-SH, SH-SY5Y IMR32, SK-N-AS, KCNR, LAN5 and SK-N-BE NB cell lines, normal human neural stem cells and neural crest progenitors but not by differentiation-committed counterparts, (i.e cerebral granule neurones) (Tacconelli et al., 2004). This suggests a tissue-specific rather than NB tumour-specific alternative splice mechanism that potentially relates to an undifferentiated neural progenitor/stem cell-like tumour cell phenotype. TrkAIII expression by NB cells does not associate with mutations or deletions within the TrkA gene, supporting its status as an alternative splice variant (Tacconelli et al., 2004).

3.3.2 Epigenetic regulation of alternative TrkAIII splicing

The association between a high TrkAI/II to TrkAIII expression ratio with low stage NB and a low TrkAI/II to TrkAIII expression ratio with high stage NB (Tacconelli et al., 2004; Cao et al., 2010), supports the hypothesis that NBs switch from TrkAI to TrkAIII expression during progression. Alternative TrkAIII splicing may, therefore, represent a regulated tumour promoting switch, through which NB tumour suppressing signals from TrkAI/II can be converted to oncogenic signals from TrkAIII. Although the mechanisms involved in alternative TrkAIII splicing remain to be fully elucidated, potential epigenetic regulation of alternative TrkAIII splicing within the hostile tumour microenvironment is supported by the promotion of alternative TrkAIII splicing in human NB cell lines by conditions that mimic tumour-associated hypoxia (Tacconelli et al., 2004). The same conditions also promote alternative TrkAIII splicing in normal neural stem cells and undifferentiated neural crest progenitors, but not in differentiation committed counterparts (Tacconelli et al., 2004), suggesting that hypoxia-regulated alternative TrkAIII splicing in NB cells may represent conservation and pathological subversion of a physiological neural stem/progenitor cell hypoxia-protection mechanism. We do not exclude, however, that alternative and/or additional mechanisms may promote alternative TrkAIII splicing in NBs.

3.3.3 Differences between TrkAI/II and TrkAIII splice variants

Comparative analysis of TrkAI and TrkAIII receptors expressed in human SH-SY5Y NB cells has revealed several differences (Table 1). These include: a) Differences in molecular size.

TrkAI is expressed as immature 110kDa and mature gp140kDa N-glycosylated proteins that reduce to a single 80kDa protein upon tunicamycin treatment, whereas TrkAIII is expressed as a single 100kDa N-glycosylated protein that reduces to 70kDa upon tunicamycin treatment; b) Differences in receptor compartmentalization. The mature gp140 TrkAI receptor is expressed predominantly at the cell surface with GN accumulation of the immature gp110TrkAI receptor, whereas TrkAIII is not expressed at the cell surface but is retained within intracellular membranes, within which it exhibits relatively equal distribution between the endoplasmic reticulum (ER), endoplasmic reticulum and Golgi intermediate (ERGIC); Golgi network (GN) and associated vesicle compartments (Tacconelli et al., 2004; Farina et al., 2009a, 2009b); c) Differences in spontaneous versus ligand-dependent activation. TrkAI exhibits ligand-dependent but not spontaneous activity, whereas TrkAIII exhibits spontaneous ligand-independent activation and does not bind neurotrophins; d) Differences in post receptor signal transduction. In response to ligand, activated TrkA receptors exhibit receptor-associated tyrosine kinase and PI3K activity, are phosphorylated on Y490, Y674/675 and Y758 residues, bind Shc, Grb2 and FRS2 adapters and signal through PI3K/Akt and Ras/MAPK, whereas spontaneously active TrkAIII exhibits tyrosine kinase and PI3K activity, is constitutively phosphorylated on Y490, Y674/675 and Y758 residues, binds only low levels of non-phosphorylated Shc, does not bind FRS2 or GRB2 and signals through IP3K/Akt but not Ras/MAPK (Tacconelli et al., 2004); and e) differences in biological activity, with TrkAI exhibiting tumour-suppressing and TrkAIII oncogenic activity in NB models (Tacconelli et al., 2004).

These differences depend upon the omission of sequences encoded within exons 6/7 and form the basis of the differential TrkAI/II tumour-suppressing and TrkAIII oncogenic activity observed (Tacconelli et al., 2004; Farina et al., 2009a, 2009b). Intracellular TrkAIII retention versus cell surface TrkAI expression may depend upon differences in extracellular domain N-glycosylation, which regulates cell surface TrkA expression (Watson et al., 1999). Spontaneous ligand-independent TrkAIII activation most likely depends upon the omission of the extracellular D4 Ig-like domain plus associated N-glycosylation sites, which prevent ligand-independent TrkA activation (Arevalo et al., 2000). Differences in adapter protein binding exhibited by ligand-activated TrkAI and spontaneously-active TrkAIII and subsequent differences in post receptor signalling most likely reflect differences in receptor localisation, with lack of post TrkAIII signalling through Ras/MAPK explained either by dislocation from caveolae-associated Ras/MAPK (Paratcha & Ibanez, 2002; Rajagopal et al., 2004), altered adapter protein binding (Tacconelli et al., 2004; Farina et al., 2009a, 2009b); TrkAIII activity below the Ras/MAPK activation threshold (Hallberg et al., 1998); and/or direct PI3K/Akt inhibition of Raf-MEK-ERK signalling (Moelling et al., 2002), the latter possibility supported by TrkAIII antagonism of NGF/TrkAI-induced ERK phosphorylation (Tacconelli et al., 2004).

Interestingly, post TrkAIII receptor signalling through PI3K/Akt but not Ras/MAPK resembles post receptor signalling from GN-associated immature gp110TrkAI trans-activated by G-protein associated A_{2A} adenosine receptors (Rajagopal et al., 2004), indicating that an intracellular location alters post TrkA receptor signalling.

The characteristics exhibited by TrkAIII of spontaneous ligand-independent activity and chronic post receptor signalling are considered to be pre-requisites for oncogenic RTK activation (Bennasruone et al., 2004). How this relates to tumour suppressing signalling from ligand-activated cell surface TrkAI is dealt with below.

	TrkAI	TrkAIII
Expressed at the cell surface in caveolae	Yes	No
Spontaneous tyrosine kinase and PI3kinase activity	No	Yes
Constitutive tyrosine phosphorylation	No	Yes
Signals through Ras/MAPK upon activation	Yes	No
NB cell differentiation	Yes	No
Inhibits NB cell proliferation	Yes	No
Binds NGF	Yes	No
NB tumour suppressing activity	Yes	No
Oncogenic activity	No	Yes

Table 1. Summary of the differences between TrkAI and TrkAIII receptors expressed in SH-SY5Y NB cells.

3.3.4 TrkAIII as a NB oncogene

In contrast to the tumour-suppressing effects of TrkAI/II receptors in NB and NB models (Tacconelli et al., 2004; Nakagawara et al., 1992; Nakagawara & Koger, 2000; Nakagawara, 2001; Brodeur et al., 2006; Tanaka et al., 1998; Suzuki et al., 1993; Cao et al., 2010), TrkAIII transforms NIH3T3 fibroblasts rendering them tumourigenic in nude mice, promotes NB tumor-spheroid growth *in vitro;* and promotes primary (Tacconelli et al., 2004) and metastatic NB xenograft growth in nude mice (Figure 3), consistent with an oncogenic and pro-metastatic function. This is supported by the engineered deletion of the TrkA D4 Ig-like domain, which also results in oncogenic activation (Arevalo et al., 2000). TrkAIII, however, is also expressed by stressed non-tumourigenic normal neural stem cells, neural crest progenitors and normal thymocytes (Tacconelli et al., 2004, 2007), suggesting that TrkAIII transforming potential, like that of many oncogenes, depends upon additional factors.

A potential link between TrkAIII expression and metastatic bone disease, suggested by the increased capacity of TrkAIII transfected SH-SY5Y NB cells to form osteolytic bone metastases in nude mice (Figure 3), is also supported by the recent report that high TrkAIII expression and a low TrkAI/II to TrkAIII expression ratio associate significantly with metastatic bone disease in advanced stage human NB (Cao et al., 2010). The possibility that TrkAIII expression within primary tumours may both indicate and be involved in metastatic bone disease is of potential diagnostic/prognostic and therapeutic importance, considering that metastatic bone disease in NB carries immediate stage 4 diagnosis, very poor prognosis and is the major cause of post therapeutic disease relapse (Mugishima & Sakurai, 2000).

It is clear that the extracellular D4 domain and associated N-glycosylation sites, encoded within *TrkA* exons 6/7, are critical for correct TrkA receptor physiological function, cell surface expression, ligand-dependent activation and preventing ligand-independent receptor oncogenic activation (Arevalo et al., 2000; Watson et al., 1999). The loss of this domain confers oncogenic potential to TrkAIII (Tacconelli et al., 2004; Arevalo et al., 2000; Watson et al., 1999; Farina et al., 2009a, 2009b).

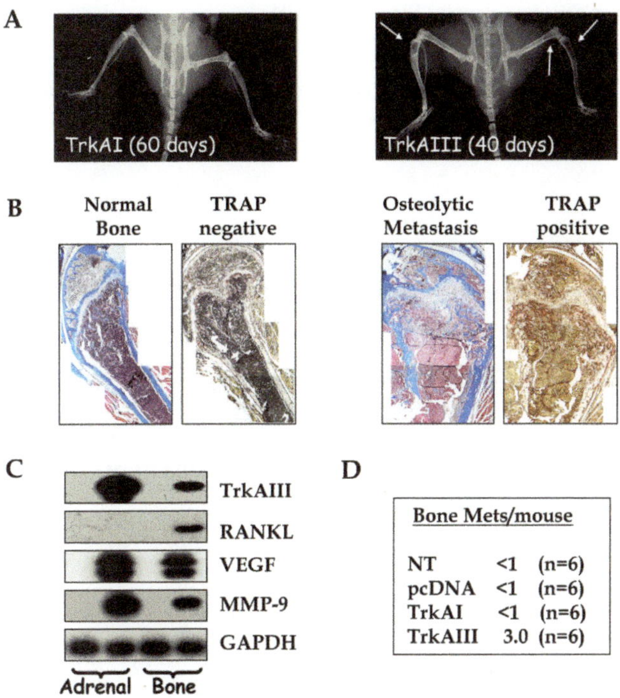

D

Bone Mets/mouse		
NT	<1	(n=6)
pcDNA	<1	(n=6)
TrkAI	<1	(n=6)
TrkAIII	3.0	(n=6)

E

Macro-Metastatic sites

	Skin	Adr	Trx	Lung	Liver	Bone	Brain	Survival (60 dy)
NT	0/6	0/6	0/6	0/6	0/6	1/6	0/6	5/6
pcDNA	0/6	0/6	0/6	0/6	0/6	1/6	0/6	6/6
TrkAI	0/6	0/6	0/6	0/6	0/6	1/6	0/6	5/6
TrkAIII	1/6	3/6	0/6	0/6	0/6	5/6	0/6	1/6

A) Radiographic appearance of normal bone and bone bearing osteolytic metastases (arrows) in representative nude mice injected via the intra-cardiac route with either TrkAI (60 days following injection) or TrkAIII (40 days following injection) transfected SH-SY5Y NB cells. B) Histological appearance of normal TRAP negative femur from a nude mouse 60 days following injection with TrkAI transfected SH-SY5Y cells and a TRAP positive osteolytic bone metastasis from a nude mouse 40 days following injection with TrkAIII transfected SH-SY5Y NB cells. C) RT-PCR Southern blot comparison of TrkAIII, RANKL, VEGF, MMP-9 and GAPDH mRNA expression in normal adrenal gland and normal bone versus adrenal and osteolytic bone metastasis from a nude mouse injected with TrkAIII expressing SH-SY5Y cells. D) The mean number of bone metastases per nude mouse 60 days following intra-cardiac injection with either non-transfected (NT), control pcDNA vector, TrkAI or TrkAIII transfected SH-SY5Y cells. E) The number and distribution of macro-metastases and 60 day survival-rate of nude mice injected via the intra-cardiac route with either non-transfected, empty pcDNA vector, TrkAI or TrkAIII transfected SH-SY5Y cells.

Fig. 3. TrkAIII Promotes osteolytic bone metastasis.

4. Getting to grips with intracellular TrkAIII

The intracellular membrane-associated retention of TrkAIII is a prerequisite for oncogenic potential and oncogenic activity in NB models. Therefore, a greater understanding of the intracellular membrane compartments within which TrkAIII locates and exhibits activity will improve our understanding of how TrkAIII exerts an oncogenic rather than tumour-suppressing function.

4.1 TrkAIII within the ER

Intracellular non-nuclear membranes are separated into the ER, ERGIC, GN, and associated transport vesicle compartments.

Ultracentrifugation fractionation of intracellular membranes, receptor pulse-labelling and indirect IF experiments clearly demonstrate that N-glycosylated immature gp110kDa TrkAI receptors move rapidly from the ER to the GN where they accumulate and mature into gp140kDa TrkA prior to being transported to the cell surface (Farina et al., 2009b). TrkAIII on the other hand, neither alters in molecular size nor reaches the cell surface but accumulates within the intracellular membrane compartment, exhibiting relatively equal steady-state distribution between ER, ERGIC, GN and vesicle membranes (Figure 4) (Farina et al., 2009a, 2009b).

TrkAIII accumulation within the ER suggests either that TrkAIII re-cycles back to the ER and/or exhibits difficulty overcoming the ER quality control (ERQC) system. The latter possibility is supported by constitutive association with between ER-associated TrkAIII and the ER chaperones Grp78/Bip and calnexin, which recognise and retain misfolded proteins within the ER as a protective measure (Gregerssen & Bross, 2010). In contrast, TrkAI interaction with these chaperones is not detected under normal conditions but is induced by conditions of ER-stress, which promote TrkAI ER-retention (Farina et al., 2009b). This implicates the TrkA D4 domain and associated N-glycosylation sites, omitted from TrkAIII, in the correct folding of TrkA within the ER and subsequent ER-exit of nascent TrkA receptors.

The possibility that TrkAIII ER-retention does not depend upon spontaneous receptor activation is supported by observations that TrkAIII is not activated throughout the ER ; that TrkAIII ER-retention is reduced by the PTPase inhibitor sodium orthovanadate in association with augmented TrkAIII activity (Figure 5) (Farina et al., 2009b), by the observation that tyrosine kinase dead Y674/675F mutated TrkAIII exhibits enhanced ER-retention and that inhibition of TrkAIII activity by the tyrosine kinase inhibitor CEP-701 promotes TrkAIII ER-retention (Farina et al., 2009a, 2009b). In contrast, cell surface gp140TrkAI but not intracellular GN-associated gp110TrkAI is activated by sodium orthovanadate. This suggests that intracellular TrkAI, unlike TrkAIII, is not maintained in an intracellular inactive state by associated PTPases (Figure 5). These observations indicate that TrkAIII within the ER exists largely in PTPase-inhibited form, complexed with Brp78/Bip and calnexin; with inactivation promoting ER-retention. The PTPases responsible for inhibiting TrkAIII within the ER remain to be elucidated.

4.2 TrkAIII within the ERGIC/GN/vesicle compartment

In SH-SY5Y NB cells, TrkAIII overcomes ERQC, confirmed by the loss of Grp78/Bip and calnexin binding by non-ER membrane-associated TrkAIII, and distributes to the ERGIC, GN and associated vesicles compartments in roughly equal steady-state levels (Farina et al., 2009a, 2009b). TrkAIII activation, on the other hand, exhibits a relatively restricted association with a peri-nuclear centralised vesicle population that closely overlaps ERGIC and GN membranes (Farina et al., 2009a), suggesting conditions favourable for spontaneous TrkAIII activation localise to a relatively specific intracellular vesicle compartment in NB cells.

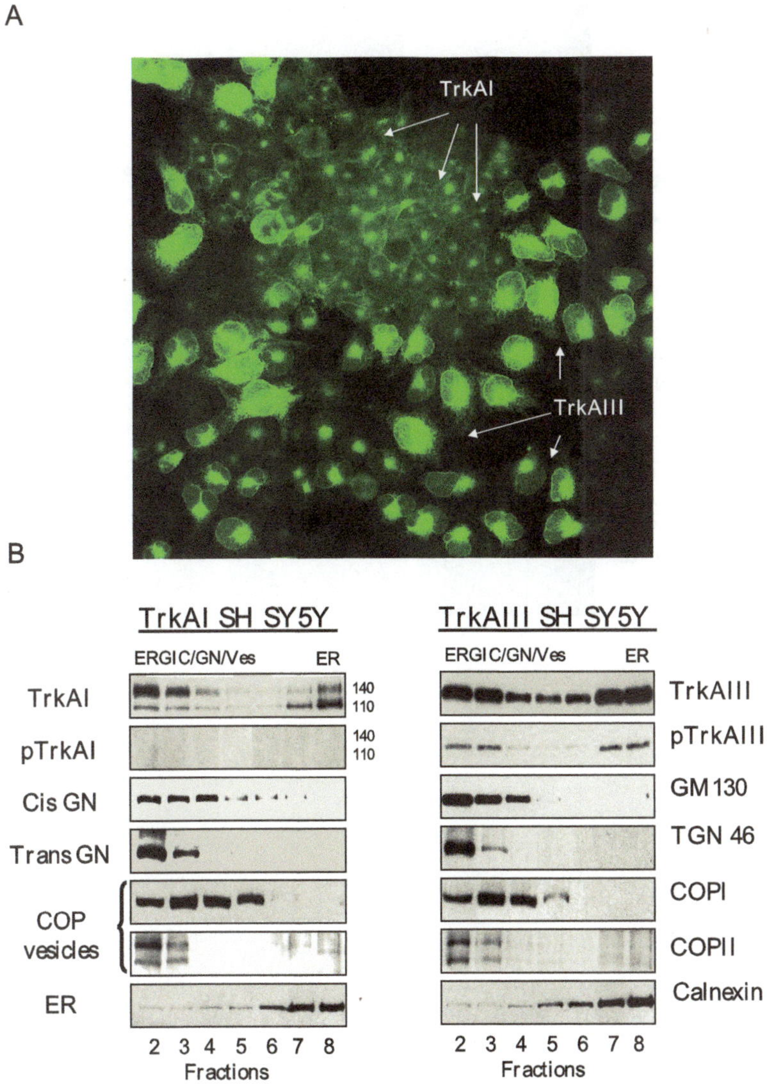

A) Indirect IF demonstrating differences in cell surface and GN-associated TrkAI expression and intracellular TrkAIII expression in a mixed population of TrkAI and TrkAIII transfected SH-SY5Y cells. B) Western blots demonstrating differences in TrkAI and TrkAIII distribution in ultracentrifugation density gradient-purified intracellular ER, GN and COP vesicle membranes from TrkAI and TrkAIII transfected SH-SY5Y cells.

Fig. 4. Comparison of TrkAI and TrkAIII localisation in SH-SY5Y cells.

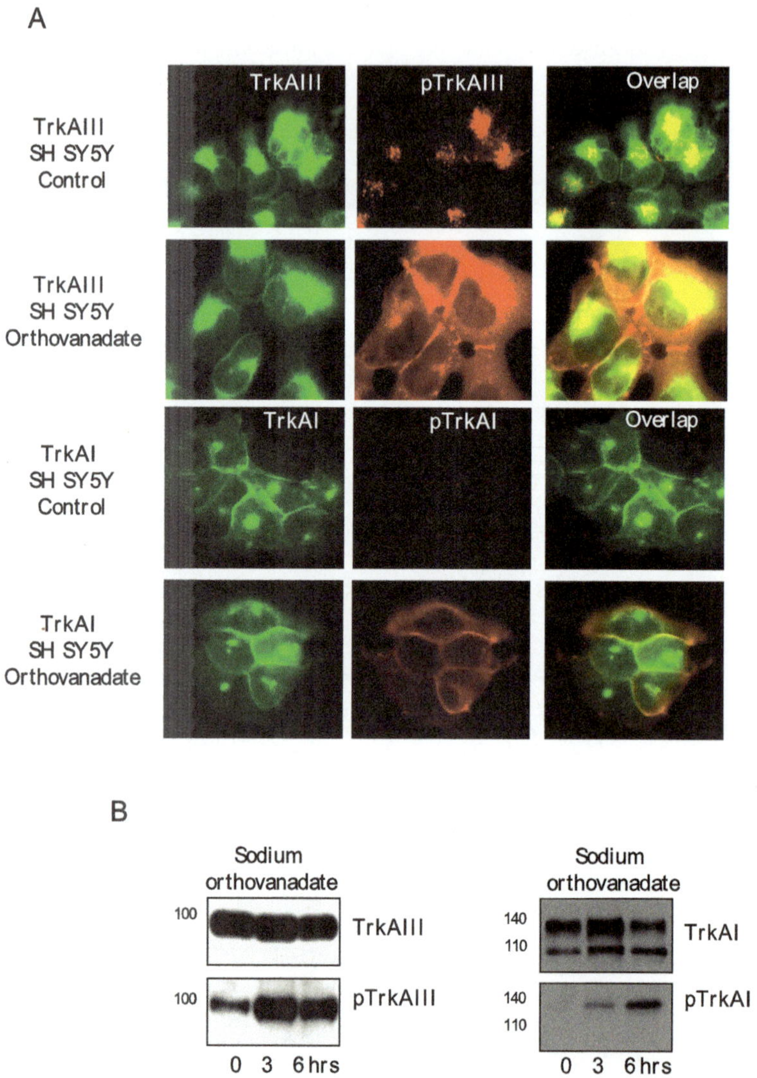

A) Indirect IF demonstrating the augmenting effect of the PTPase inhibitor sodium orthovanadate on intracellular TrkAIII tyrosine phosphorylation levels and capacity to induce tyrosine phosphorylation of cell surface gp140TrkAI but not intracellular gp110TrkAI, in stable transfected SH-SY5Y cells. B) Western blots demonstrating the augmenting effect of sodium orthovanadate upon total TrkAIII tyrosine phosphorylated levels and its capacity to induce tyrosine phosphorylation of TrkAI in stable transfected SH-SY5Y cells.

Fig. 5. Intracellular TrkAIII but not intracellular TrkAI exhibits spontaneous PTPase-regulated activity.

TrkAIII activation within this vesicle compartment is inhibited by Brefeldin A (Farina et al., 2009a, 2009b), a non-competitive inhibitor of G-protein the Arf-1 and ERGIC/GN disrupting agent (Szul et al., 2007), indicating that TrkAIII activation in SH-SY5Y cells is ARF-1 dependent and occurs within the context of full ERGIC/GN assembly.

TrkAIII activation, furthermore, is not inhibited by anti-catalytic anti-NGF antibodies nor by c-Src inhibitors or A_{2A} adenosine receptor antagonists (Farina et al., 2009a, 2009b), confirming that TrkAIII activation in this vesicle compartment is spontaneous and ligand-independent, and most likely facilitated by D4 domain omission, combined with a localised deficit in PTPase activity.

Spontaneous TrkAIII activity within the ERGIC/GN associated vesicle compartment also depends upon TrkAIII interaction with the heat shock protein ATPase "Hsp-90", and is inhibited by the Hsp90 inhibitor Geldanamycin A (GA) and its clinically relevant analogues 17-AAG and 17-DMAG, currently in clinical trials for potential use in NB (Farina et al., 2009b; Szul et al., 2007). TrkAIII can, therefore, be added to EGFRvIII, BCR-Abl, Flt3 and PDGFR oncogene Hsp90 clients that exhibit sensitivity to GA and GA-analogues (Szul et al., 2007; Xu & Neckers, 2007). However, the potential therapeutic use of GA-analogues as TrkAIII inhibitors in NB is mitigated by the observations that GA and GA-analogues also inhibit TrkAI expression, neurotrophin-mediated TrkAI activation and subsequent post-receptor signalling, suggesting potential for side-effects on normal TrkA-dependent cellular functions. Furthermore, ER-associated inactivated TrkAIII induces a protective ER-stress response that is potentially involved in increasing NB cell resistance to GA-induced cytotoxicity (Farina et al., 2009b) (see section 7.3.).

Intracellular TrkAIII activation is also restricted to interphase, lost during mitosis in association with ERGIC/GN disruption, with re-activation observed post cytokinesis in association with ERGIC/GN reassembly (Farina et al., 2009a). TrkAIII activation is, therefore, subject to cell cycle regulation and occurs within the context of a fully assembled ERGIC/GN compartment.

Intracellular TrkAIII activated within ERGIC/GN-associated vesicles exhibits cytoplasmic tyrosine kinase domain orientation (Farina et al., 2009a). This places TrkAIII within a novel substrate context, a more detailed understanding of which will be critical for more detailed elucidation TrkAIII oncogenic function. This is exemplified by the novel interaction reported between TrkAIII and the interphase centrosome (Farina et al., 2009a) (see section 7.5.), which unveils a novel alternative oncogenic mechanism to "Classical" cell surface oncogenic RTK signalling.

5. Potential TrkAIII oncogenic mechanisms

5.1 Growth and differentiation

TrkA expression is considered to be a prerequisite for NB cell differentiation and tumour regression (Nakagawara, 2001). In support of this, TrkA gene transduction restores NGF responsiveness to NB cells and induces differentiation, growth arrest and/or apoptosis (Tacconelli et al., 2004; Matsushima et al., 1990; Lavenius et al., 1995; Lucarelli et al., 1997; Eggert et al., 2002). NGF/TrkA-mediated NB cell growth arrest and differentiation has been reported to depend upon Ras/MAPK pathway activation (Pumiglia & Decker, 1997). In contrast to TrkAI, TrkAIII transduction into NB cells neither induces growth arrest nor differentiation but inhibits the differentiation-inducing effects of NGF-activated TrkAI by antagonising Ras/MAPK signalling (Tacconelli et al., 2004). This places alternative TrkAIII splicing as a potential pivotal regulator of neurotrophin-mediated NB differentiation, helping to maintain NB cells in an undifferentiated state.

5.2 Angiogenesis

Angiogenesis is essential for primary and metastatic tumour growth and results in the formation of a relatively disorganised tumor neo-vasculature, required for oxygenation and nutrition of the growing tumour mass (Folkman, 2006). In contrast to TrkAI/II which has been reported to inhibit angiogenic factor expression and reduce tumour associated angiogenesis (Eggert et al., 2000, 2002), TrkAIII stimulates tumour-associated angiogenesis in NB models and alters the angiogenic equilibrium between MMP-9, VEGF and Tsp-1, increasing VEGF and MMP-9 but reducing Tsp-1 expression (Tacconelli et al., 2004). This equilibrium is an important determinant of tumour angiogenesis, since MMP-9 triggers VEGF-mediated angiogenesis and Tsp-1 inhibits both MMP-9 activation and VEGF activity (Bergers et al., 2000; Rodriguez-Manzaneque et al., 2001). The alteration of this equilibrium by TrkAIII is PI3K but not Ras/MAPK dependent (Tacconelli et al., 2004) and provides a potential angiogenic mechanism through which TrkAIII exerts oncogenic activity.

5.3 Induction of a more stress-resistant phenotype

The attainment of a more stress-resistant phenotype is not only involved in tumour progression but is a major determinant in eventual disease relapse from a "no evidence of disease" status. TrkAIII promotes a more stress-resistant NB cell phenotype, increasing resistance to the cytotoxic effects of the chemotherapeutic agents doxorubicin (Tacconelli et al., 2004) and GA (Farina et al., 2009b). This effect may not only involve protective PI3K/Akt/NF-κB signalling (Jaboin et al., 2002) but also the pre-conditioning of cells to stress as a result of partial activation of an ER-stress response (Farina et al., 2009b).

The ER stress response, reviewed elsewhere (Ron & Walter, 2007), is caused by the accumulation of unfolded or misfolded proteins within the ER, which results in the activation of three ER transmembrane proteins IRE1α, PERK and ATF6, all of which attempt to shift the ER back to homeostasis. PERK activation impedes protein translation, IRE1α activation splices XBP1 mRNA to produce the homeostatic transcription factor XBP1s which, together with activated ATF6(n), increases the transcription of genes that augment ER size, increase ER function and protect against apoptosis. Should this adaptive response be insufficient, the ER-response switches to apoptosis-inducing mode, considered to be caused by continuous IRE1α and PERK activation (Shore et al., 2011). In human SH-SY5Y NB cells, TrkAIII induces partial activation of the ER-stress response by activating ATF6(N) and increasing the expression of Grp78/BiP but does not induced XBP1 mRNA splicing to XBP1s (Farina et al., 2009b). This modified ER-stress response pre-conditions cells to resist further stress, helping to explain why TrkAIII expressing NB cells exhibit resistance to GA-induced cytotoxicity, despite GA-inhibition of TrkAIII tyrosine kinase activity (Farina et al., 2009b). This provides an additional oncogenic mechanism through which inactive TrkAIII retained within the ER may promote NB cell survival within the stressful tumour microenvironment.

5.4 Bone metastasis: Stress resistance, angiogenesis and RANKL

TrkAIII expression in SH-SY5Y NB cells promotes the formation of osteolytic bone metastases in a nude mouse model. This effect is likely to involve the osteoclast-differentiation factor RANKL (Tanaka et al., 2005), the expression of which is induced by TrkAIII expressing NB cells within the bone metastatic environment, which together with a more angiogenic and stress-resistant phenotype results in the growth of osteolytic metastases (Figure 3). Furthermore, the relatively hypoxic bone environment would be expected to promote alternative TrkAIII splicing in NB cells arriving within the bone marrow, providing a novel potential molecular mechanism for promoting NB metastasis to bone, consistent with Paget's "Seed and Soil" hypothesis for organ specific metastasis (Paget, 1989; Cao et al., 2010). This possibility is supported by the reported association between high level TrkAIII expression and low TrkAI/II to TrkAIII expression ratio with metastatic bone disease in NB patients (Cao et al., 2010).

5.5 Centrosome amplification and genetic instability

Interphase-restricted spontaneous activation of TrkAIII within ERGIC/GN-associated vesicles, in cytoplasmic tyrosine kinase domain orientation, results in interaction between a proportion of TrkAIII and the interphase centrosome, around which the ERGIC, GN and associated vesicle compartments assemble and integrate (Farina et al., 2009a; Mazzorana et al., 2011). This interaction is characterised by TrkAIII co-purification with centrosomes; TrkAIII binding of centrosome γ-tubulin; TrkAIII-mediated tyrosine phosphorylation of centrosome components; increased centrosome interaction with polo kinase 4; decreased centrosome interaction with separase; and centrosome amplification (Farina et al., 2009a). The result of this interaction is increased genetic instability characterised by: multi-polar spindle formation; mitotic catastrophe; anaphase DNA bridging; multinuclear cell formation; polyploidy and aneuploidy (Farina et al., 2009a). Therefore, TrkAIII also acts as a novel membrane-associated centrosome tyrosine kinase, promoting centrosome amplification and increasing genetic instability, unveiling an important and novel alternative mechanism through which TrkAIII exerts oncogenic activity.

TrkAIII promotion of genetic instability, combined with increased stress-resistance and angiogenesis, suggests that TrkAIII could act early during tumour progression to promote the accumulation of genetic damage within the hostile primary tumour microenvironment, progressing malignant tumours inevitably towards eventual oncosuppressor loss.

6. The clinical significance of assessing alternative TrkAIII splicing in NB prognosis

The possibility that alternative TrkA splicing represents a novel diagnostic/prognostic factor in NB is supported by two reports (Tacconelli et al., 2004; Cao et al., 2010). In the first, TrkAI/II and TrkAIII expression assessed by densitometric RT-PCR/Southern blotting in 24 primary human NBs found predominant TrkAIII over TrkAI/II expression in 1 of 11 stage 1/2 , and in 6 of 13 stage 3/4 NBs. A significantly higher TrkAI/II to TrkAIII expression ratio was also detected in stage 1/2 compared to stage 3/4 NBs, suggesting that the TrkAI/II to TrkAIII expression ratio decreases in association with disease progression and visa versa. In the second report (Cao et al., 2010), SYBR I Green fluorescent quantitative PCR was used to quantify alternative TrkAI/II and TrkAIII splicing in 39 NBs and results used to estimate 5 year survival rates. In this study, TrkAI/II expression was found to be significantly lower in tumours of high stage and higher in tumours of low stage, whereas TrkAIII expression was low in low stage tumours and significantly higher in high stage tumours. Univariate analysis revealed that the 5 year survival rate of patients aged >1year with abdominal tumors, bone metastases and a low TrkAI/II to TrkAIII ratio was significantly lower than controls, whereas multivariate analysis demonstrated that only a low TrkAI/II to TrkAIII ratio and bone metastasis exerted a negative impact upon the 5-year survival rate. From these studies, it appears that high TrkAI/II expression characterises NBs with better prognosis, whereas high TrkAIII expression characterise NBs with poor prognosis, suggesting that early assessment of alternative TrkA splicing, combined with bone scanning, may represent an important diagnostic/prognostic parameter in NB.

7. Potential therapeutic ways of reducing TrkAIII involvement in NB

TrkAIII exhibits predominant expression in advanced stage NB and promotes oncogenesis in NB models in association with spontaneous activation and chronic post-receptor signalling through the PI3K/Akt/NF-κB but not Ras/MAPK pathway. This results in an impediment to NB cell differentiation and growth inhibition; augmented stress- resistance, increased genetic instability, and a more angiogenic and tumorigenic phenotype (Tacconelli et al., 2004; Farina et al., 2009a, 2009b). This suggests that inhibitors of TrkAIII tyrosine kinase activity and/or post TrkAIII signalling, may be an important addition to future NB therapy.

Within this context, the Trk kinase inhibitors K252α and its analogue CEP-701; the ARF inhibitor BFA and the Hsp90 inhibitor GA have all been shown to inhibit TrkAIII tyrosine kinase activity (Farina et al., 2009a, 2009b). CEP-701 reversibly inhibits TrkAIII tyrosine kinase activity and TrkAIII-induced centrosome amplification at nanomolar concentrations (Farina et al., 2009a), exhibits anti-tumor activity in NB xenograft models (Evans et al., 1999) and is in clinical trials in NB patients (Brodeur et al., 2009). The fungal macrolide BFA, a non-competitive interfacial inhibitor of the interaction between *sec7* domain-containing ARF-GEFs and ARFs 1 and 5, that disrupts the ERGIC/GN compartment by inhibiting the GDP-GTP ARF cycle necessary for vesicle assembly (Vigil et al., 2010; Pommier & Cherfils, 2005), reversibly inhibits TrkAIII tyrosine kinase activity in association with ERGIC/GN disruption (Farina et al., 2009a, 2009b). BFA exhibits anti-tumour activity that is mainly additive to standard chemotherapeutic agents in neuroendocrine tumor cells (Larsson et al., 2009), suggesting therapeutic potential for interfacial inhibitors of sec7 domain ARF-GEF/ARF interaction in reducing TrkAIII tyrosine kinase involvement in NB. The ansinomycin antibiotic, Hsp90 inhibitor, GA and its clinically relevant analogues, 17-AAG and 17-DMAG, inhibit RTK oncogene activity, NB xenograft tumour growth and are currently in clinical trials for potential future use in NB (Szul et al., 2007; Kang et al., 2006). GA and GA-analogues reversibly inhibit TrkAIII tyrosine kinase activity and inhibit proliferation of TrkAIII expressing NB cells (Farina et al., 2009a, 2009b), suggesting potential therapeutic use for reducing TrkAIII involvement in NB.

Inhibitors of TrkAIII tyrosine kinase activity, however, do not inhibit TrkAIII expression nor promote TrkAIII degradation but cause redistribution of inactive TrkAIII back to the ER, with potential to induce and/or augment a protective ER-stress response (Farina et al., 2009a, 2009b). This may explain the high level of resistance to GA-mediated cytotoxicity exhibited by TrkAIII but not TrkAI transfected NB cells, associated with an altered ER-stress response, despite GA-mediated inhibition of TrkAIII activity (Farina et al., 2009a, 2009b). Therefore, in addition to potential off-target effects, reversible TrkAIII-targeted kinase inhibitors may increase stress-resistance by promoting TrkAIII ER-retention and inducing a subsequent ER-stress response. Indeed, GA selects resistant slow growing TrkAIII expressing NB cells from mixed populations, which exhibit TrkAIII re-activation post GA removal, suggesting a potential mechanisms for post GA-therapy relapse (Farina et al., 2009b). We consider, therefore, that combined inhibition of TrkAIII expression and activity may represent a preferable therapeutic goal. For this purpose, we are currently developing specific peptide nucleic acid (PNA) inhibitors of TrkAIII expression based upon sequence at the novel exon5/exon 8 splice junction (TrkAIII PNA conjugate $(KKAA)_4$-GGCCGGGACAC) (Farina et al., 2009a, 2009b). Current TrkAIII PNA conjugates inhibit TrkAIII but not TrkAI expression at micromolar concentrations and restore sensitivity to GA-induced cytotoxicity in TrkAIII expressing NB cells (Farina et al., 2009b). We are further developing these inhibitors in order to optimise uptake and lower effective inhibitory concentrations.

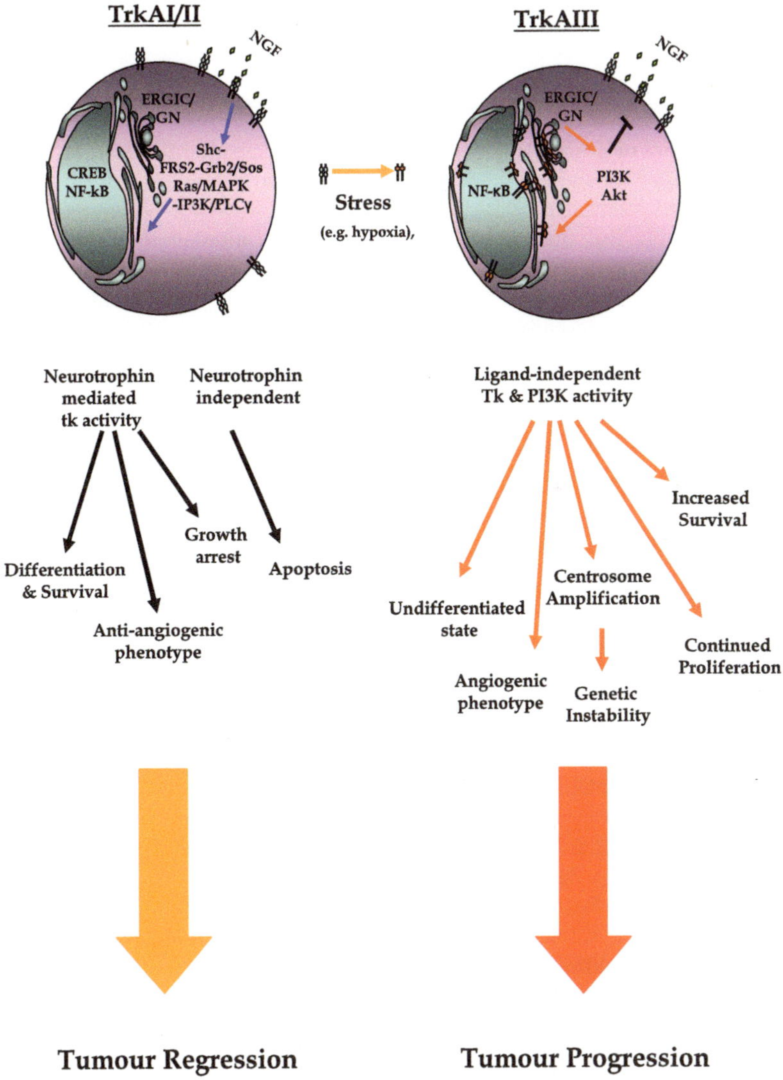

Summary of the differences in signalling, localisation and biological tumour suppressing outcome of TrkAI/II expression and tumour promoting/oncogenic outcome of stress-regulated alternative TrkAIII splicing

Fig. 6. Alternative TrkAIII splicing: a regulated NB tumour-promoting switch.

At the post receptor signalling level, PI3K/Akt pathway inhibitors reverse the pro-angiogenic effect of TrkAIII on the MMP-9/VEGF/TSP-1 equilibrium and may, therefore, be useful in reducing the pro-angiogenic TrkAIII effects, in addition to reducing protective PI3K/Akt/NF-κB signalling in TrkAIII expressing NB cells (Tacconelli et al., 2004).
The further elucidation of the molecular mechanisms responsible for promoting alternative TrkAIII splicing in NB cells may provide novel ways to reverse this process to favour tumour-suppressing TrkAI/II splicing.

8. Conclusions

The association between alternative TrkAIII splicing and advanced stage NB; the tumour-suppressing potential of TrkAI/II and oncogenic/tumour promoting potential of TrkAIII in NB models, and hypoxia up-regulation of alternative TrkAIII splicing in NB cells, suggest that stress-regulated alternative TrkAIII splicing may represent a pivotal promoter of NB tumour progression. The mechanisms through which intracellular TrkAIII exerts its oncogenic effects include: maintenance of a de-differentiated state; increased stress-resistance; increased genetic instability and the promotion of a more angiogenic and tumourigenic phenotype, and are summarised in Figure 6.
We propose that the assessment of alternative TrkA splicing in NB is of potential prognostic/diagnostic value and that the best way to limit TrkAIII and reduce its tumour promoting influence would be to combine inhibitors of TrkAIII expression (PNA and/or siRNA) and tyrosine kinase activity (CEP-701, BFA, GA-analogues), within the context of current chemotherapeutic protocols.

9. Acknowledgements

This work was supported by grants from AIRC, PRIN and the "Maugeri" Foundation.

10. References

Arevalo, J. C.; Conde, B.; Hempstead, B. I.; Chao, M. V.; Martin-Zanca, D. & Perez, P. (2001). A novel mutation within the extracellular domain of TrkA causes constitutive receptor activation. *Oncogene,* 20, 1229-1234

Arevalo, J. C.; Conde, B.; Hempstead, B. L.; Chao, M. V.; Matrin-Zanca, D. & Perez, P. (2000). TrkA immunoglobulin-like ligand binding domains inhibit spontaneous activation of the receptor. *Molecular and Cellular Biology,* 20, 5908-5916

Azar, C. G.; Scavarda, N. J.; Reynolds, C. P. & Brodeur, G. M. (1990). Multiple defects of the nerve growth factor receptor in human neuroblastomas. *Cell Growth & Differentiation,* 1, 421-428

Barker, P. A.; Lomen-Hoerth, C.; Gensch, E. M.; Meakin, S. O.; Glass, D. J. & Shooter, E. M. (1993). Tissue specific alternative splicing generates two isoforms of the TrkA receptor. *Journal of Biological Chemistry,* 268, 15150-15157

Bennasruone, A.; Gardin, A.; Aunis, D.; Cremel, G. & Hubert, P. (2004). Tyrosine kinase receptors as attractive targets of cancer therapy. *Critical Reviews in Oncology and Hematology,* 50, 23-38

Bergers, G.; Brekken, R.; McMahon, G.; Vu, T. H.; Itoh, T.; Tamaki, K.; Tanzawa, K.; Thorpe, P.; Itohara, S.; Werb, Z. & Hanahan, D. (2000). Matrix metalloproteinase-9 triggers the angiogenic switch during carcinogenesis. *Nature Cell Biology,* 2, 737-744

Bibel, M. & Barde, Y-A. (2000). Neurotrophins: key regulators of cell fate and cell shape in the vertebrate nervous system. *Genes and Development*, 14, 2919-2937

Brodeur, G. M.; Mintum, J. E.; Ho, R.; Simpson, A. M.; Iyer, R.; Varela, C. R.; Light, J. E.; Kolla, V. & Evans, A. E. (2009). Trk receptor expression and inhibition in neuroblastomas. *Clinical Cancer Research*, 15, 3244-3250

Cao, F.; Liu, X.; Zhang, J.; Wang, Y. & Zhang, N. (2010). Expression of TrkA splicing isoforms in neuroblastoma and its clinical significance. *Chinese Journal of Clinical Oncology*, 37, 1282-1285

Clary, D. O. & Reichardt, L. F. (1994). An alternative splice form of the nerve growth factor receptor confers an enhanced response to neurotrophin 3. *Proceedings of the National Academy of Science.* USA, 91, 11133-11137

Coulier, F.; Kumar, R.; Ernst, M.; Klein, R.; Martin-Zanca, D. & Barbacid, M. (1990). Human Trk oncogenes activated by point mutation, in-frame deletion, and duplication of the tryrosine kinase domain. *Molecular and Cellular Biology*, 10, 4202-4210

Cunningham, M. E.; Stephens, R. M.; Kaplan, D. R. & Greene, L. A. (1997). Autophosphorylation of activation loop tyrosines regulates signalling by the Trk nerve growth factor receptor. *Journal of Biological Chemistry*, 272, 10957- 10967

Dubus, P.; Parrens, M.; El-Mokhtari, Y.; Ferrer, J.; Groppi, A. & Merlio, J. P. (2000). Identification of novel TrkA variants with deletions in the leucine-rich motifs of the extracellular domain. *Journal of Neuroimmunology*, 107, 42-49

Eggert, A.; Grotzer, M. A.; Ikegaki, N.; Liu, X. G.; Evans, A.E. & Brodeur, G. M. (2002). Expression of the neurotrophin receptor TrkA down-regulates expression and function of angiogenic stimulators in SH-SY5Y neuroblastoma cells. *Cancer Research*, 62, 1802-1808

Eggert, A.; Ikegaki, N.; Liu, X.; Chou, T. T.; Lee, V. M.; Trojanowski, J. Q. & Brodeur, G. M. (2000). Molecular dissection of TrkA signal transduction pathways mediating differentiation in human neuroblastoma cells. *Oncogene*, 19, 2043- 2051

Ernsberger, U. (2009). Role of neurotrophin signalling in the differentiation of neurons from dorsal root ganglia and sympathetic ganglia. *Cell and Tissue Research*, 336, 349-384

Evans, A. (2000). Neuroblastoma a historical perspective, In: *Neuroblastoma*, Brodeur, G.M.; Sawada, T.; Tsuchida, S. & Voute, P. A. (Eds.), pp1-7, Elsevier Press, ISBM: 0 444 50222X, Amsterdam, Holland

Evans, A. E.; Kisselbach, K. D.; Yamashiro, D. J.; Ikegaki, N.; Camoratto, A. M.; Dionne, C. A. & Brodeur, G. M. (1999). Antitumor activity of CEP-751 (KT-6587) on human neuroblastoma and medulloblastoma xenografts. *Clinical Cancer Research*, 5:3594-3602

Farina, A. R.; Tacconelli, A.; Cappabianca, L.; Cea, G.; Chioda, A.; Romanelli, A.; Pensato, S.; Pedone, C.; Gulino, A. & Mackay, A. R. (2009b). The neuroblastoma tumour-suppressor TrkAI and its oncogenic alternative TrkAIII splice variant exhibit geldanamycin-sensitive interactions with Hsp90 in human neuroblastoma cells. *Oncogene*, 28, 4075-4094

Farina, A. R.; Tacconelli, A.; Cappabianca, L.; Cea, G.; Panella, S.; Chioda, A.; Romanelli, A.; Pedone, C.; Gulino, A. & Mackay, A. R. (2009a). The TrkAIII splice variant targets the centrosome and promotes genetic instability. *Molecular Cellular Biology*, 29, 4812-4830

Fiore, M.; Chaldakov, G. N. & Aloe, L. (2009). Nerve growth factor as a signalling molecule for nerve cells and also for the neuroendocrine-immune systems. *Reviews in Neuroscience*, 20, 133-145

Folkman, J. (2006). Angiogenesis. *Annual Reviews in Medicine*, 57, 1-18

George, D. J.; Suzuki, H.; Bova, G. S. & Isaacs, J. T. (1998). Mutational analysis of the TrkA gene in prostate cancer. *Prostate*, 36, 172-180

Greco, A.; Miranda, C. & Pierroti, M. A. (2010). Rearrangements of NTRK-1 gene in papillary thyroid carcinoma. *Molecular and Cellular Endocrinology*, 321, 44-49

Greco, A.; Villa, R. & Pierotti, M. A. (1996). Genomic organisation of the human NTRK1 gene. *Oncogene*, 13, 2463-2466

Green, L. A. & Kaplan, R. M. (1995). Early events in neurotrophin signaling via Trk and p75 receptors. *Current Opinions in Neurobiology*, 5, 579-587

Gregerssen, N. & Bross, P. (2010). Protein misfolding and cellular stress: an overview. *Methods in Molecular Biology*, 648, 3- 23

Hallberg, B.; Ashcroft, M.; Loeb, D. M. & Kaplan, R.M. (1998). Nerve growth factor induced stimulation of Ras requires Trk interaction with Shc but does not involve phosphoinositol 3-OH kinase. *Oncogene*, 17, 691-697

Hempstead, B. L.; Martin-Zanca, D.; Kaplan, D. R.; Parada, L. F. & Chao, M. V. (1991). High affinity NGF binding requires coexpression of the trk proro-oncogene and low affinity NGF receptor. *Nature*, 350, 678-683

Holden, P. H.; Asopa, V.; Robertson, A. G.; Clarke, A. R.; Tyler, S.; Bennett, G.; Brain, S. D.; Wilcock, G. K.; Allen, S. J.; Smith, S. K. & Dawbarn, D. (1997). Immunoglobulin-like domains define the nerve growth factor binding site for the TrkA receptor. *Nature Biotechnology*, 15, 668-672

Howe, C. I.; Valletta, J. S.; Rusnak, A. S. & Mobley, W. C. (2004). NGF signalling from clatherin-coated vesicles. Evidence that signalling endosomes serve as a platform for the Ras/MAPK pathway. *Journal of Neurobiology*, 58, 207- 216

Jaboin, J.; Kim, C. J.; Kaplan, D. R. & Thiele, C. J. (2002). Brain-derived neurotophic factor activation of TrkA protects neuroblastoma cells form chemotherapy-induced apoptosis via phsophatidylinositol-3 kinase pathway. *Cancer Research*, 62, 6756-6763

Jiang, M.; Stanke, J. & Lahti, J. M. (2011) The connections between neural crest development and neuroblastoma. *Current Trends in Developmental Biology*, 94, 77-127

Kalnina, Z.; Zayakin, P.; Silina, K. & Line, A. (2005). Alterations in pre-mRNA splicing in cancer. *Genes Chromosomes and Cancer*, 42, 342-357

Kang, J.; Kamal, A.; Burrows, F. J.; Evers, B. M. & Chung, D. N. (2006). Inhibition of neuroblastoma xenograft growth by Hsp90 inhibitors. *Anticancer Research*, 26, 1903-1908

Kaplan, D. R. & Miller, F. D. (2000). Neurotrophin signal transduction in the nervous system. *Current Opinions in Neurobiology*, 10, 381-391

Kaplan, D. R. & Stevens, R. M. (1994). Neurotrophin signal transduction by the Trk receptor. *Journal of Neurobiology*, 25, 1404-1417

Kaplan, D. R.; Martin-Zanca, D. & Parada, L. F. (1991). Tyrosine phosphorylation and tyrosine kinase activity of the trk proto-oncogene product induced by NGF. *Nature*, 350, 358-160

Klein, R.; Jing, S.; Nanduri, V.; O'Rourke, E. & Barbacid, M. (1991). The trk proto-oncogene encodes a receptor for nerve growth factor. *Cell*, 65, 189-197

Larsson, D. E.; Hassan, S.; Larsson, R.; Oberg, K. & Granberg, D. (2009). Combination analysis of anti-cancer drugs on neuroendocrine tumor cell lines. *Cancer Chemotherapy and Pharmacology*, 65, 5-12

Lavenius, E.; Gestblom, C.; Johansson, I.; Nanberg, E. & Pahlmen, S. (1995). Transfection of TrkA into human neuroblastoma cells restores ability to differentiate in response to nerve growth factor. *Cell Growth & Differentiation*, 6, 727-736

Lucarelli, E.; Kaplan, D. & Thiele, C.J. (1997). Activation of trk-A but not trk-B signal transduction pathway inhibits growth of neuroblastoma cells. *European Journal of Cancer*, 33, 2068-2070

Majdan, M.; Walsh, G. S.; Aloyz, R. & Miller, F. D. (2001). TrkA mediates developmental sympathetic neuron survival by silencing an ongoing p75NTR-mediated death signal. *Journal of Cell Biology*, 155, 1275-1285

Marsh, H. N.; Dubreuil, C. I.; Quevedo, C.; Lee, A.; Majdan, M.; Walsh, G. S.; Housedorn, S.; Said, F. A.; Zoueva, O.; Kozlowski, M.; Siminovitch, K.; Neel, B. G.; Miller, F. D. & Kaplan, D. R. (2003). SHP-1 negatively regulates neuronal survival by functioning as a TrkA phosphatase. *Journal of Cell Biology*, 163, 999-1010

Martin-Zanca, D.; Hughes, S. H. & Barbacid, M. (1986). A human oncogene formed by the fusion of truncated tropomyosin and protein tyrosine kinase sequences. *Nature*, 319, 743-748

Martin-Zanca, D.; Oskam, R.; Mitra, G.; Copeland, T. & Barbacid, M. (1989). Molecular and biochemical characterisation of the human Trk oncogene. *Molecular and Cellular Biology*, 9, 24-33

Matsushima, H. & Bogenmann, E. (1990). Nerve growth factor (NGF) induces neuronal differentiation in neuroblastoma cells transfected with the NGF receptor cDNA. *Molecular and Cellular Biology*, 10, 5015-5020

Mazzorana, M.; Montoya, G. & Mortuza, G. B. (2011). The centrosome a target for cancer therapy. *Current Cancer Drug Targets*. 11, 600-612

Meakin, S. O.; MacDonald, J. I. S.; Gryz, E. A.; Kubu, C. J. & Verdi, J. M. (1999). The signalling adapter FRS-2 competes with Shc for binding to the nerve growth factor receptor TrkA. A model discriminating between proliferation and differentiation. *Journal of Biological Chemistry*, 274, 9861-9870

Mischel, P. S.; Umbach, J. A.; Eskandari, S.; Smith, S. G.; Gundersen, C. B. & Zampighi, G. A. (2002). Nerve growth factor signals via pre-existing TrkA receptor oligomers. *Biophysical Journal*, 83, 968-976

Modrek, B. & Lee, C. (2005). A genomic view of alternative splicing. *Nature Genetics*. 30, 13-19

Moelling, K.; Schad, K.; Bosse, M.; Zimmermann, S. & Schweneker, M. (2002). Regulation of Raf-Akt crosstalk. *Journal of Biological Chemistry*, 277, 31099-31106

Moises, T.; Dreier, A.; Flhor, S.; Esser, M.; Brauers, E.; Reiss, K.; Merken, D.; Weis, J. & Kruttgen, A. (2007). Tracking TrkA's trafficking. NGF receptor Trafficking controls NGF receptor signalling. *Molecular Neurobiology*, 35, 151-159

Monshipouri, M.; Jiang, H. & Lazarovici, P. (2000). NGF stimulation of erk phosphorylation is impaired by a point mutation in the transmembrane domain of trkA receptor. *Journal of Molecular Neuroscience*, 14, 69-76

Mugishima, H. & Sakurai, M. (2000). Symptoms of Neuroblastoma: Paraneoplastic syndromes, In: *Neuroblastoma*, Brodeur, G.M.; Sawada, T.; Tsuchida, S. & Voute, P. A. (Eds.), pp293-301, Elsevier Press, ISBM: 0 444 50222X, Amsterdam, Holland

Nakagawara A (2004). Neural crest development and neuroblastoma: the genetic and biological link. *Progress in Brain Research*,146, 233-242

Nakagawara, A (2001). Trk receptor tyrosine kinases: a bridge between cancer and neural development. *Cancer Letters*, 169, 107-114

Nakagawara, A. & Koger, P. (2000). Expression and function of Trk and its related genes in human neuroblastoma. In: *Neuroblastoma,* Brodeur, G.M.; Sawada, T.; Tsuchida, S. & Voute, P. A. (Eds.), pp147-157, Elsevier Press, ISBM: 0 444 50222X, Amsterdam, Holland

Nakagawara, A.; Arima, M.; Azar, C. G.; Scavarla, N. J. & Brodeur, G. M. (1992). Inverse relationship between trk expression and N-myc amplification in human neuroblastoma. *Cancer Research*, 52, 1364-1368

Ninkina, N.; Grashchuk, M.; Buchman, V. L. & Davies, A. M. (1997). TrkA variants with deletions in the leucine-rich motifs of the extracellular domain. *Journal of Biological Chemistry*, 272, 13019-13025

Nykjaer, A.; Willnow, T. E. & Peterson, C. M. (2005). P75NTR- live or let die. *Current Opinions in Neurobiology*, 15, 49-57

Obermeier, A.; Bradshaw, R. A.; Seedorf, K.; Choidas, A.; Schlessinger, J. & Ullrich, A. (1994). Neuronal differentiation signals are controlled by nerve growth factor receptor/Trk binding sites for SHC and PLCγ. *EMBO Journal*. 13, 1585-1590

Obermeier, A.; Haltre, H.; Weismuller, K. H.; Jung, G.; Schlessinger, J. & Ullrich, A. (1993). Tyrosine 785 is a major determinant of Trk-substrate interaction. *EMBO Journal*, 12, 933-941

Obermeier, A.; Lammares, R.; Weismuller, K. H.; Jung, G.; Schlessinger, J. & Ullrich, A. (1993). Identification of Trk binding sites for SHC and phosphatidylinositol 3-kinase and formation of a multimeric signalling complex. *Journal of Biological Chemistry*. 268, 22963-22966

Oppenheim, R. W. (1991). Cell death during development of the nervous system. *Annual Reviews in Neuroscience*, 14, 453- 501

Ostman, A. & Bohmer, F. D. (2001). Regulation of receptor tyrosine kinase signalling by protein tyrosine phosphatases. *Trends in Cell Biology*. 11, 258-266

Paget, S. (1989). The distribution of secondary growths in cancer of the breast. 1889. *Cancer Metastasis Reviews*, 8, 98-101

Paratcha, G. & Ibanez, C. F. (2002). Lipid rafts and the control of neurotrophin signalling in the nervous system: variations on a theme. *Current Opinions in Neurobiology*, 12, 524-549

Parrens, M.; Labouyrie, E.; Groppi, A.; Dubus, P.; Carles, D.; Velley, J. F.; deMascarel, A. & Merlio, J. P. (1998). Expression of NGF receptors in normal and pathological human thymus. *Journal of Neuroimmunology*, 85, 11-21

Patapoutian, A. & Reichardt, L. F. (2001). Trk receptors: mediators of neurotrophin action. *Current Opinions in Neurobiology*, 11, 272-280

Peng, X.; Greene, L. A.; Kaplan, D. R. & Stephens, R. M. (1995). Deletion of a conserved juxtamembrane sequence in Trk abolishes NGF-promoted neuritogenesis. *Neuron*, 15, 395-406

Pommier, Y. & Cherfils, J. (2005). Interfacial inhibition of macromolecular interactions: nature's paradigm for drug discovery. *Trends in Pharmacological Science*, 26, 138-145

Pumiglia, K. M. & Decker, S. J. (1997). Cell cycle arrest mediated by the MEK/mitogen activated protein kinase pathway. *Proceedings of the National Academy of Science USA*, 94, 448-452

Rajagopal, R.; Chen, Z. Y.; Lee, F. S. & Chao, M. V. (2004). Transactivation of Trk neurotrophin receptors by G-protein- coupled receptor ligands occurs on intracellular membranes. *Journal of Neuroscience*, 24, 6650-6658

Reuther, G. W.; Lambert, Q. T.; Caligiuri, M. A. & Der, C. J. (2000). Identification and characterisation of an activating TrkA deletion mutation in acute myeloid leukaemia. *Molecular and Cellular Biology*, 20, 8655-8666

Rodriguez-Manzaneque, J. C.; Lane, T. F.; Ortega, M. A.; Hynes, R. O.; Lawler, J. & Iruela-Arispe, M. L. (2001). Thrombospondin-1 suppresses spontaneous tumor growth and inhibits activation of metalloproteinase-9 and mobilisation of vascular endothelial cell growth factor. *Proceedings of the National Academy of Sciences USA*, 98, 12485-12490

Ron, D. & Walter, P. (2007). Signal integration in the endoplasmic reticulum unfolded protein response. *Nature Reviews in Molecular and Cellular Biology*, 8, 519-529

Sastry, S. K. & Elferink, L. A. (2011). Checks and balances: interplay of RTKs and PTPs in cancer progression. *Biochemical Pharmacology*, Article ahead of print (doi:10.1016/j.bcp.2011.06.016)

Scaruffi, P.; Cusano, R.; Dagnino, M. & Tonini GP. (1999). Detection of DNA polymorphisms and point mutations of high affinity nerve growth factor receptor (TrkA) in human neuroblastoma. *International Journal of Oncology*, 14, 935- 938

Segal, R. A.; Battachararyya, A.; Rua, L. A.; Alberta, J. A.; Stephens, R. M.; Kaplan, D. R. & Stiles, C. D. (1996). Differential utilization of Trk autophosphorylation sites. *Journal of Biological Chemistry*, 271, 20175-20181

Shore, G. C.; Papa, F. R. & Oakes, S. A. (2011). Signaling cell death from the endoplasmic reticulum stress response. *Current Opinions in Cell Biology*, 23, 143-149

Sugimoto, T.; Kuroda, H.; Horii, Y.; Moritake, H.; Tanaka, T. & Hattori, S. (2001). Signal transduction pathways through TRK-A and TRK-B receptors in human neuroblastoma cells. *Japanese Journal of Cancer Research*, 92, 152-160

Suzuki, T.; Bogenmann, E.; Shimada, H.; Stram, D. & Seeger, R. C. (1993). Lack of high-affinity nerve growth factor receptors in aggressive neuroblastomas. *Journal of the National Cancer Institute*, 85, 377-384

Szul, T.; Grabski, R.; Lyons, S.; Morohashi, Y.; Shestopal, S.; Lowe, M. & Sztul, E. (2007). Dissecting the role of the ARF guanine nucleotide exchange factor GBF1 in Golgi biogenesis and protein trafficking. *Journal of Cell Science*, 120, 3929-3940

Tacconelli, A.; Farina, A. R.; Cappabianca, L.; Cea, G.; Panella, S.; Chioda, A.; Gallo, R.; Cinque, B.; Sferra, R.; Vetuschi, A.; Campese, A. F.; Screpanti, I.; Gulino, A. & Mackay, A. R. (2007). TrkAIII expression in the thymus. *Journal of Neuroimmunology*, 183, 151-161

Tacconelli, A.; Farina, A. R.; Cappabianca, L.; DeSantis, G.; Tessitore, A.; Vetuschi.; A.; Sferra, R.; Rucci, N.; Argent, B.; Screpanti, I.; Gulino, A. & Mackay, A. R. (2004). TrkA alternative splicing: A regulated tumor-promoting switch in human neuroblastoma. *Cancer Cell*, 6, 347-360

Takita, J.; Hyashi, Y.; Takei, K.; Yamaguchi, N.; Hanada, R.; Yamamoto, K. & Yokota, J. (2000). Allelic imbalance on chromosome 18 in neuroblastoma. *European Journal of Cancer*, 36, 508-513

Tanaka, S.; Nakamura, K.; Takahasi, N. & Suda, T. (2005). Role of RANKL in physiological and pathological bone resorption and therapeutics targeting the RANKL-RANK signalling system. *Immunology Reviews*, 208, 30-49

Tanaka, T.; Sugimoto, T. & Sawada, T. (1998). Prognostic discrimination among neuroblastomas according to Ha-ras/trk A gene expression: a comparison of the profiles of neuroblastomas detected clinically and those through mass screening. *Cancer*, 83, 1626-1633

Valdez, G.; Akmentin, W.; Philippidou, P.; Kuruvilla, R.; Ginty, D. & Halegoua, S. (2003). Picher-mediated macro- endocytosis underlies retrograde signalling by neurotrophin receptors. *Journal of Neuroscience*, 25, 5236-5247

Vega, J. A.; Garcia-Suarez, O.; Hannestad, J.; Perez-Perez, M. & Germana, A. (2003). Neurotrophins and the immune system. *Journal of Anatomy*, 203, 1-19

Vigil, D.; Cherfils, A.; Rossman, K. L. & Derr, C. J. (2010). Ras superfamily GEFs and GAPs, validated and tractable targets for cancer therapy. *Nature Reviews in Cancer*, 10, 842-857

Watson, F. L.; Porcionatto, M. A.; Bhattacharyya, A.; Stiles, C. & Segal, R. A. (1999). TrkA glycosylation regulates localisation and activity. *Journal of Neurobiology*, 39, 323-336

Weier, H-U. G.; Rhein, A. P.; Shadravan, F.; Collins, C. & Polikoff, D. (1995). Rapid physical mapping of the human protoncogene (NTRK1) to human chromosome 1q21-q22 by P1 clone selection, fluorescence in situ hybridisation (FISH), and computer-assisted microscopy. *Genomics*, 26, 390-393

Wiesman, C.; Muller, Y. A. & de Vos, A. M. (2000). Ligand binding sites in Ig-like domains of receptor tyrosine kinases. *Journal of Molecular Medicine*, 78, 247-260

Windisch, J. M.; Marksteiner, R. & Schneider, R. (1995). Nerve growth factor binding site on TrkA mapped to a single 24- amino acid rich leucine-rich motif. *Journal of Biological Chemistry*, 270, 28133-28136

Xu, W. & Neckers, L. (2007). Targeting the molecular chaperone heat shock protein 90 provides a multifaceted effect on diverse cell signalling pathways of cancer cells. *Clinical Cancer Research*, 13, 1625-1629

Yao, R. & Cooper, G. M. (1995). Requirement for phosphoinositol-3 kinase in the prevention of apoptosis by nerve growth factor. *Science*, 267, 2003-2005

Zaccaro, M. C.; Ivanisevic, L.; Perez, P.; Meakin, S. O. & Saragovi, H. U. (2002). P75 coreceptors regulate ligand dependent and ligand independent Trk receptor activation, in part by altering trk docking subdomains. *Journal of Biological Chemistry*, 276, 31023-31029

6

Interplay Between Protein Kinase C Isoforms Alpha and Epsilon, Neurofibromin, and the Ras/MAPK Pathway in Neuroblastoma Differentiation

George Leondaritis[1,*], Xenia Koliou[1], Shalini Johnson[1], Chengjun Li[1], Andreas Florakis[1], Konstantinos Dimas[2], Nikos Sakellaridis[2] and Dimitra Mangoura[1,*]
[1]Neurosciences, Biomedical Research Foundation of the Academy of Athens (BRFAA) Athens,
[2]Department of Pharmacology, Medical School, University of Thessaly, Larissa, Greece

1. Introduction

Neuroblastoma (NB) [1] is the most common extracranial tumor in childhood and accounts for nearly half of neoplasms diagnosed during infancy (Maris, 2010; Brodeur, 2003). A striking feature of these tumors has been their heterogeneous course, which ranges from spontaneous regression to inevitable progression and death (Brodeur, 2003). Current pharmacological approaches in the treatment of NBs include standard combination chemotherapy using dose-intensive cycles of carboplatin, etoposide, cyclophosphamide, and doxorubicin, with the addition of topoisomerase I inhibitors. For intermediate-risk NB, a high rate of survival among patients may still be achieved with significant reduction of doses and duration of chemotherapy (Baker et al., 2010). The retinoic acid analogue isotretinoin (13-cis-retinoic acid) is additionally used in high-risk NB patients with progressive or recurrent disease (Maris, 2010; Reynolds et al., 2003).
Animal cancer models have offered valuable preclinical testing systems for studying the impact of specific genes in the appearance and the progress of the disease as well as the efficacy of novel therapeutic regimes. Animal models of NB have been developed by subcutaneous inoculation (xenografting) of established human NB cell lines in immunocompromised mice; for instance, the cell line SK-N-BE2c was successfully used to develop an animal model and test the effects of imatinib (Meco et al., 2005). Yet, the major

* Corresponding Authors (George Leondaritis, Dimitra Mangoura)
[1] Abbreviations used: ERK, extracellular signal-regulated kinase; GAP, GTPase-activating protein; GEF, guanine nucleotide exchange factor; DAG, diacylglycerol; TH, tyrosine hydroxylase; GAP43, growth-associated protein 43; NPY, neuropeptide Y; TPA, 12-O-tetradecanoyl-phorbol-13-acetate; dBcAMP, dibutyryl cAMP; BrdU, 5-bromo-2-deoxyuridine.

drawback was the lack of metastases. Pseudometastatic models were next developed by tail-vein injections of human NB cell lines in athymic mice (Pastorino et al., 2010). A clinically relevant model should, however, reflect the characteristics of advanced NB in children, that is large adrenal gland tumors and multiple small metastatic lesions. Such models have been generated only in nude mice with murine NB cells (NXS2) or by allografting human NB cell lines (Pastorino et al., 2010). Spontaneous adrenal neuroblastomas may be developed, yet rarely, in experimental animals (Rice, 2004), while, neither carcinogen-induced nor genetically engineered animal NB models have been successfully generated thus far.

Therefore, the development of novel therapeutic strategies, including both new targets and models, is urgently needed. Progress is expected through elucidation of the key molecular pathways that drive NB proliferation, differentiation, or apoptosis. Clinical trial data have also suggested that induced differentiation may be an alternative therapeutic approach, and retinoic acid analogues have been introduced in the clinical practice (Reynolds & Lie, 2000; Brodeur, 2003). The clinical observation of spontaneous differentiation into benign ganglioneuromas has provided the basis for studying neuronal differentiation of NB cells in culture (Reynolds & Lie, 2000; Edsjo et al., 2003; Hahn et al., 2008), and such studies have provided invaluable mechanistic insight into the fundamental mechanisms of neuronal differentiation and neurotransmitter phenotype acquisition (Mangoura et al., 2006b; Edsjo et al., 2007). The agents, mostly used to study NB cell differentiation in culture are phorbol esters, membrane permeable non-hydrolyzable cAMP analogues, and the clinically relevant vitamin A metabolite retinoic acid, alone or in combination with specific neurotrophic and growth factors (Table 1). These agents target distinct proximal signalling pathways: phorbol esters activate novel and conventional protein kinase C (PKC) isoforms, cAMP analogues activate protein kinase A (PKA) and exchange proteins activated by cAMP (Epacs), while retinoic acid acts as a ligand for nuclear hormone receptors/transcription factors (RARs) (Table 1). Yet, a significant level of crosstalk amongst these agents has been demonstrated in the induction of NB differentiation. Activation of PKCs and the ensuing Ras/ERK signalling cascade have been highlighted as central modulators of NB differentiation, with novel (PKCε) and conventional (PKCα) PKC isoforms critically controlling the signalling output and dynamics of MAPKs (Griner & Kazanietz, 2007). The importance of the PKC/Ras/ERK pathway is further emphasized by recent studies showing that neurofibromin, a prominent tumor suppressor and a neuronal RasGAP protein (a) is a PKCα and PKCε substrate (Mangoura et al., 2006a) actively phosphorylated during phorbol ester-induced differentiation (Leondaritis et al., 2009) and (b) provides responsiveness to retinoic acid (Holzel et al., 2010). In these studies, the role of PKCα and PKCε may be viewed as differential and even opposing, with PKCε emerging as a crucial, neuronal differentiation-specific PKC isoform.

In this chapter, we introduce the basic aspects of the PKC/NF1/Ras/ERK pathway and its implications in neuronal differentiation, we discuss critical findings from studies with NB cells that highlight the importance of this pathway in NB differentiation, and present original experiments that further expand current knowledge. Finally, we propose that agents promoting NB differentiation via distinct primary targets may actually converge on establishing a balance between PKCα and PKCε activities that coordinates neurofibromin (NF1)-dependent Ras/ERK activation and NB differentiation.

2. PKC isoforms, NF1, and the Ras/ERK pathway in differentiation of neuroblastoma cells

2.1 The PKC/NF1/Ras/ERK pathway

2.1.1 The PKC family: Structure, regulation, and substrates

The PKC family of serine/threonine protein kinases consists of at least ten isoforms that are classified into three subgroups based on their structure and specific cofactor requirements. Conventional PKCs (cPKCs: α, βI, βII and γ) are activated by the second messengers Ca^{2+} and DAG, while novel PKCs (nPKCs: δ, ε, η and θ) are activated only by DAG. In contrast to conventional and novel, atypical PKCs (aPKCs: ζ and λ/ι) are insensitive to both Ca^{2+} and DAG, but responsive to the Par6–Cdc42 complex (Parker & Murray-Rust, 2004; Rosse et al., 2010). PKCs are considered hubs for the transduction of signals from G protein-coupled and tyrosine kinase receptors (Parker & Murray-Rust, 2004; Griner and Kazanietz 2007), having long been recognized as a link between receptor-dependent generation of DAG by phospholipases C and D, and the key event for enganging the ERK pathway, the activation of Ras and Raf (Mangoura and Dawson, 1993; Marais et al., 1998). Attesting to the widespread effects of PKC activation, numerous studies have investigated the involvement of all PKC isoforms in oncogenesis and cellular differentiation, proliferation, polarity, migration, apoptosis, and survival (Bosco et al., 2011; Rosse et al., 2010; Larsson, 2006).

PKCs are founding members of the AGC kinase group and share a common structure consisting of a conserved C-terminal kinase catalytic domain and a more divergent N-terminal regulatory region. The regulatory region contains C1 and C2-domains (cPKC and nPKCs) that recognize the second messengers DAG/phospholipids or Ca^{2+}/phospholipids, respectively, and a pseudosubstrate sequence that serves in autoinhibition by interacting with the substrate-binding pocket of the catalytic domain. Binding of second messengers or allosteric effectors on the C1/C2-domains of the regulatory region results in stabilized interaction with the plasma membrane and activation (Parker & Murray-Rust, 2004; Griner and Kazanietz 2007). PKCs are additionally regulated by specific phosphorylation events that "prime" the kinase for activation. As for all AGC kinases, PDK1 phosphorylates threonines (Thr) in the activation loop (Thr566 in PKCε). Residues in the turn motif (Thr710 in PKCε) and the C-terminal hydrophobic motif of c/nPKCs (Ser729 in PKCε) are often phosphorylated by the mTORC2 complex (Freeley et al., 2011). These phosphorylations critically depend on the occupation of the catalytic site by ATP, stabilize the active conformation of PKCs, and result in a fully primed kinase (Cameron et al., 2009). Additional auto- or in-trans phosphorylation events by other PKC isoforms may have more subtle effects, such as modulation of catalytic activity, protein stability, or binding to other proteins (Freeley et al., 2011). Specifically for PKCε, phosphorylation on Ser368 in the regulatory region by cPKCs suggests a high level of functional crosstalk within members of the PKC family (Durgan et al., 2008).

By the acute and reversible post-translational modification of phosphorylation, PKCs regulate the activity and subcellular localization of several of their protein substrates. PKCs phosphorylate an array of substrates that include transcription factors, receptors, ion channels, and cytoskeletal proteins (Mangoura and Dawson 1993; Mangoura, 1997; Parker & Murray-Rust, 2004; Larsson, 2006; Mangoura et al., 2006a). In many cases, however, proof of direct PKC phosphorylation of substrates in vivo has remained limited, with several molecules representing remote "PKC targets". PKCs also act as scaffols, as they interact with other proteins independently of their enzymatic properties as kinases (e.g. Saurin et al.,

2008; Valcova et al., 2007). Mechanistically and pharmacologically important PKC-binding proteins are the RACKs (receptors for activated C-kinases), which stabilize the interaction of activated PKCs with plasma membrane (Schechtman & Mochly-Rosen, 2001). Studies of the PKC-RACK interactions by Mochly-Rosen and co-workers, have shown that isoform-specific activators or inhibitors may be rationally designed, from unique 7-8 amino acid sequences in each PKC or in their respective RACKs (Budas et al., 2007; Csukai & Mochly-Rosen, 1999). As such, εV1-2 and ψεRACK peptides, specific inhibitor and activator peptides for PKCε, respectively, and analogous peptides for other PKCs have been used in numerous studies in culture and in vivo with great success (Asimaki and Mangoura, 2011; Asimaki et al., 2011).

2.1.2 The Ras/ERK pathway and modulation by PKCs

Ras GTPases, are key molecules for growth and neurotrophic factor signalling through the three kinase MAPK module, consisting of Rafs (MAPKKK), MEK1/2 (MAPKK), and ERK1/2 (MAPK) (Raman et al., 2007 and refs. therein). All Ras proteins, namely H-, N- and K-Ras, cycle between active GTP-bound and inactive GDP-bound states; activation of guanine nucleotide exchange factors (GEFs) after membrane receptor stimulation promotes the exchange of GDP for GTP and activation of Ras (Buday & Downward, 2008). The opposite event is controlled by GTPase-activating proteins (GAPs) that activate the intrinsic GTPase activity of Ras and lead to GTP hydrolysis and Ras inactivation (Scheffzek et al., 1998). Ras-GTP recruits Raf to the membrane and together with other kinases activates Raf kinase activity (Stokoe and McCormick, 1997). Subsequently, relay phosphorylations through MEKs result in phosphorylation and activation of ERK, which is considered as the terminal effector of the pathway (Raman et al., 2007). The Ras/ERK pathway controls various cellular processes such as proliferation, migration, and differentiation. A recent review by Katz et al., provides an overview of the Ras/ERK pathway impact on cellular differentiation and oncogenesis (Katz et al., 2007). Our focus is the PKC input on the regulation and dynamics of activation of Ras and ERK.

Mechanistically, PKC activation is necessary for the formation of Ras and activated Raf-1 complexes (Marais et al. 1998; Hamilton et al., 2001). PKCs may directly phosphorylate Raf (Ueda et al., 1996), RasGEFs (Ebinu et al. 1998; Roose et al., 2005; Zheng et al., 2005), and RasGAPs (Izawa et al., 1996; Mangoura et al., 2006a; Leondaritis et al., 2009), hence regulating the output of Ras/ERK signalling at multiple levels. PKCs on GEFs: Members of the GRP family of RasGEFs possess C1-domains that "recognize" DAG produced by phospholipases in the membrane upon membrane receptor stimulation, and through these interactions translocate to the membranes too (Ebinu et al. 1998). The GEF activity of RasGRP1,3 is greatly enhanced by concurrent phosphorylation by DAG-activated nPKCs, at least in T- and B-cells (Roose et al., 2005; Zheng et al., 2005). PKCs may also activate SOS1, the other major RasGEF, directly by phosphorylation (Rubio et al., 2006) or indirectly, by recruiting Grb2/SOS1 complexes via the Syk tyrosine kinase (Kawakami et al., 2003). PKCs on RasGAPs: Most of the cellular RasGAP activity is attributed to p120GAP and neurofibromin, and earlier studies have suggested a PKC-dependent inhibition of RasGAP activity in certain cell types (Downward et al., 1990). PKCs indirectly modulate the GAP activity of p120GAP via its interaction with RACK1 (Koehler & Moran, 2001), and neurofibromin, the main neuronal RasGAP, is directly regulated by PKC. Neurofibromin is phosphorylated by PKCs in vitro, particularly at the C-terminal domain (Izawa et al., 1996). Evidence for direct PKCα and PKCε-dependent neurofibromin phosphorylation was documented later in cultured neurons, and neuroblastoma and glioma cell lines (Mangoura et al., 2006a). Moreover, phosphorylation of neurofibromin results in both its increased association with actin and enhancement of its GAP activity (Mangoura et al., 2006a). PKC-phosphorylation sites on neurofibromin are present in the N-terminal CSRD domain (Mangoura et al., 2006a) and in the C-terminal domain (Leondaritis et al., 2009). The residue Ser2808 in the C-tail of neurofibromin is indeed a PKC-specific site and its phosphorylation correlates well with enhanced signalling through the Ras/ERK pathway in TPA-treated SH-SY5Y cells (Leondaritis et al., 2009). Interestingly, studies with glioblastoma cell lines or tumors have indicated that PKCα may promote proteasome-dependent neurofibromin proteolysis, hence insufficient neurofibromin RasGAP activity to control Ras and accelerated cellular proliferation (McGillicuddy et al., 2009). Whether neurofibromin phosphorylation on Ser2808 (or other sites) is directly involved is, however, unknown. In sharp contrast, phosphorylation of neurofibromin in-non tumor cellular contexts has been correlated with increased stability of the protein, at least in melanocytes (Kaufmann et al., 1999) and neurons (Mangoura et al., 2006a). In conclusion, PKCs have the potential to directly impact on the activation state of Ras by modulating the activity of both GEFs and GAPs in a variety of ways. It should be also noted that in certain cell lines, PKC-dependent ERK activation may occur independently of Ras, since the dominant-negative form of Ras (RasS17N) that resists GEF-dependent activation does not inhibit TPA-induced ERK activation (Ueda et al., 1996; Rubio et al., 2008 and refs. therein). Overall, c/nPKCs like PKCα, PKCη, PKCδ and PKCε and aPKCs have been suggested to provide an activatory input on ERK pathway mostly at the level of Raf (Ueda et al., 1996; Schönwasser et al., 1998; Paruchuri et al., 2002).

2.1.3 NF1 and PKCε in neuronal differentiation

All major transduction molecules of the Ras/ERK pathway, namely Ras and Raf, are also potent inducers of differentiation and neuritic outgrowth in several neuronal cell lines (Wood et al., 1993; Olsson & Nanberg, 2001; Hynds et al., 2003). Moreover, it is the intensity and duration of Ras/ERK activation that determines the biological outcome. Seminal observations were first made in PC12 cells treated with EGF or NGF. Both growth factors activate the same Ras/ERK pathway, yet, transient ERK activation by EGF induces cell proliferation, whereas a sustained ERK activation by NGF induces neurite outgrowth and differentiation (Marshall, 1995 and refs. therein). The reasons for these fundamental differences are still debated (Santos et al., 2007; von Kriegsheim et al., 2009). At any rate, both nPKCs (for example PKCδ, Santos et al., 2007) and neurofibromin (von Kriegsheim et al., 2009) may actively mediate the long-lasting ERK activation that drives PC12 cell differentiation.

Neurofibromin is highly expressed in neurons with lower levels of expression detected in oligodendrocytes, Schwann cells, astrocytes, and other cell types (Li et al., 2001 and refs therein). Support for a specific role of neurofibromin in neuronal differentiation derives from several studies which show that its expression is developmentally regulated in the CNS and dorsal root ganglia in mouse and chick embryos, and that its peaks in expression coincide with the onset of neuronal differentiation (Vogel et al., 1995; Li et al., 2001). Studies in mice where neurofibromin has null expression after genetic ablation of central exons that render the protein unstable (functional knockout) have revealed an essential role for neurofibromin in the dependence of PNS neurons to neurotrophins (Vogel et al., 1995). Specifically, larger numbers of sensory and sympathetic neurons survive and continue to differentiate in the absence of NGF in culture (Vogel et al., 1995; Vogel et al., 2000; Zhu et al., 2001), in a Ras-depended manner (Vogel et al., 2000). Interestingly, functional ablation of neurofibromin in CNS neurons via a synapsin-Cre approach does not result in altered morphology or survival rates (Zhu et al., 2001). Analysis in the PC12 cell model, utilizing siRNA-downregulation or overexpression of neurofibromin dominant-negative construct approaches, has yielded somewhat contradictory results. In one study, neurofibromin silencing did not affect NGF-induced differentiation, yet, it enabled EGF to partially promote differentiation (von Kriegsheim et al., 2009). In other studies, overexpression of a neurofibromin-based dominant negative construct, known to increase Ras-GTP and p-ERK levels, or siRNA-silencing of neurofibromin resulted in inhibition of NGF-induced differentiation (Ynoue et al., 2003; Patrakitkomjorn et al. 2008). These disparing results may stem from differences in the time period of siRNA silencing, extent of neurofibromin downregulation, and concentrations and times of NGF treatment. Nonetheless, these data attest to a developmental time-dependent function of neurofibromin during neuronal differentiation.

Many studies in neuronal cell lines and primary neurons have implicated most of PKC isoforms in survival and differentiation mechanisms (Mangoura et al., 1993; Hundle et al., 1997; Lallemend et al., 2005; Shirai et al., 2008). In their majority, PKCs have been shown to have a positive role in neuritic outgrowth; yet, in a recent large-scale analysis in hippocampal neurons PKCι and PKCη scored as potent negative neurite growth regulators (Buchser et al., 2010). PKCε on the other hand is regarded as the isoform involved in differentiation of both CNS and PNS neurons (Mangoura et al., 1993; Larsson, 2006; Mangoura, 1997; Hundle et al., 1997; Shirai et al., 2008). In fact, in the developing chick brain, it is the major isoform found in early post-mitotic, just starting to differentiate neurons (Mangoura et al., 1993). A significant number of studies on the pro-differentiation role of PKCε have been actually performed on NB cell lines, as will be presented in more detail in the following sections.

2.2 Neuroblastoma differentiating agents and underlying signalling mechanisms

2.2.1 Retinoids

Agents, neurotransmitters, growth factors, and neurotrophic factors used in culture models of NB differentiation are summarized in Table 1. Typical differentiating agents are the retinoids all trans-RA, 13-cis RA, and N-(4-hydroxyphenyl) retinamide (4-HPR, or fenretidine) (Reynolds & Lie, 2000), which cause growth arrest concomitantly with downregulation of MYCN expression, upregulation of an array of neuronal markers (neuron-specific enolase, neuropeptide Y, GAP43, MAP2, neurofilament-M, and synaptophysin), induction of neurite outgrowth, and increases in neurotransmitter biosynthetic enzyme activity and expression. The neurotransmitter phenotype induced by RA depends on the cell line, with cells developing sympathetic noradrenergic or cholinergic phenotypes (Edsjo et al., 2007 and refs. therein). Efforts to establish a consensus on what constitutes the RA-induced differentiation has recently led to recognition of a set of 10 genes as a potential signature and a more general yet reliable predictor of differentiation in NBs (Hahn et al., 2008). Moreover, a gene-expression high-throughput screening of small molecule libraries revealed a synergistic action of RA (all trans RA and 13-cis RA) and histone deacetylase inhibitors towards induction of NB differentiation, both in culture and in vivo (Hahn et al., 2008).

Agent	Phenotype/Markers	Signalling pathway	Cell lines/Comments/ References
Retinoids			
all-trans RA/13-cis RA	growth arrest, ↑ neuronal markers, morphology	RAR, PKCs, ATM, ERK (inconclusive)	Most NB cell lines, resistance, heterogeneity (see text)
4-HPR (fenretinide)	growth arrest apoptosis/necrosis variable differentiation	RAR-independent, ceramide, PKCs, ROS	RA-sensitive and resistant NB cell lines (1-3)
Phorbol esters			
TPA (12-O-tetradecanoyl-phorbol-13-acetate)	growth retardation ↑ neuronal markers morphology	PKCs (ERK, RARs)	best studied in SH-SY5Y (also SK-N-SH, SK-N-SN) (see text)
cAMP analogues			
dBcAMP	growth arrest ↑ neuronal markers morphology	PKA/Epac, CREB, PI3K/ERK	Most NB cell lines (see text)
Growth factors			
IGF-1/bFGF	↑ neuronal markers morphology	PKCs, ERK, RARβ	SH-SY5Y (4-5)
NGF	↑ neuronal markers morphology	TrkA, PKCs	TrkA/SH-SY5Y, IMR32 (5)
GDNF	growth inhibition cell cycle arrest ↑ neuronal markers	RET/TrkA	SH-SY5Y, LA-N-5 (6)
GPCR agonists			
Adenosine	↑ neuronal markers morphology	PKC, ERK, PKA (receptor-specific)	SH-SY5Y (7)
PACAP	↑ neuronal markers morphology	cAMP, ERK/p38	SH-SY5Y (8)
Other			
Uridine	growth retardation ↑ neuronal markers morphology	PKCε	LAN-5 (9)

Table 1. NB differentiating agents and signalling mechanisms studied; growth retardation refers to decreased proliferation rate; morphology refers to increased neuritic outgrowth measured as a percentage of neurite-bearing cells or average neurite length; neuronal markers refer to increases in neuron-specific enolase, NPY, GAP43, synaptophysin, and TH (mRNA or protein level); signalling pathway implication has been derived mostly by pharmacological and genetic manipulation studies. Only selected pathways are presented to best serve the focus of this chapter. Details of some of the experiments are discussed in the text and further information may be found in the respective references [1-3, (Edsjo et al., 2007; Janardhanan et al., 2009; Reynolds & Lie, 2000); 4-5, (Perez-Juste & Aranda, 1999; Fagerstrom et al., 1996); 6, (Peterson & Bogenmann, 2004); 7, (Canals et al., 2005); 8, (Monaghan et al., 2008); 9, (Silei et al., 2000)].

Studies with NB cell lines are subjected to some degree of heterogeneity in the response which may stem from: the passage number, culture conditions, concentration of agents, length of treatment, and certainly the read-out assay system. Thus conflicting reports are not rare, for example the NB cell line IMR32 has been described as resistant (Joshi et al., 2007), sensitive (Holzel et al., 2010), or weakly responsive to RA (Guzhova et al., 2001). Similarly, SK-N-BE2 cells have been characterized as RA-resistant in a long-term 25-30 day colony formation assay (Holzel et al., 2010), and as sensitive when increased neuritic outgrowth was recorded after 2-4 days of exposure (Zeidman et al., 1999a, 2002). For RA, in particular, this is a significant issue, since prediction of resistance to retinoid therapy is very important in the clinical setting. Until recently, no predictive markers of RA responsiveness were established for clinical use. A connection with amplification of MYCN has been suggested (Reynolds et al., 2000), yet, MYCN-overexpressing stable SK-N-SH cells retain their capacity to differentiate in response to a variety of agents, including RA (Edsjo et al., 2004). Several other genes investigated in NBs have not come through as predictors, and even RARs have been questioned, because RA-resistant cells are sensitive to fenretinide (N-(4-hydroxyphenyl) retinamide), the synthetic retinoid that acts independently of RARs (Reynolds et al., 2000; Reynolds and Lie, 2000). More recently, neurofibromin deficiency in NB cells was proposed as a strong predictor of RA responsiveness, as shRNA silencing of neurofibromin was shown to confer resistance to retinoic acid independently of MYCN expression. Neurofibromin-deficient cells continue to proliferate in the presence of low concentrations of RA, bypassing check points for growth arrest and induction of differentiation, and exhibiting reduced expression of RA-target genes, Ret included (Holzel et al., 2010). Expression of Ret, the GDNF receptor, is very important for differentiation of NB cells (Peterson & Bogenmann, 2004; Esposito et al., 2008), especially through its action on upregulation of TrkA, a powerful and favorable prognostic marker in NB tumors (Edsjo et al., 2007; Brodeur, 2003).

The need for prognostic markers and therapeutic targets has strongly driven research on the signalling mechanisms that regulate RA-induced NB differentiation. Apparently RARs constitute a major requirement for the action of RA, as RA confers a significant upregulation of RARβ that drives gains in growth arrest and morphological NB differentiation (Maden, 2007). Besides the well-appreciated role of RARβ, other key signalling pathways appear to contribute to or modulate the RA-induced NB differentiation. These pathways are rapidly engaged upon addition of RA and often persist over a long time period. Thus, RA added to SH-SY5Y or SK-N-BE rapidly (within 20 min) activates the ATM kinase (Fernandes et al., 2007), which is a component of the DNA damage signal transduction pathway. ATM's autophosphorylation persists for over 4 days and correlates with enhanced ATM-dependent CREB phosphorylation and cell differentiation (Fernandes et al., 2007). Importantly, ATM inhibition or depletion does not prevent RA-induced upregulation of target genes, rather impairs cell survival (Fernandes et al., 2007).

A large body of evidence suggests a positive role of Ras, Raf, and prolonged ERK activation in neuronal differentiation in PC12 cells and several other cellular models (see section 2.1.2), but the situation is certainly more complicated when RA-induced NB differentiation is concerned. ERK is invariably activated by RA in the short- (Delaune et al., 2008) or long-term (Lee & Kim, 2004; Miloso et al., 2004), yet inhibition of the ERK activating kinase MEK by U0126 or PD98059 has yielded contradictory results on whether RA-induced ERK activation is necessary for neuritic outgrowth in SH-SY5Y and SK-N-BE(2)C cells (Miloso et al., 2004; Lee & Kim, 2004). Stable overexpression of RKIP (Raf kinase inhibitor protein), a scaffold protein crucial for Raf and ERK pathway activation, accelerated the rate of neuritic outgrowth and increased the expression of neuronal markers in response to RA in SH-SY5Y cells, all concurrent with sustained ERK activation (Hellmann et al., 2010). Furthermore, in

SH-SY5Y and LA-N-5 cells, ERK mediates an early (within 1h) RA-induced formation of promyelocytic leukemia nuclear bodies, an event associated with NB differentiation (Delaune et al., 2008). Apparently, ERK activity may impinge differentially on early and late gene regulation and inhibitor studies have not always addressed these issues with sufficient detail (Miloso et al., 2004; Lee & Kim, 2004; Delaune et al., 2008; Holzel et al., 2010). In addition, evidence from the various differentiation protocols and agents suggests that the transcription programs for neuritic outgrowth or expression of neuron-specific genes may be independently regulated in NB cells. In all, ERK activity appears to be crucial for the expression of neuron-specific genes, in the absence of a positive signalling stimulus for the induction of neuritic outgrowth (see below in section 2.2.2).

Besides its role as a differentiating agent, 13-cis-RA antagonizes significantly the cytotoxic effects of agents like etoposide and cisplatin (Hadjidaniel & Reynolds, 2010), which suggests another mechanism of impact of the RA responsiveness, this time involving the Ras/ERK pathway. For example, an inverse correlation between resistance to doxorubicin and ERK pathway activation has been suggested in SK-N-SH cells (Mattingly et al., 2001), while NFkB activation by doxorubicin and etoposide in SH-SY5Y cells, thought to be required for drug-induced toxicity, depends also on Ras and MEK activities (Armstrong et al., 2006). With the newly established role of neurofibromin in RA responsiveness and its direct implication in signalling through the Ras/ERK pathway for neuronal differentiation, neurofibromin may indeed contribute to some extent in (the prevention of) cytotoxic responses, an aspect not yet considered.

Experimental evidence from chemical inhibition or overexpression of dominant-negative mutants studies has implicated several PKC isoforms, mostly nPKCs, in RA-induced differentiation. RA-induced ERK activation in SH-SY5Y cells was significantly reduced in the presence of the c/nPKC inhibitor GF1092303X, as well as the RA-induced cell survival and neuritic outgrowth (Miloso et al., 2004). A peptide derived from the actin-binding site of PKCε has been shown to attenuate RA-induced neuritic outgrowth in SK-N-BE(2), while RA induced an increase of the cytoskeleton-associated PKCε pool (Zeidman et al., 2002). Besides PKCε, PKCθ and PKCδ have also been suggested to play a role in RA-induced differentiation (Nitti et al, 2010). In LAN-5 cells, RA-induced differentiation is inhibited by PKCθ-antisense oligonucleotides (Sparatore et al., 2000), while in SH-SY5Y cells, modulation of PKCδ activity by inhibition with rottlerin or overexpression of dominant-negative PKCδ suggested a positive role of PKCδ activity in SH-SY5Y differentiation via the function of NADPH oxidase system (Nitti et al, 2010).

2.2.2 Phorbol esters

Long-term treatment of SH-SY5Y cells with the phorbol ester 12-O-tetradecanoyl-phorbol-13-acetate (TPA) has been extensively studied as a NB and human sympathetic neuron differentiation model, providing instrumental insights on the role of PKC in NB differentiation. TPA, acting as a DAG analog, directly binds and activates c/nPKCs, the main transducers of the TPA differentiation signal. Treatment of SH-SY5Y cells with low nanomolar concentrations of TPA results in the acute activation of PKCs and progressively drives cells towards a well-described sympathetic phenotype. This phenotype is characterized by increased neuritic outgrowth and upregulation of neuron-specific genes, such as GAP-43, neuropeptide Y, and tyrosine hydroxylase (Pahlman et al. 1981; Troller et al. 2001; Olsson & Nanberg 2001), increases in noradrenaline content (Pahlman et al., 1984;

Heikkila et al. 1993), and development of membrane excitability (Jalonen & Akerman, 1988). Besides SH-SY5Y and the parental cell lines SK-N-SH and SK-N-SN, IMR32 cells also respond to TPA treatment with induction of neuronal genes that specify neurotransmitter phenotypes (Mangoura et al., 2006b). PKC activation may mediate significant crosstalk with the RARs, as TPA induces the upregulation of RARβ expression in an nPKC/Ras/Raf-dependent manner (Perez-Juste & Aranda, 1999). Also in IMR32 cells, a synergistic transcriptional action of PKC and Ras with NF1 has been demonstrated in the induction of TH expression by TPA (Mangoura et al., 2006b).

The prominent role of PKCs in TPA-induced SH-SY5Y differentiation has been established in many studies and the most important aspects have been reviewed by Larsson, Pahlman, and co-workers (Larsson, 2006; Edsjo et al., 2007), where they note that PKCε is primarily responsible for TPA-induced differentiation, in particular for the induction of neuritic outgrowth. Characteristically, transfections with PKC constructs have suggested a dominant role of the PKCε regulatory domain as well as of its, unique amongst other PKCs, actin-binding properties in inducing neuritic outgrowth (Zeidman et al., 1999a, Zeidman et al., 2002) [2]. Thus, the PKCε pro-differentiating effects may involve mechanisms that do not directly implicate its kinase activity (Zeidman et al., 1999a). The kinase activity is also very important, as c/nPKC inhibitors, such as GF1092303X and Ro-318220, have been repeatedly shown to effectively inhibit TPA-induced ERK activation (Olsson et al., 2000; Troller et al., 2001; Leondaritis et al., 2009), neurofibromin phosphorylation (Leondaritis et al., 2009), and, TPA-induced neuritic outgrowth, expression of neuronal markers, and increase of neurotransmitter content (Heikkila et al., 1993; Fagerstrom et al., 1996; Troller et al., 2001; Olsson et al., 2000). Yet, further elucidation of the roles of individual PKCs would greatly benefit from more specific ATP-targeted inhibitors of cPKCs and nPKCs (Way et al., 2000). In this context, studies that used long-term inhibition of cPKCs with Go6976 to assess proliferation and survival of NB cells need to be re-evaluated, in lieu of recent studies suggesting that (a) Go6976 is a highly potent inhibitor of Aurora A and B kinases (Stolz et al., 2009), (b) Aurora A is overexpressed in most NB cell lines and stage 3-4 NB tumors and (c) Aurora A inhibitors have broad anti-NB activity (Maris, 2010 and refs therein).

An important feature of TPA-induced differentiation of SH-SY5Y cells is the apparent bifurcation of proximal signalling requirements for neuritic outgrowth or neuronal marker expression. Indeed, inhibition of ERK activation by PD98059 abolishes TPA-induced upregulation of neuropeptide Y and GAP-43, but has no effect on neuritic outgrowth (Olsson & Nanberg, 2001). In agreement, inhibition of PKCβI by LY379196 reduces TPA-induced ERK activation, and expression of GAP43 and neuropeptide Y, yet has no effect on neuritic outgrowth (Troller et al., 2001). Collectively, most studies converge on two important aspects: (i) the occurrence of an active cPKCα and cPKCβI-ERK axis in regulation of the early (within 24h) induction of neuronal markers and (ii) the mandatory role of PKCε, via both catalytic and scaffolding mechanisms, in the later induction of neuritic outgrowth and maintenance of differentiation.

2.2.3 Cyclic AMP analogues

cAMP analogues, such as bi-butyryl-cAMP (dbcAMP), have been long used, often in combination with bromodeoxyuridine (BrdU), to induce NB differentiation. Many neuronal

[2]Florakis et al., 2006, Federation of European Neuroscience Societies (FENS) Forum 3:A051.5

cell lines, like PC12 and NB cells (SH-SY5Y and IMR32), respond to these powerful intracellular signal transducers with increased neuritic outgrowth and upregulation of neuronal markers, such as GAP43 and TH (e.g Christensen et al., 2003; Birkeland et al., 2009). The effect of cAMP analogues may also be reproduced with forskolin, a direct activator of adenylyl cyclase (AC). Forskolin models the established ability of many GPCR agonists coupled to Gs/AC activation to drive differentiation via increased production of cAMP in various NB and other cellular contexts (Monaghan et al., 2008; Canals et al., 2005). Two major pathways serve as proximal transducers of the cAMP signal: the Epac1/2 (exchange protein activated by cAMP)/Rap GTPase and the PKA pathways (Bos, 2006), both of which may contribute to differentiation (Christensen et al., 2003; Birkeland et al., 2009). In addition to PKA and Epac, PI3K has also been implicated in cAMP-induced differentiation of NB cells as well as in the maintenance of elongated neurites (Sanchez et al., 2004).

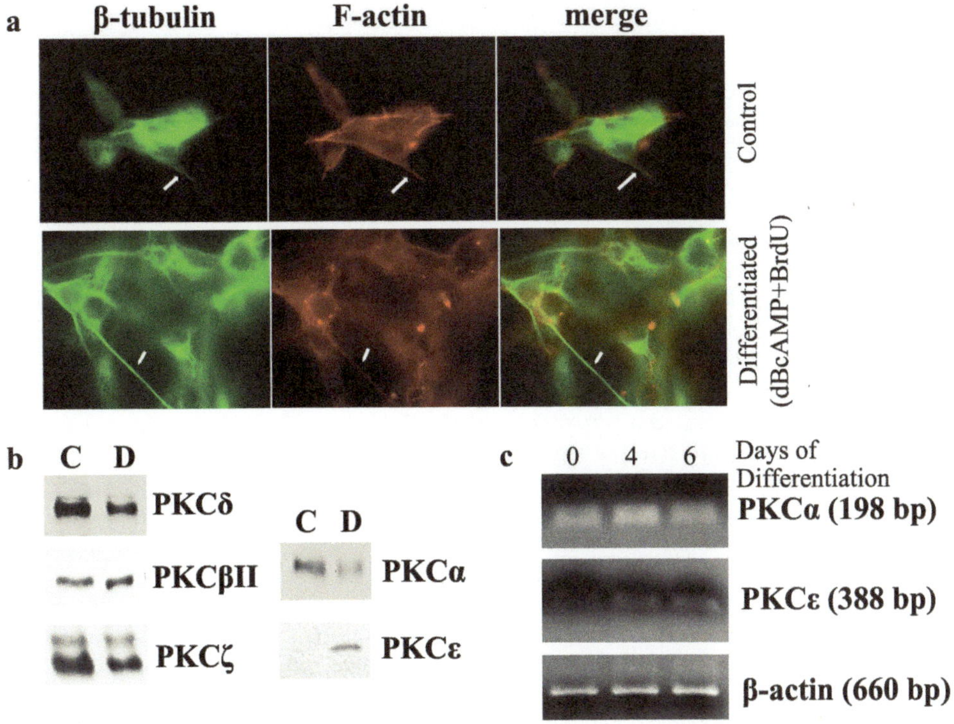

Fig. 1. Upregulation of PKCε and downregulation of PKCα during cAMP-induced differentiation of IMR32 cells. Cells were incubated in MEM plus 10% heat-inactivated FBS in the absence (control, C) or presence (D) of dBcAMP+ BrdU. Fixation, antibodies, immunostaining, and microscopy (a), as well as Western blotting (b) and RT-PCR (c) were performed as described (e. g., Mangoura et al., 1993; Li et al., 2001; Mangoua et al., 2006b; Leondaritis et al., 2009)

A typical example of cAMP-differentiated IMR32 cells is illustrated in Fig. 1a. After 4-6 days of 1 mM dBcAMP and 2.5 μM BrdU cells have acquired pyramidal-shaped cell bodies and elongated neurites that often extend up to 4-5 times the cell body length. Double staining for F-actin and βIII-tubulin reveals the extended organization of microtubules into organized, axon-like bundles, quite rich in F-actin (Fig. 1a, arrows in upper versus arrows in lower panels). PKCs have not been widely implicated in cAMP-induced NB differentiation, yet our analysis of the protein levels of PKC isoforms reveals great differences in control and differentiated cells (Fig. 1b). Specifically, the levels of the cPKC βII, and nPKC δ or ζ remain unaltered, cPKCα is extensively downregulated and nPKCε upregulated (Fig. 1b). Downregulation of PKCα is probably a post-translational event, as its mRNA levels remain constant throughout dBcAMP+BrdU exposure (Fig. 1c, 0 versus 4 and 6 days). In contrast, PKCε mRNA expression is significantly and progressively upregulated over the same time period (Fig. 1c). From these observations it is clear that cPKCα and nPKCε may impinge on cAMP-differentiation pathways, in a similar manner to that described for RA and TPA-differentiation pathways in sections 2.2.1 and 2.2.2.

2.3 Aspects of PKC regulation in neuroblastoma differentiation

2.3.1 cPKCs vs nPKCs and differentiation

Ample evidence exists for PKC requirement in NB differentiation by TPA and RA (Table 1, sections 2.2.1 and 2.2.2). Furthermore, PKC activity is implicated in NB differentiation mechanisms set in motion by growth factors, neurotrophic factors, and GPCR agonists (Fagerstrom et al., 1996; Silei et al., 2000; Canals et al., 2005; Monaghan et al., 2008) (Table 1). In some instances, PKCε has been identified as the crucial isoform (e.g. Silei et al., 2000; Fagerstrom et al., 1996), but there is still some controversy for the contribution of other nPKCs, namely PKC δ and θ. PKCθ, expressed occasionally in NB cells or tumors (Zeidman et al., 1999b), may contribute to apoptotic pathways in SK-N-BE(2) and SH-SY5Y cells (Schultz & Larsson, 2004; Schultz et al., 2003). Unlike θ, δ is commonly expressed (Zeidman et al., 1999b), yet again, transfection studies with full-length, catalytically inactive, or active PKCδ variants have revealed a pro-apoptotic role (Schultz et al., 2003; Schultz & Larsson, 2004). A major role of PKCδ in the sensitization of NB cells (SH-SY5Y and SK-N-BE(2C)) to etoposide (Marengo et al., 2011) was just recently described, validating similar observations in other cell types (Griner and Kazanietz, 2007). The function of aPKCs in NB differentiation is not clear at present, except recent indications that inhibition of PKCι has pro-apoptotic, and antiproliferative effects (Pilai et al., 2011).

The balance between abundance and activity of cPKCs versus nPKCs during initiation (early responses) or maintenance of NB differentiation has emerged as an important question. cPKCs are thought to be involved in early responses, such as induction of neuronal markers and commitment of NB cells to survival pathways. nPKCs appear to control the long term phenotypic result consisting of elaboration of dentrites, as well as stabilization of the transcriptional networks that specify differentiation and neurotransmitter phenotype acquisition. This distinct mode of action may be best appreciated by the altered regulation of expression levels of the cPKC α and the nPKC ε during cAMP-induced differentiation of IMR32 cells (Fig. 1). This shift in balance of PKCα/PKCε expression during differentiation has been repeatedly observed in developmental studies and the analysis of the periods of neurogenesis and neurodifferentiation, or in culture models that recapitulate these periods (Mangoura et al., 1993; Battaini et al., 1994). Furthermore, it has been suggested that growth factor-induced differentiation of SH-SY5Y may occur even when PKCα is ablated after treatment with high (1 μM) TPA concentrations (Fagerstrom et al., 1996). Remarkably, experiments in IMR32 cells directly corroborate and expand this notion. As shown in Fig. 2, direct, specific downregulation of PKCα expression with phosphorothioate-modified antisense oligonucleotides (5'-GGGACCATGGCTGACGT-3', 15 μg/mL x 5 days) results in a differentiated phenotype, indistinguishable from that caused by dBcAMP+BrdU (Fig. 1). Thus, suppression of PKCα alone may suffice for the induction of morphological differentiation in NB cell lines.

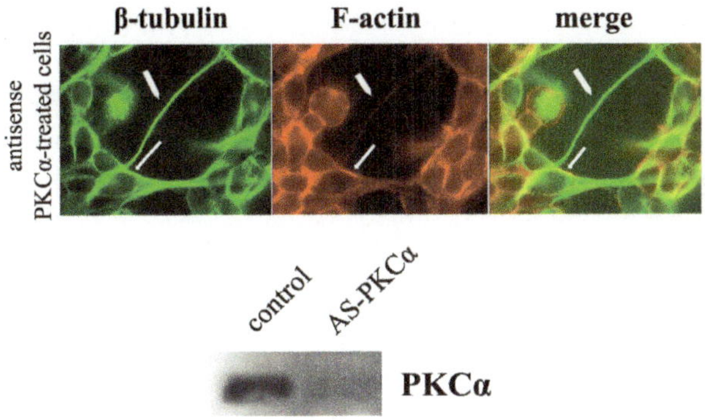

Fig. 2. Specific downregulation of PKCα induces differentiation in IMR32 cells. PKCα translation was silenced with antisense-PKCα oligonucleotides. Arrows indicate different long, tubulin-rich processes and intense cortical actin staining (upper panel). Downregulation of PKCα protein levels was confirmed by Western blotting (lower panel). Methods were performed as in Fig. 1

2.3.2 PKCs and cytoskeletal changes during NB differentiation

The input of PKC activation on cytoskeletal changes associated with neuritic outgrowth during NB differentiation in all three cytoskeleton systems, namely microtubules, F-actin, and intermediate filaments is well established. The F-actin cortical cytoskeleton may be viewed, in a general sense, as a direct target of the differentiation process (Mangoura et al., 1997). Among prominent PKC substrates of particular relevance are proteins that directly bind to F-actin, such as MARCKS, GAP43, adducin, fascin, and ERM proteins (Larsson, 2006). MARCKS and GAP43 have a pivotal role in remodeling the F-actin cytoskeleton during neurite outgrowth, growth cone motility, and synapse formation (Laux et al., 2000; Larsson, 2006). Neurofibromin is another PKC substrate that may associate with the F-actin cytoskeleton in neurons and SH-SY5Y cells (Li et al., 2001; Mangoura et al., 2006a).

Analysis of cytoskeletal protein localization after a prolonged (24h) treatment of IMR32 cells with TPA reveals also a sustained recruitment of neurofibromin in Triton X-100 insoluble fractions (HP lanes, Fig. 3) where cortical cytoskeleton proteins reside; concurrently, neurofibromin is not detected in the urea-soluble fractions (UF lanes, Fig. 3), where cytosolic organelle and nuclear proteins are found. At the same time, there is substantial loss of the intermediate filament protein vimentin in Triton X-100-soluble (cytosol) and -insoluble fractions (T2 and HP lanes, respectively), consistent with its downregulation upon differentiation of NB cells (Yabe et al., 2003). In parallel, vinculin, an F-actin binding protein and developmentally-regulated (Cheng et al., 2000) PKC substrate (Mangoura, 1997),

becomes enriched in cytoplasmic actin fractions (T2 lanes), suggestive of the extended reorganization of the actin cytoskeleton at the onset of neuritic outgrowth.
PKCs may serve also as upstream regulators of other signalling modules that modify cortical actin cytoskeleton proteins. For example, nPKCs, and specifically PKCε, are necessary for Src/FAK-dependent formation of active Cas/Crk complexes in differentiated SH-SY5Y cells (Fagerstrom et al., 1998; Bruce-Staskal & Bouton, 2001) and in neurons (Mangoura, 1997). Importantly, Src activation and phosphorylation is a PKCε-sensitive, long lasting (>16h) event during TPA- and IGF1/bFGF-induced differentiation of SH-SY5Y cells, suggesting the engagement of this pathway in the extensive remodeling of actin cytoskeleton during elongation and elaboration of neurites (Fagerstrom et al., 1998). Notably, PKCε was recently shown to organize a proximal signalling protein complex containing Src and Fyn tyrosine kinases, essential for downstream ERK activation in neurons (Asimaki & Mangoura, 2011), and in SH-SY5Y cells (Asimaki et al., 2007).

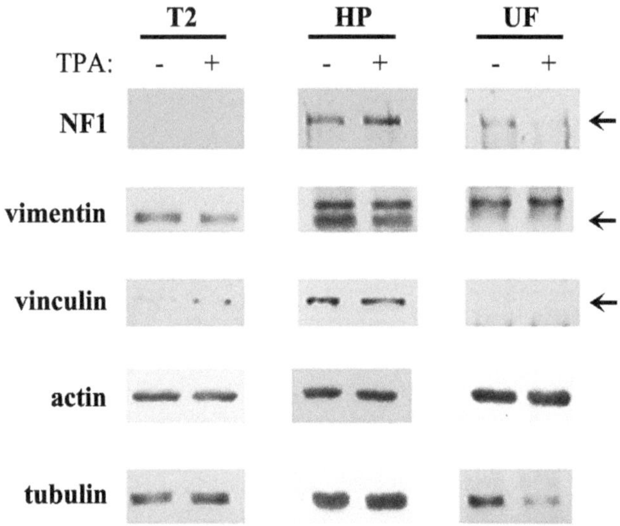

Fig. 3. Changes in cytoskeletal protein localization during early phases of TPA-induced differentiation in IMR32 cells. Cells were treated with 100 nM TPA for 24 h and cell lysates were fractionated into Triton X 100-soluble cytoplasmic actin fractions (T2), Triton X 100-insoluble cortical actin fractions (HP), and urea-soluble fractions (UF, representing also nuclear proteins), as described (Fox et al., 1993). Protein abundance in the fractions was analysed using Western blotting and the indicated antibodies (Mangoura, 1997; Li et al., 2000; Mangoura et al., 2006a).

Independent studies on gene expression profiles in advanced NB tumors have shown that many genes involved in Fyn signalling and organization of the F-actin cytoskeleton are downregulated (Berwanger et al., 2002). The importance of Fyn, in particular, was further validated when expression of active Fyn elicited differentiation and growth arrest in NB cells (Berwanger et al., 2002). These studies collectively highlight the tight inter-regulation between the abundance and activation of PKCε and Src/Fyn, and the re-organization of the

F-actin cytoskeleton during NB differentiation. Further support for this aspect is lend by the high concentration of PKCε in growth cones of differentiated SH-SY5Y and SK-N-BE(2) cells (Fagerstrom et al., 1996; Zeidman et al., 1999a, 2002).

2.3.3 Differentiating agents regulate a functional PKCα/PKCε balance that controls neurofibromin phosphorylation and downstream ERK signalling in neuroblastoma cells

Neurofibromin is currently emerging as an important signalling protein positioned at the intersection of NB differentiation pathways, as A, it acts as a rheostat for the activation of the Ras/ERK pathway (Cichowski et al., 2003; Mangoura et al., 2006a, b), B, it is a NB tumor suppressor with only 50% of NB cell lines bearing two normal alleles, and 6% of primary NBs bearing genomic NF1 aberrations (Holzel et al., 2010), C, it is a PKC substrate (Mangoura et al., 2006a) and it is extensively and persistently phosphorylated at a PKC-specific site, the C-terminal Ser2808, in TPA-differentiated SH-SY5Y cells (Leondaritis et al., 2009), D, it provides responsiveness to RA (Holzel et al., 2010). Neurofibromin has been also implicated in cAMP signalling in other cell types (Rubin & Gutman, 2005) and this suggests that it may impinge on cAMP-induced NB differentiation as well. Yet, the effects of NB differentiating agents on neurofibromin abundance (Cichowski et al., 2003), phosphorylation (Izawa et al., 1996; Mangoura et al., 2006a; Leondaritis et al., 2009), and RasGAP activity (Mangoura et al., 2006a), all critical aspects of its function as a Ras/ERK pathway modulator, have not been thoroughly addressed with the exception of TPA-differentiated SH-SY5Y (Leondaritis et al., 2009). Long-term treatment of SH-SY5Y with TPA or RA results in differentiation with variations in the acquired neurotransmitter phenotypes (Pahlman et al., 1984), yet morphologically, all cells long extensions, heavily decorated with β-tubulin (Fig. 4a, arrows) and F-actin in their growing neuritic tips (Fig. 4a, arrowheads), these features are virtually absent in control cells (Fig. 4a, upper panel).

It is a striking event that neurofibromin is significantly phosphorylated (2-3 fold over control) at the PKC-specific, C-terminal Ser2808 site in SH-SY5Y cells even after 8 day of differentiation with TPA or RA (Fig. 4b). Thus, persistent PKC-specific neurofibromin phosphorylation appears to be a common feature of both TPA- and RA-differentiated SH-SY5Y cells. Neurofibromin may be acutely phosphorylated after stimulation by EGF or TPA by either PKCα or PKCε in neurons (Mangoura et al., 2006a). In SH-SY5Y cells, TPA-dependent, acute neurofibromin Ser2808-phosphorylation appears to be mediated primarily by cPKCs (Leondaritis et al., 2009). In the long term, PKCα mRNA levels are modestly increased in TPA- and RA-differentiated cells (2-3 fold over control), concurrently with extensive upregulation of PKCε mRNA levels (>10-fold over control) (Fig. 4c). At the protein level, however, differentiation is accompanied by reciprocal changes in PKCα and PKCε abundance and activity: PKCα protein levels are substantially downregulated, while PKCε protein levels are significantly upregulated, at least in RA-differentiated cells (Fig. 4d). Most importantly, phosphorylation of PKCε at Ser729, the hydrophobic motif residue, which is essential for priming the catalytic competence of PKCε (Cameron et al., 2009; Freeley et al., 2011), is significantly increased in both TPA- and RA-differentiated cells (Fig. 4d). Furthermore, phosphorylation of MARCKS, which can reliably serve as a proxy marker for total PKC activity, is also significantly increased in TPA- and RA-differentiated cells (Fig. 4d).

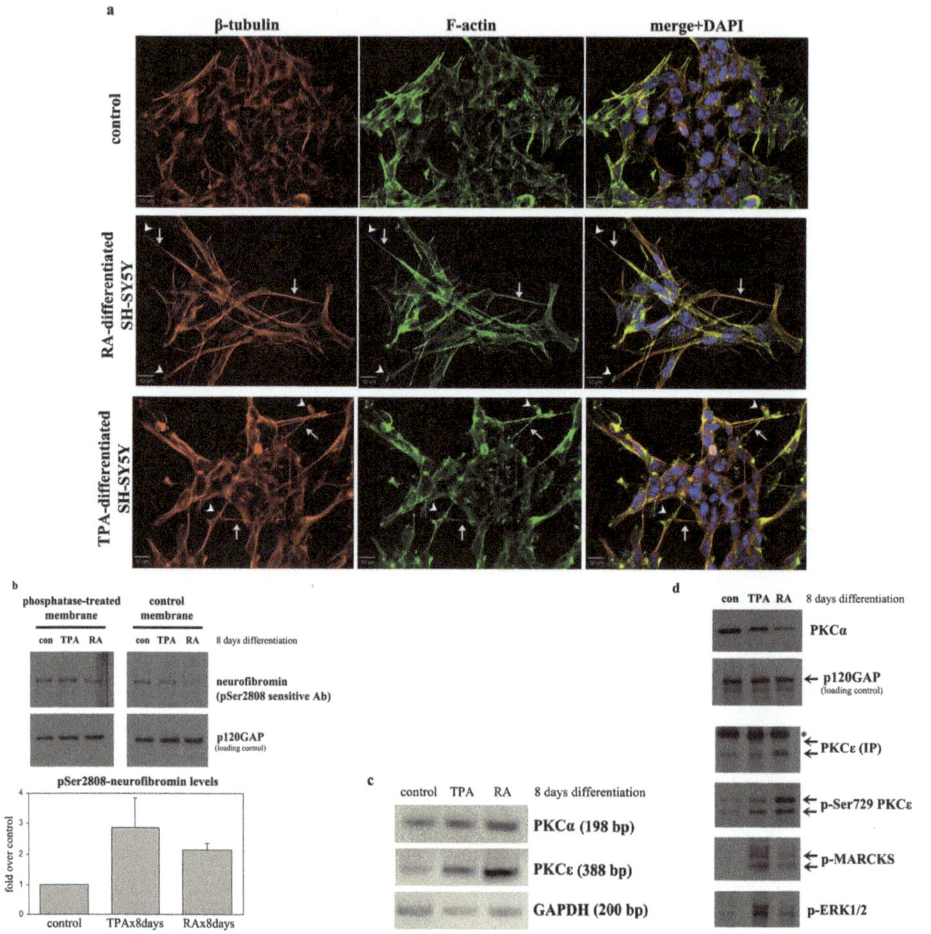

a. Cells were incubated in RPMI+10% HI-FBS in the absence (control, upper panel) or presence of 10 μM RA (middle panel), or 20 nM TPA (lower panel) for 8 days. Fixation and staining was performed as in Fig. 1. Images are projections of 5 0.5μm Z-stacks, deconvoluted with the nearest-neighbor algorithm (Slidebook software, Neurosciences Imaging Facility). b. Ser2808 phosphorylation of neurofibromin was studied with the use of sc-67 antibody in Western blot-phosphatase assays as described (Leondaritis et al., 2009). Note the significant gains in immunoreactivity to sc-67 in TPA- and RA-treated samples on membranes treated with phosphatase (left panel) that define the level of phosphorylation of neurofibromin on Ser2808. Quantification suggests a 2-3 fold increase of neurofibromin's Ser2808 phosphorylation in differentiated cells (lower panel). c) mRNA levels of PKCα, PKCε, and GAPDH were measured as described previously (Mangoura et al., 2006b). d) Abundance and phosphorylated forms of indicated proteins were assayed by Western blotting in total cell lysates; IP indicates that PKCε was immunoprecipitated from cell lysates and asterisk a crossreactive protein in the immunoprecipitates. Antibodies for p120GAP, p-Ser729 PKCε, p-MARCKS and p-ERK1/2 were as in Leondartis et al., 2009 and Asimaki & Mangoura, 2011.

Fig. 4. TPA and RA-differentiated SH-SY5Y cells exhibit similar patterns of morphology, neurofibromin phosphorylation, PKCα/PKCε expression and activation, and PKC downstream signalling.

Thus, differentiation in SH-SY5Y cells is characterized by intense, PKCε-dependent signalling; this may impact directly on phosphorylation and activation of downstream targets, such as neurofibromin (Fig. 4b) and ERK (Fig. 4d). In aggregate, this experimental evidence suggests that PKCε activation, neurofibromin Ser2808-phosphorylation, and ERK activation are all long-term effects, clearly associated with NB differentiation. Amongst these signal transduction, transcriptional, and translational events, regulation of PKCε arises as a nodal and fundamental feature of the differentiation process itself.

3. Conclusions

Regulation of long-term signalling that confers long lasting gene expression, and elicits and maintains differentiation in NB cells has yet to be fully explored. Moreover, the acute versus prolonged changes in posttranslational modifications of proteins within a signalling pathway that would support the fine tuning of pathway's output towards cell differentiation are still largely unresolved. NB cells constitute a unique model to address these issues, in hope that understanding the differentiation mechanism may provide predictors for NB therapy and clues for novel druggable targets or for increased efficacy of existing drugs. In this chapter we focused on PKCs (PKCε), neurofibromin, and the ERK pathway as important components of the action of differentiating agents in NB cells. Our experimental observations may well apply to most NB cells as the two cell lines used, IMR32 and SH-SY5Y, do not share a common pattern of genetic alterations: IMR32 cells are MYCN-positive and have wild-type ALK, while SH-SY5Y are MYCN-negative and have an activating mutation in ALK. Another focal point discussed for its important clinical implications, is the involvement of the tumor suppressor neurofibromin in RA- and TPA-induced differentiation.

PKCε is expected to impact significantly on NB differentiation through both its catalytic and scaffolding properties which may operate simultaneously. Apparently, cPKCs and nPKCs may be important for NB cell proliferation and apoptosis, and these may be regulated by PKCε. Also of clinical importance is the possibility that nPKCs (PKCδ, ε or others) may modulate NB cell responses to cytotoxic drugs. A second point concerning PKCε is its characterization as an oncogene in non-neural tumors (Basu & Sivaprasad, 2008). This PKCε eccentricity is shared with other members of the signaling mechanisms involved in NB differentiation, for example with H-Ras, a well-known oncogene when mutated, yet a favorable prognostic marker in MYCN-negative NB tumors when overexpressed, or TrkA, an oncogene and yet a favorable predictor when highly expressed in NBs (Brodeur, 2003). Both latter proteins are crucial for neuronal differentiation and survival in different cellular models, as PKCε. Therefore, we post the hypothesis that increases in PKCε in non NB tumors may reflect the cell's response to increase its differentiation.

In summary, novel approaches to treat NB in future are likely to be based on the continuing elucidation of the underlying signalling pathways that govern NB cell proliferation, apoptosis and differentiation, including, but not limited to, the PKC/ neurofibromin/ Ras/ ERK pathway. Combinatorial and multimodal therapies towards maximum efficacy and low toxicity will critically depend on the integration and implementation of this knowledge in further preclinical and clinical studies.

4. Acknowledgements

We wish to thank Sophia Karouzaki for help with PKCε immunoprecipitation. This work was supported by National Institutes of Health HD09402 and Greek Secretariat of Research & Technology PENED 03ED778 grants to D.M.

5. References

Armstrong, M.B., Bian, X., Liu, Y., Subramanian, C., Ratanaproeksa, A.B., Shao, F., Yu, V.C., Kwok, R.P., Opipari, A.W., & Castle, V.P. (2006). Signaling from p53 to NF-kappa B determines the chemotherapy responsiveness of neuroblastoma. *Neoplasia,* 8, 11, 964-974.

Asimaki, O., Sakellaridis, N., & Mangoura, D. (2007). Transactivation of Epidermal Growth Factor Receptor EGFR by CB1 cannabinoid receptor agonists. 8th Symposium of the Hellenic Society of Pharmacology, p17-18.

Asimaki, O., & Mangoura, D. (2011). Cannabinoid receptor 1 induces a biphasic ERK activation via multiprotein signaling complex formation of proximal kinases PKCε, Src, and Fyn in primary neurons. *Neurochem Int,* 58, 2, 135-144.

Asimaki, O., Leondaritis, G., Lois, G., Sakellaridis, N., & Mangoura , D. (2011). CB1R-dependent transactivation of FGFR 1 emanates from lipid rafts and amplifies ERK1/2 activation in embryonic cortical neurons. *J Neurochem,* 116, 5, 866-873.

Baker, D.L., Schmidt, M.L., Cohn, S.L., Maris, J.M., London, W.B., Buxton, A., Stram, D., Castleberry, R.P., Shimada, H., Sandler, A., Shamberger, R.C., Look, A.T., Reynolds, C.P., Seeger, R,C., Matthay, K.K.; Children's Oncology Group. (2010). Outcome after reduced chemotherapy for intermediate-risk neuroblastoma. *N Engl J Med,* 363, 14, 1313-1323.

Basu, A., & Sivaprasad, U. (2008) Protein kinase Cε makes the life and death decision. *Cell Signal,* 19, 8, 1633–1642.

Battaini, F., Garbillo, G., Bergamaschi, S., Parenti, M., Wetsel, W.C., Govoni, S., & Trabucchi, M. (1994) Regulation of protein kinase C in NG108-15 cell differentiation. *Biochem Biophys Res Commun,* 201, 1, 135-42.

Berwanger, B., Hartmann, O., Bergmann, E., Bernard, S., Nielsen, D., Krause, M., Kartal, A., Flynn, D., Wiedemeyer, R., Schwab, M., Schäfer, H., Christiansen, H., & Eilers, M. (2002) Loss of a FYN-regulated differentiation and growth arrest pathway in advanced stage neuroblastoma. *Cancer Cell,* 2, 5, 377-386.

Birkeland, E., Nygaard, G., Oveland, E., Mjaavatten, O., Ljones, M., Doskeland S.O., Krakstad, C., & Selheiml, F. (2009). Epac-induced Alterations in the Proteome of Human SH-SY5Y Neuroblastoma Cells. *J Proteomics Bioinform* 2, 6, 244-254.

Bos, J.L. (2006). Epac proteins: multi-purpose cAMP targets. *Trends Biochem Sci,* 31, 12, 680-686.

Brodeur, G.M. (2003). Neuroblastoma: biological insights into a clinical enigma. *Nat Rev Cancer,* 3, 3, 203-216.

Bruce-Staskal, P.J., & Bouton, A.H. (2001). PKC-dependent activation of FAK and src induces tyrosine phosphorylation of Cas and formation of Cas-Crk complexes. *Exp Cell Res,* 264, 2, 296-306.

Buchser, W.J., Slepak, T.I., Gutierrez-Arenas, O., Bixby, J.L., & Lemmon, V.P. (2010). Kinase/phosphatase overexpression reveals pathways regulating hippocampal neuron morphology. *Mol Syst Biol*, 6, 391.

Budas, G.R., Koyanagi, T., Churchill, E.N., & Mochly-Rosen, D. (2007). Competitive inhibitors and allosteric activators of protein kinase C isoenzymes: a personal account and progress report on transferring academic discoveries to the clinic. *Biochem Soc Trans*, 35, Pt 5,1021-1026.

Buday, L., & Downward, J. (2008). Many faces of Ras activation. *Biochim Biophys Acta*, 1786, 2, 178-187.

Cameron, A.J., Escribano, C., Saurin, A.T., Kostelecky, B., & Parker, P.J. (2009). PKC maturation is promoted by nucleotide pocket occupation independently of intrinsic kinase activity. *Nat Struct Mol Biol*, 16, 6, 624-630.

Canals, M., Angulo, E., Casadó, V., Canela, E.I., Mallol, J., Viñals, F., Staines, W., Tinner, B., Hillion, J., Agnati, L., Fuxe, K., Ferré, S., Lluis, C., & Franco, R. (2005). Molecular mechanisms involved in the adenosine A and A receptor-induced neuronal differentiation in neuroblastoma cells and striatal primary cultures. *J Neurochem*, 92, 2, 337-348.

Christensen, A.E., Selheim, F., de Rooij, J., Dremier, S., Schwede, F., Dao, K.K., Martinez, A., Maenhaut, C., Bos, J.L., Genieser, H.G., & Døskeland, S.O. (2003). cAMP analog mapping of Epac1 and cAMP kinase. Discriminating analogs demonstrate that Epac and cAMP kinase act synergistically to promote PC-12 cell neurite extension. *J Biol Chem*, 278, 37, 35394-35402.

Cheng, Y., Leung, S., & Mangoura, D. (2000). Transient suppression of cortactin ectopically induces large telencephalic neurons towards a GABAergic phenotype. *J Cell Sci.* 113, 18, 3161-3172.

Cichowski, K., Santiago, S., Jardim, M., Johnson, B. W. & Jacks, T. (2003). Dynamic regulation of the Ras pathway via proteolysis of the NF1 tumor suppressor. *Genes Dev*, 17, 4, 449–454.

Csukai, M., & Mochly-Rosen, D. (1999). Pharmacologic modulation of protein kinase C isozymes: the role of RACKs and subcellular localisation. *Pharmacol Res*, 39, 4, 253-259.

Delaune, A., Corbière, C., Benjelloun, F.D., Legrand, E., Vannier, J.P., Ripoll, C., & Vasse, M. (2008). Promyelocytic leukemia-nuclear body formation is an early event leading to retinoic acid-induced differentiation of neuroblastoma cells. *J Neurochem*, 104, 1, 89-99.

Downward, J., Graves, J.D., Warne, P.H., Rayter, S., & Cantrell, D.A. (1990). Stimulation of p21ras upon T-cell activation. *Nature*, 346, 6286, 719-723.

Durgan, J., Cameron, A.J., Saurin, A.T., Hanrahan, S., Totty, N., Messing, R.O., & Parker, P.J. (2008). The identification and characterization of novel PKCepsilon phosphorylation sites provide evidence for functional cross-talk within the PKC superfamily. *Biochem J*, 411, 2, 319-331.

Ebinu, J.O., Bottorff, D.A., Chan, E.Y., Stang, S.L., Dunn, R.J., & Stone, J.C. (1998). RasGRP, a Ras guanyl nucleotide- releasing protein with calcium- and diacylglycerol-binding motifs. *Science*, 280, 5366, 1082-1086.

Edsjö, A., Lavenius, E., Nilsson, H., Hoehner, J,C., Simonsson, P., Culp, L.A., Martinsson, T., Larsson, C., Påhlman, S. (2003). Expression of trkB in human neuroblastoma in relation to MYCN expression and retinoic acid treatment. *Lab Invest*, 83, 6, 813-823.

Edsjö, A., Nilsson, H., Vandesompele, J., Karlsson, J., Pattyn, F., Culp, L.A., Speleman, F., & Påhlman, S. (2004). Neuroblastoma cells with overexpressed MYCN retain their capacity to undergo neuronal differentiation *Lab Invest*, 84, 4, 406–417.

Edsjö, A., Holmquist, L., & Påhlman, S. (2007). Neuroblastoma as an experimental model for neuronal differentiation and hypoxia-induced tumor cell dedifferentiation. *Semin Cancer Biol*, 17, 3, 248-256.

Esposito, C.L., D'Alessio, A., de Franciscis, V., & Cerchia, L. (2008). A Cross-Talk between TrkB and Ret Tyrosine Kinases Receptors Mediates Neuroblastoma Cells Differentiation. *PLoS ONE*, 3, 2, e1643.

Fagerström, S., Påhlman, S., Gestblom, C., & Nånberg, E. (1996). Protein kinase C-epsilon is implicated in neurite outgrowth in differentiating human neuroblastoma cells. *Cell Growth Differ*, 7, 6, 775-785.

Fagerström, S., Påhlman, S., & Nånberg, E. (1998). Protein kinase C-dependent tyrosine phosphorylation of p130cas in differentiating neuroblastoma cells. *J Biol Chem*, 273, 4, 2336-2343.

Fernandes,N.D., Sun, Y., & Price, B.D. (2007). Activation of the Kinase Activity of ATM by Retinoic Acid Is Required for CREB-dependent Differentiation of Neuroblastoma Cells. *J Biol Chem*, 282, 22, 16577–16584.

Fox, J.E., Lipfert, L., Clark, E.A., Reynolds, C.C., Austin, C.D., & Brugge, J.S. (1993). On the role of the platelet membrane skeleton in mediating signal transduction. Association of GP IIb-IIIa, pp60c-src, pp62c-yes, and the p21ras GTPase-activating protein with the membrane skeleton. *J Biol Chem*, 268, 34, 25973-25984.

Freeley, M., Kelleher, D., & Long A. (2011). Regulation of Protein kinase C function by phosphorylation on conserved and non-conserved sites. *Cell Signal*, 23, 5, 753-762.

Griner, E.M., & Kazanietz, M.G. (2007). Protein kinase C and other diacylglycerol effectors in cancer. *Nat Rev Cancer*, 7, 4, 281-294.

Guzhova, I., Hultquist, A., Cetinkaya, C., Nilsson, K., Påhlman, S., & Larsson. L.G. (2001). Interferon-gamma cooperates with retinoic acid and phorbol ester to induce differentiation and growth inhibition of human neuroblastoma cells. *Int J Cancer*, 1, 94, 97-108.

Hadjidaniel, M.D., & Reynolds, C.P. (2010). Antagonism of cytotoxic chemotherapy in neuroblastoma cell lines by 13-cis-retinoic acid is mediated by the antiapoptotic Bcl-2 family proteins. *Mol Cancer Ther*, 9, 12, 3164-3174.

Hahn, C.K,. Ross, K.N., Warrington, I.M., Mazitschek, R., Kanegai, C.M., Wright, R.D., Kung, A.L., Golub, T.R., Stegmaier, K. (2008). Expression-based screening identifies the combination of histone deacetylase inhibitors and retinoids for neuroblastoma differentiation. *Proc Natl Acad Sci U S A*, 105, 28, 9751-9756.

Hamilton, M., Liao, J., Cathcart, M.K., & Wolfman, A. (2001). Constitutive association of c-N-Ras with c-Raf-1 and protein kinase C epsilon in latent signaling modules. *J Biol Chem*, 276, 31, 29079-29090.

Heikkila, J., Jalava, A., & Eriksson K. (1993). The selective protein kinase C inhibitor GF109203X inhibits phorbol ester-induced morphological and functional differentiation of SH-SY5Y human neuroblastoma cells. *Biochem Biophys Res Commun*, 197, 3, 1185–1193.

Hellmann, J., Rommelspacher, H., Mühlbauer, E., & Wernicke, C. (2010). Raf kinase inhibitor protein enhances neuronal differentiation in human SH-SY5Y cells. *Dev Neurosci*, 32, 1, 33-46.

Hölzel, M., Huang, S., Koster, J., Ora, I., Lakeman, A., Caron, H., Nijkamp, W., Xie, J., Callens, T., Asgharzadeh, S., Seeger, R.C., Messiaen, L., Versteeg, R., & Bernards, R. (2010). NF1 is a tumor suppressor in neuroblastoma that determines retinoic acid response and disease outcome. *Cell*, 142, 2, 218-29.

Hundle, B., McMahon, T., Dadgar, J., Chen, C.H., Mochly-Rosen, D., & Messing, R.O. (1997). An Inhibitory Fragment Derived from Protein Kinase Ce Prevents Enhancement of NGF Responses by Ethanol and Phorbol Esters. *J Biol Chem*, 272, 23, 15028-15035.

Hynds, D.L., Spencer, M.L., Andres, D.A., & Snow, D.M. (2003). Rit promotes MEK-independent neurite branching in human neuroblastoma cells. *J Cell Sci*, 116, Pt 10, 1925-1935.

Izawa, I., Tamaki, N., & Saya, H. (1996). Phosphorylation of neurofibromatosis type 1 gene product (neurofibromin) by cAMP-dependent protein kinase. *FEBS Lett*, 382, 1-2, 53-59.

Jalonen, T., & Akerman, K.E. (1988). Single transient potassium channels in human neuroblastoma cells induced to differentiate in vitro. *Neurosci Lett*, 86, 1, 99–104.

Janardhanan, R., Banik, N.L., & Ray, S.K. (2009). N-Myc down regulation induced differentiation, early cell cycle exit, and apoptosis in human malignant neuroblastoma cells having wild type or mutant p53. *Biochem Pharmacol*, 78, 9, 1105-1114.

Joshi, S., Guleria, R.S., Pan, J., Dipette, D., & Singh, U.S. (2007). Heterogeneity in retinoic acid signaling in neuroblastomas: Role of matrix metalloproteinases in retinoic acid-induced differentiation. *Biochim Biophys Acta*, 1772, 9, 1093-1102.

Katz, M., Amit, I., & Yarden, Y. (2007). Regulation of MAPKs by growth factors and receptor tyrosine kinases. *Biochim Biophys Acta*, 1773, 8, 1161-1176.

Kaufmann, D., Junge, I., Bartelt, B., Lattke, H., & Müller, R. (1999). On the lysosomal degradation of neurofibromin and its phosphorylation in cultured melanocytes. *Biol Chem*, 380, 9, 1071-1078.

Kawakami, Y., Kitaura, J., Yao, L., McHenry, R.W., Kawakami, Y., Newton, A.C., Kang, S., Kato, R.M., Leitges, M., Rawlings, D.J., & Kawakami, T. (2003). A Ras activation pathway dependent on Syk phosphorylation of protein kinase C. *Proc Natl Acad Sci U S A*, 100, 16, 9470-5.

Koehler, J.A., & Moran, M. F. (2001). RACK1, a protein kinase C scaffolding protein, interacts with the PH domain of p120GAP. *Biochem Biophys Res Commun*, 283, 4, 888-895.

Lallemend, F., Hadjab, S., Hans, G., Moonen, G., Lefebvre, P.P., & Malgrange, B. (2005). Activation of protein kinase CbetaI constitutes a new neurotrophic pathway for deafferented spiral ganglion neurons. *J Cell Sci*, 118, Pt 19, 4511-4525.

Larsson, C. (2006). Protein kinase C and the regulation of the actin cytoskeleton. *Cell Signal*, 18, 3, 276-284.

Laux, T., Fukami, K., Thelen, M., Golub, T., Frey, D. & Caroni P. (2000). GAP43, MARCKS and CAP23 modulate PI(4,5)P2 at plasmalemmal rafts and regulate cell cortex actin dynamics through a common mechanism. *J Cell Biol*, 149, 7, 1455–1472.

Lee, J.H., & Kim K.T. (2004). Induction of cyclin-dependent kinase 5 and its activator p35 through the extracellular-signal-regulated kinase and protein kinase A pathways during retinoic-acid mediated neuronal differentiation in human neuroblastoma SK-N-BE(2)C cells. *J Neurochem*, 91, 634–647

Leondaritis, G., Petrikkos, L., & Mangoura, D. (2009). Regulation of the Ras-GTPase activating protein neurofibromin by C-tail phosphorylation: implications for protein kinase C/Ras/extracellular signal-regulated kinase ½ pathway signaling and neuronal differentiation. *J Neurochem*, 109, 2, 573-583.

Li, C., Cheng, Y., Gutmann, D.A., & Mangoura D. (2001). Differential localization of the neurofibromatosis 1 (NF1) gene product, neurofibromin, with the F-actin or microtubule cytoskeleton during differentiation of telencephalic neurons. *Brain Res Dev Brain Res*, 130, 2, 231-248.

Maden, M. (2007). Retinoic acid in the development, regeneration and maintenance of the nervous system. *Nat Rev Neurosci*, 8, 10, 755-765.

Mangoura, D., & Dawson, G. (1993). Opioid peptides activate phospholipase D and protein kinase C-epsilon in chicken embryo neuron cultures. *Proc Natl Acad Sci U S A*, 90, 7, 2915-2919.

Mangoura, D., Sogos, V., & Dawson, G. (1993). PKC-e is a developmentally regulated, neuronal isoform in the chick embryo CNS. *J Neurosci Res*, 35, 5, 488-498.

Mangoura, D. (1997). mu-Opioids activate tyrosine kinase focal adhesion kinase and regulate cortical cytoskeleton proteins cortactin and vinculin in chick embryonic neurons. *J Neurosci Res*, 50, 3, 391-401.

Mangoura, D., Pelletiere, C., Leung, S., Sakellaridis, N., & Wang DX. (2000). Prolactin concurrently activates src-PLD and JAK/Stat signaling pathways to induce proliferation while promoting differentiation in embryonic astrocytes. *Int J Dev Neurosci*, 18, 7, 693-704.

Mangoura, D., Sun, Y., Li, C., Singh, D., Gutmann, D.H., Flores, A., Ahmed, M., & Vallianatos, G. (2006a). Phosphorylation of neurofibromin by PKC is a possible molecular switch in EGF receptor signaling in neural cells. *Oncogene*, 25, 5, 735-745.

Mangoura, D., Theofilopoulos, S., Karouzaki, S., & Tsirimonaki, E. (2006b). 12-O-tetradecanoyl-phorbol-13-acetate-dependent up-regulation of dopaminergic gene expression requires Ras and neurofibromin in human IMR-32 neuroblastoma. *J Neurochem*, 97, Suppl 1, 97-103.

Marais, R., Light, Y., Mason, C., Paterson, H., Olson, M.F. & Marshall C.J. (1998). Requirement of Ras-GTP-Raf complexes for activation of Raf-1 by protein kinase C. *Science*, 280, 109-112.

Marengo, B., De Ciucis, C., Ricciarelli, R., Passalacqua, M., Nitti, M., Zingg, J.M., Marinari, U.M., Pronzato, M.A., & Domenicotti, C. (2011). PKCδ sensitizes neuroblastoma cells to L-buthionine-sulfoximine and etoposide inducing reactive oxygen species overproduction and DNA damage. *PLoS One*, 6, 2, e14661

Maris, J.M. (2010). Recent advances in neuroblastoma. *N Engl J Med*, 362, 23, 2202-2211

Marshall, C.J. (1995). Specificity of receptor tyrosine kinase signalling: transient versus sustained extracellular signal-regulated kinase activation. *Cell*, 80, 2, 179-185.

Mattingly, R.R., Milstein, M.L., & Mirkin, B.L. (2001). Down-regulation of growth factor-stimulated MAP kinase signaling in cytotoxic drug-resistant human neuroblastoma cells. *Cell Signal*, 13, 7, 499-505.

McGillicuddy, L.T., Fromm, J.A., Hollstein, P.E., Kubek, S., Beroukhim, R., De Raedt, T., Johnson, B.W., Williams, S.M., Nghiemphu, P., Liau, L.M., et al. (2009). Proteasomal and genetic inactivation of the NF1 tumor suppressor in gliomagenesis. *Cancer Cell*, 16, 1, 44-54.

Meco, D., Riccardi, A., Servidei, T., Brueggen, J., Gessi, M., Riccardi, R., & Dominici, C. (2005). Antitumor activity of imatinib mesylate in neuroblastoma xenografts. *Cancer Lett*, 228, 1-2, 211-219.

Miloso, M., Villa, D., Crimi, M., Galbiati, S., Donzelli, E., Nicolini, G., & Tredici, G. (2004). Retinoic acid-induced neuritogenesis of human neuroblastoma SH-SY5Y cells is ERK independent and PKC dependent. *J Neurosci Res*, 75, 2, 241-252.

Monaghan, T.K., Mackenzie, C.J., Plevin, R., & Lutz, E.M. (2008). PACAP-38 induces neuronal differentiation of human SH-SY5Y neuroblastoma cells via cAMP-mediated activation of ERK and p38 MAP kinases. *J Neurochem*, 104, 1, 74-88.

Nitti, M., Furfaro, A.L., Cevasco, C., Traverso, N., Marinari, U.M., Pronzato, M.A., & Domenicotti, C. (2010). PKC delta and NADPH oxidase in retinoic acid-induced neuroblastoma cell differentiation. *Cell Signal*, 22, 5, 828-835.

Olsson, A.K. & Nanberg, E. (2001). A functional role for ERK in gene induction but not in Olsson, A.K., Vadhammar, K., & Nånberg, E. (2000). Activation and protein kinase C-dependent nuclear accumulation of ERK in differentiating human neuroblastoma cells. *Exp Cell Res*, 256, 2, 454-467. neurite outgrowth in differentiating neuroblastoma cells. *Exp Cell Res*, 265, 1, 21–30.

Påhlman, S., Odelstad, L., Larsson, E., Grotte, G. & Nilsson, K. (1981). Phenotypic changes of human neuroblastoma cells in culture induced by 12-O-tetradecanoyl-phorbol-13-acetate. *Int J Cancer*, 28, 5, 583–589.

Påhlman, S., Ruusala, A.I., Abrahamsson, L., Mattsson, M.E., & Esscher, T. (1984). Retinoic acid-induced differentiation of cultured human neuroblastoma cells: a comparison with phorbolester-induced differentiation. *Cell Differentiation*, 14, 2, 135-144.

Parker, P.J., & Murray-Rust, J. (2004). PKC at a glance. *J Cell Sci*, 117, Pt 2, 131-132.

Paruchuri, S., Hallberg, B., Juhas, M., Larsson, C., & Sjölander, A. (2002). Leukotriene D(4) activates MAPK through a Ras-independent but PKCepsilon-dependent pathway in intestinal epithelial cells. *J Cell Sci*, 115, Pt 9, 1883-1893.

Pastorino, F., Loi, M., Sapra, P., Becherini, P., Cilli, M., Emionite, L., Ribatti, D., Greenberger, L.M., Horak, I.D., & Ponzoni, M. (2010) Tumor regression and curability of preclinical neuroblastoma models by PEGylated SN38 (EZN-2208), a novel topoisomerase I inhibitor. *Clin Cancer Res*, 16, 19, 4809-4821.

Patrakitkomjorn, S., Kobayashi, D., Morikawa, T., Wilson, M.M., Tsubota, N., Irie, A., Ozawa, T., Aoki, M., Arimura, N., Kaibuchi, K., Saya, H. & Araki N. (2008). Neurofibromatosis type 1 (NF1) tumor suppressor, neurofibromin, regulates the neuronal differentiation of PC12 cells via its associating protein CRMP-2. *J Biol Chem*, 283, 14, 9399-9413.

Perez-Juste, G., & Aranda, A. (1999). Differentiation of neuroblastoma cells by phorbol esters and insulin-like growth factor 1 is associated with induction of retinoic acid receptor beta gene expression. *Oncogene*, 18, 39, 5393-5402.

Peterson, S., & Bogenmann, E. (2004). The RET and TRKA pathways collaborate to regulate neuroblastoma differentiation. *Oncogene*, 23, 1, 213-225.

Pillai, P., Desai, S., Patel, R., Sajan, M., Farese, R., Ostrov, D., & Acevedo-Duncan, M. (2011). A novel PKC-ι inhibitor abrogates cell proliferation and induces apoptosis in neuroblastoma. *Int J Biochem Cell Biol*, 43, 5, 784-794.

Raman, M., Chen, W., & Cobb, M.H. (2007). Differential regulation and properties of MAPKs. *Oncogene* 26, 22, 3100-3112.

Reynolds, C.P., & Lie, S.O. (2000) Retinoid therapy of neuroblastoma. In *Neuroblastoma*. Brodeur, G.M., Sawada, T., Tsuchida, Y., & Voute, P.A., pp 519-539, Elsevier Science BV.

Reynolds,C.P., Wang, Y., Melton, L.J., Einhorn, P.A., Slamon, D.J, & Maurer, B.J. (2000). Retinoic-acid-resistant neuroblastoma cell lines show altered MYC regulation and high sensitivity to fenretinide. *Medical and Pediatric Oncology*, 35,6, 597–602.

Reynolds, C.P., Matthay, K.K., Villablanca, J.G., & Maurer, B.J. (2003) Retinoid therapy of high-risk neuroblastoma. *Cancer Lett*, 197, 1-2, 185-192.

Rice, J.M. (2004). Causation of nervous system tumors in children: insights from traditional and genetically engineered animal models. *Toxicol Appl Pharmacol*, 199, 2, 175-191

Roose, J.P., Mollenauer, M., Gupta, V.A., Stone, J., & Weiss, A.A. (2005). Diacylglycerol-protein kinase C-RasGRP1 pathway directs Ras activation upon antigen receptor stimulation of T cells. *Mol Cell Biol*, 25, 11, 4426-4441.

Rosse, C., Linch, M., Kermorgant, S., Cameron, A.J., Boeckeler, K., & Parker, P.J. (2010). PKC and the control of localized signal dynamics. *Nat Rev Mol Cell Biol*, 11, 2, 103-112.

Rubin, J.B., Gutmann, D.H. (2005). Neurofibromatosis type 1 - a model for nervous system tumour formation? *Nat Rev Cancer*, 5, 7, 557-564.

Rubio, I., Rennert, K., Wittif, U., Beer, K., Durst, M., Stang, S. L., Stone, J. & Wetzker R. (2006). Ras activation in response to phorbol ester proceeds independently of the EGFR via an unconventional nucleotide-exchange factor system in COS-7 cells. *Biochem J*, 398, 2, 243–256.

Sánchez, S., Jiménez, C., Carrera, A.C., Diaz-Nido, J., Avila, J., & Wandosell, F. (2004). A cAMP-activated pathway, including PKA and PI3K, regulates neuronal differentiation. *Neurochem Int*, 44, 4, 231-242.

Santos, S.D., Verveer, P.J., & Bastiaens, P.I. (2007). Growth factor-induced MAPK network topology shapes Erk response determining PC-12 cell fate. *Nat Cell Biol*, 9, 3, 324-330.

Saurin, A.T., Durgan, J., Cameron, A.J., Faisal, A., Marber, M.S., & Parker, P.J. (2008). The regulated assembly of a PKCepsilon complex controls the completion of cytokinesis. *Nat Cell Biol*, 10, 8, 891-901.

Schechtman, D., & Mochly-Rosen, D. (2001). Adaptor proteins in protein kinase C-mediated signal transduction. *Oncogene*, 20, 44, 6339-6347.

Scheffzek, K., Ahmadian, M.R., & Wittinghofer, A. (1998). GTPase-activating proteins: helping hands to complement an active site. *Trends Biochem Sci*, 23, 257-262

Schönwasser, D.C., Marais, R.M., Marshall, C.J., & Parker, P.J. (1998). Activation of the mitogen-activated protein kinase/extracellular signal-regulated kinase pathway by conventional, novel, and atypical protein kinase C isotypes. *Mol Cell Biol*, 18, 2, 790-798.

Schultz, A., Jönsson, J.I., & Larsson, C. (2003). The regulatory domain of protein kinase Ctheta localises to the Golgi complex and induces apoptosis in neuroblastoma and Jurkat cells. *Cell Death Differ*, 10, 6, 662-675.

Schultz, A., & Larsson, C. (2004). Ceramide influences neurite outgrowth and neuroblastoma cell apoptosis regulated by novel protein kinase C isoforms. *J Neurochem*, 89, 6, 1427-1435.

Shirai, Y., Adachi, N., & Saito, N. (2008). Protein kinase Cepsilon: function in neurons. *FEBS J*, 275, 16, 3988-3994.

Silei, V., Politi, V., & Lauro, G.M. (2000). Uridine induces differentiation in human neuroblastoma cells via protein kinase C epsilon. *J Neurosci Res*, 61, 2, 206-211.

Sparatore, B., Patrone, M., Passalacqua, M., Pedrazzi, M., Pontremoli, S., & Melloni, E. (2000). Human neuroblastoma cell differentiation requires protein kinase C-theta. *Biochem Biophys Res Commun*, 279, 2, 589-594.

Stokoe, D., & McCormick, F. (1997). Activation of c-Raf-1 by Ras and Src through different mechanisms: activation in vivo and in vitro. *EMBO J*, 16, 9, 2384-2396.

Stolz, A., Vogel, C., Schneider, V., Ertych, N., Kienitz, A., Yu, H., & Bastians, H. (2009). Pharmacologic abrogation of the mitotic spindle checkpoint by an indolocarbazole discovered by cellular screening efficiently kills cancer cells. *Cancer Res*, 69, 9, 3874-3883.

Troller, U., Zeidman, R., Svensson, K. & Larsson C. (2001). A PKCbeta isoforms mediates phorbol ester-induced activation of Erk1/2 and expression of neuronal differentiation genes in neuroblastoma cells. *FEBS Lett*, 508, 1, 126–130.

Ueda, Y., Hirai, S., Osada, S., Suzuki, A., Mizuno, K., & Ohno S. (1996). Protein kinase C activates the MEK-ERK pathway in a manner independent of Ras and dependent on Raf. *J Biol Chem*, 271, 38, 23512-23519.

Valkova, C., Maerz, S., Imhof, D., & Liebmann, C. (2007). Protein kinase Cepsilon may act as EGF-inducible scaffold protein for phospholipase Cgamma1. *Cell Signal*, 19, 9, 1830-1843.

Vogel, K.S., Brannan, C.I., Jenkins, N.A., Copeland, N.G., & Parada, L.F. (1995). Loss of Neurofibromin Results in Neurotrophin-Independent Survival of Embryonic Sensory and Sympathetic Neurons. *Cell*, 82, 5, 733-742.

Vogel, K.S., El-Afandi, M., & Parada, L.F. (2000). Neurofibromin Negatively Regulates Neurotrophin Signaling through p21ras in Embryonic Sensory Neurons. *Mol Cell Neurosci*, 15, 4, 398-407.

von Kriegsheim, A., Baiocchi, D., Birtwistle, M., Sumpton, D., Bienvenut, W., Morrice, N., Yamada, K., Lamond, A., Kalna, G., Orton, R., Gilbert, D., & Kolch, W. (2009). Cell fate decisions are specified by the dynamic ERK interactome. *Nat Cell Biol*, 11, 12, 1458-1464.

Way, K.J., Chou, E., & King, G.L. (2000). Identification of PKC-isoform-specific biological actions using pharmacological approaches. *Trends Pharmacol Sci*, 21, 5, 181-187.

Wood, K.W., Qi, H., D'Arcangelo, G., Armstrong, R.C., Roberts, T.M., & Halegoua, S. (1993). The cytoplasmic raf oncogene induces a neuronal phenotype in PC12 cells: a potential role for cellular raf kinases in neuronal growth factor signal transduction. *Proc Natl Acad Sci U S A*, 90, 11, 5016-5020.

Yabe, J.T., Chan, W.K., Wang, F.S., Pimenta, A., Ortiz, D.D., & Shea, T.B. (2003). Regulation of the transition from vimentin to neurofilaments during neuronal differentiation. *Cell Motil Cytoskeleton*, 56, 3, 193-205.

Yunoue, S., Tokuo, H., Fukunaga, K., Feng, L., Ozawa, T., Nishi, T., Kikuchi, A., Hattori, S., Kuratsu, J., Saya, H. & Araki N. (2003). Neurofibromatosis type I tumor suppressor regulates neuronal differentiation via its GTPase-activating protein function toward Ras. *J Biol Chem*, 278, 29, 26958-26969.

Zeidman, R., Löfgren, B., Pâhlman, S., & Larsson, C. (1999a). PKCepsilon, via its regulatory domain and independently of its catalytic domain, induces neurite-like processes in neuroblastoma cells. *J Cell Biol*, 145, 4, 713-726.

Zeidman, R., Pettersson, L., Sailaja, P.R., Truedsson, E., Fagerström, S., Påhlman, S., & Larsson, C. (1999b). Novel and classical protein kinase C isoforms have different functions in proliferation, survival and differentiation of neuroblastoma cells. *Int J Cancer*, 81, 3, 494-501.

Zeidman, R., Trollér, U., Raghunath, A., Påhlman, S., & Larsson, C. (2002). Protein Kinase Cε Actin-binding Site Is Important for Neurite Outgrowth during Neuronal Differentiation. *Mol Biol Cell*, 13, 1, 12–24.

Zheng, Y., Liu, H., Coughlin, J., Zheng, J., Li, L., & Stone, J.C. (2005). Phosphorylation of RasGRP3 on threonine 133 provides a mechanistic link between PKC and Ras signaling systems in B cells. *Blood*, 105, 9, 3648-3654.

Zhu, Y., Romero, M.I., Ghosh, P., Ye, Z., Charnay, P., Rushing, E.J., Marth, J.D., & Parada, L.F. (2001). Ablation of NF1 function in neurons induces abnormal development of cerebral cortex and reactive gliosis in the brain. *Genes Dev*, 15, 7, 859-876.

7

Bioactive Sphingolipids in Neuroblastoma

Mehrdad Rahmaniyan, Amr Qudeimat and Jacqueline M. Kraveka
Division of Pediatric Hematology Oncology
Hollings Cancer Center and Darby Children's Research Institute
Medical University of South Carolina
USA

1. Introduction

Neuroblastoma is a solid tumor cancer that originates in the nerve tissue of the neck, chest, abdomen, or pelvis, but most commonly in the adrenal gland. It is the third most common pediatric cancer and accounts for ~15% of all childhood cancer deaths. Neuroblastoma has one of the lowest survival rates of all pediatric cancers. It is the most common solid tumor diagnosed during infancy. This tumor may involute spontaneously in infants, or it may sometimes mature to a benign ganglioneuroma. On the other hand, older children often present with advanced stage disease at the time of diagnosis. While survival in patients with favorable biological features may exceed 90%; the survival rates for children with high risk neuroblastoma have historically been under 40%. However, advances made in recent years in understanding the biology of neuroblastoma have led to the identification of patient groups with higher risk disease and to the rise of new modalities for combating this disease. Patients with high-risk neuroblastoma undergo aggressive multi-modal therapies including, chemotherapy, immunotherapy, surgery, stem cell transplantation, and radiation. Survivors also experience many treatment related toxicities and long term side effects. Therefore, new approaches are needed for these patients (Maris, 2010)

One of the molecules that can stimulate differentiation of neuroblastoma cells is Ceramide (Fig. 1), a biologically active effector molecule composed of a fatty acyl chain bound to a sphingoid backbone via an amide linkage (Kraveka & Hannun, 2009). The study and modulation of sphingolipids and their effects has emerged as an attractive therapeutic target due to their potent anti-proliferative effects (Hannun & Obeid, 2008). Ceramide is the central building block for sphingolipids. It serves as a precursor for the synthesis of more complex sphingolipids, and is generated by multiple pathways (Fig. 2). Sphingolipids comprise a class of lipids that share the presence of a sphingosine (or related sphingoid) base in the backbone of their structures. Research in the past two decades has shown that sphingolipids, in addition to their roles as structural components of cell membranes, play important roles as regulators of signal transduction in cell differentiation, cell proliferation, inflammation and apoptosis. Ceramide mediates important cellular activities such as induction of cell differentiation, growth arrest, senescence, and apoptosis. Sphingosine-1-phosphate has the opposite effect of ceramide stimulating cell proliferation and is involved in angiogenesis and inflammation (Kolesnick, 2002). In this chapter we will review the roles these bioactive sphingolipids and their related enzymes play in cancer pathogenesis and how their regulation is a novel target for neuroblastoma therapy.

2. Sphingolipids

2.1 Background

Sphingolipids were first discovered in the late 1800s. Sphingolipids such as cerebroside and sphingomyelin were first isolated from brain tissues by J. L. W. Thudichum (van Echten-Deckert & Herget, 2006). He named these compounds after the Sphinx because of their enigmatic properties. For a long time, sphingolipids had been identified as biologically inert components of cell membranes. However, advances in biochemistry and molecular biology have demonstrated that these lipids play key roles in the regulation of several fundamental biological processes such as signal transduction, cell proliferation, migration, and apoptosis (Ogretmen & Hannun, 2004). These regulations are mediated by many enzymes involved in sphingolipid metabolism (Hannun & Luberto, 2000).

2.2 Structure and metabolism of sphingolipids

Sphingolipids are composed of a long chain sphingoid base that is acylated with a fatty acid via an amide linkage, and a polar head group (Fig 1.). In contrast to ceramide, complex sphingolipids contain hydrophilic groups such as phosphate, phosphocholine, or sugar residues. Based on the head group, sphingolipids may be divided into three groups: ceramides, sphingomyelins, and glycosphingolipids. Ceramide is the central building block for sphingolipids and has a hydroxyl group at position 1, sphingomyelin has phosphocholine, and glycosphingolipids have carbohydrate groups. The latter are further subdivided into cerebrosides, gangliosides, and sulfatides (Jana & Pahan, 2010; Sietsma et al., 2002). Gangliosides, such as GD2, are composed of a gylcosphingolipid (ceramide and oligosaccharide) with one or more sialic acids such as n-acytlneuraminic acid liked to the sugar.

The metabolic pathways of sphingolipids are very complex (Fig 2.). Sphingolipid metabolism is regulated at several different levels such as the expression of regulating enzymes, post-translational modifications, or allosteric mechanisms (Futerman & Hannun, 2004). There are multiple pathways for the generation and regulation of bioactive Sphingolipids (Figure 2). Many of these pathways reside in specific sub-cellular compartments and respond to various extra- and intra-cellular stimuli. Most enzymes of sphingolipid metabolism have specific sub-cellular localization(s), thereby exerting profound effects on the signaling and regulatory functions of the generated sphingolipid in a specific compartment. The best studied of these pathways are the *de-novo* pathway, the sphingomyelinase pathway, and the salvage/recycling pathway (Kraveka & Hannun, 2009).

The *de-novo* pathway pathway of ceramide synthesis starts at the cytosolic surface of the endoplasmic reticulum (ER) where a series of enzymes generate ceramides with different acyl chain lengths from non-sphingolipid precursors (Futerman & Hannun, 2004; Gault et al., 2010; Kok et al., 1997; Merrill, 2002) . This pathway is initiated by condensation of serine with palmitoyl-CoA, and catalyzed by the rate-limiting enzyme serine palmitoyl transferase, resulting in the formation of 3-ketosphinganine. The latter is reduced in an NADPH-dependent reaction by the enzyme 3-ketosphinganine reductase to sphinganine, which is then acylated into dihydroceramide by (dihydro)-ceramide synthases (Fig. 3) (Saddoughi et al., 2008, van Echten-Deckert, 2006). A desaturation follows by the enzyme dihydroceramide desaturase (DES-1/DEGS-1) to insert a double bond between carbons 4-5 in the sphingosine backbone of dihydroceramide to generate ceramide (Michel et al., 1997). Ceramide synthases (Fig. 3) are also referred to as Lass (longevity-assurance homologue) family members. Six mammalian ceramide synthases have been identified molecularly, and each ceramide synthases protein exerts specificity for the generation of distinct endogenous dihydroceramides and ceramides with fatty-acid chain length specificity (Ogretmen, 2006; Pewzner-Jung et al., 2006).

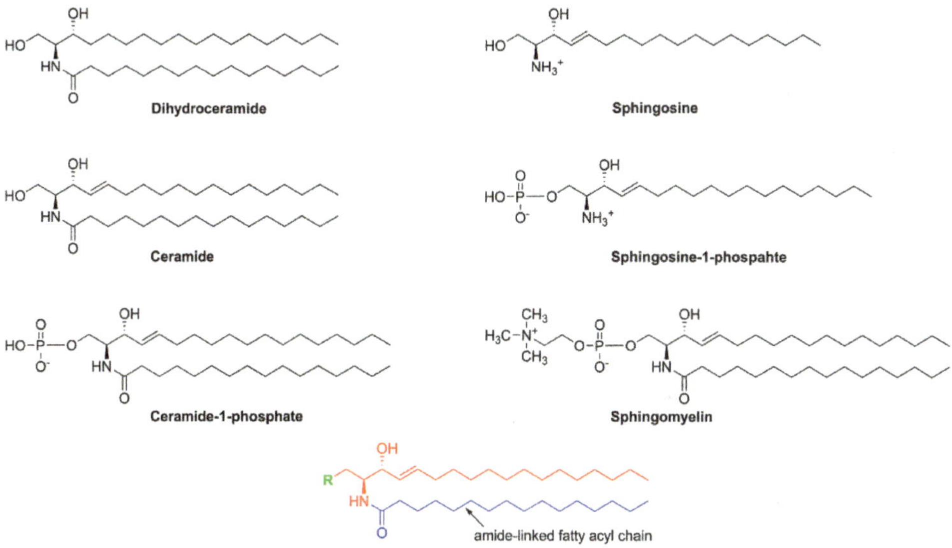

Ceramide is composed of a sphingoid base (18 carbons) and an amide linked fatty acid (14-26 carbons). Complex sphingolipids are composed of a hydrophilic head group (R) attached to the lipophilic ceramide backbone. These head groups may be phosphocholine in sphingomyelin or sugars in glycosphingolipids.

Fig. 1. Bioactive sphingolipids.

The *de novo* pathway is localized to the ER and continues in the Golgi apparatus where the enzymes glucosylceramide synthase and sphingomyelin synthase are localized (Pettus et al., 2002) . Once ceramide is generated, it can be glycosylated by glucosylceramide synthase to form glucosylceramide on the cytoplasmic surface of Golgi. Glucosylceramide then serves as the precursor for glycosphingolipids. Ceramide may also be galactosylated to galactosylceramide by galactosylceramide synthase in the ER. Sulfatides and Gala-series glycosphingolipids are formed from galactosylceramide synthase. In turn, glycosphingolipids are hydrolyzed by β-glucosidases and galactosidases to regenerate ceramide (Tettamanti, 2004). Gangliosides such as GD-2, are structurally and biochemically derived from lactosylceramide which is formed by transfer of a galactosyl residue to glucosylceramide. Sequential addition of one, two or three sialic acids to lactosylceramide results in formation of GM3, GD3 and GT3 (Bektas & Spiegel, 2004). In addition, ceramide can be converted into a number of other bioactive sphingolipids, including ceramide-1-phosphate, sphingosine, and sphingosine-1-phosphate.

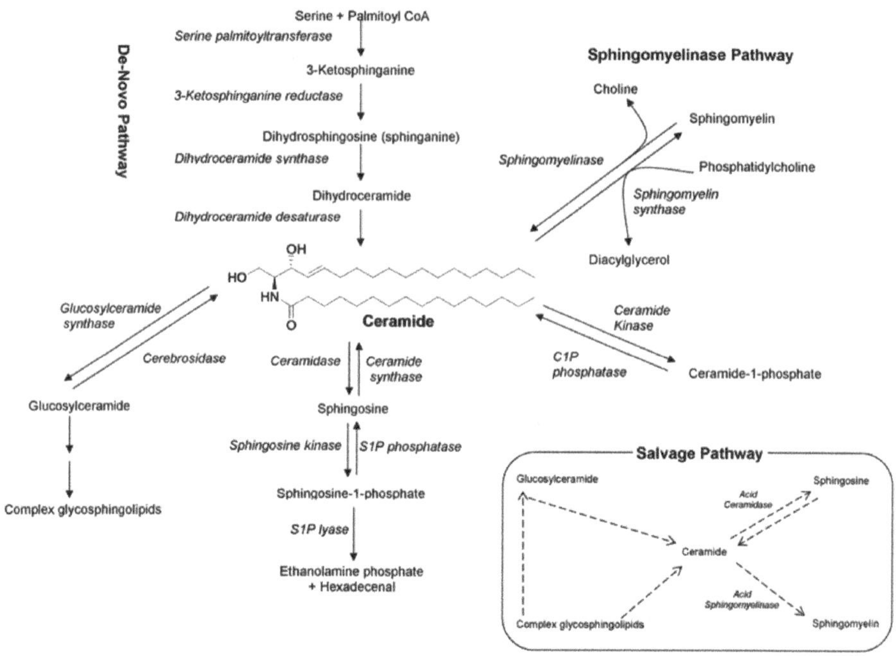

Ceramide is the central building block for complex sphingolipids. Enzymes are shown in italics.

Fig. 2. Sphingolipid Metabolism.

In the sphingomyelinase pathway, ceramide is generated from hydrolysis of sphingomyelin through the action of either acid or neutral sphingomyelinases (Clarke & Hannun, 2006; Marchesini & Hannun, 2004). These enzymes break down sphingomyelin to produce ceramide and phosphocholine, and are stimulated in response to TNF-α (Luberto et al., 2002; Schwandner et al., 1998), Fas ligand (Lin et al., 2000), or oxidative stress (Goldkorn et al., 1998). The sphingomyelinase mediated hydrolysis of sphingomyelin has emerged as a major pathway of stress-induced ceramide generation. Conversely, sphingomyelin synthase transfers the headgroup of phosphatidylcholine to ceramide and generates sphingomyelin and diacylglycerol in the process. This pathway has been suggested to regulate the levels of not only sphingomyelin and ceramide, but also diacylglycerol (Villani et al., 2008) as well as the activation of NFκB (Hailemariam et al., 2008; Luberto et al., 2000).

The sphingolipid recycling or salvage pathway refers to the various mechanisms of ceramide generation from the catabolism of complex sphingolipids which are broken down into sphingosine, which is then reused through reacylation to produce ceramide (Kitatani et al., 2008). This pathway involves a number of key enzymes that include sphingomyelinases, cerebrosidases, ceramidases, and ceramide synthases. It has been estimated to contribute from 50% to 90% of sphingolipid biosynthesis. Degradation of sphingolipids and glycosphingolipids takes place mostly in the acidic subcellular compartments, the late endosomes and the lysosomes. Sphingomyelin is converted to ceramide by acid sphingomyelinases. Ceramide can be deacylated with loss of the fatty acid from the amide bond through the action of acid ceramidases to yield sphingosine. Sphingosine can then translocate across the lysosome where it can be either re-acylated to ceramide or phosphorylated by sphingosine kinase 1 or 2 to generate sphingosine-1-phosphate. Sphingosine-1-phosphate can be cleared by the action of specific phosphatases that regenerate sphingosine or by the action of a lyase that cleaves sphingosine-1-phosphate into ethanolamine-1-phosphate and a C_{16}-fatty-aldehyde.

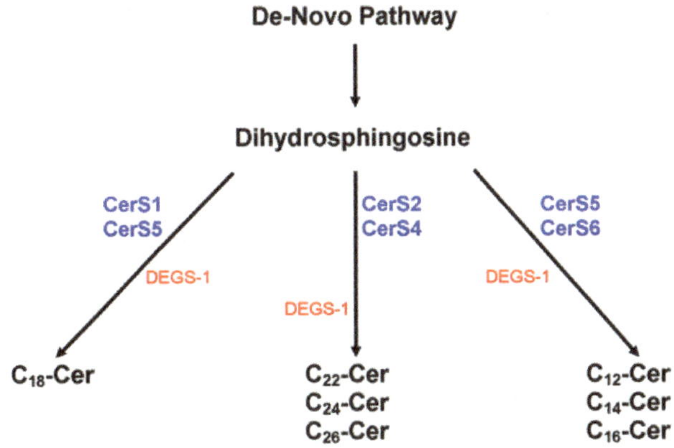

Fig. 3. Ceramide Synthases.

Ceramide synthases (CerS) acylate dihydrosphingosine to form dihydroceramide. In mammalian cells, each CerS protein exerts specificity for the generation of endogenous ceramides with distinct fatty-acid chain lengths. (Adapted from Ogretmen B, *FEBS Lett*, 2006)

3. Role of sphingolipids in cancer cell proliferation, cell differentiation, senescence and apoptosis

Sphingolipids play essential roles in cell growth, survival, and death (Birbes et al., 2002; Ogretmen & Hannun, 2004). These regulatory properties of sphingolipids allowed them to be extensively studied in cancer pathogenesis, cancer treatment, and multidrug resistance. In sphingolipid metabolism the precursors and products are biologically not inert, but they are effectors to mediate specific cell regulatory actions. These regulatory actions are mediated by interaction of sphingolipids with cell surface receptors, modulation of lipid rafts, and intracellular actions (Billich & Baumruker, 2008). The most studied bioactive sphingolipids are ceramide, ceramide-1-phospate, sphingosine, and sphingosine-1-phosphate.

3.1 Ceramide

Ceramide exerts its downstream effects via activation of ceramide-activated serine–threonine phosphatases such as protein phosphates 1 and 2 (PP1 and PP2A) (Dobrowsky et al., 1993; Wolff et al., 1994) In addition, ceramide has been shown to activate PKCζ, the kinase KSR, and cathepsin D (Conway et al., 2000; Heinrich et al., 1999; Lozano et al., 1994). Different stimuli can activate ceramide formation. Chemotherapeutic agents such as daunorubicin, etoposide, camptothecin, fludarabine, and gemcitabine activate the *de-novo* pathway of ceramide generation. Other agents such as cytarabine, actinomycin D, etoposide, cisplatin (Biswal et al., 2000; Bose et al., 1995; Chalfant et al., 2002; Gomez del Pulgar et al., 2002; Lacour et al., 2004;

Perry et al., 2000; Strum et al., 1994; Suzuki et al., 1997) actívate the sphinomyelinase pathways. TNF-α, UV, and γ radiation have been shown to activate sphingomyelinases (Haimovitz-Friedman et al., 1994; Kim et al., 1991; Liu et al., 1998; Zhang et al., 2001)

Ceramide has been widely implicated in the regulation of programmed cell death via numerous stimuli. Ceramide triggers apoptosis via mitochondrial, ER-stress and lysosomal pathways (Hannun & Obeid, 2011; Huang et al.; Mullen et al., 2011). Ceramide is able to induce G0/G1 cell cycle arrest by acting on different targets. It induces dephosphorylation of retinoblastoma (Rb) protein by the activation of protein phosphatase 1 (PP1) (Dbaibo et al., 1995; Jayadev et al., 1995; Kraveka et al., 2007). Additionally, ceramide specifically inactivates cyclin-dependent kinase 2 (CDK2) through dephosphorylation (Lee et al., 2000), or by up-regulation of CDK inhibitors p21 and p27 through activation of protein phosphatase 2A (PP2A) (Adibhatla & Hatcher, 2010).

Ceramide also can be increased by administration of short chain cell-permeable ceramides (Huang *et al.*, 2011; Ryland et al., 2011). However, the effect of systemic application of these exogenous ceramides is reduced due to precipitation and minimal membrane transport. Nanotechnology has been developed to encapsulate short-chain ceramides for systemic delivery. The nanotechnology includes nanoliposomes, nanocolloids, and nanodendrimers (Ryland *et al.*, 2011). Encapsulation of the exogenous ceramides into nanoliposomes reduces the systemic side effects when applied via intravenous or intraperintoneal routes. Exogenous C_2-ceramide treatment of neuroblastoma cell line SH-SY5Y induced apoptosis by inactivation of Akt and translocation of apoptosis-inducing factor (AIF) to the nucleus and neuronal cell death by a mitochondrial pathway (Kim et al., 2007).

The involvement of ceramide in senescence is supported by the fact that ceramide levels increased in human fibroblasts as they became senescent. Additional studies showed that treatment of low-passage-number human fibroblasts with exogenous short ceramide was able to induce morphological and biological changes associated with senescence such as dephosphorylation of Rb protein and inhibition of cyclin dependent kinases. The underlying mechanisms for these changes were the inhibition of phospholipase D (PLD), diacylglycerol generation, and PKC activity (Venable et al., 1995).

Our group has provided another direct link between ceramide and senescence by involvement of ceramide in the regulation of telomerase activity and telomere length (Kraveka et al., 2003). Telomeres contain long stretches of tandemly repeated 5′-TTAGGG-3′ sequences found at chromosome ends in mammals to protect chromosomes. Progressive shortening of telomeres during cell division triggers the onset of events leading to senescence and/or cell death. However, telomeres are more stable in immortalized and cancer cells. This stabilization is achieved by the activity of telomerase, an RNA-dependent DNA polymerase, whose activity is detected in most cancer cells, allowing them to escape senescence and acquire immortality. Treatment of human neuroblastoma cell lines, SK-N-SH and SK-N-AS, with all trans retinoic acid (ATRA) inhibited telomerase activity and increased the endogenous levels of $C_{24:0}$ and $C_{24:1}$ ceramides). The relation between ceramide and telomerase was supported by the fact that treatment of cells with ATRA in the presence of myriocin, a serine palmitoyl transferase inhibitor, significantly blocked the accumulation of ceramide, and presence of myriocin prevented in part the inhibition of telomerase. Mechanistically, inhibition of telomerase by endogenous ceramide in response to ATRA treatment involved, at least in part, down-regulation of the expression of telomerase reverse transcriptase (hTERT) mRNA. The regulation of telomerase expression by ceramide involves the inactivation of c-MYC transcription factor through increased ubiquitin-proteasome-mediated proteolysis (Ogretmen et al., 2001). Additionally, ceramide mediates rapid shortening of telomeres, involving the inhibition of nuclear localization and the telomere-binding function of glyceraldehydes-3-phosphate dehydrogenase (Sundararaj et al., 2004). These data suggest that ceramide is one of the upstream regulators of telomerase activity and telomere length and has a key role in induction of senescence.

3.2 Dihydroceramide

Dihydroceramide, an intermediate in *de novo* pathway, is synthesized from sphinganine. Dihydroceramides were thought to be biologically inactive. Previous studies on the biological activity of dihydroceramides using their short chain analogs concluded that dihydroceramides were inactive in inducing cell death and apoptosis (Ahn & Schroeder, 2002; Bielawska et al., 1993; Sugiki et al., 2000). However, recent studies have shown dihydroceramides to be involved in important cellular responses such as cell cycle arrest, apoptosis, ceramide channel formation, autophagy, and oxidative stress (Idkowiak-Baldys et al., 2010; Kraveka et al., 2007; Signorelli et al., 2009; Stiban et al., 2006; Wang et al., 2008; Zheng et al., 2006). These studies indicate the significance of endogenous levels of dihydroceramides in cell regulatory processes, and they suggest that the enzyme dihydroceramide desaturase has the potential to regulate cell function through both ceramide and dihydroceramide their respective sphingolipid metabolites. We will discuss dihydroceramides more in depth later in the chapter.

3.3 Sphingosine and sphingosine-1-phosphate

Sphingosine, was the first bioactive sphingolipid to be identified (Hannun et al., 1986). It is the product of ceramide degradation by ceramidases, acts like ceramide to exerting apoptotic effects in multiple cell lines (Ekiz & Baran, 2010). Other studies also showed that sphingosine interferes with multidrug resistance mechanisms in cancer cells. These mechanisms were ineffective against sphingosine-induced cell death. Sphingosine interacts with protein kinase C (PKC), ERK, akt/Protein Kinase B (akt/PKB) to induce apoptosis (Chang et al., 2001; Jarvis et al., 1997). Additionally, sphingosine causes the release of cytochrome c from mitochondrial membrane followed by activation of caspases (Cuvillier et al., 2001). In murine Neuro-2A neuroblastoma cells, sphingosine induced differentiation (Riboni, et al., 1998).

Sphingosine-1-phosphate acts not only as anti-apoptotic agent, but also is implicated in angiogenesis, adhesion, migration, and inflammation (Chalfant & Spiegel, 2005; van Echten-Deckert & Herget, 2006). It can function as an extracellular first messenger and also as intracellular second messenger. Intracellularly, it serves as second messenger regulating calcium mobilization, cell proliferation and survival (Ling et al., 2011). Extracellularly, sphingosine-1-phosphate exerts most of its actions as a specific ligand for a family of nine G-protein-couples receptors (GPCRs) called sphingosine-1-phosphate -R_{1-5} and Gpr63 (Argraves et al., 2010), contributing to physiological and pathological processes such as angiogenesis which is a critical factor for tumor progression (Ling *et al.*, 2011). Mechanistically, the proliferative effect of sphingosine-1-phosphate may be mediated by mitogen-activated protein kinase (MAPK) pathway (Shu et al. 2002). It also stimulates cell survival pathways, such as nuclear factor κB (NF-κB) (Xia et al., 2002) and the Akt/PI3K (Phosphatidylinositol 3-kinase) pathway (Banno et al., 2001). Growth factors and cytokines

including vascular endothelial growth factor (VEGF) and platelet derived growth factor (PDGF) induce spingosine kinase leading to elevation of sphingosine-1-phosphate.
Sphingosine kinase-1 inhibition can sensitize cells toward the action of radiation, to ceramide, and to cytotoxic agents such as doxorubicin, etoposide, imatinib, and cicplatin (Billich & Baumruker, 2008). There are currently several sphingosine kinase-1 and 2 inhibitors available and in development. Sphingosine kinase is an attractive target in cancer treatment because blockage of its product, sphingosine-1-phosphate inhibits proliferation and induces apoptosis in cancer cells (French et al., 2006). Another approach is the use of the anti-sphingosine-1-phosphate receptor monoclonal antibodies. These antibodies can induce tumor progression in murine xenograft and allograft models (Saddoughi et al., 2008). They also can prevent sphingosine-1-phosphate induced cell proliferation and the release of pro-angiogenic cytokines. This pathway presents an important target for cancer treatment.

3.4 Ceramide-1-phosphate

Ceramide-1-phosphate, another product of ceramide by phosphorylation ceramide kinase (CERK), shows pro-survival effects by inducing DNA synthesis, blocking caspases, suppressing acid sphingomyelinase, and promoting phagasome formation (Chalfant & Spiegel, 2005; Gomez-Munoz, 2004; Gomez-Munoz et al., 1995; Gomez-Munoz et al., 2004; Hinkovska-Galcheva et al., 2005). It is involved in mast cell degranulation (Mitsutake et al., 2004). It has been shown to also serve as an activator of cytosolic phospholipase A2 (cPLA2a) (Pettus et al., 2004), and thus may function as a key regulator of eicosanoid synthesis. ATRA has been reported to inhibit CERK transcription in SH-SY-5Y neuroblastoma cells (Murakami et al., 2010)

3.5 Glucosylceramide

Glucosylceramides have proliferative effects and are implicated in the development of drug resistance in cancer cells (Lucci et al., 1998; Messner & Cabot, 2010; Ogretmen & Hannun, 2004). Numerous studies showed that glucosylceramide synthase overexpression is associated with multidrug resistance in many cancers including breast cancer (Zhang et al., 2011), leukemia (Xie et al., 2008) colon cancer (Liu et al., 2010b), and glioblastoma (Barth et al., 2010). One study showed that glucosylceramide synthase regulates MDR1 expression through cSrc and β-catenin signaling (Liu *et al.*, 2010b). In leukemia cells overexpression glucosylceramide synthase gene is correlated with Bcl-2 signal transduction (Liu et al., 2010a). In glioblastoma and neuroblastoma cells, glucosylceramide synthase mediated drug resistance is via inhibition of NADPH oxidase (NOX), thus blocking ROS generation and limiting apoptosis (Barth et al., 2010). A new mixed-backbone oligonucleotide (MBO-asGCS), that specifically suppresses overexpressed human glucosylceramide synthase gene, can restore drug sensitivity in multidrug resistant cancer cells leading to apoptosis (Patwardhan et al., 2009). Additionally, co-Inhibition of MRD1 gene and glucosylceramide synthase by siRNA can restore sensitivity in multidrug resistant breast cancer cells (Zhang *et al.*, 2011). Inhibition of glucosylceramide synthase by 1-Phenyl-2-decanolyamino-3-morpholino-1-propanol (PDMP) inhibited cell growth in murine neuroblastoma cells (Uemura et al., 1991). Taken together, these data suggest the involvement of glucosylceramide synthase in multidrug resistance and pharmacological targeting of glucosylceramide synthase is an important goal to restore sensitivity of multidrug resistant cancer cells to cytotoxic agents and improve their efficacy.

4. Ceramide levels and sphingolipid expression in cancer

Total ceramide levels and the amounts of individual ceramide species have been shown to be altered in tumor samples. Total ceramide content was decreased in ovarian tumors compared to normal ovarian tissue (Rylova et al., 1998). High grade astrocytomas also had lower levels of ceramide (Riboni et al., 2002). Utilizing liquid chromatography/mass spectrometry (LC/MS) to identify individual ceramide species has yielded some interesting results. Defects in the ceramide synthase 1 dependent generation of C_{18}-ceramide (Figure 3) have been implicated in the pathogenesis of squamous cell carcinomas of the head and neck (HNSCC) (Koybasi et al., 2004). The data showed that the levels of C_{16}-, C_{24}-, $C_{24:1}$-ceramides were significantly elevated in the majority of tumor tissues compared to their normal tissues, while the levels of only C_{18}-ceramide were significantly decreased. Further experiments showed that overexpression of ceramide synthase 1, which is responsible for C_{18}- generation, resulted in the inhibition of HNSCC cell growth, and enhanced chemotherapy-induced apoptosis in UMSCC22A HNSCC cells *in situ*, and in HNSCC xenografts *in vivo* (Senkal et al., 2007). More recent work from Dr. Ogretmen's group showed that knockdown of ceramide synthase 6/C_{16}-ceramide induced endoplasmic reticulum stress-mediated apoptosis (Senkal et al., 2010). A study by Schiffmann (Schiffmann et al., 2009) measured endogenous ceramide levels in 43 malignant breast tumors and 21 benign breast biopsies via LC/MS. The levels of C_{16}-, $C_{24:1}$- and $C_{24:0}$-ceramides were significantly elevated in malignant tumors as compared to benign and normal tissue. As expected, increased mRNA expression of ceramide synthases 2, 4, and 6 was detected. In breast cancer elevated levels of C_{16} ceramide were associated with metastatic disease.

In summary, these recent reports appear contradictory to many of the older cell-based studies in which *in-vitro* treatments with ceramide or agents that stimulate ceramide generation induced apoptosis. However, these newer studies suggest that the levels of specific ceramide species and/or the activity and expression enzymes of sphingolipid metabolism play an important role in cancer pathogenesis. These studies suggest a relationship between certain long-chain ceramides and malignant transformation (Ponnusamy et al., 2010; Ryland *et al.*, 2011). Studies also suggest that *de novo* generated ceramides differing in their fatty acid chain length may have opposing roles in promotion/suppression of tumors. These facts show that the biological function of ceramide may vary by its carbon chain length. Studies are currently underway in our laboratory examining sphingolipid species content and expression of sphingolipid enzymes in "low/intermediate risk" and "high risk" neuroblastoma tumor samples.

The cellular ratio of ceramide/sphingosine-1-phosphate determines the cell fate and response to chemotherapy. Several studies suggest that sphingosine-1-phosphate regulates survival, migration, and proliferation of cancer cells. Elevated sphingosine-1-phosphate levels are associated with resistance to apoptosis and poor prognosis in cancer (Ryland *et al.*, 2011). Lung, colon, kidney, breast, ovary, stomach, and uterine cancers showed increased levels of sphingosine kinase 1 protein and mRNA (Ogretmen & Hannun, 2004). Sphingosine kinase 2 overexpression has been reported in neuroblastoma (Li et al., 2011).

Acid ceramidase, another enzyme in sphingolipid metabolism that hydrolyzes ceramide into sphingosine, may be dysregulated in some cancers. Acid ceramidase was overexpressed in leukemic T-cell large granular lymphocyte leukemia and its inhibition induced apoptosis in these cells (Shah et al., 2008). One study showed that acid ceramidase was induced by genistein (a phytoestrogen isoflavone) contributing to growth in MCF-7 breast cancer cells (Lucki & Sewer, 2011). Daunorubicin treatment in hepatoma cell line increased acid ceramidase levels leading to protection of these cells from daunorubicin-induced apoptosis (Morales et al., 2007). Acid ceramidase overexpression lead to resistance of prostate cancer cells to chemotherapy and radiation. In these cells acid ceramidase overexpression was associated with increased autophagy and lysosomal density leading to higher resistance by rapidly metabolizing ceramide (Mahdy et al., 2009; Turner et al., 2011). These results demonstrate that inhibitors to sphingolipid pathway enzymes have great potential in the treatment of malignancies.

5. The dihydroceramide desaturase enzyme: Implications for neuroblastoma therapy

5.1 Desaturase enzymes

Dihydroceramide desaturase family members, consisting of DES1 and DES2, belong to the desaturase/hydroxylase superfamily. Dihydroceramide desaturase 1, is encoded by DES1 (degenerative spermatocyte homologue 1) gene, and it is myristoylated at N-terminus (Beauchamp et al., 2007)). A family of sphingolipid Δ4-desaturases (homologues of the *Drosophila melanogaster* degenerative spermatocyte gene-1 (*des-1*)) were identified via a bioinformatics approach (Ternes et al., 2002). These proteins contain three His-containing consensus motifs that are characteristic of a group of membrane fatty acid desaturases. The human homologue of *des-1* is now referred to as *DEGS-1*, although it was first cloned in 1997 and named as Membrane Lipid Desaturase (MLD) since its physiologic substrate was not determined at the time (Cadena et al., 1997). DEGS-1 is the only dihydroceramide desaturase reported to be present in human cells, and its mouse homologue (mDES1) was shown to have desaturase activity (Omae et al., 2004). hDES2, the human homologue of the mouse DES2 (mDes2) gene, like mDES2 has dihydroceramide hydroxylase activity (Mizutani et al., 2004). While mDES2 has been reported to have both desaturase and hydroxylase activity, no desaturase activity was detected in HEK 293 human embryonic kidney cells overexpressing hDES2 (Mizutani *et al.*, 2004). DES2 is responsible for biosynthesis of phytosphingoglycolipids in the microvilli of intestinal epithelial cells, kidney, and skin (Omae et al., 2004).

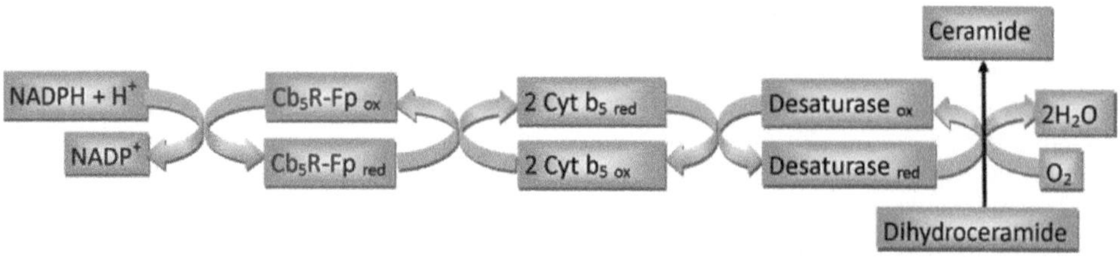

Dihydroceramide synthesized by de novo pathway is desaturated by the multi-enzyme complex consisting of a flavoprotein-containing cytochrome b5 reductase (Cb5R-Fp), a cytochrome (cyt) b5, and a desaturase. (Adapted from Geeraert L, et al., Biochem J 1997)

Fig. 4. Dihydroceramide Desaturase Complex.

The dihydroceramide desaturase complex consists of flavin-containing cytochrome b_5 reductase, a heme-containing cytochrome b_5, and a non heme-containing desaturase (Causeret et al., 2000; Geeraert et al., 1997).

5.2 Role of dihydroceramide desaturase on cell growth, cell cycle, and endogenous ceramide and dihydroceramide levels in neuroblastoma

We investigated the role of dihydroceramide desaturase as a key enzyme in the *de novo* pathway of ceramide generation using human neuroblastoma SMS-KCNR cells (Kraveka *et al.*, 2007). This study included the use of a novel *in situ* assay for desaturase activity using pyridinum conjugated water-soluble dihydroceramide analogues. The dihydroceramidoid (C_{12}-dhCCPS) was as substrate to measure the activity of the enzyme by monitoring the conversion of C_{12}-dhCCPS to C_{12}-CCPS via LC/MS. Our results showed that dihydroceramide desaturase was an active enzyme in neuroblastoma cells and the assay provided a powerful method to study the dihydroceramide desaturase activity and the effects of related inhibitors on dihydroceramide desaturase activity.

The effect of dihydroceramide desaturase inhibition by siRNA on endogenous ceramide and dihydroceramides was studied. There was approximately a 13-fold increase of endogenous dihydroceramides whereas endogenous ceramides decreased by 25% compared to untreated cells. No significant changes were seen in other sphingolipids. Desaturase inhibition resulted in growth inhibition and cell cycle arrest at G0/G1. Phosphorylated Rb (pRb) is critical for cell cycle progression by regulating the G1/S phase restriction point, thus controlling entry into the S phase. There was more than 50% decrease in pRb in cells treated with dihydroceramide desaturase siRNA, whereas no change in total Rb level was seen. To determine the involvement of protein phosphate 1 or 2A (PP1 and PP2A) in Rb dephosphorylation, cells were pre-treated with either okadaic acid, a specific PP2A inhibitor, or tautomycin, a specific PP1 inhibitor. Tautomycin was able to inhibit Rb hypophosphorylation whereas okadaic acid showed minimal effect, indicating involvement of PP1.

Next, the effect of the synthetic retinoid, *N*-(4-hydroxyphenyl)retinamide (4-HPR), also known as fenretinide, on dihydroceramide desaturase activity was studied. This retinoid had been reported to increase ceramide levels via *de-novo* synthesis within 6 hours of treatment (Wang et al., 2001). We therefore initially aimed at testing if the inhibition of DEGS-1 by siRNA would block the 4-HPR induced ceramide generation and the anti-tumor effects of 4-HPR. Previously, 4-HPR had been reported to generate ceramide. However, some of the limitations of these earlier studies were due to the method used for the quantitation of ceramide levels in which ceramide was measured by enzymatic or labeling methods where it was difficult to differentiate ceramide from dihydroceramide species. Sphingolipid levels were measured by LC/MS. Increasing concentrations of 4-HPR were directly proportional to increases in endogenous dihydroceramide levels. There was no elevation but rather a modest decrease in endogenous ceramide levels. All-trans-retinoic acid had no effect on desaturase activity. The *in situ* assay for desaturase activity showed inhibition of desaturase activity in cells treated with 4-HPR. There was no change in mRNA as well as protein levels of dihydroceramide desaturase indicating that 4-HPR may be a direct and/or posttranslational inhibitor of dihydroceramide desaturase.

Indeed, we recently demonstrated that dihydroceramide desaturase is a direct in vitro target for fenretinide (see below) (Rahmaniyan et al., 2011). Taken together, these observations reveal that 4-HPR is a potent and rapid inhibitor of dihydroceramide desaturase which

induces dihydroceramide generation. In agreement with our study, it was recently reported that inhibition of dihydroceramide desaturase in cultured keratinocytes contributes to increases in dihydroceramide and phytoceramides while ceramide levels decrease (Brodesser & Kolter, 2011). Additionally, Wang et al showed that 4-HPR works synergistically with *D*-erythro-*N,N*-dimethylsphingosine (DMS), a sphingosine kinase inhibitor, resulting in increased intracellular sphinganine and dihydroceramide (Wang *et al.*, 2008).
Furthermore, treament of 4-HPR with the synthetic sphingolipid protein kinase C inhibitor, l-*threo*-dihydrosphingosine (safingol) was synergistic in neuroblastoma, melanoma, prostate, ewings sarcoma, colon, breast, and lung cancer cell lines (Batra et al., 2004; Maurer et al., 2000). Of importance for neuroblastoma is that neuroblastoma cell lines resistant to cis-retinoic acid are sensitive to 4-HPR (Reynolds et al., 2000). Together with our findings, these data suggest that dihydroceramides have a novel biological function involving cell growth and cell cycle, and they may play a role as targets for cytotoxic agents in cancer cells.

6. Dihydroceramide desaturase inhibitors

6.1 Background on enzyme Inhibition

Before discussing the inhibitors for dihydroceramide desaturase , it is helpful to review the basic biochemistry of enzyme kinetics and types of inhibition. In general, enzyme inhibitors mediate their inhibitory actions either via affecting the gene expression of the enzyme of interest or via posttranslational modification of the enzyme, which are an indirect effect. Another mode of inhibition is to act directly on the enzyme itself, for instance binding to the active center of the enzyme and thus blocking the activity. Direct acting inhibitors may inhibit the enzyme activity reversibly or irreversibly. The reversible inhibition is divided into competitive, non-competitive, and uncompetitive inhibition. In competitive inhibition the inhibitor and the substrate compete to bind to the pools of free enzyme molecules (Fig. 5). While most likely inhibitor and substrate compete for a common binding pocket (i.e. active site), they could bind to separate sites on the enzyme molecule exerting a negative regulation on each other. Thus, the apparent K_m value increases with increasing inhibitor concentrations, but the V_{max} value stays constant at all inhibitor concentrations (Copeland, 2005). The dissociation constant K_m represents the substrate's affinity for the enzyme and K_i represents the inhibitor's affinity for the enzyme. The smaller these values, the higher the binding's affinity for the enzyme. A non-competitive inhibitor binds to both the free enzyme and the enzyme-substrate (ES) complex (Fig. 5). This type of inhibitor has two different dissociation constants, one for binary enzyme-inhibitor (EI) complex (K_i) and one for the ternary enzyme-substrate-inhibitor (ESI) complex (αK_i). Thus, Vmax decreases with increasing inhibitor concentrations, but K_m value depends on the α values. If $\alpha > 1$, the inhibitor binds preferentially to the free enzyme, and K_m increases with increasing inhibitor concentrations. If $\alpha<1$ the inhibitor binds preferentially to the ES complex, and K_m value decreases with increasing inhibitor concentrations. If $\alpha=1$, the inhibitor binds with equal affinity to both the free enzyme and the ES complex, thus the K_m values is constant. Unlike competitive inhibitors, non-competitive inhibitors can't be overcome by high substrate concentrations.
An uncompetitive inhibitor binds exclusively to the ES complex (Fig. 5). The formation of ES complex augments the inhibitor affinity for the ES complex contributing to decreased apparent values of both K_m and V_{max} with increasing substrate concentrations. Irreversible inhibitors or inactivators are characterized by the formation of covalent bonds with enzyme

molecules. The rate of covalent bond formation (rate of enzyme inactivation) will be slow (Copeland, 2005). Thus, irreversible inhibitors display time-dependent inhibition. This is because the amount of active enzyme at a given concentration of irreversible inhibitor depends on pre-incubation time of the inhibitor with the enzyme. The inactivation rate of the system is determined by the pseudo-first-order rate constant K_{obs} (Adam et al., 2001; Copeland, 2005). Irreversible inhibitors form initially a reversible non-covalent complex with the enzyme (EI or ESI) and this then reacts to produce the covalently modified "dead-end complex" EI*. The rate at which EI* is formed is called the inactivation rate or k_{inact}. The binding and inactivation steps of this reaction are investigated by incubating the enzyme with inhibitor and assaying the amount of activity remaining over time. The activity will decrease in a time-dependent manner (Maurer & Fung, 2000). In this section some of the dihydroceramide desaturase inhibitors will be discussed which act directly or indirectly on the enzyme.

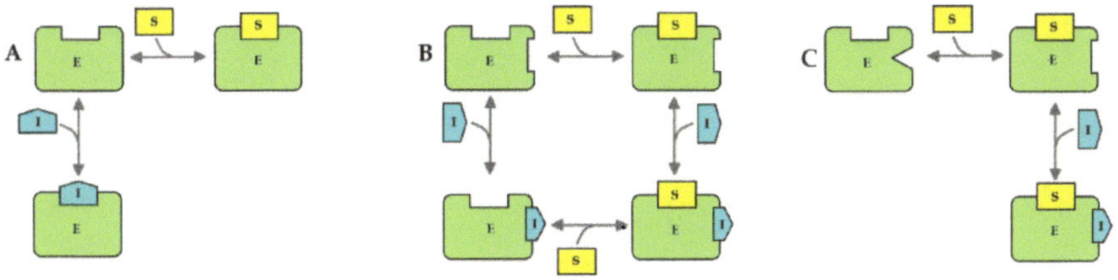

Fig. 5. Types of Enzyme Inhibition.

(A) Competitive inhibition, the enzyme (E) can bind either the substrate (S) or the inhibitor (I); (B) Non-competitive inhibition, the inhibitor can bind to both the free enzyme and ES complex; (C) Uncompetitive inhibition, the inhibitor binds only to the ES complex.

6.2 Direct acting agents: Retinoids and ceramide analogues

Retinoids are natural and synthetic derivatives of vitamin A which include all-trans retinloic acid (ATRA), 13-cis retinoic acid, (13-cis-RA), and 4-HPR. They have been used in neuroblastoma treatment due to their effects on cell differentiation, proliferation, and apoptosis (Formelli & Cleris, 2000; Reynolds, 2000; Reynolds & Lemons, 2001). Treatment with 13-cis retinoic acid is now standard of care for patients with high risk neuroblastoma following stem cell transplant (Matthay et al., 2009; Matthay et al., 1999). Some of retinoids mediate their effects through the binding to retinoic acid receptors (RAR) and retinoid X receptors (RXR). Their toxicity has limited their clinical use. For this reason, a large number of synthetic analogues of retinoids has been developed and used in pre-clinical and clinical settings (Villani et al., 2006). ATRA has been shown to modulate sphingolipid metabolizing enzymes. In a recent study, it has been shown that ATRA induces growth arrest in estrogen receptor-positive MCF-7 cells by increased ceramide levels through neutral sphingomyelinase-2. P70 ribosomal S6 kinase (S6K) was identified as downstream effector of ATRA and neutral sphingomyelinase-2. In the same study, ATRA contributed to 3-fold upregulation of dihydroceramide desaturase mRNA (Clarke et al., 2011). 4-HPR is a synthetic retinoid with low toxicity in humans compared to its parent compound ATRA. This difference is believed to be a result of the substitution of an amide-linked 4-hydroxyphenyl moiety for the carbonyl functional group of ATRA (Fig 6). In addition, this change markedly reduces 4-HPR's binding affinity for nuclear retinoid receptors, supporting the fact that 4-HPR's anticancer activity is independent of retinoid receptors (Hail et al., 2010). The hydroxyl functional group of 4-HPR has been demonstrated to have essential roles in 4-HPR-promoting cytotoxic effects. This functional group also mediates its uptake in cancer cells. In addition, the hydroxyl functional group of 4-HPR triggers ROS production by a mechanism requiring the mitochondrial enzyme dihydroorotate dehydrogenase, an enzyme associated with the mitochondrial electron transport chain and required for *de novo* pyrimidine synthesis.

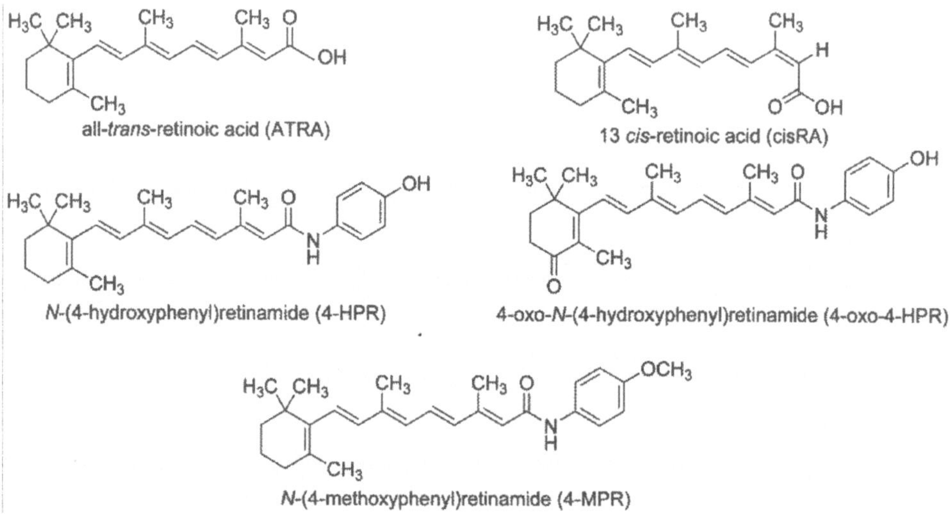

Fig. 6. The Chemical Structures of ATRA, cisRA, 4-HPR and its metabolites 4-oxo-4-HPR and 4-MPR.

4-HPR has been used in clinical trials as chemopreventive and chemotherapeutic agent for various cancers including breast, prostate, head and neck, pancreas, oral leukoplakia, and neuroblastoma. 4-HPR reduced the incidence of contralateral breast cancer and ipsilateral breast cancer recurrence (Torrisi et al., 2001). At low levels, 4-HPR induces apoptosis; at higher levels it shows necrosis as well (Lovat et al., 2004). The precise mechanism of its apoptotic action is not fully understood. Unlike most retinoids, 4-HPR has low affinity for retinoid receptors and its mediated apoptosis is RAR independent (Mershon et al., 2007). 4-HPR induces alkaline ceramidase 2 leading to increased dihydrosphingosine (sphinganine) levels (Mao et al., 2010). Besides its ability to generate ROS (Jiang et al., 2011, Lovat et al., 2005), 4-HPR may increase ceramide levels via induction of ceramide synthase (Fig. 7) (Jiang et al., 2004; Wang et al., 2001) and acidic sphingomyelinase (Corazzari et al., 2005; Lovat *et al.*, 2004) . 4-HPR-enhanced ceramide is subsequently metabolized via glycosphingolipids and GD3 synthase to the ganglioside GD3 which activates 12-lypoxygenase (12-LOX). 12-LOX then mediates ROS generation with subsequent growth arrest and DNA damage-inducible transcription factor GADD153 and the Bcl-2 related protein BAK (Fig. 7) (Lovat et al., 2005) resulting in release of cytochrome c and activation of caspases-9 and-3 and ultimately apoptosis. In addition, in neuroblastoma cells 4-HPR induces the proapoptotic gene BBC3, a BH3-only family member of Bcl-2, which initiates the mitochondrial apoptotic pathway (Wei et al., 2005). All mentioned mechanisms are p53-independent, indicating that all cancers with p53 mutation are sensitive to cytotoxic effects of 4-HPR.

4-HPR has a very broad range (0.7- 10 μM) of cytotoxicity and may have different effects dependent on the concentration and type of cancer cell used (Formelli et al., 2008). In neuroblastoma cells, high concentrations of 4-HPR (>5 μM) have been shown to induce apoptosis and necrosis (Wang *et al.*, 2001a) while lower concentrations (< 3 μM) of 4-HPR have been reported to induce G_1-S arrest and hypophosphorylation of Rb (DiPietrantonio et al., 1998; Kraveka *et al.*, 2007; Wu et al., 2001). For neuroblastoma patients enrolled on a Phase I pediatric trial the mean plasma steady-state concentration on day 7 was as 9.9 μmol/L with the maximal tolerated dosage of 2,475 mg/m^2 per day (Villablanca et al., 2006). One of the difficulties with 4-HPR treatment in patients is its low absorption. Another more recent pediatric Phase I study using a new formulation of 4-HPR to improve bioavailability (4HPR/Lym-X-Sorb oral powder), reported the day 7 mean peak plasma concentrations to be 19.7 μM at the recommended dose of 1700 mg/m2 per day (Marachelian et al., 2009). These doses safely achieved levels active against neuroblastoma in vivo with minimal toxicity.

We recently determined that the enzyme dihydroceramide desaturase is a direct target for 4-HPR *in-vitro* using rat liver microsomes as enzyme source (Rahmaniyan et al., 2011). 4-HPR inhibited the enzyme dihydroceramide desaturase in a time-dependent manner and a dilution experiment showed almost no recovery of the enzyme activity suggesting that 4-HPR may inhibit the dihydroceramide desaturase activity irreversibly (Rahmaniyan et al., 2011).

Two major metabolites of 4-HPR have been identified: *N*-(4-methoxyphenyl)retinamide (4-MPR) and 4-oxo-*N*-(4-hydroxyphenyl)retinamide (4-oxo-4-HPR). 4-MPR is an inactive metabolite (Fig 6) with no apoptotic effects that can be used in cancer cells as a biomarker to predict response of cells to 4-HPR (Mehta et al., 1998). 4-MPR has longer plasma half-life than 4-HPR indicating that 4-MPR and 4-HPR have distinct tissue uptake and metabolism (Hail et al., 2010). 4-oxo-4-HPR, a very active and polar metabolite, is able to inhibit 4-HPR resistant cell growth and to act synergistically with the parent drug (Tiberio et al., 2010). In ovarian carcinoma cells 4-oxo-4-HPR is formed by induction of CYP26A1 (Villani et al., 2004). Mechanistically, 4-oxo-4-HPR induces cell cycle arrest at G2/M, increases ceramide levels, and caspase-dependent apoptosis (Villani *et al.*, 2006). It generates ROS and causes mitotic arrest via inhibition of tubulin polymerization. ROS generation is independent from mitotic arrest and occurs earlier (Tiberio et al., 2010). In our *in vitro* model, we showed that 4-oxo-4-HPR is also a direct inhibitor of dihydroceramide desaturase as well, exhibiting lower K_i and IC_{50} than 4-HPR, indicating that 4-oxo-4-HPR is more potent than the parent drug. 4-MPR showed only very little inhibitory effect on dihydroceramide desaturase activity (Rahmaniyan et al., 2011).

Another direct inhibitor of dihydroceramide desaturase is ceramide analogue, C_8-cyclopropenyl-ceramide (C_8CPPC or GT11) (Triola et al., 2001) which is a competitive inhibitor of dihydroceramide desaturase. It was used in our *in vitro* studies and served as positive control to validate the assay (Rahmaniyan et al., 2011). At higher concentrations, GT11 loses its specificity where it also inhibits serine palmitoyl transferase in cells but not in vitro. In addition, it inhibits sphingosine lyase activity contributing to sphingosine-1-phosphate accumulation (Triola et al., 2004). Together, these data indicate that the enzyme dihydroceramide desaturase may be a direct target for chemotherapeutic agents and exploring the type of bonds in enzyme-inhibitor complex could be of further interest.

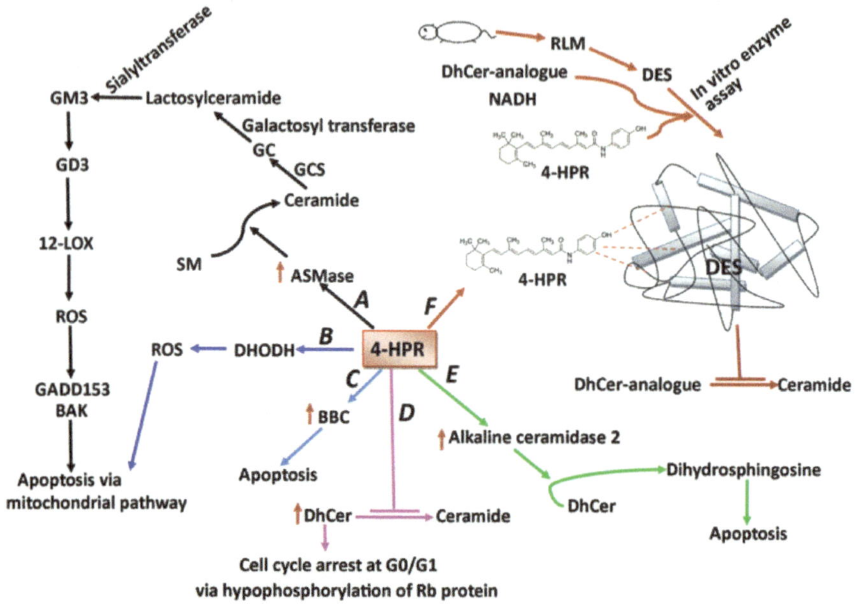

(A) Enhanced ceramide by activation of acid sphinomyelinase (ASMase) can lead to formation of gangliosides GM3 and GD3 resulting in reactive oxygen species (ROS) generation via 12-Lipoxygenase (12-LOX). ROS induces the transcription factor GADD153 and BAK protein resulting in mitochondrial apoptosis; (B) Dihydroorotate dehydrogenase (DHODH) is a required component for 4-HPR-mediated ROS generation in certain tissues resulting in mitochondrial apoptosis; (C) The proapoptotic gene BBC3, a BH-3 only protein member of Bcl-2 family, can mediate apoptosis in response to 4-HPR; (D) inhibition of dihydroceramide desaturase (DES) by 4-HPR accumulates dihydroceramides (dhCer) in cells resulting in cell cycle arrest at G0/G1 by a mechanism involving pRb; (E) Increased dihydrosphingosine resulting from activation of alkaline ceramidase-2 by 4-HPR can initiate apoptosis; (F) In addition to above mentioned *in vivo* mechanisms, 4-HPR also has an *in vitro* effects. *In vitro* enzyme assay using rat liver miocrosomes (RLM) as protein source for DES, dhCer-analogue as substrate, and NADH as cofactor demonstrates that 4-HPR inhibits the conversion of dhCer-analogue into ceramide supporting the fact that 4-HPR binds directly to the DES enzyme itself.

Fig. 7. Sphingolipid Mediated Mechanisms of Action of Fenretinide (4-HPR):

6.3 Indirect acting agents: Oxidative stress, celecoxib, and resveratrol

Dihydroceramide desaturase activity can be modulated by oxidative stress contributing to accumulation of dihydroceramides (Idkowiak-Baldys *et al.*, 2010). We have reported that H_2O_2, tert-butylhydroperoxide, and the intracellular ROS inducer menadione contribute to dihydroceramide desaturase inhibition in breast and lung cancers as well as neuroblastoma. In these cells, accumulation of dihydroceramides was observed with little change in ceramide levels. The *in vitro* assay using cell lysates obtained from cells treated with H_2O_2 showed inactivation of dihydroceramide desaturase. However, in the direct *in vitro* assay using rat liver microsomes or cell homogenates, H_2O_2 did not show a significant effect on dihydroceramide desaturase activity indicating that H_2O_2 inhibits dihydroceramide desaturase indirectly. The multi-enzyme complex of dihydroceramide desaturase (Fig. 4) is involved in coupled reactions responsible for electron transport from NADPH to terminal desaturase that reduces oxygen. However, NADPH is added to the reaction and is present in both RLMs and cell homogenates. These results suggest that dihydroceramide desaturase inhibition by H_2O_2 is mediated by modulating the redox status of the cell.

Another indirect-acting dihydroceramide desaturase inhibitor is the COX-2 inhibitor celecoxib. Celecoxib has been reported to inhibit neuroblastoma growth and induce apoptosis (Chen et al., 2011; Ponthan et al., 2007). One study showed that treatment of various cancer cells with celecoxib has increased dihydroceramide species such as C_{16}-, $C_{24:0}$- and $C_{24:1}$- dihydroceramidse by dihydroceramide desaturase inhibition, whereas very long chain ceramides such as $C_{24:0}$- and $C_{24:1}$-ceramides were decreased. The anti-proliferative effect of celecoxib were related to dihydroceramide desaturase inhibition which was COX-2-independent (Schiffmann et al., 2009).

Resveratrol is a natural product found in grape skin, red wine, cranberries, blueberries, and peanuts. It is a phytochemical with anti-oxidant, anti-inflammatory and cardioprotective properties. It also causes apoptotic effects on cancer cells, including neuroblastoma (Soto et al., 2011; van Ginkel et al., 2007). In leukemia cell line HL-60 the apoptotic effect is mediated by ceramide accumulation via induction of CerS/LASS genes and down-regulation of SK1 and GCS genes (Cakir et al., 2011). Additionally, it induces autophagy in HGC-27 gastric cancer cells without apoptosis. In this study, autophagy was mediated by the inhibition of dihydroceramide desaturase (Signorelli *et al.*, 2009) by resveratrol. However, our *in vitro* assay neither celecoxib or resveratrol inhibited dihydroceramide desaturase. They had some inhibition at higher concentrations, supporting the fact that both agents may act indirectly on the enzyme (unpublished observations). Additionally, photodynamic therapy (Separovic et al., 2009), γ-tocopherol (Jiang *et al.*, 2004), and XM462 (Munoz-Olaya et al., 2008) may function as indirect inhibitors of dihydroceramide desaturase by modulating the redox status of the cells as in case of hydrogen peroxide.

7. Conclusions and future directions

In cancer cells there is an underlying defect in apoptosis due to either overexpression of anti-apoptotic genes, or mutations in pro-apoptotic genes (Ogretmen & Hannun, 2004) leading to escape of apoptotic signaling and ultimately tumorogenesis (Huang et al., 2011). Thus, cancer is a disease characterized by imbalance between cell division and cell death. (Corazzari et al., 2005). Ceramide, the central molecule of sphingolipids, has been identified as mediator for differentiation, cell cycle arrest, cellular senescence, and apoptosis. Dysregulated enzymes and metabolites in sphingolipid metabolism, are associated with development and pathogenesis of various types of cancers. Sphingolipid metabolism is characterized by interconversion of one metabolite into another. For instance, ceramide can be degraded by ceramidase into sphingosine, which is further phosphorylated into sphingosine-1-phosphate. This and other pathways in sphingolipid metabolism create a network regulating individual molecules. A dysregulation in this network by altered levels of bioactive metabolites and enzymes in cancer indicates the importance of sphingolipids in pathogenesis and progression of cancer (Ogretmen & Hannun, 2004).

As discussed before, accumulating evidence shows involvement of sphingolipid signaling in development of human cancers. Angiogenesis is an essential factor for tumor growth and metastasis. The process of angiogenesis is regulated by many angiogenic factors, such as

VEGF (Eggert et al., 2000). In neuroblastoma, tumor vascularity correlates with an aggressive phenotype. It has been demonstrated that VEGF is highly overexpressed in neuroblastoma, which is associated with poor prognosis (Li et al., 2011). Sphingosine-1-phosphate signaling pathway is known to be involved in angiogenesis, which shows a close interaction with VEGF (Heo et al., 2009). Li and colleagues found that spingosine kinase 2 is highly expressed in neuroblastoma cells and tissues. The product of this enzyme, sphingosine-1-phosphate, induces VEGF expression in neuroblastoma cells via HIF-1-α independent pathway. The same study showed that among sphingosine-1-phosphate receptors, S1P-receptor 2 ($S1P_2$) correlates with VEGF mRNA expression suggesting that $S1P/S1P_2$/VEGF signaling pathway may promote neuroblastoma growth and angiogenesis. This observation was supported by the fact that blockade of sphingosine-1-phosphate $_2$ by sphingosine-1-phosphate antagonist JTE-013 resulted in inhibition of tumor growth and angiogenesis. Taken together, these data suggest that sphingolipid signaling pathway is involved in angiogenesis and poor prognosis in neuroblastoma and modulation of sphingolipid signaling pathway may provide an effective approach to control neuroblastoma.

Neuroblastomas originate from embryonic neural crest tissue, and are characterized by failure in differentiation. Spontaneous regression may result from maturation of neoplastic cells into terminally differentiated ganglion cells. Neuroblastoma is known to undergo spontaneous regression by differentiation and apoptosis to a benign phenotype, almost half of cases are aggressive with tendency to metastasize. The ability of neuroblastoma to spontaneously regress through differentiation has generated considerable interest in agents to induce this important biological process (Lovat et al., 2000). Previous studies demonstrated that ceramide positively influences neurite outgrowth, which is one aspect of neuronal differentiation, either as a mediator of nerve growth factor signaling through p75 in hippocampal neurons (Schultz & Larsson, 2004), or upon direct application to neuroblastoma cells in culture such as Neuro2a cells (Prinetti et al., 1997; Riboni et al., 1998; Riboni et al., 1995). Riboni and colleagues showed that agents such as ATRA, or conditions leading to increase in cellular ceramide levels contribute to neuroblastoma differentiation. ATRA induced ceramide increase was also augmented by exogenous administration of sphingomyelin, sphingosine, or L-serine. Additionally, ATRA contributed to activation of neutral sphingomyelinase. The resulting increase in ceramide content contributed to differentiation in neuroblastoma cells. Mechanistically, ceramide-induced differentiation has been mediated by PP2A. An isoform of protein kinase C (PKC), namely PKCε, was also shown to be involved in both ATRA and growth factor induced morphological changes during neuroblastoma differentiation (Schultz & Larsson, 2004). It was also shown that in Neuro2a cells, exogenously administered sphingosine can be rapidly metabolized by degradation or N-acylation, where N-acylation largely dominates over degradation. This results in increase cellular levels of ceramide and, consequently, in differentiation of neuroblastoma cells. These data suggest that ceramide is involved in the regulation of neuroblastoma differentiation, which may offer a new strategy in neuroblastoma treatment.

Spontaneous regression may also result from programmed cell death or apoptosis. Schaefer and colleagues showed that ceramide treatment of five neuroblastoma cell lines results in apoptosis. Although these neuroblastoma cells express CD95 receptors (a TNF receptor family member), they are resistant to apoptosis stimulated by anti-CD95 antibody or by CD95 ligand. However, ceramide treatment of these cells leads to apoptosis, suggesting that ceramide may act downstream of the CD95-death inducing signaling complex (DISC)

(Schaefer et al., 2000). Ceramide is also able to induce apoptosis in neuroblastoma cells by inactivation of Akt pathway and translocation of apoptotic-inducing factor (AIF) from the mitochondria (Kim et al., 2007). Administration of short chain C_2 ceramide to cultured neuroblastoma cells causes apoptosis by activation of intrinsic pathway (Movsesyan et al., 2002). As reported before, dihydroceramide accumulation in neuroblastoma cells causes cell cycle arrest as a result of dihydroceramide desaturse inhibition (Kraveka et al., 2007). Taken together, these data provide evidence in support of a role of sphingolipids in neuronal apoptosis, which might result in spontaneous regression in neuroblastoma, and this will open a new avenue in the therapeutic treatment of neuroblastoma.

A dynamic sphingolipid equilibrium has been described. This equilibrium is characterized by a balance between pro-apoptotic and pro-survival sphingolipids (Cuvillier et al., 1996; Fox et al., 2006), for example the balance between ceramide and sphingosine-1-phosphate. If this balance shifts to ceramide, it can lead to cellular death or cell cycle arrest. If it shifts to sphingosine-1-phosphate, it can result in cell proliferation. The regulation of ceramidases and sphingosine kinases may help to regulate the dynamic balance between these two metabolites. However, this may not sufficient because there are other sphingolipid metabolites such ceramide-1-phosphate and glycosphingolipids that are also in balance with ceramide. Thus, it is necessary to study all sphingolipid metabolites and their regulating enzymes. Processes, which enhance the intracellular accumulation of ceramide, will provide favorable pro-apoptotic outcome in chemotherapy. Yet another way to increase ceramide levels are to administer exogenous short chain ceramides and metabolic precursors of ceramide (palmitate, sphingosine, and C_6-ceramide). These can be used in combination with chemotherapeutics to augment their effects.

Dihydroceramide desaturase is an important enzyme that has the potential to modulate the dihydroceramide /ceramide ratio in the cell. However, the regulation of dihydroceramide desaturase activity has not been well characterized. Dihydroceramide had been considered primarily as an inactive precursor of ceramide. However, recent studies including our work have demonstrated that dihydroceramides have a novel biological functions including cell cycle arrest, apoptosis, ceramide channel formation, autophagy and oxidative stress. These studies indicate the significance of endogenous levels of dihydroceramides in cell regulatory processes, and they suggest that dihydroceramide desaturase has the potential to regulate cell function through both ceramide and dihydroceramide (Kraveka et al., 2007, Rahmaniyan et al., 2011). These observations have implications for the mechanism of action of 4-HPR and for a potential role for dihydroceramide desaturase as a target for chemotherapeutic agents (Rahmaniyan et al., 2011). Thus, the development of new drugs which augment ceramide and dihydroceramide levels will induce cell toxicity and apoptosis in cancer cells. Inhibition of dihydroceramide desaturase is a novel target for cancer therapy. The balance of ceramides and dihydroceramides within a cell may be key to cancer cell proliferation.

8. Acknowledgements

We dedicate this chapter to our patients and their families. We would like to thank the members of the Kraveka Laboratory, Dr. Li Li, Dr. Leslie Wooten-Blanks and Dr. Heather Escoto. We would like to thank Dr. Lina Obeid, Dr. Yusuf Hannun, and Dr. Besim Ogretmen for their mentorship, support, and helpful discussions. We thank the Lipidomics Core Facility in the Department of Biochemistry and Molecular Biology at the Medical University of South Carolina, especially Dr. Alicja Bielawska, Dr. Jacek Bielawski, Dr. Zdzislaw M.

Szulc, Barbara Rembiesa and Jason Pierce. We thank the Children's Oncology Group Neuroblastoma Committee and the Children's Oncology Group Neuroblastoma Tumor Bank for providing us with neuroblastoma tumor samples. This work was supported by National Institutes of Health Grants: K01-CA100767 and P20-RR17677, a CureSearch Research Fellowship Award, and by grants from the Rally Foundation for Childhood Cancer Research, St. Baldrick's Foundation, National Philoptochos Children's Medical Fund, Hyundai Hope on Wheels, Monica Kreber Golf Tournament, and Chase After a Cure Foundation.

9. References

Adam, G.C.; Cravatt, B.F. & Sorensen, E.J. (2001) Profiling the specific reactivity of the proteome with non-directed activity-based probes. *Chem Biol,* Vol.8, No.1, pp.81-95

Adibhatla, R.M. & Hatcher, J.F. (2010) Protection by d609 through cell-cycle regulation after stroke. *Mol Neurobiol,* Vol.41, No.2-3, pp.206-17

Ahn, E.H. & Schroeder, J.J. (2002) Sphingoid bases and ceramide induce apoptosis in ht-29 and hct-116 human colon cancer cells. *Exp Biol Med (Maywood),* Vol.227, No.5, pp.345-53

Argraves, K.M.; Wilkerson, B.A. & Argraves, W.S. (2010) Sphingosine-1-phosphate signaling in vasculogenesis and angiogenesis. *World J Biol Chem,* Vol.1, No.10, pp.291-7

Barth, B.M.; Gustafson, S.J.; Young, M.M.; Fox, T.E.; Shanmugavelandy, S.S.; Kaiser, J.M.; Cabot, M.C.; Kester, M. & Kuhn, T.B. (2010) Inhibition of nadph oxidase by glucosylceramide confers chemoresistance. *Cancer biology & therapy,* Vol.10, No.11, pp.1126-36

Batra, S.; Reynolds, C.P. & Maurer, B.J. (2004) Fenretinide cytotoxicity for ewing's sarcoma and primitive neuroectodermal tumor cell lines is decreased by hypoxia and synergistically enhanced by ceramide modulators. *Cancer research,* Vol.64, No.15, pp.5415-24

Beauchamp, E.; Goenaga, D.; Le Bloc'h, J.; Catheline, D.; Legrand, P. & Rioux, V. (2007) Myristic acid increases the activity of dihydroceramide delta4-desaturase 1 through its n-terminal myristoylation. *Biochimie,* Vol.89, No.12, pp.1553-61

Bektas, M. & Spiegel, S. (2004) Glycosphingolipids and cell death. *Glycoconj J,* Vol.20, No.1, pp.39-47

Bielawska, A.; Crane, H.M.; Liotta, D.; Obeid, L.M. & Hannun, Y.A. (1993) Selectivity of ceramide-mediated biology. Lack of activity of erythro-dihydroceramide. *J Biol Chem,* Vol.268, No.35, pp.26226-32

Billich, A. & Baumruker, T. (2008) Sphingolipid metabolizing enzymes as novel therapeutic targets. *Subcell Biochem,* Vol.49, 487-522

Birbes, H.; El Bawab, S.; Obeid, L.M. & Hannun, Y.A. (2002) Mitochondria and ceramide: Intertwined roles in regulation of apoptosis. *Adv Enzyme Regul,* Vol.42, 113-29

Biswal, S.S.; Datta, K.; Acquaah-Mensah, G.K. & Kehrer, J.P. (2000) Changes in ceramide and sphingomyelin following fludarabine treatment of human chronic b-cell leukemia cells. *Toxicology,* Vol.154, No.1-3, pp.45-53

Bose, R.; Verheij, M.; Haimovitz-Friedman, A.; Scotto, K.; Fuks, Z. & Kolesnick, R. (1995) Ceramide synthase mediates daunorubicin-induced apoptosis: An alternative mechanism for generating death signals. *Cell,* Vol.82, No.3, pp.405-14

Brodesser, S. & Kolter, T. (2011) Dihydroceramide desaturase inhibition by a cyclopropanated dihydroceramide analog in cultured keratinocytes. *Journal of lipids,* Vol.2011, 724015

Cadena, D.L.; Kurten, R.C. & Gill, G.N. (1997) The product of the mld gene is a member of the membrane fatty acid desaturase family: Overexpression of mld inhibits egf receptor biosynthesis. *Biochemistry,* Vol.36, No.23, pp.6960-7

Cakir, Z.; Saydam, G.; Sahin, F. & Baran, Y. (2011) The roles of bioactive sphingolipids in resveratrol-induced apoptosis in hl60: Acute myeloid leukemia cells. *Journal of cancer research and clinical oncology,* Vol.137, No.2, pp.279-86

Causeret, C.; Geeraert, L.; Van Der Hoeven, G.; Mannaerts, G.P. & Van Veldhoven, P.P. (2000) Further characterization of rat dihydroceramide desaturase: Tissue distribution, subcellular localization, and substrate specificity. *Lipids,* Vol.35, No.10, pp.1117-25

Chalfant, C.E.; Rathman, K.; Pinkerman, R.L.; Wood, R.E.; Obeid, L.M.; Ogretmen, B. & Hannun, Y.A. (2002) De novo ceramide regulates the alternative splicing of caspase 9 and bcl-x in a549 lung adenocarcinoma cells. Dependence on protein phosphatase-1. *J Biol Chem,* Vol.277, No.15, pp.12587-95

Chalfant, C.E. & Spiegel, S. (2005) Sphingosine 1-phosphate and ceramide 1-phosphate: Expanding roles in cell signaling. *J Cell Sci,* Vol.118, No.Pt 20, pp.4605-12

Chang, H.C.; Tsai, L.H.; Chuang, L.Y. & Hung, W.C. (2001) Role of akt kinase in sphingosine-induced apoptosis in human hepatoma cells. *J Cell Physiol,* Vol.188, No.2, pp.188-93

Chen, Y.; Tsai, Y.H. & Tseng, S.H. (2011) Combined valproic acid and celecoxib treatment induced synergistic cytotoxicity and apoptosis in neuroblastoma cells. *Anticancer research,* Vol.31, No.6, pp.2231-9

Clarke, C.J. & Hannun, Y.A. (2006) Neutral sphingomyelinases and nsmase2: Bridging the gaps. *Biochim Biophys Acta,* Vol.1758, No.12, pp.1893-901

Clarke, C.J.; Mediwala, K.; Jenkins, R.W.; Sutton, C.A.; Tholanikunnel, B.G. & Hannun, Y.A. (2011) Neutral sphingomyelinase-2 mediates growth arrest by retinoic acid through modulation of ribosomal s6 kinase. *The Journal of biological chemistry,* Vol.286, No.24, pp.21565-76

Conway, A.; Pyne, N.J. & Pyne, S. (2000) Ceramide-dependent regulation of p42/p44 mitogen-activated protein kinase and c-jun n-terminal-directed protein kinase in cultured airway smooth muscle cells. *Cell Signal,* Vol.12, No.11-12, pp.737-43

Copeland, R.A. (2005) *Evaluation of enzyme inhibitors in drug discovery: A guide for medicinal chemists and pharmacologists* (0471686964 edn) (Hoboken, Wiley intersciences).

Corazzari, M.; Lovat, P.E.; Oliverio, S.; Di Sano, F.; Donnorso, R.P.; Redfern, C.P. & Piacentini, M. (2005) Fenretinide: A p53-independent way to kill cancer cells. *Biochemical and biophysical research communications,* Vol.331, No.3, pp.810-5

Cuvillier, O.; Nava, V.E.; Murthy, S.K.; Edsall, L.C.; Levade, T.; Milstien, S. & Spiegel, S. (2001) Sphingosine generation, cytochrome c release, and activation of caspase-7 in doxorubicin-induced apoptosis of mcf7 breast adenocarcinoma cells. *Cell Death Differ,* Vol.8, No.2, pp.162-71

Cuvillier, O.; Pirianov, G.; Kleuser, B.; Vanek, P.G.; Coso, O.A.; Gutkind, S. & Spiegel, S. (1996) Suppression of ceramide-mediated programmed cell death by sphingosine-1-phosphate. *Nature,* Vol.381, No.6585, pp.800-3

Dbaibo, G.S.; Pushkareva, M.Y.; Jayadev, S.; Schwarz, J.K.; Horowitz, J.M.; Obeid, L.M. & Hannun, Y.A. (1995) Retinoblastoma gene product as a downstream target for a ceramide-dependent pathway of growth arrest. *Proceedings of the National Academy of Sciences of the United States of America,* Vol.92, No.5, pp.1347-51

Dipietrantonio, A.M.; Hsieh, T.C.; Olson, S.C. & Wu, J.M. (1998) Regulation of g1/s transition and induction of apoptosis in hl-60 leukemia cells by fenretinide (4hpr). *Int J Cancer,* Vol.78, No.1, pp.53-61

Dobrowsky, R.T.; Kamibayashi, C.; Mumby, M.C. & Hannun, Y.A. (1993) Ceramide activates heterotrimeric protein phosphatase 2a. *J Biol Chem,* Vol.268, No.21, pp.15523-30

Eggert, A.; Sieverts, H.; Ikegaki, N. & Brodeur, G.M. (2000) P75 mediated apoptosis in neuroblastoma cells is inhibited by expression of trka. *Med Pediatr Oncol,* Vol.35, No.6, pp.573-6

Ekiz, H.A. & Baran, Y. (2010) Therapeutic applications of bioactive sphingolipids in hematological malignancies. *Int J Cancer,* Vol.127, No.7, pp.1497-506

Formelli, F.; Cavadini, E.; Luksch, R.; Garaventa, A.; Villani, M.G.; Appierto, V. & Persiani, S. (2008) Pharmacokinetics of oral fenretinide in neuroblastoma patients: Indications for optimal dose and dosing schedule also with respect to the active metabolite 4-oxo-fenretinide. *Cancer Chemother Pharmacol,* Vol.62, No.4, pp.655-65

Formelli, F. & Cleris, L. (2000) Therapeutic effects of the combination of fenretinide and all-trans-retinoic acid and of the two retinoids with cisplatin in a human ovarian carcinoma xenograft and in a cisplatin-resistant sub-line. *Eur J Cancer,* Vol.36, No.18, pp.2411-9

Fox, T.E.; Finnegan, C.M.; Blumenthal, R. & Kester, M. (2006) The clinical potential of sphingolipid-based therapeutics. *Cellular and molecular life sciences : CMLS,* Vol.63, No.9, pp.1017-23

French, K.J.; Upson, J.J.; Keller, S.N.; Zhuang, Y.; Yun, J.K. & Smith, C.D. (2006) Antitumor activity of sphingosine kinase inhibitors. *J Pharmacol Exp Ther,* Vol.318, No.2, pp.596-603

Futerman, A.H. & Hannun, Y.A. (2004) The complex life of simple sphingolipids. *EMBO Rep,* Vol.5, No.8, pp.777-82

Gault, C.R.; Obeid, L.M. & Hannun, Y.A. (2010) An overview of sphingolipid metabolism: From synthesis to breakdown. *Adv Exp Med Biol,* Vol.688, 1-23

Geeraert, L.; Mannaerts, G.P. & Van Veldhoven, P.P. (1997) Conversion of dihydroceramide into ceramide: Involvement of a desaturase. *Biochem J,* Vol.327 (Pt 1), 125-32

Goldkorn, T.; Balaban, N.; Shannon, M.; Chea, V.; Matsukuma, K.; Gilchrist, D.; Wang, H. & Chan, C. (1998) H2o2 acts on cellular membranes to generate ceramide signaling and initiate apoptosis in tracheobronchial epithelial cells. *J Cell Sci,* Vol.111 (Pt 21), 3209-20

Gomez Del Pulgar, T.; Velasco, G.; Sanchez, C.; Haro, A. & Guzman, M. (2002) De novo-synthesized ceramide is involved in cannabinoid-induced apoptosis. *Biochem J,* Vol.363, No.Pt 1, pp.183-8

Gomez-Munoz, A. (2004) Ceramide-1-phosphate: A novel regulator of cell activation. *FEBS Lett,* Vol.562, No.1-3, pp.5-10

Gomez-Munoz, A.; Duffy, P.A.; Martin, A.; O'brien, L.; Byun, H.S.; Bittman, R. & Brindley, D.N. (1995) Short-chain ceramide-1-phosphates are novel stimulators of DNA synthesis and cell division: Antagonism by cell-permeable ceramides. *Mol Pharmacol,* Vol.47, No.5, pp.833-9

Gomez-Munoz, A.; Kong, J.Y.; Salh, B. & Steinbrecher, U.P. (2004) Ceramide-1-phosphate blocks apoptosis through inhibition of acid sphingomyelinase in macrophages. *J Lipid Res,* Vol.45, No.1, pp.99-105

Hail, N., Jr.; Chen, P.; Kepa, J.J.; Bushman, L.R. & Shearn, C. (2010) Dihydroorotate dehydrogenase is required for n-(4-hydroxyphenyl)retinamide-induced reactive oxygen species production and apoptosis. *Free radical biology & medicine,* Vol.49, No.1, pp.109-16

Hailemariam, T.K.; Huan, C.; Liu, J.; Li, Z.; Roman, C.; Kalbfeisch, M.; Bui, H.H.; Peake, D.A.; Kuo, M.S.; Cao, G.; Wadgaonkar, R. & Jiang, X.C. (2008) Sphingomyelin synthase 2 deficiency attenuates nf{kappa}b activation. *Arterioscler Thromb Vasc Biol,*

Haimovitz-Friedman, A.; Kan, C.C.; Ehleiter, D.; Persaud, R.S.; Mcloughlin, M.; Fuks, Z. & Kolesnick, R.N. (1994) Ionizing radiation acts on cellular membranes to generate ceramide and initiate apoptosis. *J Exp Med,* Vol.180, No.2, pp.525-35

Hannun, Y.A.; Loomis, C.R.; Merrill, A.H., Jr. & Bell, R.M. (1986) Sphingosine inhibition of protein kinase c activity and of phorbol dibutyrate binding in vitro and in human platelets. *J Biol Chem,* Vol.261, No.27, pp.12604-9

Hannun, Y.A. & Luberto, C. (2000) Ceramide in the eukaryotic stress response. *Trends Cell Biol,* Vol.10, No.2, pp.73-80

Hannun, Y.A. & Obeid, L.M. (2008) Principles of bioactive lipid signalling: Lessons from sphingolipids. *Nat Rev Mol Cell Biol,* Vol.9, No.2, pp.139-50

Hannun, Y.A. & Obeid, L.M. (2011) Many ceramides. *The Journal of biological chemistry,* Vol.286, No.32, pp.27855-62

Heinrich, M.; Wickel, M.; Schneider-Brachert, W.; Sandberg, C.; Gahr, J.; Schwandner, R.; Weber, T.; Saftig, P.; Peters, C.; Brunner, J.; Kronke, M. & Schutze, S. (1999) Cathepsin d targeted by acid sphingomyelinase-derived ceramide. *Embo J,* Vol.18, No.19, pp.5252-63

Heo, K.; Park, K.A.; Kim, Y.H.; Kim, S.H.; Oh, Y.S.; Kim, I.H.; Ryu, S.H. & Suh, P.G. (2009) Sphingosine 1-phosphate induces vascular endothelial growth factor expression in endothelial cells. *BMB reports,* Vol.42, No.10, pp.685-90

Hinkovska-Galcheva, V.; Boxer, L.A.; Kindzelskii, A.; Hiraoka, M.; Abe, A.; Goparju, S.; Spiegel, S.; Petty, H.R. & Shayman, J.A. (2005) Ceramide 1-phosphate, a mediator of phagocytosis. *J Biol Chem,* Vol.280, No.28, pp.26612-21

Huang, W.C.; Chen, C.L.; Lin, Y.S. & Lin, C.F. (2011) Apoptotic sphingolipid ceramide in cancer therapy. *J Lipids,* Vol.2011, 565316

Idkowiak-Baldys, J.; Apraiz, A.; Li, L.; Rahmaniyan, M.; Clarke, C.J.; Kraveka, J.M.; Asumendi, A. & Hannun, Y.A. (2010) Dihydroceramide desaturase activity is modulated by oxidative stress. *Biochem J,* Vol.427, No.2, pp.265-74

IJana, A. & Pahan, K. (2010) Sphingolipids in multiple sclerosis. *Neuromolecular Med,* Vol.12, No.4, pp.351-61

Jarvis, W.D.; Fornari, F.A., Jr.; Auer, K.L.; Freemerman, A.J.; Szabo, E.; Birrer, M.J.; Johnson, C.R.; Barbour, S.E.; Dent, P. & Grant, S. (1997) Coordinate regulation of stress- and mitogen-activated protein kinases in the apoptotic actions of ceramide and sphingosine. *Mol Pharmacol,* Vol.52, No.6, pp.935-47

Jayadev, S.; Liu, B.; Bielawska, A.E.; Lee, J.Y.; Nazaire, F.; Pushkareva, M.; Obeid, L.M. & Hannun, Y.A. (1995) Role for ceramide in cell cycle arrest. *The Journal of biological chemistry,* Vol.270, No.5, pp.2047-52

Jiang, Q.; Wong, J.; Fyrst, H.; Saba, J.D. & Ames, B.N. (2004) Gamma-tocopherol or combinations of vitamin e forms induce cell death in human prostate cancer cells by interrupting sphingolipid synthesis. *Proc Natl Acad Sci U S A,* Vol.101, No.51, pp.17825-30

Kim, M.Y.; Linardic, C.; Obeid, L. & Hannun, Y. (1991) Identification of sphingomyelin turnover as an effector mechanism for the action of tumor necrosis factor alpha and gamma-interferon. Specific role in cell differentiation. *J Biol Chem,* Vol.266, No.1, pp.484-9

Kim, N.H.; Kim, K.; Park, W.S.; Son, H.S. & Bae, Y. (2007) Pkb/akt inhibits ceramide-induced apoptosis in neuroblastoma cells by blocking apoptosis-inducing factor (aif) translocation. *J Cell Biochem,* Vol.102, No.5, pp.1160-70

Kitatani, K.; Idkowiak-Baldys, J. & Hannun, Y.A. (2008) The sphingolipid salvage pathway in ceramide metabolism and signaling. *Cell Signal,* Vol.20, No.6, pp.1010-8

Kok, J.W.; Nikolova-Karakashian, M.; Klappe, K.; Alexander, C. & Merrill, A.H., Jr. (1997) Dihydroceramide biology. Structure-specific metabolism and intracellular localization. *J Biol Chem,* Vol.272, No.34, pp.21128-36

Kolesnick, R. (2002) The therapeutic potential of modulating the ceramide/sphingomyelin pathway. *J Clin Invest,* Vol.110, No.1, pp.3-8

Koybasi, S.; Senkal, C.E.; Sundararaj, K.; Spassieva, S.; Bielawski, J.; Osta, W.; Day, T.A.; Jiang, J.C.; Jazwinski, S.M.; Hannun, Y.A.; Obeid, L.M. & Ogretmen, B. (2004) Defects in cell growth regulation by c18:0-ceramide and longevity assurance gene 1 in human head and neck squamous cell carcinomas. *J Biol Chem,* Vol.279, No.43, pp.44311-9

Kraveka, J.M. & Hannun, Y.A. (2009) Bioactive sphingolipids: An overview on ceramide, ceramide 1-phosphate dihydroceramide, sphingosine, sphingosine 1-phosphate, in: A. Lajtha (Ed.) *Handbook of neurochemistry and molecular neurobiology.* (vol. XVI) 3rd ed. (New York, NY, Springer), 373-384.

Kraveka, J.M.; Li, L.; Bielawski, J.; Obeid, L.M. & Ogretmen, B. (2003) Involvement of endogenous ceramide in the inhibition of telomerase activity and induction of morphologic differentiation in response to all-trans-retinoic acid in human neuroblastoma cells. *Arch Biochem Biophys,* Vol.419, No.2, pp.110-9

Kraveka, J.M.; Li, L.; Szulc, Z.M.; Bielawski, J.; Ogretmen, B.; Hannun, Y.A.; Obeid, L.M. & Bielawska, A. (2007) Involvement of dihydroceramide desaturase in cell cycle progression in human neuroblastoma cells. *J Biol Chem,* Vol.282, No.23, pp.16718-28

Lacour, S.; Hammann, A.; Grazide, S.; Lagadic-Gossmann, D.; Athias, A.; Sergent, O.; Laurent, G.; Gambert, P.; Solary, E. & Dimanche-Boitrel, M.T. (2004) Cisplatin-induced cd95 redistribution into membrane lipid rafts of ht29 human colon cancer cells. *Cancer Res,* Vol.64, No.10, pp.3593-8

Lee, J.Y.; Bielawska, A.E. & Obeid, L.M. (2000) Regulation of cyclin-dependent kinase 2 activity by ceramide. *Experimental cell research,* Vol.261, No.2, pp.303-11

Li, M.H.; Hla, T. & Ferrer, F. (2011) Sphingolipid modulation of angiogenic factor expression in neuroblastoma. *Cancer Prev Res (Phila),*

Lin, T.; Genestier, L.; Pinkoski, M.J.; Castro, A.; Nicholas, S.; Mogil, R.; Paris, F.; Fuks, Z.; Schuchman, E.H.; Kolesnick, R.N. & Green, D.R. (2000) Role of acidic sphingomyelinase in fas/cd95-mediated cell death. *J Biol Chem,* Vol.275, No.12, pp.8657-63

Ling, B.; Chen, L.; Alcorn, J.; Ma, B. & Yang, J. (2011) Sphingosine-1-phosphate: A potential therapeutic agent against human breast cancer. *Invest New Drugs,* Vol.29, No.2, pp.396-9

Liu, B.; Andrieu-Abadie, N.; Levade, T.; Zhang, P.; Obeid, L.M. & Hannun, Y.A. (1998) Glutathione regulation of neutral sphingomyelinase in tumor necrosis factor-alpha-induced cell death. *J Biol Chem,* Vol.273, No.18, pp.11313-20

Liu, Y.; Xie, K.M.; Yang, G.Q.; Bai, X.M.; Shi, Y.P.; Mu, H.J.; Qiao, W.Z.; Zhang, B. & Xie, P. (2010a) Gcs induces multidrug resistance by regulating apoptosis-related genes in k562/ao2 cell line. *Cancer chemotherapy and pharmacology,* Vol.66, No.3, pp.433-9

Liu, Y.Y.; Gupta, V.; Patwardhan, G.A.; Bhinge, K.; Zhao, Y.; Bao, J.; Mehendale, H.; Cabot, M.C.; Li, Y.T. & Jazwinski, S.M. (2010b) Glucosylceramide synthase upregulates mdr1 expression in the regulation of cancer drug resistance through csrc and beta-catenin signaling. *Molecular cancer,* Vol.9, 145

Lovat, P.E.; Corazzari, M.; Di Sano, F.; Piacentini, M. & Redfern, C.P. (2005) The role of gangliosides in fenretinide-induced apoptosis of neuroblastoma. *Cancer letters,* Vol.228, No.1-2, pp.105-10

Lovat, P.E.; Di Sano, F.; Corazzari, M.; Fazi, B.; Donnorso, R.P.; Pearson, A.D.; Hall, A.G.; Redfern, C.P. & Piacentini, M. (2004) Gangliosides link the acidic sphingomyelinase-mediated induction of ceramide to 12-lipoxygenase-dependent apoptosis of neuroblastoma in response to fenretinide. *J Natl Cancer Inst,* Vol.96, No.17, pp.1288-99

Lovat, P.E.; Ranalli, M.; Annichiarrico-Petruzzelli, M.; Bernassola, F.; Piacentini, M.; Malcolm, A.J.; Pearson, A.D.; Melino, G. & Redfern, C.P. (2000) Effector mechanisms of fenretinide-induced apoptosis in neuroblastoma. *Exp Cell Res,* Vol.260, No.1, pp.50-60

Lozano, J.; Berra, E.; Municio, M.M.; Diaz-Meco, M.T.; Dominguez, I.; Sanz, L. & Moscat, J. (1994) Protein kinase c zeta isoform is critical for kappa b-dependent promoter activation by sphingomyelinase. *J Biol Chem,* Vol.269, No.30, pp.19200-2

Luberto, C.; Hassler, D.F.; Signorelli, P.; Okamoto, Y.; Sawai, H.; Boros, E.; Hazen-Martin, D.J.; Obeid, L.M.; Hannun, Y.A. & Smith, G.K. (2002) Inhibition of tumor necrosis factor-induced cell death in mcf7 by a novel inhibitor of neutral sphingomyelinase. *J Biol Chem,* Vol.277, No.43, pp.41128-39

Luberto, C.; Yoo, D.S.; Suidan, H.S.; Bartoli, G.M. & Hannun, Y.A. (2000) Differential effects of sphingomyelin hydrolysis and resynthesis on the activation of nf-kappa b in normal and sv40-transformed human fibroblasts. *J Biol Chem,* Vol.275, No.19, pp.14760-6

Lucci, A.; Cho, W.I.; Han, T.Y.; Giuliano, A.E.; Morton, D.L. & Cabot, M.C. (1998) Glucosylceramide: A marker for multiple-drug resistant cancers. *Anticancer research,* Vol.18, No.1B, pp.475-80

Lucki, N.C. & Sewer, M.B. (2011) Genistein stimulates mcf-7 breast cancer cell growth by inducing acid ceramidase (asah1) gene expression. *The Journal of biological chemistry,* Vol.286, No.22, pp.19399-409

Mahdy, A.E.; Cheng, J.C.; Li, J.; Elojeimy, S.; Meacham, W.D.; Turner, L.S.; Bai, A.; Gault, C.R.; Mcpherson, A.S.; Garcia, N.; Beckham, T.H.; Saad, A.; Bielawska, A.; Bielawski, J.; Hannun, Y.A.; Keane, T.E.; Taha, M.I.; Hammouda, H.M.; Norris, J.S. & Liu, X. (2009) Acid ceramidase upregulation in prostate cancer cells confers resistance to radiation: Ac inhibition, a potential radiosensitizer. *Molecular therapy : the journal of the American Society of Gene Therapy,* Vol.17, No.3, pp.430-8

Mao, Z.; Sun, W.; Xu, R.; Novgorodov, S.; Szulc, Z.M.; Bielawski, J.; Obeid, L.M. & Mao, C. (2010) Alkaline ceramidase 2 (acer2) and its product dihydrosphingosine mediate the cytotoxicity of n-(4-hydroxyphenyl)retinamide in tumor cells. *The Journal of biological chemistry,* Vol.285, No.38, pp.29078-90

Marachelian, A.; Kang, M.H.; Hwang, K.; Villablanca, J.G.; Groshen, S.; Matthay, K.K.; Maris, J.; Desantes, K.B.; Reynolds, C.P. & Maurer, B.J. (2009) Phase i study of fenretinide (4-hpr) oral powder in patients with recurrent or resistant neuroblastoma: New approaches to neuroblastoma therapy (nant) consortium trial. *J Clin Oncol.* 27:15s, Abstract 10009.

Marchesini, N. & Hannun, Y.A. (2004) Acid and neutral sphingomyelinases: Roles and mechanisms of regulation. *Biochem Cell Biol,* Vol.82, No.1, pp.27-44

Maris, J.M. (2010) Recent advances in neuroblastoma. *The New England journal of medicine,* Vol.362, No.23, pp.2202-11

Matthay, K.K.; Reynolds, C.P.; Seeger, R.C.; Shimada, H.; Adkins, E.S.; Haas-Kogan, D.; Gerbing, R.B.; London, W.B. & Villablanca, J.G. (2009) Long-term results for children with high-risk neuroblastoma treated on a randomized trial of myeloablative therapy followed by 13-cis-retinoic acid: A children's oncology group study. *Journal of clinical oncology : official journal of the American Society of Clinical Oncology,* Vol.27, No.7, pp.1007-13

Matthay, K.K.; Villablanca, J.G.; Seeger, R.C.; Stram, D.O.; Harris, R.E.; Ramsay, N.K.; Swift, P.; Shimada, H.; Black, C.T.; Brodeur, G.M.; Gerbing, R.B. & Reynolds, C.P. (1999) Treatment of high-risk neuroblastoma with intensive chemotherapy, radiotherapy, autologous bone marrow transplantation, and 13-cis-retinoic acid. Children's cancer group. *The New England journal of medicine,* Vol.341, No.16, pp.1165-73

Maurer, B.J.; Melton, L.; Billups, C.; Cabot, M.C. & Reynolds, C.P. (2000) Synergistic cytotoxicity in solid tumor cell lines between n-(4-hydroxyphenyl)retinamide and modulators of ceramide metabolism. *Journal of the National Cancer Institute,* Vol.92, No.23, pp.1897-909

Maurer, T. & Fung, H.L. (2000) Comparison of methods for analyzing kinetic data from mechanism-based enzyme inactivation: Application to nitric oxide synthase. *AAPS PharmSci,* Vol.2, No.1, pp.E8

Mehta, R.R.; Hawthorne, M.E.; Graves, J.M. & Mehta, R.G. (1998) Metabolism of n-[4-hydroxyphenyl]retinamide (4-hpr) to n-[4-methoxyphenyl]retinamide (4-mpr) may serve as a biomarker for its efficacy against human breast cancer and melanoma cells. *European journal of cancer,* Vol.34, No.6, pp.902-7

Merrill, A.H., Jr. (2002) De novo sphingolipid biosynthesis: A necessary, but dangerous, pathway. *J Biol Chem,* Vol.277, No.29, pp.25843-6

Mershon, S.M.; Anding, A.L.; Chapman, J.S.; Clagett-Dame, M.; Stonerock, L.A. & Curley, R.W., Jr. (2007) Solid phase-assisted synthesis and screening of a small library of n-

(4-hydroxyphenyl)retinamide (4-hpr) analogs. *Bioorg Med Chem Lett,* Vol.17, No.3, pp.836-40

Messner, M.C. & Cabot, M.C. (2010) Glucosylceramide in humans. *Advances in experimental medicine and biology,* Vol.688, 156-64

Michel, C.; Van Echten-Deckert, G.; Rother, J.; Sandhoff, K.; Wang, E. & Merrill, A.H., Jr. (1997) Characterization of ceramide synthesis. A dihydroceramide desaturase introduces the 4,5-trans-double bond of sphingosine at the level of dihydroceramide. *J Biol Chem,* Vol.272, No.36, pp.22432-7

Mitsutake, S.; Kim, T.J.; Inagaki, Y.; Kato, M.; Yamashita, T. & Igarashi, Y. (2004) Ceramide kinase is a mediator of calcium-dependent degranulation in mast cells. *J Biol Chem,* Vol.279, No.17, pp.17570-7

Mizutani, Y.; Kihara, A. & Igarashi, Y. (2004) Identification of the human sphingolipid c4-hydroxylase, hdes2, and its up-regulation during keratinocyte differentiation. *FEBS Lett,* Vol.563, No.1-3, pp.93-7

Morales, A.; Paris, R.; Villanueva, A.; Llacuna, L.; Garcia-Ruiz, C. & Fernandez-Checa, J.C. (2007) Pharmacological inhibition or small interfering rna targeting acid ceramidase sensitizes hepatoma cells to chemotherapy and reduces tumor growth in vivo. *Oncogene,* Vol.26, No.6, pp.905-16

Movsesyan, V.A.; Yakovlev, A.G.; Dabaghyan, E.A.; Stoica, B.A. & Faden, A.I. (2002) Ceramide induces neuronal apoptosis through the caspase-9/caspase-3 pathway. *Biochem Biophys Res Commun,* Vol.299, No.2, pp.201-7

Mullen, T.D.; Jenkins, R.W.; Clarke, C.J.; Bielawski, J.; Hannun, Y.A. & Obeid, L.M. (2011) Ceramide synthase-dependent ceramide generation and programmed cell death: Involvement of salvage pathway in regulating postmitochondrial events. *J Biol Chem,* Vol.286, No.18, pp.15929-42

Munoz-Olaya, J.M.; Matabosch, X.; Bedia, C.; Egido-Gabas, M.; Casas, J.; Llebaria, A.; Delgado, A. & Fabrias, G. (2008) Synthesis and biological activity of a novel inhibitor of dihydroceramide desaturase. *ChemMedChem,* Vol.3, No.6, pp.946-53

Murakami, M.; Ito, H.; Hagiwara, K.; Yoshida, K.; Sobue, S.; Ichihara, M.; Takagi, A.; Kojima, T.; Tanaka, K.; Tamiya-Koizumi, K.; Kyogashima, M.; Suzuki, M.; Banno, Y.; Nozawa, Y. & Murate, T. (2010) Atra inhibits ceramide kinase transcription in a human neuroblastoma cell line, sh-sy5y cells: The role of coup-tfi. *Journal of neurochemistry,* Vol.112, No.2, pp.511-20

Ogretmen, B. (2006) Sphingolipids in cancer: Regulation of pathogenesis and therapy. *FEBS Lett,* Vol.580, No.23, pp.5467-76

Ogretmen, B. & Hannun, Y.A. (2004) Biologically active sphingolipids in cancer pathogenesis and treatment. *Nat Rev Cancer,* Vol.4, No.8, pp.604-16

Ogretmen, B.; Kraveka, J.M.; Schady, D.; Usta, J.; Hannun, Y.A. & Obeid, L.M. (2001) Molecular mechanisms of ceramide-mediated telomerase inhibition in the a549 human lung adenocarcinoma cell line. *The Journal of biological chemistry,* Vol.276, No.35, pp.32506-14

Omae, F.; Miyazaki, M.; Enomoto, A.; Suzuki, M.; Suzuki, Y. & Suzuki, A. (2004) Des2 protein is responsible for phytoceramide biosynthesis in the mouse small intestine. *Biochem J,* Vol.379, No.Pt 3, pp.687-95

Patwardhan, G.A.; Zhang, Q.J.; Yin, D.; Gupta, V.; Bao, J.; Senkal, C.E.; Ogretmen, B.; Cabot, M.C.; Shah, G.V.; Sylvester, P.W.; Jazwinski, S.M. & Liu, Y.Y. (2009) A new mixed-backbone oligonucleotide against glucosylceramide synthase sensitizes multidrug-resistant tumors to apoptosis. *PloS one,* Vol.4, No.9, pp.e6938

Perry, D.K.; Carton, J.; Shah, A.K.; Meredith, F.; Uhlinger, D.J. & Hannun, Y.A. (2000) Serine palmitoyltransferase regulates de novo ceramide generation during etoposide-induced apoptosis. *J Biol Chem,* Vol.275, No.12, pp.9078-84

Pettus, B.J.; Bielawska, A.; Subramanian, P.; Wijesinghe, D.S.; Maceyka, M.; Leslie, C.C.; Evans, J.H.; Freiberg, J.; Roddy, P.; Hannun, Y.A. & Chalfant, C.E. (2004) Ceramide 1-phosphate is a direct activator of cytosolic phospholipase a2. *J Biol Chem,* Vol.279, No.12, pp.11320-6

Pettus, B.J.; Chalfant, C.E. & Hannun, Y.A. (2002) Ceramide in apoptosis: An overview and current perspectives. *Biochim Biophys Acta,* Vol.1585, No.2-3, pp.114-25

Pewzner-Jung, Y.; Ben-Dor, S. & Futerman, A.H. (2006) When do lasses (longevity assurance genes) become cers (ceramide synthases)?: Insights into the regulation of ceramide synthesis. *J Biol Chem,* Vol.281, No.35, pp.25001-5

Ponnusamy, S.; Meyers-Needham, M.; Senkal, C.E.; Saddoughi, S.A.; Sentelle, D.; Selvam, S.P.; Salas, A. & Ogretmen, B. (2010) Sphingolipids and cancer: Ceramide and sphingosine-1-phosphate in the regulation of cell death and drug resistance. *Future oncology,* Vol.6, No.10, pp.1603-24

Ponthan, F.; Wickstrom, M.; Gleissman, H.; Fuskevag, O.M.; Segerstrom, L.; Sveinbjornsson, B.; Redfern, C.P.; Eksborg, S.; Kogner, P. & Johnsen, J.I. (2007) Celecoxib prevents neuroblastoma tumor development and potentiates the effect of chemotherapeutic drugs in vitro and in vivo. *Clinical cancer research : an official journal of the American Association for Cancer Research,* Vol.13, No.3, pp.1036-44

Prinetti, A.; Bassi, R.; Riboni, L. & Tettamanti, G. (1997) Involvement of a ceramide activated protein phosphatase in the differentiation of neuroblastoma neuro2a cells. *FEBS Lett,* Vol.414, No.2, pp.475-9

Rahmaniyan, M.; Curley, R.W., Jr.; Obeid, L.M.; Hannun, Y.A. & Kraveka, J.M. (2011) Identification of dihydroceramide desaturase as a direct in vitro target for fenretinide. *The Journal of biological chemistry,*

Reynolds, C.P. (2000) Differentiating agents in pediatric malignancies: Retinoids in neuroblastoma. *Current oncology reports,* Vol.2, No.6, pp.511-8

Reynolds, C.P. & Lemons, R.S. (2001) Retinoid therapy of childhood cancer. *Hematology/oncology clinics of North America,* Vol.15, No.5, pp.867-910

Reynolds, C.P.; Wang, Y.; Melton, L.J.; Einhorn, P.A.; Slamon, D.J. & Maurer, B.J. (2000) Retinoic-acid-resistant neuroblastoma cell lines show altered myc regulation and high sensitivity to fenretinide. *Medical and pediatric oncology,* Vol.35, No.6, pp.597-602

Riboni, L.; Bassi, R.; Caminiti, A.; Prinetti, A.; Viani, P. & Tettamanti, G. (1998) Metabolic fate of exogenous sphingosine in neuroblastoma neuro2a cells. Dose-dependence and biological effects. *Ann N Y Acad Sci,* Vol.845, 46-56

Riboni, L.; Campanella, R.; Bassi, R.; Villani, R.; Gaini, S.M.; Martinelli-Boneschi, F.; Viani, P. & Tettamanti, G. (2002) Ceramide levels are inversely associated with malignant progression of human glial tumors. *Glia,* Vol.39, No.2, pp.105-13

Riboni, L.; Prinetti, A.; Bassi, R.; Caminiti, A. & Tettamanti, G. (1995) A mediator role of ceramide in the regulation of neuroblastoma neuro2a cell differentiation. *J Biol Chem,* Vol.270, No.45, pp.26868-75

Ryland, L.K.; Fox, T.E.; Liu, X.; Loughran, T.P. & Kester, M. (2011) Dysregulation of sphingolipid metabolism in cancer. *Cancer Biol Ther,* Vol.11, No.2, pp.138-49

Rylova, S.N.; Somova, O.G. & Dyatlovitskaya, E.V. (1998) Comparative investigation of sphingoid bases and fatty acids in ceramides and sphingomyelins from human ovarian malignant tumors and normal ovary. *Biochemistry. Biokhimiia,* Vol.63, No.9, pp.1057-60

Saddoughi, S.A.; Song, P. & Ogretmen, B. (2008) Roles of bioactive sphingolipids in cancer biology and therapeutics. *Subcell Biochem,* Vol.49, 413-40

Schaefer, J.T.; Barthlen, W. & Schweizer, P. (2000) Ceramide induces apoptosis in neuroblastoma cell cultures resistant to cd95 (fas/apo-1)-mediated apoptosis. *Journal of pediatric surgery,* Vol.35, No.3, pp.473-9

Schiffmann, S.; Sandner, J.; Birod, K.; Wobst, I.; Angioni, C.; Ruckhaberle, E.; Kaufmann, M.; Ackermann, H.; Lotsch, J.; Schmidt, H.; Geisslinger, G. & Grosch, S. (2009) Ceramide synthases and ceramide levels are increased in breast cancer tissue. *Carcinogenesis,*

Schultz, A. & Larsson, C. (2004) Ceramide influences neurite outgrowth and neuroblastoma cell apoptosis regulated by novel protein kinase c isoforms. *J Neurochem,* Vol.89, No.6, pp.1427-35

Schwandner, R.; Wiegmann, K.; Bernardo, K.; Kreder, D. & Kronke, M. (1998) Tnf receptor death domain-associated proteins tradd and fadd signal activation of acid sphingomyelinase. *J Biol Chem,* Vol.273, No.10, pp.5916-22

Senkal, C.E.; Ponnusamy, S.; Bielawski, J.; Hannun, Y.A. & Ogretmen, B. (2010) Antiapoptotic roles of ceramide-synthase-6-generated c16-ceramide via selective regulation of the atf6/chop arm of er-stress-response pathways. *The FASEB journal : official publication of the Federation of American Societies for Experimental Biology,* Vol.24, No.1, pp.296-308

Senkal, C.E.; Ponnusamy, S.; Rossi, M.J.; Bialewski, J.; Sinha, D.; Jiang, J.C.; Jazwinski, S.M.; Hannun, Y.A. & Ogretmen, B. (2007) Role of human longevity assurance gene 1 and c18-ceramide in chemotherapy-induced cell death in human head and neck squamous cell carcinomas. *Mol Cancer Ther,* Vol.6, No.2, pp.712-22

Separovic, D.; Bielawski, J.; Pierce, J.S.; Merchant, S.; Tarca, A.L.; Ogretmen, B. & Korbelik, M. (2009) Increased tumour dihydroceramide production after photofrin-pdt alone and improved tumour response after the combination with the ceramide analogue lcl29. Evidence from mouse squamous cell carcinomas. *Br J Cancer,* Vol.100, No.4, pp.626-32

Shah, M.V.; Zhang, R.; Irby, R.; Kothapalli, R.; Liu, X.; Arrington, T.; Frank, B.; Lee, N.H. & Loughran, T.P., Jr. (2008) Molecular profiling of lgl leukemia reveals role of sphingolipid signaling in survival of cytotoxic lymphocytes. *Blood,* Vol.112, No.3, pp.770-81

Sietsma, H.; Dijkhuis, A.J.; Kamps, W. & Kok, J.W. (2002) Sphingolipids in neuroblastoma: Their role in drug resistance mechanisms. *Neurochem Res,* Vol.27, No.7-8, pp.665-74

Signorelli, P.; Munoz-Olaya, J.M.; Gagliostro, V.; Casas, J.; Ghidoni, R. & Fabrias, G. (2009) Dihydroceramide intracellular increase in response to resveratrol treatment mediates autophagy in gastric cancer cells. *Cancer Lett,* Vol.282, No.2, pp.238-43

Soto, B.L.; Hank, J.A.; Van De Voort, T.J.; Subramanian, L.; Polans, A.S.; Rakhmilevich, A.L.; Yang, R.K.; Seo, S.; Kim, K.; Reisfeld, R.A.; Gillies, S.D. & Sondel, P.M. (2011) The anti-tumor effect of resveratrol alone or in combination with immunotherapy in a neuroblastoma model. *Cancer immunology, immunotherapy : CII,* Vol.60, No.5, pp.731-8

Stiban, J.; Fistere, D. & Colombini, M. (2006) Dihydroceramide hinders ceramide channel formation: Implications on apoptosis. *Apoptosis,* Vol.11, No.5, pp.773-80

Strum, J.C.; Small, G.W.; Pauig, S.B. & Daniel, L.W. (1994) 1-beta-d-arabinofuranosylcytosine stimulates ceramide and diglyceride formation in hl-60 cells. *J Biol Chem,* Vol.269, No.22, pp.15493-7

Sugiki, H.; Hozumi, Y.; Maeshima, H.; Katagata, Y.; Mitsuhashi, Y. & Kondo, S. (2000) C2-ceramide induces apoptosis in a human squamous cell carcinoma cell line. *Br J Dermatol,* Vol.143, No.6, pp.1154-63

Sundararaj, K.P.; Wood, R.E.; Ponnusamy, S.; Salas, A.M.; Szulc, Z.; Bielawska, A.; Obeid, L.M.; Hannun, Y.A. & Ogretmen, B. (2004) Rapid shortening of telomere length in response to ceramide involves the inhibition of telomere binding activity of nuclear glyceraldehyde-3-phosphate dehydrogenase. *J Biol Chem,* Vol.279, No.7, pp.6152-62

Suzuki, A.; Iwasaki, M.; Kato, M. & Wagai, N. (1997) Sequential operation of ceramide synthesis and ice cascade in cpt-11-initiated apoptotic death signaling. *Exp Cell Res,* Vol.233, No.1, pp.41-7

Ternes, P.; Franke, S.; Zahringer, U.; Sperling, P. & Heinz, E. (2002) Identification and characterization of a sphingolipid delta 4-desaturase family. *J Biol Chem,* Vol.277, No.28, pp.25512-8

Tettamanti, G. (2004) Ganglioside/glycosphingolipid turnover: New concepts. *Glycoconj J,* Vol.20, No.5, pp.301-17

Tiberio, P.; Cavadini, E.; Abolafio, G.; Formelli, F. & Appierto, V. (2010) 4-oxo-n-(4-hydroxyphenyl)retinamide: Two independent ways to kill cancer cells. *PloS one,* Vol.5, No.10, pp.e13362

Torrisi, R.; Decensi, A.; Formelli, F.; Camerini, T. & De Palo, G. (2001) Chemoprevention of breast cancer with fenretinide. *Drugs,* Vol.61, No.7, pp.909-18

Triola, G.; Fabrias, G.; Dragusin, M.; Niederhausen, L.; Broere, R.; Llebaria, A. & Van Echten-Deckert, G. (2004) Specificity of the dihydroceramide desaturase inhibitor n-[(1r,2s)-2-hydroxy-1-hydroxymethyl-2-(2-tridecyl-1-cyclopropenyl)ethyl]o ctanamide (gt11) in primary cultured cerebellar neurons. *Molecular pharmacology,* Vol.66, No.6, pp.1671-8

Triola, G.; Fabrias, G. & Llebaria, A. (2001) Synthesis of a cyclopropene analogue of ceramide, a potent inhibitor of dihydroceramide desaturase *Angew Chem Int Ed Engl,* Vol.40, No.10, pp.1960-1962

Turner, L.S.; Cheng, J.C.; Beckham, T.H.; Keane, T.E.; Norris, J.S. & Liu, X. (2011) Autophagy is increased in prostate cancer cells overexpressing acid ceramidase and enhances resistance to c6 ceramide. *Prostate cancer and prostatic diseases,* Vol.14, No.1, pp.30-7

Uemura, K.; Sugiyama, E. & Taketomi, T. (1991) Effects of an inhibitor of glucosylceramide synthase on glycosphingolipid synthesis and neurite outgrowth in murine neuroblastoma cell lines. *Journal of biochemistry,* Vol.110, No.1, pp.96-102

Van Echten-Deckert, G. & Herget, T. (2006) Sphingolipid metabolism in neural cells. *Biochim Biophys Acta,* Vol.1758, No.12, pp.1978-94

Van Ginkel, P.R.; Sareen, D.; Subramanian, L.; Walker, Q.; Darjatmoko, S.R.; Lindstrom, M.J.; Kulkarni, A.; Albert, D.M. & Polans, A.S. (2007) Resveratrol inhibits tumor growth of human neuroblastoma and mediates apoptosis by directly targeting mitochondria. *Clinical cancer research : an official journal of the American Association for Cancer Research,* Vol.13, No.17, pp.5162-9

Venable, M.E.; Lee, J.Y.; Smyth, M.J.; Bielawska, A. & Obeid, L.M. (1995) Role of ceramide in cellular senescence. *J Biol Chem,* Vol.270, No.51, pp.30701-8

Villablanca, J.G.; Krailo, M.D.; Ames, M.M.; Reid, J.M.; Reaman, G.H. & Reynolds, C.P. (2006) Phase i trial of oral fenretinide in children with high-risk solid tumors: A report from the children's oncology group (ccg 09709). *Journal of clinical oncology : official journal of the American Society of Clinical Oncology,* Vol.24, No.21, pp.3423-30

Villani, M.; Subathra, M.; Im, Y.B.; Choi, Y.; Signorelli, P.; Del Poeta, M. & Luberto, C. (2008) Sphingomyelin synthases regulate production of diacylglycerol at the golgi. *Biochem J,*

Villani, M.G.; Appierto, V.; Cavadini, E.; Bettiga, A.; Prinetti, A.; Clagett-Dame, M.; Curley, R.W. & Formelli, F. (2006) 4-oxo-fenretinide, a recently identified fenretinide metabolite, induces marked g2-m cell cycle arrest and apoptosis in fenretinide-sensitive and fenretinide-resistant cell lines. *Cancer Res,* Vol.66, No.6, pp.3238-47

Villani, M.G.; Appierto, V.; Cavadini, E.; Valsecchi, M.; Sonnino, S.; Curley, R.W. & Formelli, F. (2004) Identification of the fenretinide metabolite 4-oxo-fenretinide present in human plasma and formed in human ovarian carcinoma cells through induction of cytochrome p450 26a1. *Clin Cancer Res,* Vol.10, No.18 Pt 1, pp.6265-75

Wang, H.; Maurer, B.J.; Liu, Y.Y.; Wang, E.; Allegood, J.C.; Kelly, S.; Symolon, H.; Liu, Y.; Merrill, A.H., Jr.; Gouaze-Andersson, V.; Yu, J.Y.; Giuliano, A.E. & Cabot, M.C. (2008) N-(4-hydroxyphenyl)retinamide increases dihydroceramide and synergizes with dimethylsphingosine to enhance cancer cell killing. *Mol Cancer Ther,* Vol.7, No.9, pp.2967-76

Wang, H.; Maurer, B.J.; Reynolds, C.P. & Cabot, M.C. (2001) N-(4-hydroxyphenyl)retinamide elevates ceramide in neuroblastoma cell lines by coordinate activation of serine palmitoyltransferase and ceramide synthase. *Cancer research,* Vol.61, No.13, pp.5102-5

Wei, J.S.; Whiteford, C.C.; Cenacchi, N.; Son, C.G. & Khan, J. (2005) Bbc3 mediates fenretinide-induced cell death in neuroblastoma. *Oncogene,* Vol.24, No.54, pp.7976-83

Wolff, R.A.; Dobrowsky, R.T.; Bielawska, A.; Obeid, L.M. & Hannun, Y.A. (1994) Role of ceramide-activated protein phosphatase in ceramide-mediated signal transduction. *J Biol Chem,* Vol.269, No.30, pp.19605-9

Wu, J.M.; Dipietrantonio, A.M. & Hsieh, T.C. (2001) Mechanism of fenretinide (4-hpr)-induced cell death. *Apoptosis,* Vol.6, No.5, pp.377-88

Xie, P.; Shen, Y.F.; Shi, Y.P.; Ge, S.M.; Gu, Z.H.; Wang, J.; Mu, H.J.; Zhang, B.; Qiao, W.Z. & Xie, K.M. (2008) Overexpression of glucosylceramide synthase in associated with multidrug resistance of leukemia cells. *Leukemia research,* Vol.32, No.3, pp.475-80

Zhang, X.; Wu, X.; Li, J.; Sun, Y.; Gao, P.; Zhang, C.; Zhang, H. & Zhou, G. (2011) Mdr1 (multidrug resistence 1) can regulate gcs (glucosylceramide synthase) in breast cancer cells. *J Surg Oncol,*

Zhang, Y.; Mattjus, P.; Schmid, P.C.; Dong, Z.; Zhong, S.; Ma, W.Y.; Brown, R.E.; Bode, A.M.; Schmid, H.H. & Dong, Z. (2001) Involvement of the acid sphingomyelinase pathway in uva-induced apoptosis. *J Biol Chem,* Vol.276, No.15, pp.11775-82

Zheng, W.; Kollmeyer, J.; Symolon, H.; Momin, A.; Munter, E.; Wang, E.; Kelly, S.; Allegood, J.C.; Liu, Y.; Peng, Q.; Ramaraju, H.; Sullards, M.C.; Cabot, M. & Merrill, A.H., Jr. (2006) Ceramides and other bioactive sphingolipid backbones in health and disease: Lipidomic analysis, metabolism and roles in membrane structure, dynamics, signaling and autophagy. *Biochim Biophys Acta,* Vol.1758, No.12, pp.1864-84

8

The *NBPF* Gene Family

Vanessa Andries, Karl Vandepoele and Frans van Roy
Department for Molecular Biomedical Research, VIB
Department of Biomedical Molecular Biology, Ghent University
Belgium

1. Introduction

Neuroblastoma is one of the most intensely studied solid malignancies that affect children (Maris & Matthay, 1999). These tumours are heterogeneous biologically and clinically. One subset of neuroblastoma is susceptible to spontaneous apoptosis with little or no therapy and another subset differentiates over time, but most of these tumours are difficult to cure with current treatments. A relatively high proportion of affected children die due to resistance of the neuroblastoma to therapy (Van Roy *et al.*, 2009). Every step in the identification or functional understanding of the genes that play important roles in this cancer could bring us closer to understanding the molecular mechanism and could help to develop more effective therapy.

We will describe the novel *NBPF* gene family and its role in neuroblastoma. The *NBPF* gene family was originally identified by the disruption of one of its members in a neuroblastoma patient (Vandepoele *et al.*, 2008). This gene was named *NBPF1*, for Neuroblastoma Breakpoint Family, member 1. Several reports indicate that the *NBPF* gene family might play an important role in neuroblastoma and possibly in other cancers as well. Additionally, this evolutionarily recent gene family has been involved as an important player in human evolution.

2. Identification of *NBPF1* during the positional cloning of a constitutional translocation in a neuroblastoma patient

In 1983, karyotypic analysis of fibroblasts from a Belgian neuroblastoma patient revealed a *de novo*, constitutional translocation between chromosomes 1p36.2 and 17q11.2 (Laureys *et al.*, 1990; Laureys *et al.*, 1995). These two chromosomal regions are often rearranged in sporadic neuroblastoma tumours (Savelyeva *et al.*, 1994). So it was believed that the translocation had predisposed the patient to neuroblastoma by disrupting one or more genes. Although previous cytogenetic experiments indicated that the translocation was balanced, analysis of the breakpoint sequences showed greater complexity (Figure 1). First, in both derivative chromosomes, a few nucleotides of unknown origin were inserted between the chromosome 1 and 17 sequences (Vandepoele *et al.*, 2008). Such insertions are frequently observed in reciprocal constitutional translocations (Willett-Brozick *et al.*, 2001). Second, on chromosome 1, the translocation resulted in the deletion of a genomic fragment of 5,215 base pairs that is present in the human genome reference sequence (Vandepoele *et al.*, 2008). However, numerous reports describe structural variation at this locus (see below), which makes it impossible to determine the precise size of the deletion in this neuroblastoma patient. No deletions or insertions of genomic regions were observed on chromosome 17, which means that the translocation at this level is indeed balanced. Notably, both translocation breakpoints are located in LINE repeats, classified as type L1-PA4 for chromosome 1 and as type L2 for chromosome 17, but no significant sequence homology between these two LINE repeats was found. Therefore, most probably these repeats do not participate in the mechanism of this translocation (Vandepoele *et al.*, 2008).

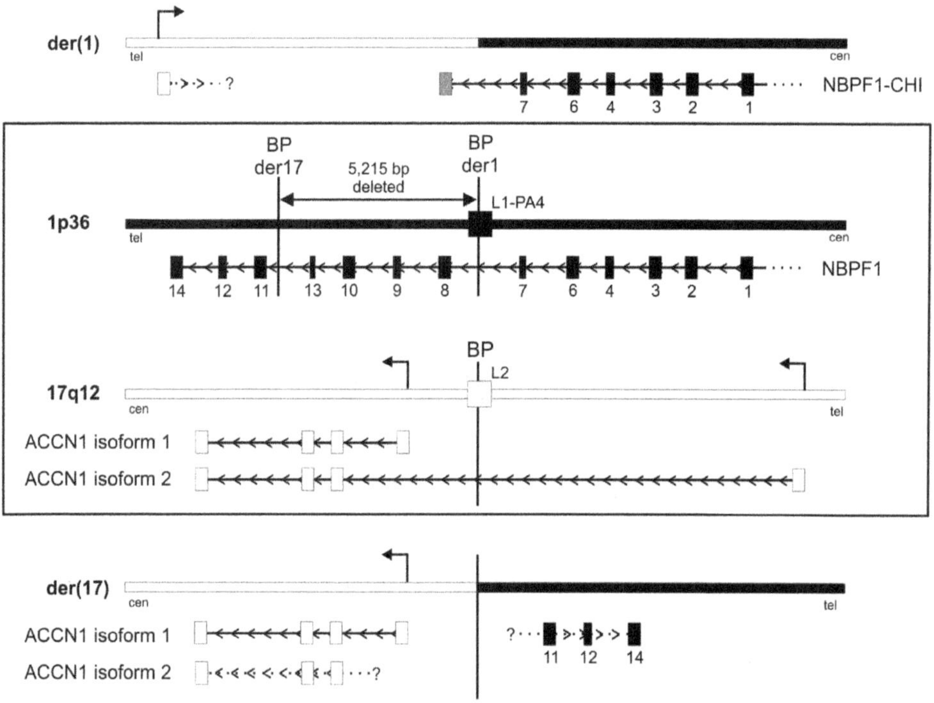

Fig. 1. Genomic overview of the translocation breakpoint of the der(1) and der(17) chromosomes.

Central box: Normal 1p36 and 17q12 chromosomes. Both translocation breakpoints (BP) on chromosome 1 are located in intronic regions of the *NBPF1* gene, and the translocation results in deletion of 5,215 bp. The translocation breakpoint on chromosome 17 is located in the *ACCN1* gene and disrupts only isoform 2. **Top**: On the der(1) chromosome, the translocation gives rise to two chimeric transcripts of *NBPF1* sequences (NBPF1-CHI) fused to sequences derived from chromosome 17 (grey box), thereby extending the open reading frame. Translocation of the promoter and the first exon of *ACCN1* isoform 2 might result in chimeric transcripts on der(1), but so far no transcripts have been isolated (question mark with dotted line). **Bottom**: On the der(17) chromosome, isoform 2 of the *ACCN1* gene is probably no longer expressed due to loss of its promoter and first exon (dotted line with question mark), whereas the last three *NBPF1* exons are translocated to the der(17) chromosome (exon types 11, 12 and 14) (Modified after Vandepoele *et al.*, 2008).

On chromosome 17, the translocation disrupts *ACCN1*, a potential glioma tumour suppressor gene (Vila-Carriles *et al.*, 2006). *ACCN1* encodes a member of the superfamily of amiloride-sensitive degenerin/epithelial sodium channels (DEG/ENaC) and is also known as MDEG (Waldmann *et al.*, 1996), BNaC1 (Garcia-Anoveros *et al.*, 1997) and ASIC2 (Waldmann *et al.*, 1997). *ACCN1* is expressed primarily in the brain, where it might play a role in neurotransmission (Garcia-Anoveros *et al.*, 1997). Alternative initiation of transcription results in two variants encoding distinct isoforms differing in their N-terminal domains (Lingueglia *et al.*, 1997). The translocation in the neuroblastoma patient disrupts only isoform 2 of the *ACCN1* gene. Translocation of the promoter and the first exon of *ACCN1* isoform 2 could result in chimeric transcripts from the derivative chromosome 1 (der(1)), but no such transcripts could be identified. Isoform 2 is probably not expressed from derivative chromosome 17 (der(17)) due to the loss of its promoter and first exon (Figure 1) (Vandepoele *et al.*, 2008).

Oncomine expression analysis (Rhodes *et al.*, 2007) of *ACCN1* showed that it is expressed at significantly lower levels in neuroblastoma tumours with *MYCN* amplification, in higher stage tumours, and in tumours with 1p36 loss of heterozygosity. These findings indicate that *ACCN1* plays a role in tumour aggressiveness (Vandepoele *et al.*, 2008). ACCN1 also has a role in oncogenesis of glioma cells, in which functional restoration of ACCN1 at the plasma membrane decreases cell migration (Vila-Carriles *et al.*, 2006). Gain of chromosome 17q is the most frequent genetic alteration observed in neuroblastoma, but the biological basis is complex because dosage alterations involve genes localised on both sides of the 17q breakpoints. It has been suggested that genes mapping between 17cen and 17q12 suppress tumour progression, whereas genes mapping between 17q23.1 and 17qter promote its progression (Lastowska *et al.*, 2002). These findings further stress the possible role of *ACCN1* as a tumour suppressor of neuroblastoma.

Cloning of the chromosome 1 breakpoint identified a novel gene that is disrupted by this translocation. This gene was named *NBPF1*, for Neuroblastoma Breakpoint Family, member 1. *NBPF1* is a member of a newly discovered gene family with an intricate genomic structure (see section 3.1). The translocation truncates *NBPF1* and gives rise to two chimeric transcripts of *NBPF1* sequences fused to sequences derived from chromosome 17, thereby extending the open reading frame with either 34 or 11 additional codons. The breakpoint of the der(1) chromosome is located in an intron between exon types 7 and 8 (Figure 1). The translocation breakpoint of the der(17) chromosome is also intronic, but it is located between exon types 13 and 11, which results in deletion of a part of the *NBPF1* gene, as described above. The three last *NBPF1* exons, of type 11, 12 and 14, are translocated to the der(17) chromosome, but so far no chimeric transcripts have been described (Figure 1) (Vandepoele *et al.*, 2008).

We determined the expression level of *NBPF1* in 32 neuroblastoma cell lines. This profiling showed that *NBPF1* expression varied widely between the different samples, in line with a previous expression analysis of the total *NBPF* family (Vandepoele *et al.*, 2008). Interestingly, we did not observe complete loss of *NBPF1* expression in any cell line, as has been reported for other genes located in the 1p36 region (Janoueix-Lerosey *et al.*, 2004; Fransson *et al.*, 2007). Statistical analysis of these data revealed a significantly lower expression level of *NBPF1* in cell lines with a heterozygous deletion of the *NBPF1* locus than in cell lines without *NBPF1* loss ($p<0.05$), indicating that *NBPF1* could be a tumour suppressor gene (TSG) in neuroblastoma. Although this decreased expression of *NBPF1* might be explained by the lower gene copy number, it is striking that such downregulation was observed for only 15-20% of the genes affected by hemizygosity of this region (Janoueix-Lerosey *et al.*, 2004). Therefore, in addition to loss of heterozygosity, other mechanisms probably play a role in downregulation of some of these genes. It has been proposed that the combined decrease in the expression of these genes, rather than the inactivation of one single classical TSG, could cause the unfavourable outcome associated with 1p deletions in neuroblastoma (Fransson *et al.*, 2007). Oncomine analysis (Rhodes *et al.*, 2007) showed that in two studies there was no significant difference in *NBPF* expression between different tumour grades or INSS stages but one study showed decreased *NBPF* levels in neuroblastoma tumours that relapsed within five years, which also indicates that *NBPF1* might suppress the development of neuroblastoma. More importantly, induced *NBPF1* expression in human colon cancer cells decreased their clonal growth in a soft agar assay, demonstrating that NBPF1 can act as a TSG, at least in colon cancer (Vandepoele *et al.*, 2008). Like neuroblastoma, colon cancer is characterised by frequent deletions or translocations of 1p36 (Schwab *et al.*, 1996). Indeed several reports indicate that the same TSG might be implicated in both neuroblastoma and colon cancer (Kong *et al.*, 1997; Reyes-Mugica *et al.*, 1998).

3. The *NBPF* gene family

3.1 Structure of the *NBPF* gene family

The cloning of the breakpoints of the constitutional translocation in a neuroblastoma patient revealed that this translocation had disrupted *NBPF1* (see section 2). This gene is a member of the *NBPF* gene family, which is located primarily on duplicated regions of chromosome 1 (Figure 2A). In neuroblastoma, these regions frequently contain aberrations. For instance, one third of primary neuroblastoma tumours carry a deletion of the 1p36 region (White *et al.*, 2005). The *NBPF* genes have a repetitive structure with high intergenic and intragenic sequence similarity, both in coding and non-coding regions (Vinogradova *et al.*, 2002; Vandepoele *et al.*, 2005). The *NBPF1* gene consists of 25 coding exons, but on the basis of their high sequence identities, these exons can be classified into 14 different exon types (Figure 2B). All other *NBPF* genes contain variable numbers of some or all of the exon types present in *NBPF1*, but some genes also contain exons without significant homology to the *NBPF1* exons. The *NBPF* gene family consists of 24 members located primarily on three regions of chromosome 1, namely, 1p36, 1p12 and 1q21, but two members, *NBPF21P* and *NBPF22P*, are located on chromosomes 3p and 5q, respectively.
Several members of this gene family are abundantly expressed in different human cell lines and human tissues, but no discernable orthologs could be found in the genomes of mouse or rat. Nevertheless, the *NBPF* genes do not appear to be restricted to primates because sequences with low but significant homology to *NBPF* have been identified in bovine and canine genomes (Vandepoele *et al.*, 2005).
We previously analysed the genomic organisation of the *NBPF* gene family (Vandepoele *et al.*, 2005). For that analysis, we used the reference sequence of the human genome of the NCBI build 35, which is an improvement over the first release because it contains only 341 gaps (IHGSC 2004) instead of the 150,000 gaps that were present in the first draft version. However, the *NBPF* genes are located in regions that are refractory to all standard sequencing efforts. In this analysis, we obtained numerous small contigs that contained only partial *NBPF* genes. To provide an up-to-date description of the *NBPF* genes in the human genome reference sequence, we now report on the analysis of *NBPF* sequences in the current human genome release (Build 37.2).

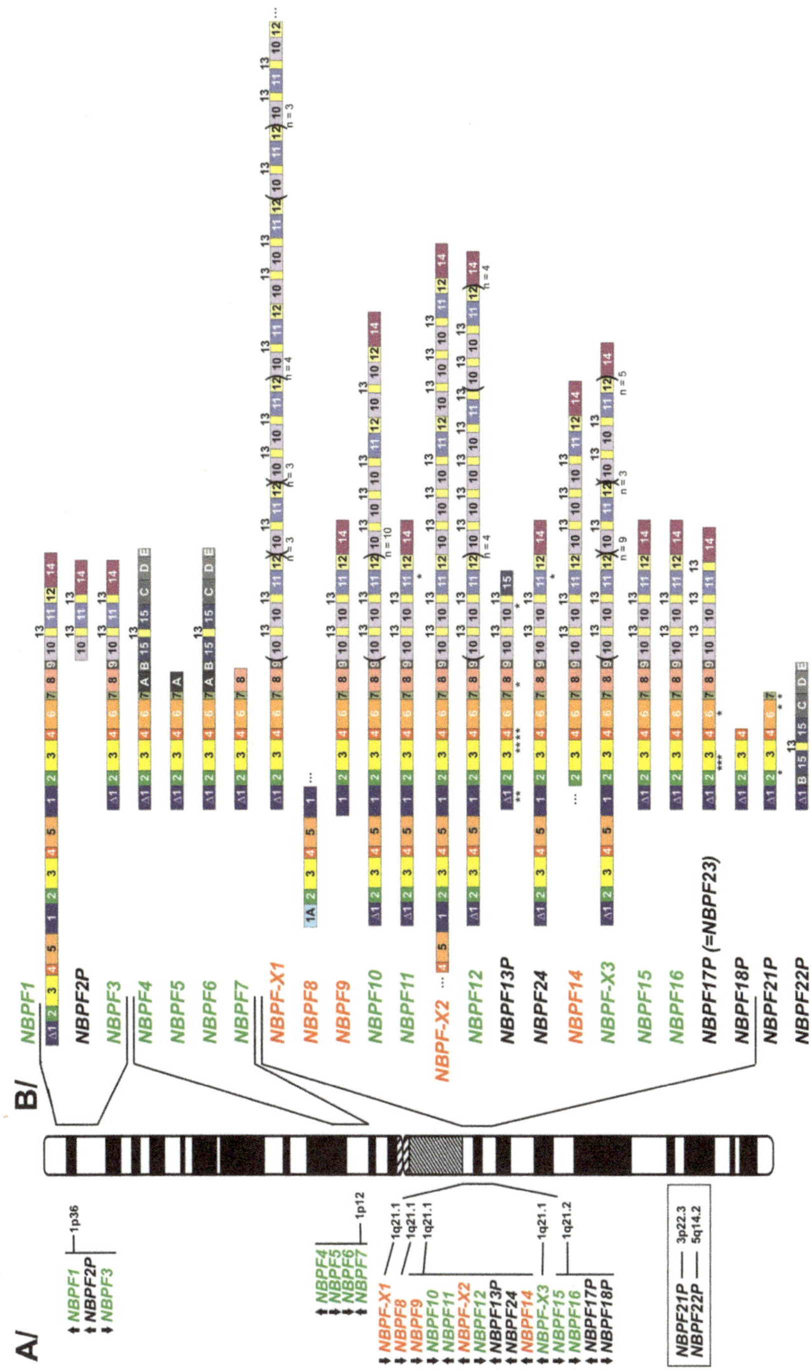

Fig. 2. Genomic overview of the *NBPF* gene family.

Legend to figure 2: Genomic overview of the *NBPF* gene family. A/ Ideogram of human chromosome 1 showing the localisation of the *NBPF* genes. The arrow in front of each gene indicates its orientation in the chromosome. The colour of the gene symbol indicates whether it is full-length (green; start and stop codons present in one continuous ORF in the predicted cDNA), partial (red; due to gaps in the genomic sequence), or a pseudogene (black, P). Vertical lines indicate whether genes are present in a single genomic contig of the human genome assembly (NCBI Build 37.2). The two genes not linked to the ideogram, *NBPF21P* and *NBPF22P*, are located on other chromosomes. B/ The open reading frames of the different *NBPF* genes were assembled *in silico* based on cDNA sequences. *NBPF4* to *NBPF6* and *NBPF22P* contain exons with no significant homology to exons present in *NBPF1*. These are shown as gray boxes with letters instead of numbers. *NBPF8* contains a deletion of two nucleotides in the first coding exon, which results in a frameshift mutation. Due to skipping of the type-2 exon in several *NBPF8* transcripts, this frameshift often does not result in a premature stop. *NBPF-X* sequences are new *NBPF* members that still lack an official gene symbol. Frameshift and nonsense mutations in pseudogenes are indicated by asterisks. Three consecutive dots indicate the presence of gaps in the current genomic assembly (Updated from Vandepoele *et al.*, 2005).

In addition to the 22 *NBPF* genes we identified before (Vandepoele *et al.*, 2005), two additional *NBPF* genes are currently present in GenBank: *NBPF23* and *NBPF24*. Copy number variations of *NBPF23* were recently shown to be involved in neuroblastoma (see below) (Diskin *et al.*, 2009). In our previous analysis, we only focused on the coding exons, and so the 5'UTR was not properly annotated in the databases. However, the *NBPF23* sequences are upstream of the *NBPF17P* encoding exons at a similar distance as the 5'UTR exons of *NBPF1* are from its coding sequences. We therefore believe that the *NBPF23* gene is not a novel gene but is the 5'UTR of *NBPF17P*. We described *NBPF17P* as a pseudogene because it contains nonsense mutations in the normal coding sequence (Vandepoele *et al.*, 2005). In view of that, it is interesting that Diskin *et al.* (2009) found that this sequence is strongly expressed in several tissues, which indicates that this "pseudogene" might have a function. The other new *NBPF* member in GenBank is *NBPF24*, but this is still a hypothetical sequence predicted from a fragment of genomic DNA (see below).
The short arm of chromosome 1 contains two regions that harbour *NBPF* genes. The 1p36 locus contains the *NBPF1* gene. Additionally, one functional gene (*NBPF3*) and a partial duplication of this gene (*NBPF2P*) are located proximal to *NBPF1*. Closer to the centromere on 1p12, there is a second cluster of *NBPF* genes (*NBPF4* to *NBPF7*). These genes are very similar to each other and make up a separate branch of the *NBPF* evolutionary tree (Vandepoele *et al.*, 2005). The sequences of these two clusters were not changed in the most recent human genome reference sequence. The updated version of the human genome reference sequence has undergone numerous changes in chromosome 1q. Overall, it now contains more *NBPF* sequences than the previously published sequence. The *NBPF8* gene was the most proximal *NBPF* gene in our old analysis, but it is now preceded by a novel *NBPF* member, which we call *NBPF-X1*. This is the longest *NBPF* gene we have observed so far, with a size of 77 kb and a cDNA of 11 kb. As there is still a gap in the genomic sequence on the 5' side of *NBPF-X1*, the gene and its derived cDNA are presumably even longer. Distal to *NBPF-X1*, *NBPF8* is an aberrant member of the *NBPF* gene family. Deletion of two nucleotides in its first coding exon causes a frameshift. However, this frameshift can be rescued by an alternative splicing event that excludes the second coding exon from the mature mRNA. *NBPF9*, *NBPF10* and *NBPF11* are identical to those in the old analysis. Like

NBPF-X1, NBPF10 contains numerous repeats of the 3′ exons. *NBPF11* contains a frameshift mutation in one of its last exons, but this gene is nevertheless expressed in a variety of tissues, and hence, we consider it a functional gene. *NBPF11* is followed by a second new *NBPF* gene, *NBPF-X2*. As the 5′ end of this gene is located near a gap in the contig, only a partial sequence is available. In our previous analysis, the sequence of the *NBPF12* gene was incomplete, with only nine consecutive exons in an uninterrupted contig. In the current genome sequence, the complete *NBPF12* gene is present and contains 77 exons. This is followed by *NBPF13P*, a pseudogene with numerous nonsense mutations in different exons, and the new *NBPF24*. Interestingly, *NBPF24* is an almost identical copy of *NBPF11* and contains the same frameshift mutation in one of its last exons. The following gene, *NBFP14*, has not changed in the current assembly, but it is followed by the last new *NBPF* gene, *NBPF-X3*. Like other new members, *NBPF-X3* is also composed of many repetitions of the standard NBPF exon types. The identical *NBPF15* and *NBPF16* genes are contained in the last contig on chromosome 1q, together with the *NBPF17P* and *NBPF18P* pseudogenes. In our previous analysis, *NBPF19* and *NBPF20* were not positioned on chromosome 1. In the current assembly, these sequences are no longer represented. Since the 1q21 region is prone to copy number variation and the human genome reference sequence is derived from different haplotypes, it is possible that *NBFP19* and *NBPF20* are not true paralogs of the current *NBPF* genes, but simply variants of other *NBPF* genes in another haplotype.

In addition to the NBPF sequences on chromosome 1, two other regions in the human genome contain NBPF-like sequences: 3p22.3 (*NBPF21P*) and 5q14.2 (*NBPF22P*). These sequences have only limited homology to the *NBPF* genes on chromosome 1 but share a common origin and are hence included in the *NBPF* family.

Analysis of the predicted protein sequences showed that several pairs of exon types encode a novel protein domain, called the NBPF repeat. The NBPF repeat comprises a PFAM protein domain of unknown function, called DUF1220 (Vandepoele *et al.*, 2005), and we will refer to this repeat as the NBPF/DUF1220 repeat. It is always built of two exons and is present in multiple copies in the different NBPF proteins. It is also present as a single copy with lower homology in the human *PDE4DIP* gene encoding myomegalin (Figure 3) (Verde *et al.*, 2001). Myomegalin is a centrosomal protein and contains, besides its NBPF/DUF1220 domain, some regions that show homology to *CDK5RAP2*, a gene that lacks NBPF/DUF1220 sequences. Mutation of *CDK5RAP2* has been implicated in microcephaly (Bond & Woods, 2006). There is recent evidence for involvement of the NBPF/DUF1220 repeat in human evolutionary adaptation, cognitive function, and disease, including neuroblastoma (see below). Other than the novel NBPF/DUF1220 repeat, there are no known protein domains in the NBPF proteins.

3.2 The *NBPF* gene family and human evolution

Several regions on chromosome 1 consist of recently duplicated sequences, and the *NBPF* gene family is located primarily on such segmental duplications (Vandepoele *et al.*, 2005). Segmental duplications, also known as low copy repeats, are duplicated blocks of genomic DNA longer than 1 kbp and with high sequence identity, and they typically map to two or more locations in the genome (Marques-Bonet *et al.*, 2009b). The number of base pairs mapping to high-identity duplications are similar in the human and mouse genomes, but the segmental duplications in mouse are tandemly organised, whereas in humans most of them are interspersed (She *et al.*, 2008). Additionally, human segmental duplications tend to

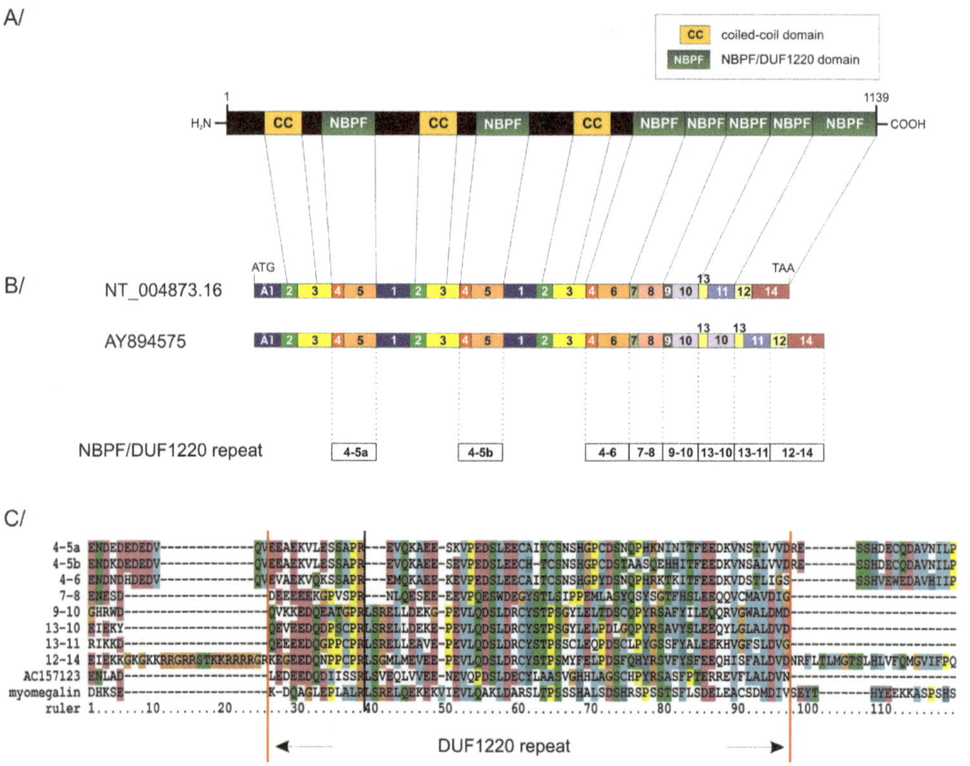

Fig. 3. Exon organisation of the *NBPF1* gene and the predicted domain structure of the translated NBPF1 protein.

A/ Analysis of the predicted NBPF protein sequences showed that each of several pairs of exon types encodes a novel protein domain, called the NBPF repeat. The NBPF repeat comprises a PFAM protein domain of unknown function, called DUF1220 (see C). It is always built of two exons and is present in multiple copies in the different NBPF proteins. Three coiled-coil regions were predicted in the N-terminal domain of the NBPF1 protein. Each coiled-coil is encoded by a combination of the type-2 exon and a part of the type-3 exon. B/ Schematic representation of the open reading frame of the *NBPF1* gene as predicted from the human genome sequence (NT_004873.16) and present in an isolated cDNA sequence (AY894575) derived from this gene. The isolated cDNA contains multiple copies of exon types 10, 11, 12 and 13, which are present only once in the genomic sequence. The several exon couples that constitute the NBPF/DUF1220 repeat are shown in white boxes at the bottom. C/ Amino acid alignment of the different NBPF repeats present in the NBPF1 protein. A homologous sequence was isolated from the draft version of the bovine genome and assembled *in silico* (depicted as AC157123). The bottom sequence is derived from one of the human homologs of rat myomegalin (AB007923; AA 1564-1654). The black line denotes the exon boundaries, whereas the red lines denote the PFAM protein domain of unknown function, DUF1220 (Adapted from Vandepoele *et al.*, 2005, Oxford Journals (2005), reproduced by permission).

be enriched in spliced transcripts (She *et al.*, 2008) and show a higher sequence identity (Marques-Bonet & Eichler, 2009). It has been shown that segmental duplications, together with retrotransposons, account for the large-scale structural variations in primate genomes. Humans and other great apes share interspersed duplications, but a burst of segmental duplications also occurred in the common ancestor of humans and African great apes (Marques-Bonet *et al.*, 2009a).

As segmental duplications appeared quite recently, it is presumed that genes residing in these regions played a role in evolution. The *morpheus* gene family, for example, is found only in humans and African apes and is located in segmental duplications on chromosome 16 (Johnson *et al.*, 2001). These genes were repeatedly duplicated and positively selected for during primate evolution and, therefore, presumably played a role in speciation events. Amino acid replacements in putative protein-encoding exons of this gene family occurred after the separation of human/great-ape lineages from orangutan and after the divergence of human and chimpanzee lineages. This points to adaptive evolution of the *morpheus* gene family during the emergence of humans and African apes (Johnson *et al.*, 2001). It is becoming clear that lineage-specific gains and losses in gene copy number have emerged as an important aspect of primate genetic variation (Cheng *et al.*, 2005). An array-based comparative genomic hybridisation that surveyed gene duplication and losses across 10 primate species identified over 4,000 genes that show lineage-specific copy-number gains and losses (Dumas *et al.*, 2007). Those genes exhibiting lineage-specific copy number changes are likely involved in the phenotypic differences that distinguish these primate lineages. Interestingly, NBPF/DUF1220 sequences show human lineage-specific copy number increases (Dumas *et al.*, 2007), consistent with previous reports (Fortna *et al.*, 2004; Vandepoele *et al.*, 2005; Popesco *et al.*, 2006). Different experiments indicated that the number of NBPF/DUF1220 repeats was very large in humans, reduced in African great apes, further reduced in orangutan and Old World monkeys, single-copy in non-primate mammals, and absent in non-mammalian species (Popesco *et al.*, 2006). The dramatically elevated copy number in humans indicates the importance of the NBPF/DUF1220 repeat in human evolution. Moreover, comparison of the human chromosome 1 with that of chimpanzee revealed a remarkable human 3-mer higher order repeat (HOR) organisation based on an ~1.6-kbp primary repeat unit fully embedded within the *NBPF* genes (Figure 4A). This HOR pattern is not found in chimpanzee and shows some peculiarities, namely that the repeat unit is much longer than most primary repeat units identified so far and that the HOR is fully embedded within a gene. Additionally, the total absence of tandem repeats of NBPF HOR copies in chimpanzees while 47 tandem repeat HOR copies are present in human genomes reflects a human accelerated HOR pattern that distinguishes humans from nonhuman primates (Figure 4B) (Paar *et al.*, 2011).

It has been shown that genes with an important contribution to human evolution, like the *NBPF* gene family, are located in human segmental duplications, which are frequently organised around core duplicons (Jiang *et al.*, 2007). Comparison of chimpanzee and man shows that new lineage-specific segmental duplications map preferentially near shared ancestral duplications, a phenomenon called duplication shadowing (Cheng *et al.*, 2005). Unique genes mapping near these duplication blocks have a ten-fold higher probability of becoming duplicated than other randomly distributed regions. The NBPF/DUF1220 domains are among the few core duplicons that exist in the human genome and appear to be responsible for much of the duplicated sequences in the pericentromeric region of chromosome 1 (Jiang *et al.*, 2007). These large, high-identity duplication blocks are prone to rearrangements that lead to the formation of both harmless and pathogenic copy number variations, as discussed in the following section.

A/

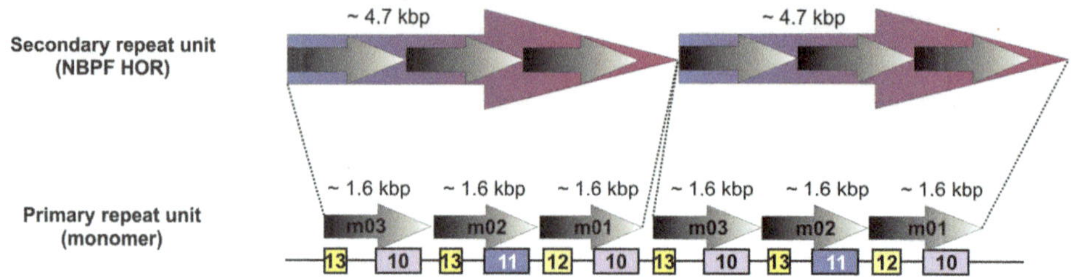

B/

Species	NBPF monomers	Number of NBPF HOR copies	Number of tandem NBPF HOR copies
Human	165	57	47
Chimpanzee	48	14	0
Orangutan	17	7	0
Rhesus macaque	7	2	0
Mouse	0	0	0

Fig. 4. Schematic illustration of the NBPF HOR copy.
A/ The NBPF HOR copy consists of three 1.6-kbp primary repeat units organised into ~4,770-bp secondary repeat units. The divergence between the three consensus monomers (m01, m02 and m03) is between 15 and 20%, whereas the average divergence between the 3-mer HOR copies is mostly below 0.5%, which is characteristic of a well-developed HOR pattern. Figure not drawn to scale. B/ The total number of NBPF monomers and the number of NBPF HOR copies (both tandemly organised and dispersed) gradually increases with evolutionary development, but the tandem repetition of the NBPF HOR copies is exclusive to humans (Modified after Paar *et al.*, 2011, Oxford Journals (2011), reproduced by permission).

3.3 The *NBPF* gene family shows frequent copy number variations that are sometimes associated with pathologies, including neuroblastoma

As previously discussed, primate segmental duplications are larger, more complex and more interspersed than those in other mammalian genomes. This pattern promotes genomic instability and leads to considerable copy number variation (Bailey & Eichler, 2006). A copy number variation (CNV) is a structurally variable region of DNA longer than 1 kbp present in the genomes of humans (Redon *et al.*, 2006), primates and many other species (Graubert *et al.*, 2007; Chen *et al.*, 2009). In these genomes, the DNA region is present in various copy numbers due to gains and losses of genomic DNA. Surprisingly, as much as 12% of the human genome is copy number variable, and despite efficient DNA repair, the rates of *de novo* CNVs are at least 100 to 10,000 fold greater than rates of point mutations (Lupski, 2007).

Nonallelic homologous recombination between low-copy repeats that flank unique genomic segments changes the organisation of the genome and is thought to be one of the main mechanisms that give rise to CNVs (Inoue & Lupski, 2002). Several studies indicate that the

NBPF gene family is polymorphic within the human population (Database of Genomic Variants). Analysis of the copy number differences between the genomes of 159 human individuals showed that the *NBPF* gene family is one of the most variable gene families in humans (Sudmant *et al.*, 2010). Sudmant *et al.* (2010) also showed that the *NBPF* gene duplicates are underrepresented in the human reference genome because no individual examined exhibited a copy number less than or equal to the copy number in the reference genome. Paralog-specific copy number genotyping distinguished two distinct classes of paralogs: one group is mostly copy-invariant in humans, and the other group is extensively copy number variable with some bias toward gain or loss. The *NBPF* gene family showed a paralog-specific copy number variation, and certain paralogs (*NBPF1*) were frequently amplified, extremely variable, and stratified by population, whereas other paralogs (*NBPF7*) were nearly fixed and diploid (Sudmant *et al.*, 2010). Taken together, these data clearly show that the *NBPF* gene family is polymorphic in the human population.

The functional implications of these structural variations in the human genome can be of great importance: not only are they an important source of genetic diversity between individuals, they can also affect an individual's susceptibility to disease. Several diseases, such as lupus with glomerulonephritis and Crohn's disease, have been linked to CNV of *FCGR3B* and *HBD-2*, respectively. It has been shown that a low copy number of *FCGR3B* (Fc fragment of IgG, low affinity IIIb, receptor) predisposes to glomerulonephritis, an immunologically mediated renal disease (Aitman *et al.*, 2006), whereas individuals with less than three copies of the human *beta-defensin 2* (*HBD-2*) gene have a significantly higher risk of developing Crohn's disease than individuals with four or more copies (Fellermann *et al.*, 2006). In neuroblastoma, an inherited copy number variation was shown to be associated with this childhood cancer. Indeed, Diskin *et al.* (2009) found that a common deletion polymorphism spanning less than 145 kbp at 1q21.1 is associated with neuroblastoma. Validation by quantitative PCR, fluorescent *in situ* hybridisation, and analysis of matched tumour specimens showed that this CNV is a heritable genetic variation. Interestingly, the 5'UTR of *NBPF17P* (*NBPF23*; see above) is located in this CNV. Quantitative PCR showed that this *NBPF* paralog is expressed in a variety of fetal and adult tissues, but the strongest expression was observed in fetal brain and fetal sympathetic nervous tissue. Importantly, these experiments showed that the expression level was strictly correlated with the CNV state in neuroblastoma cells (Diskin *et al.*, 2009). Recently, it has become clear that CNVs in the 1q21.1 region are associated not only with neuroblastoma, but also with an increasing number of other pathologies. Intriguingly, these copy number gains or losses either encompassed or flanked members of the *NBPF* gene family, emphasising the possible involvement of the *NBPF* gene family in human disease. CNVs at these genomic loci have been found in patients with mental retardation and congenital anomalies (Mefford *et al.*, 2008), autism (Sharp *et al.*, 2006; Szatmari *et al.*, 2007) and schizophrenia (Stefansson *et al.*, 2008). Autism and schizophrenia can be described as diametric conditions because reciprocal variants of the same genomic sequences, namely duplication and deletion, represent risk factors for these respective psychiatric conditions. Additionally, autism and schizophrenia are associated with developmentally enhanced and reduced brain growth, respectively (Crespi *et al.*, 2009). A study of 1q21.1 CNVs and brain size found that deletions of the 1q21 region are associated with microcephaly, which is characterised by an abnormally small head, whereas duplications of this region are associated with macrocephaly, which is characterised by an abnormally large head (Brunetti-Pierri *et al.*, 2008). Notably, the most striking trend in human evolution is the rapid increase in brain size over the past 3–4 million years, and the associated increase in complexity and cognitive capacity (Mekel-Bobrov *et al.*, 2007). Because NBPF/DUF1220 is present in remarkably more copies in the human genome than in other primates (Vandepoele *et al.*, 2005; Popesco *et al.*, 2006), it was hypothesised that the NBPF/DUF1220 copy number is correlated with brain size (Dumas & Sikela, 2009). Moreover, these data support the hypothesis that NBPF/DUF1220 domains are involved in the difference in brain size between autistic and schizophrenic populations and between macrocephalic and microcephalic populations. Therefore, NBPF/DUF1220 repeats could have played an important role in human evolution and in the associated increase in brain size. On the other hand, the selective advantage conferred by the increased number of NBPF/DUF1220 domains might have favored retention of the highly unstable 1q21.1 region, resulting in many recurrent rearrangements and leading to a spectrum of disorders of the human brain and to developmental defects (Dumas & Sikela, 2009).

4. *NBPF* promoter analysis

Gene duplication has generally been viewed as a primary mechanism for the origin of evolutionary novelties (Ohno, 1970). In most cases, duplication is not limited to the coding sequence but encompasses the regulatory region as well. Alternatively, new genes can acquire a regulatory region from a nonhomologous gene (Usakin *et al.*, 2005). We found evidence that the regulatory region of the *NBPF1* gene was obtained from an unrelated gene, called *EVI5* (ecotropic viral integration site 5) (Vandepoele *et al.*, 2009). *EVI5* was originally identified through its involvement in a constitutional chromosome translocation in a patient with stage 4S neuroblastoma (Roberts *et al.*, 1998). EVI5 is a centrosomal protein during interphase, but it relocalises to the midbody during late phases of mitosis. Its disruption leads to incomplete cell division and formation of multinucleate cells (Faitar *et al.*, 2005). EVI5 also exists in a protein complex with GTP-bound Rab11 and functions as a GTPase-activating protein for this small GTPase (Dabbeekeh *et al.*, 2007). Additionally, EVI5 is critical during interphase for the regulation of cyclin accumulation. It functions by stabilising the anaphase-promoting complex inhibitor, Emi1. RNA interference with EVI5 levels resulted in cell-cycle arrest and abnormal centrosome numbers *in vivo*, suggesting that EVI5 might not only regulate cyclin accumulation during interphase but also contribute to timing mechanisms to ensure mitotic fidelity (Eldridge *et al.*, 2006).

The human *EVI5*, located on chromosome 1p22, is transcribed as two isoforms differing in their transcription initiation sites and first exons. Intriguingly, the promoter of *NBPF1* shows homology only to the promoter used to control the expression of human isoform 2 of *EVI5* (called $EVI5_{NBPF}$), but not the promoter of isoform 1 (called $EVI5_{ALT}$) (Figure 5) (Vandepoele *et al.*, 2009).

The extensive sequence homology in the promoter regions of different *NBPF* paralogs shows that the recruitment of the promoter from $EVI5_{NBPF}$ occurred before expansion of the *NBPF* gene family. Phylogenetic analysis of the NBPF and $EVI5_{NBPF}$ core promoter sequences showed that promoter duplication occurred after the split between simians and prosimians, but before divergence between Old World and New World monkeys, and that positive selection played a role in the evolution of the *NBPF1* promoter in simians (Vandepoele *et al.*, 2009).

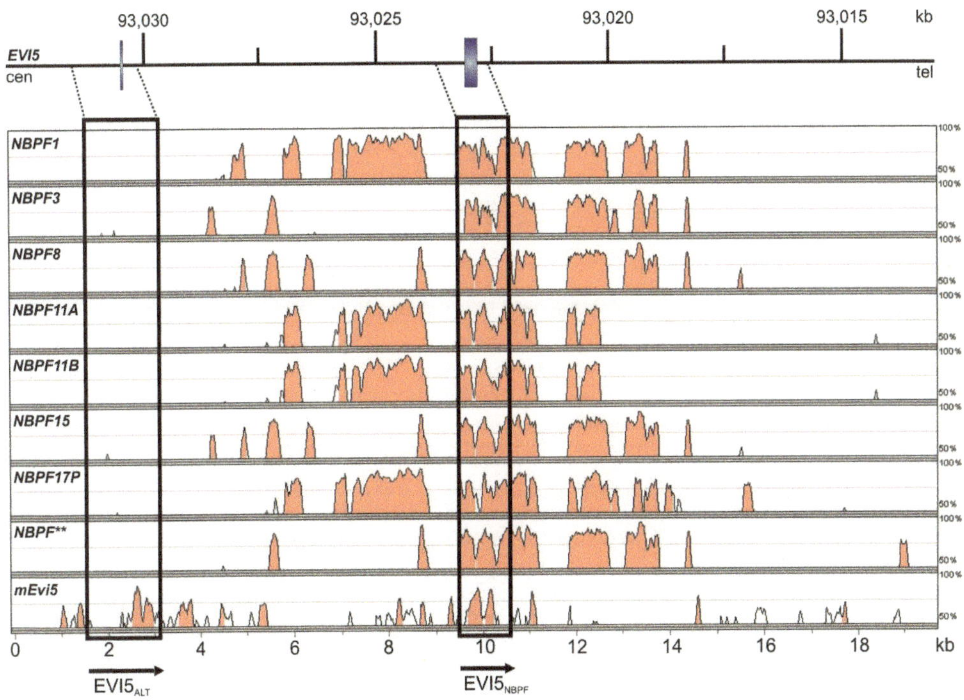

Fig. 5. Sequence homology between the promoter regions of different *NBPF* paralogs and the promoter regions of *EVI5*. Expression of the human EVI5 gene is controlled by two promoters: $EVI5_{ALT}$ controls the expression of isoform 1 and $EVI5_{NBPF}$ controls the expression of isoform 2. Arrows indicate the positions of these transcription initiation sites on the reverse strand of chromosome 1, and their first exons are represented by blue boxes on the top line. A region of 20 kbp flanking the transcription initiation site of human and mouse $EVI5_{NBPF}$ and different *NBPF* paralogs was aligned by the AVID algorithm in the Vista Genome browser. The promoter of *NBPF1* and its paralogs shows homology only with the promoter of human EVI5 that is used to control the expression of isoform 2 ($EVI5_{NBPF}$) but not the one for isoform 1 ($EVI5_{ALT}$). The homology between the human and mouse EVI5 sequences is confined mainly to the two regions corresponding to the putative promoter regions. No official gene symbol is available for NBPF** (Adapted from Vandepoele et al., 2009, Oxford Journals (2009), reproduced by permission).

The expression patterns of *NBPF* and *EVI5* in a panel of human cell lines are very similar, and the expression of both genes was decreased in neuroblastoma cell lines in which there is 1p36 loss of heterozygosity. Nevertheless, the mechanism of this decreased expression level was due to use of a different transcriptional and posttranscriptional regulation. Whereas *EVI5* was epigenetically silenced, treatment of the neuroblastoma cell lines with puromycin, an inhibitor of nonsense-mediated decay, indicated that mutation of the *NBPF* transcripts was probably responsible for decreasing the expression levels. These data together show that despite the almost identical promoter sequences and very similar expression patterns, regulation of *NBPF* and *EVI5* genes in neuroblastoma cell lines can occur by different mechanisms (Vandepoele *et al.*, 2009).

5. NBPF-interacting proteins

Many genes perform their functions by interaction of their encoded proteins with other proteins. The search for NBPF-interacting proteins revealed two hits so far: chibby and clusterin, which together can form a tri-molecular complex with NBPF1 (Vandepoele *et al.*, 2010). Interestingly, both NBPF1 and clusterin are candidate tumour suppressors for neuroblastoma (Vandepoele *et al.*, 2008; Chayka *et al.*, 2009). This suggests that the interactions between these three proteins are functionally important.

5.1 Chibby

Chibby (Cby) is a 15-kDa protein that has been strongly conserved throughout evolution from fly to human. It was originally identified as an inhibitor of the canonical Wnt-β-catenin pathway (Takemaru *et al.*, 2003). Cby interacts with the C-terminal activation domain of β-catenin and blocks its transcriptional activation potential by two mechanisms. First, it competes with T cell factor/lymphoid-enhancer factor (TCF/LEF) transcription factors for binding with β-catenin (Takemaru *et al.*, 2003). Second, in cooperation with 14-3-3 adaptor proteins, it facilitates nuclear export of β-catenin (Li *et al.*, 2008). Inhibition of the Wnt-β-catenin pathway is necessary for cardiomyocyte differentiation, proliferation and repair, and Cby has been implicated in facilitating cardiomyocyte differentiation (Singh *et al.*, 2007). Additionally, several molecules of the Wnt-β-catenin pathway play important roles in the inhibition of adipogenesis, and different findings indicate that Cby is required for adipocyte differentiation (Li *et al.*, 2007). Cby also plays a role in other processes. Reports on the binding of Cby to polycystin-2 (Hidaka *et al.*, 2004) and on the Cby knockout mouse (Voronina *et al.*, 2009; Love *et al.*, 2010) implicate Cby in the development of motile airway cilia. Germline inactivation of *Cby* resulted in complete absence of mucociliary transport due to scarcity of motile cilia in the nasal epithelium (Voronina *et al.*, 2009). In a follow-up study, characterisation of the lung morphology of Cby knockout mice showed that $Cby^{-/-}$ lungs were normal at birth, but alveolar airspace became enlarged, proliferation became reduced, and lung epithelial cells differentiated abnormally, which together affected pulmonary function (Love *et al.*, 2010). Both the lungs and nasal epithelia of Cby knockout mice showed increased expression of two direct β-catenin target genes, namely *Axin2* and *CyclinD1*, but it is not clear whether the ciliary phenotypes are related to the modest elevation of these Wnt related genes, since no change in the localisation of certain components of the Wnt-β-catenin pathway was observed. Presence of endogenous Cby at the base of cilia and the phenotypes related to the loss of Cby show that Cby is important in ciliogenesis (Voronina *et al.*, 2009; Love *et al.*, 2010).

Neuroblastoma is a disease of the sympathoadrenal lineage of the neural crest, and these tumours can develop anywhere in the sympathetic nervous system. At least three key pathways regulate the formation, migration and differentiation of the neural crest cells: the bone morphogenetic protein (BMP) pathway (Barembaum & Bronner-Fraser, 2005), the fibroblast growth factor pathway (Sauka-Spengler & Bronner-Fraser, 2008) and the Wnt signalling pathway (Crane & Trainor, 2006). Wnt signalling plays an important role in neural crest cells. For example, mouse embryos in which Wnt1 and Wnt3 were knocked out displayed severe loss of neural crest cells (Varga & Wrana, 2005). In addition, conditioned medium of cells overexpressing wingless (*Drosophila* homolog of Wnt1) could induce avian neural crest cells (Garcia-Castro *et al.*, 2002). Aberrant regulation of the embryonic developmental Wnt pathway has been implicated in many solid childhood tumours (reviewed in Koesters & Doeberitz, 2003), but a clear role for Wnt signalling in neuroblastoma has remained elusive. Nevertheless, there is mounting evidence that the Wnt pathway is involved in neuroblastoma (Table 1).

The MSX1 homeobox transcription factor functions as an intermediate between the BMP and Wnt signalling pathways to ensure proper differentiation of the neural crest cells. Elevated expression of BMP in non-neuronal ectoderm switches on the neural crest differentiation program and induces the expression of MSX1, which leads to induction of the expression of BMP and Wnt in neural crest cells (Ramos & Robert, 2005). Msx genes might regulate *Wnt1* expression at the dorsal midline of the neural tube (Bach *et al.*, 2003). Additionally, MSX1 overexpression in the *MYCN*-amplified neuroblastoma cell line SJNB8 induced the expression of four Wnt inhibitor genes: Dickkopf 1 (DKK1), Dickkopf 2 (DKK2) and Dickkopf 3 (DKK3) and secreted frizzled-related protein 1 (SFRP-1) (Revet *et al.*, 2010). Analysis of the expression profiles of MSX1, DKK1, -2, -3 and SFRP-1 in a series of neuroblastic tumours showed a significant and positive correlation between MSX1 and DKK2 expression and between MSX1 and DKK3 expression. Additionally, stronger DKK2 and DKK3 expression correlated with a significantly better prognosis. Expression profiling of neuroblastic tumours and cell lines for the different Wnt family genes showed that both the canonical Wnt3a and the non-canonical Wnt5 were strongly expressed and that they could activate upstream Wnt signalling in neuroblastoma cells by phosphorylating the dishevelled co-receptor DVL3 (Revet *et al.*, 2010). The importance of DKK3 in neuroblastoma was already shown in previous reports, in which DKK3 was implicated as a marker for neuroblastic tumour maturation and was shown to be down-regulated by *MYCN* (Bell *et al.*, 2007; Koppen *et al.*, 2008).

Additionally, β-catenin has been shown to be strongly expressed and aberrantly localised in the nucleus in high-risk neuroblastoma cells without *MYCN* amplification (Liu *et al.*, 2008). Expression profiling of primary neuroblastoma tumours demonstrated increased expression of *WNT* ligands (*WNT1, WNT6, WNT7A, WNT10B*), *DVL1* and *TCF7* in high-risk neuroblastoma tumours without *MYCN* amplification. Also several β-catenin target genes,

Gene	Function	Neuroblastoma
DKK1	interacts with co-receptor LRP	induced upon overexpression of Msx1 in NB cell line
DKK2	interacts with co-receptor LRP	
DKK3	interacts with co-receptor LRP	induced upon overexpression of Msx1 in NB cell line and downregulated by *MYCN*
SFRP1	secreted antagonist	induced upon overexpression of Msx1 in NB cell line
Wnt3a	ligand	strongly expressed in neuroblastic tumors and cell lines
Wnt5	ligand	
B-catenin	key mediator	localised in the nucleus in NB cells without MNA
Wnt1	ligand	increased expression in primary NB tumors without MNA
Wnt6	ligand	increased expression in primary NB tumors without MNA
Wnt7A	ligand	
Wnt10B	ligand	
DVL1	co-receptor	
TCF7	transcription factor	
Myc	target gene	
CD44	target gene	
FZD1	seven-transmembrane receptor	increased expression in chemoresistant NB cell lines and in relapsed patients
MDR1	target gene	

Table 1. Wnt signalling is important in neuroblastoma tumourigenesis and chemoresistance.Schematic representation of different Wnt signalling components implicated in neuroblastoma. NB: neuroblastoma; MNA: *MYCN* amplification. See text for references.

e.g. *MYC* and *CD44*, were found to be coordinately upregulated in high-risk neuroblastomas without *MYCN* amplification in comparison to high-risk *MYCN*-amplified or intermediate-risk neuroblastomas (Liu *et al.*, 2008).

Another study implicated the Wnt-β-catenin pathway in neuroblastoma chemoresistance (Flahaut *et al.*, 2009). Gene expression profiling of two doxorubicin-resistant neuroblastoma cell lines identified the frizzled1 Wnt receptor (*FZD1*) gene as the most strongly overexpressed transcript in both cell lines in comparison with their sensitive parental cell lines. FZD1 silencing resulted in significant restoration of drug sensitivity and induced a parallel strong decrease in the expression of MDR1 (Flahaut *et al.*, 2009), another β-catenin target gene frequently associated with the resistance of neuroblastoma tumours to chemotherapeutic drugs (Haber *et al.*, 1997). Moreover, FZD1 and/or MDR1 expression was significantly enhanced in the group of relapsed patients after chemotherapy, whereas no significant increase in expression was measured in the group of non-relapsed patients (Flahaut *et al.*, 2009).

These data indicate that Wnt signalling is important in neuroblastoma tumourigenesis and chemoresistance (overview in Table 1). Therefore, we hypothesise that important players in the Wnt-β-catenin pathway might play important roles in neuroblastoma. But nothing is known yet about the role of Cby in neuroblastoma tumourigenesis or chemoresistance, and further investigation is needed.

5.2 Clusterin

Clusterin (CLU), also known as apolipoprotein J, is a heterodimeric sulfated glycoprotein that is expressed in most human tissues and body fluids and is associated with many biological activities, including regulation of apoptosis and cancer (Trougakos & Gonos, 2002). Research on *CLU* function and its relation to tumourigenesis has been intensive, but many contradictory data have been reported. These contradictions can be explained mainly by the existence of three protein isoforms with different sub-cellular localisations and biological functions (Rizzi & Bettuzzi, 2010).

The most extensively studied form of CLU is the secreted form (sCLU), which is a glycosylated heterodimer present in almost all physiological fluids. sCLU is exported from the cell and released in secretions, in which it acts as an extracellular chaperone (Humphreys *et al.*, 1999). Cytoplasmic clusterin has been shown to inhibit apoptosis by interfering with Bax activation in the mitochondria (Zhang *et al.*, 2005). Clusterin binds and stabilises the Ku70-Bax protein complex and serves as a cytosolic retention factor for Bax. Depletion of clusterin disrupts the Ku70-Bax complex and triggers Bax activation and its relocalisation to the mitochondria (Trougakos *et al.*, 2009). Cytoplasmic clusterin also promotes tumour cell survival by cooperating with c-Myc during transformation (Zhang *et al.*, 2005). Additionally, a large amount of CLU confers resistance to cytotoxic agents on different cancer cell types (Lourda *et al.*, 2006). However, a nuclear form of clusterin originating from an alternative translation start site has been shown to be proapoptotic in prostate cancer cells (Moretti *et al.*, 2007), breast cancer cells (Leskov *et al.*, 2003) and neuroblastoma (Yang *et al.*, 2000).

The main question is whether clusterin is a positive or negative modulator of mammalian tumourigenesis. It is becoming clear that *CLU* can act either as a tumour suppressor (Caporali *et al.*, 2004; Chayka *et al.*, 2009) or as a tumour promoter (Lourda *et al.*, 2006), but the time-course of the disease and the selection pressures imposed on the cancer by chemotherapy or other treatments have to be taken into account.

Clusterin knockout mice are more prone to autoimmune myocarditis (McLaughlin *et al.*, 2000) and to transformation of the prostate epithelium (Bettuzzi *et al.*, 2009). In homozygous knockout mice, the normal portion of prostate tissue is characterised by stronger expression of the proliferation marker Ki67 and shows activated NF-κB signalling, but this was not observed in wild type mice (Bettuzzi *et al.*, 2009). Additionally, in TRAMP mice, a transgenic animal model of prostate cancer (Greenberg *et al.*, 1995), the *CLU* gene is dramatically downregulated during onset and progression of prostate cancer (Caporali *et al.*, 2004). Crossing of these TRAMP mice with the clusterin knockout mice led to development of a more advanced invasive disease in the progeny, confirming the role of *CLU* as a negative tumour modulator in prostate cancer (Bettuzzi *et al.*, 2009).

On the contrary, overexpression of clusterin in LNCaP prostate cancer cells conferred resistance to both androgen ablation *in vivo* and cytotoxic chemotherapy (Miyake *et al.*, 2000c). Additionally, the administration of clusterin antisense oligonucleotides in prostate cancer xenograft models delayed progression to androgen independence and enhanced chemosensitivity (Miyake *et al.*, 2000b). A human clusterin antisense oligonucleotide (OGX-011) synergistically enhanced the cytotoxic effects of paclitaxel in human xenografts of prostate cancer (Miyake *et al.*, 2000a). This antisense oligonucleotide is currently undergoing clinical trials for tumour therapy. The phase I trial demonstrated that OGX-011 is well tolerated and that it inhibits clusterin expression in prostate cancer (Chi *et al.*, 2005). The phase II trial assessed the effects of combined therapy with androgen ablation and OGX-011 given prior to radical prostatectomy in patients with metastatic castration-resistant prostate cancer. This study showed that the combined therapy was associated with improved survival (Chi *et al.*, 2010).

The biological role of clusterin is controversial in both prostate cancer and neuroblastoma. Indeed, also in neuroblastoma it has been shown that clusterin can function both as a tumour suppressor gene and as an oncogene. Overexpression of clusterin impaired the invasion of neuroblastoma cell lines by inhibiting the NF-κB activity by stabilising IκBs, the inhibitors of NF-κB signalling (Santilli *et al.*, 2003). Additionally, Oncomine expression analysis (Rhodes *et al.*, 2007) showed a lower expression level of the *CLU* gene in primary human neuroblastomas with *MYCN* amplification, and further investigation demonstrated that MYCN acts as a negative regulator of clusterin expression by inducing transcription of the 17-5p~92 microRNA cluster (Chayka *et al.*, 2009). This polycistronic cluster encodes six microRNAs (miR-17-5p, -18a, -19a, -19b, -20a and -92) and is homologous to the miRNA 106a~92 cluster (Mestdagh *et al.*, 2010b). Most miRNAs encoded by this cluster are expressed at higher levels in neuroblastoma cell lines overexpressing *MYCN* or carrying *MYCN* amplification. MYCN transcriptionally induces the expression of the miRNA 17-5p~92 cluster by directly binding to its promoter. The therapeutic potential of this miRNA cluster was demonstrated by injecting a miR-17-5p-specific antagomir into nude mice that had been injected with a neuroblastoma cell line with *MYCN* amplification. Tumour growth *in vivo* was reduced substantially, and this reduction was associated with down-modulation of miR-17-5p activity and with a reciprocal increase of both p21 and BIM protein levels. Nevertheless, the expression pattern of miR-17-5p in primary tumours is complex, because high levels of miR-17-5p expression were detected in both *MYCN*-amplified and non *MYCN*-amplified tumours (Fontana *et al.*, 2008). Additionally, it has been demonstrated that miR-17-5p~92 dampens TGF-β signalling by acting both upstream and downstream of pSMAD2/SMAD4 (Mestdagh *et al.*, 2010a). This finding further underscores its ability to regulate multiple components of the same pathway.

When *MYCN*-transgenic mice were crossed with clusterin knockout mice, the progeny showed reduced tumour-free survival, active NF-κB signalling, and epithelial to mesenchymal transition (Chayka *et al.*, 2009); this resembles the phenotype of TRAMP mice in which CLU was homozygously deleted (Bettuzzi *et al.*, 2009). These data indicate that clusterin functions as a TSG for neuroblastoma, even though several reports indicate that it can promote neuroblastoma. Treatment with histone deacetylase inhibitors (HDACIs) resulted in upregulation of clusterin in different cancer cell lines, including neuroblastoma (Liu *et al.*, 2009; Subramanian *et al.*, 2011). Suppression of clusterin in combination with high-dose HDACIs synergistically enhanced HDACI-induced cell death through cytochome-c-mediated apoptosis in HDACI-resistant cancer cells. Additionally, combining OGX-011 with low-dose HDACIs enhanced HDACI-induced growth arrest in both HDACI-sensitive and -resistant cancer cell lines. Moreover, in mice xenografted with neuroblastoma cells, combining OGX-011 and valproate (the only HDACI proven to be safe in young children) synergistically inhibited tumour growth *in vivo*, whereas neither OGX-011 nor valproate alone had an effect on tumour progression (Liu *et al.*, 2009).

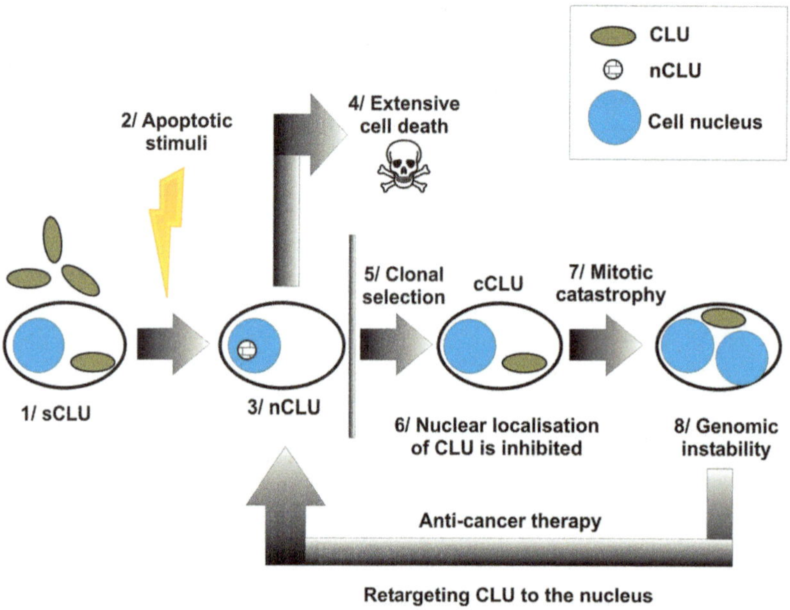

Fig. 6. Proposed model for CLU in tumourigenesis.
In normal cells and under physiological conditions the basal expression level of *CLU* in benign cells is low and confined to the secreted form of CLU (sCLU) (1). Several apoptotic stimuli (2) lead to the production of nuclear CLU (nCLU) (3), which in turn induces extensive cell death (4). In the early phases of tumourigenesis, genetic lesions lead to acquisition of survival advantages and consequent clonal selection (5). A key step in the transformation process is prevention of CLU from entering the nucleus. Cells with high levels of cytoplasmic CLU are then selected for, which results in acquisition of a death-resistant phenotype (6). This phenotype is associated with impaired mitosis (7), which leads eventually to genomic instability (8) (Modified after Rizzi & Bettuzzi, 2010, Society for Endocrinology (2010), reproduced by permission).

Based on these findings, which were observed in both prostate cancer and neuroblastoma, a role for clusterin in tumourigenesis has been proposed (Figure 6). This model proposes that clusterin acts as a tumour suppressor in the early stages of cancer but can become a tumour promoter in the more malignant and advanced stages, namely when tumours become resistant to therapy (Rizzi & Bettuzzi, 2010). Under physiological conditions, the basal expression level of *CLU* in benign cells is low and confined to the secreted form of CLU (sCLU). Several apoptotic stimuli lead to the production of nuclear CLU (nCLU), which in turn induces extensive cell death. At the onset of cancer, early genetic lesions disrupt or inactivate apoptotic pathways or lead to the activation of other survival pathways. Under these conditions of clonal selection, a key step in the transformation process would be the prevention of CLU from entering the nucleus in order to prevent induction of apoptosis. At this point, cancer cells are characterised by strong expression of cytoplasmic CLU (cCLU) and are therefore resistant to death by cytotoxic therapeutic agents. This resistant phenotype can promote cell transformation that leads to late cancer stages associated with impaired mitosis, which causes further genomic instability (Rizzi & Bettuzzi, 2010).

5.3 NBPF1, Chibby and clusterin can form a tri-molecular complex

A yeast two-hybrid screening with an N-terminal fragment of the NBPF11 protein identified Cby as a binding partner of NBPF11 (Vandepoele *et al.*, 2010). This interaction is not exclusive to NBPF11 but is common to other NBPF members. For instance, Cby can also interact with NBPF1. The interaction was confirmed by other techniques, such as co-immunoprecipitation and mitochondrial recruitment (Vandepoele *et al.*, 2010). It was shown that the coiled-coil region in the N-terminal domain of NBPF interacts with the coiled-coil region in the C-terminal domain of Cby. This C-terminal portion of Cby harbours not only the binding site for NBPF, but also the binding site for most other known interaction partners of Cby, such as β-catenin (Takemaru *et al.*, 2003), polycystin-2 (Hidaka *et al.*, 2004) and TC1 (Jung *et al.*, 2006).

Functional analysis of the interaction showed that NBPF did not influence Cby-mediated Wnt signalling, nor did it compete with β-catenin binding to Cby. This indicates the presence of two different pools of Cby, one binding to β-catenin and the other binding to NBPF, or alternatively, a dimeric Cby complex that can bind simultaneously to β-catenin and NBPF. Besides its repressor function in the Wnt pathway, Cby can also play an important role in ciliogenesis, as shown in the Cby knockout mouse (see section 5.1). The role of NBPF in the formation of cilia remains uncertain, as NBPF1 overexpression did not interfere with the formation of primary cilia (Vandepoele *et al.*, 2010). An additional yeast two-hybrid screen identified clusterin as a new binding partner for Cby and showed that the C-terminus of CLU, which contains a coiled-coil domain, interacts with both the N-terminal and C-terminal domains of Cby. Additionally, co-immunoprecipitation experiments in HEK293T cells demonstrated that NBPF1, Cby and clusterin can form a tri-molecular complex (Figure 7), because all three proteins were co-purified in every setting.

Since intracellular CLU can be found both in the nucleus and in the cytoplasm (see section 5.2), the effect of Cby or NBPF or their combination on the subcellular localisation of CLU was further investigated, but no difference was observed (Vandepoele *et al.*, 2010).

The identification of two proteins that interact with NBPF is a clue to the functions of NBPF, but further investigation is needed. Anyway, the identification within the complex of two proteins (NBPF1 and CLU) as candidate tumour suppressor genes linked to neuroblastoma (Vandepoele *et al.*, 2008; Chayka *et al.*, 2009) is intriguing and warrants further scrutiny.

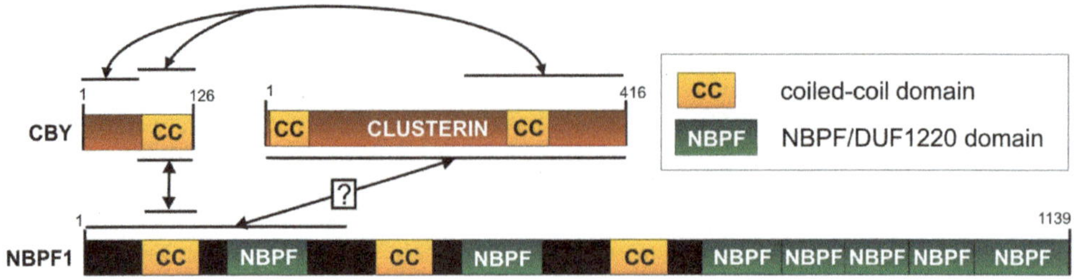

Fig. 7. NBPF1, Cby and CLU form a tri-molecular complex.

An overview of the mutual interactions between NBPF1, Cby and CLU. The coiled-coil region in the N-terminus of NBPF1 interacts with the coiled-coil region in the cytoplasmic domain of Cby. The C-terminus of CLU interacts with the full-length Cby protein, as interactions with both the N-terminus and C-terminus are observed. It is uncertain whether CLU and NBPF1 interact directly (boxed question mark) (Modified after Vandepoele *et al.*, 2010, Elsevier (2010), reproduced by permission).

6. Conclusion

In this chapter we summarise the growing evidence for the recent emergence of the *NBPF* gene family and for its role in human evolution. The NBPF/DUF1220 domains in particular seem to have been important in this context. This evidence is based on the large increase in copy number of the NBPF/DUF1220 domain in humans. On the other hand, *NBPF* genes seem to be involved in cancer and in brain and developmental disorders due to their location in unstable high-identity duplication blocks, which leads to recurrent chromosomal rearrangements. One case of particular interest is neuroblastoma. Evidence for the involvement of *NBPF* genes in this type of cancer comes not only from disruption of *NBPF1* in a neuroblastoma patient, but also from gene expression studies and the association with neuroblastoma of a copy number variation of an *NBPF* paralog. Additionally, the regulatory elements and the identification of NBPF-interacting proteins indicate that the *NBPF* gene family plays a role in neuroblastoma. Involvement of *NBPF* genes in neuroblastoma and possibly as well in other cancers points to the value of studying this gene family further. Every step in the functional understanding of these genes could bring us closer to unravelling the molecular mechanisms underlying neuroblastoma development and could help us to develop more effective therapy. Such studies could also shed light on the impact these novel genes had on recent primate evolution.

7. Acknowledgments

We thank Dr. Amin Bredan for critically editing the manuscript.
Research supported by the Fund for Scientific Research, Flanders (FWO), the Foundation against Cancer, Belgium, and the Queen Elisabeth Medical Foundation (G.S.K.E.), Belgium.

8. References

Aitman, T.J., Dong, R., Vyse, T.J., Norsworthy, P.J., Johnson, M.D., Smith, J., Mangion, J., Roberton-Lowe, C., Marshall, A.J., Petretto, E., Hodges, M.D., Bhangal, G., Patel, S.G., Sheehan-Rooney, K., Duda, M., Cook, P.R., Evans, D.J., Domin, J., Flint, J.,

Boyle, J.J., Pusey, C.D. & Cook, H.T. (2006). Copy number polymorphism in Fcgr3 predisposes to glomerulonephritis in rats and humans. *Nature*, 439: 851-855.

Bach, A., Lallemand, Y., Nicola, M.A., Ramos, C., Mathis, L., Maufras, M. & Robert, B. (2003) Msx1 is required for dorsal diencephalon patterning. *Development*, 130: 4025-4036.

Bailey, J.A. & Eichler, E.E. (2006). Primate segmental duplications: crucibles of evolution, diversity and disease. *Nature Reviews Genetics*, 7: 552-564.

Barembaum, M. & Bronner-Fraser, M. (2005). Early steps in neural crest specification. *Seminars in Cell & Developmental Biology*, 16: 642-646.

Bell, E., Lunec, J. & Tweddle, D.A. (2007). Cell cycle regulation targets of MYCN identified by gene expression microarrays. *Cell Cycle*, 6: 1249-1256.

Bettuzzi, S., Davalli, P., Davoli, S., Chayka, O., Rizzi, F., Belloni, L., Pellacani, D., Fregni, G., Astancolle, S., Fassan, M., Corti, A., Baffa, R. & Sala, A. (2009). Genetic inactivation of ApoJ/clusterin: effects on prostate tumourigenesis and metastatic spread. *Oncogene*, 28: 4344-4352.

Bond, J. & Woods, C.G. (2006). Cytoskeletal genes regulating brain size. *Current Opinion in Cell Biology*, 18: 95-101.

Brunetti-Pierri, N., Berg, J.S., Scaglia, F., Belmont, J., Bacino, C.A., Sahoo, T., Lalani, S.R., Graham, B., Lee, B., Shinawi, M., Shen, J., Kang, S.H., Pursley, A., Lotze, T., Kennedy, G., Lansky-Shafer, S., Weaver, C., Roeder, E.R., Grebe, T.A., Arnold, G.L., Hutchison, T., Reimschisel, T., Amato, S., Geragthy, M.T., Innis, J.W., Obersztyn, E., Nowakowska, B., Rosengren, S.S., Bader, P.I., Grange, D.K., Naqvi, S., Garnica, A.D., Bernes, S.M., Fong, C.T., Summers, A., Walters, W.D., Lupski, J.R., Stankiewicz, P., Cheung, S.W. & Patel, A. (2008). Recurrent reciprocal 1q21.1 deletions and duplications associated with microcephaly or macrocephaly and developmental and behavioral abnormalities. *Nature Genetics*, 40: 1466-1471.

Caporali, A., Davalli, P., Astancolle, S., D'Arca, D., Brausi, M., Bettuzzi, S. & Corti, A. (2004). The chemopreventive action of catechins in the TRAMP mouse model of prostate carcinogenesis is accompanied by clusterin over-expression. *Carcinogenesis*, 25: 2217-2224.

Chayka, O., Corvetta, D., Dews, M., Caccamo, A.E., Piotrowska, I., Santilli, G., Gibson, S., Sebire, N.J., Himoudi, N., Hogarty, M.D., Anderson, J., Bettuzzi, S., Thomas-Tikhonenko, A. & Sala, A. (2009). Clusterin, a haploinsufficient tumour suppressor gene in neuroblastomas. *Journal of the National Cancer Institute*, 101: 663-677.

Chen, W.K., Swartz, J.D., Rush, L.J. & Alvarez, C.E. (2009). Mapping DNA structural variation in dogs. *Genome Research*, 19: 500-509.

Cheng, Z., Ventura, M., She, X., Khaitovich, P., Graves, T., Osoegawa, K., Church, D., DeJong, P., Wilson, R.K., Paabo, S., Rocchi, M. & Eichler, E.E. (2005). A genome-wide comparison of recent chimpanzee and human segmental duplications. *Nature*, 437: 88-93.

Chi, K.N., Eisenhauer, E., Fazli, L., Jones, E.C., Goldenberg, S.L., Powers, J., Tu, D. & Gleave, M.E. (2005). A phase I pharmacokinetic and pharmacodynamic study of OGX-011, a 2'-methoxyethyl antisense oligonucleotide to clusterin, in patients with localised prostate cancer. *Journal of the National Cancer Institute*, 97: 1287-1296.

Chi, K.N., Hotte, S.J., Yu, E.Y., Tu, D., Eigl, B.J., Tannock, I., Saad, F., North, S., Powers, J., Gleave, M.E. & Eisenhauer, E.A. (2010). Randomized phase II study of docetaxel and prednisone with or without OGX-011 in patients with metastatic castration-resistant prostate cancer. *Journal of Clinical Oncology*, 28: 4247-4254.

Crane, J.F. & Trainor, P.A. (2006). Neural crest stem and progenitor cells. *Annual Review of Cell and Developmental Biology*, 22: 267-286.

Crespi, B., Stead, P. & Elliot, M. (2009). Evolution in health and medicine Sackler colloquium: Comparative genomics of autism and schizophrenia. *Proceedings of the National Academy of Sciences of the United States of America*, 107: 1736-1741.

Dabbeekeh, J.T., Faitar, S.L., Dufresne, C.P. & Cowell, J.K. (2007). The EVI5 TBC domain provides the GTPase-activating protein motif for RAB11. *Oncogene*, 26: 2804-2808.

Database of genomic variants. A curated catalogue of structural variation in the human genome. http://projects.tcag.ca/variation/

Diskin, S.J., Hou, C.P., Glessner, J.T., Attiyeh, E.F., Laudenslager, M., Bosse, K., Cole, K., Mosse, Y.P., Wood, A., Lynch, J.E., Pecor, K., Diamond, M., Winter, C., Wang, K., Kim, C., Geiger, E.A., McGrady, P.W., Blakemore, A.I.F., London, W.B., Shaikh, T.H., Bradfield, J., Grant, S.F.A., Li, H.Z., Devoto, M., Rappaport, E.R., Hakonarson, H. & Maris, J.M. (2009). Copy number variation at 1q21.1 associated with neuroblastoma. *Nature*, 459: 987-U112.

Dumas, L. & Sikela, J.M. (2009). DUF1220 domains, cognitive disease, and human brain evolution. *Cold Spring Harbor Symposia on Quantitative Biology*, 74: 375-382.

Dumas, L., Kim, Y.H., Karimpour-Fard, A., Cox, M., Hopkins, J., Pollack, J.R. & Sikela, J.M. (2007). Gene copy number variation spanning 60 million years of human and primate evolution. *Genome Research*, 17: 1266-1277.

Eldridge, A.G., Loktev, A.V., Hansen, D.V., Verschuren, E.W., Reimann, J.D. & Jackson, P.K. (2006). The evi5 oncogene regulates cyclin accumulation by stabilizing the anaphase-promoting complex inhibitor emi1. *Cell*, 124: 367-380.

Faitar, S.L., Dabbeekeh, J.T.S., Ranalli, T.A. & Cowell, J.K. (2005). EVI5 is a novel centrosomal protein that binds to alpha- and gamma-tubulin. *Genomics*, 86: 594-605.

Fellermann, K., Stange, D.E., Schaeffeler, E., Schmalzl, H., Wehkamp, J., Bevins, C.L., Reinisch, W., Teml, A., Schwab, M., Lichter, P., Radlwimmer, B. & Stange, E.F. (2006). A chromosome 8 gene-cluster polymorphism with low human beta-defensin 2 gene copy number predisposes to Crohn disease of the colon. *The American Journal of Human Genetics*, 79: 439-448.

Flahaut, M., Meier, R., Coulon, A., Nardou, K.A., Niggli, F.K., Martinet, D., Beckmann, J.S., Joseph, J.M., Muhlethaler-Mottet, A. & Gross, N. (2009). The Wnt receptor FZD1 mediates chemoresistance in neuroblastoma through activation of the Wnt/beta-catenin pathway. *Oncogene*, 28: 2245-2256.

Fontana, L., Fiori, M.E., Albini, S., Cifaldi, L., Giovinazzi, S., Forloni, M., Boldrini, R., Donfrancesco, A., Federici, V., Giacomini, P., Peschle, C. & Fruci, D. (2008). Antagomir-17-5p abolishes the growth of therapy-resistant neuroblastoma through p21 and BIM. *PLoS One*, 3: 2236.

Fortna, A., Kim, Y., MacLaren, E., Marshall, K., Hahn, G., Meltesen, L., Brenton, M., Hink, R., Burgers, S., Hernandez-Boussard, T., Karimpour-Fard, A., Glueck, D.,

McGavran, L., Berry, R., Pollack, J. & Sikela, J.M. (2004). Lineage-specific gene duplication and loss in human and great ape evolution. *PLoS Biology*, 2: 207.

Fransson, S., Martinsson, T. & Ejeskar, K. (2007). Neuroblastoma tumours with favorable and unfavorable outcomes: Significant differences in mRNA expression of genes mapped at Ip36.2. *Genes, Chromosomes and Cancer*, 46: 45-52.

Garcia-Anoveros, J., Derfler, B., Neville-Golden, J., Hyman, B.T. & Corey, D.P. (1997). BNaC1 and BNaC2 constitute a new family of human neuronal sodium channels related to degenerins and epithelial sodium channels. *Proceedings of the National Academy of Sciences of the United States of America*, 94: 1459-1464.

Garcia-Castro, M.I., Marcelle, C. & Bronner-Fraser, M. (2002). Ectodermal Wnt function as a neural crest inducer. *Science*, 297: 848-851.

Graubert, T.A., Cahan, P., Edwin, D., Selzer, R.R., Richmond, T.A., Eis, P.S., Shannon, W.D., Li, X., McLeod, H.L., Cheverud, J.M. & Ley, T.J. (2007). A high-resolution map of segmental DNA copy number variation in the mouse genome. *PLoS Genetics*, 3:3.

Greenberg, N.M., DeMayo, F., Finegold, M.J., Medina, D., Tilley, W.D., Aspinall, J.O., Cunha, G.R., Donjacour, A.A., Matusik, R.J. & Rosen, J.M. (1995). Prostate cancer in a transgenic mouse. *Proceedings of the National Academy of Sciences of the United States of America*, 92: 3439-3443.

Haber, M., Bordow, S.B., Haber, P.S., Marshall, G.M., Stewart, B.W. & Norris, M.D. (1997). The prognostic value of MDR1 gene expression in primary untreated neuroblastoma. *European Journal of Cancer*, 33: 2031-2036.

Hidaka, S., Konecke, V., Osten, L. & Witzgall, R. (2004). PIGEA-14, a novel coiled-coil protein affecting the intracellular distribution of polycystin-2. *Journal of Biological Chemistry*, 279: 35009-35016.

Humphreys, D.T., Carver, J.A., Easterbrook-Smith, S.B. & Wilson, M.R. (1999). Clusterin has chaperone-like activity similar to that of small heat shock proteins. *The Journal of Biological Chemistry*, 274: 6875-6881.

IHGSC (2004). Finishing the euchromatic sequence of the human genome. *Nature*, 431: 931-945.

Inoue, K. & Lupski, J.R. (2002). Molecular mechanisms for genomic disorders. *Annual Reviews of Genomics and Human Genetics*, 3: 199-242.

Janoueix-Lerosey, I., Novikov, E., Monteiro, M., Gruel, N., Schleiermacher, G., Loriod, B., Nguyen, C. & Delattre, O. (2004). Gene expression profiling of 1p35-36 genes in neuroblastoma. *Oncogene*, 23: 5912-5922.

Jiang, Z., Tang, H., Ventura, M., Cardone, M.F., Marques-Bonet, T., She, X., Pevzner, P.A. & Eichler, E.E. (2007). Ancestral reconstruction of segmental duplications reveals punctuated cores of human genome evolution. *Nature Genetics*, 39: 1361-1368.

Johnson, M.E., Viggiano, L., Bailey, J.A., Abdul-Rauf, M., Goodwin, G., Rocchi, M. & Eichler, E.E. (2001). Positive selection of a gene family during the emergence of humans and African apes. *Nature*, 413: 514-519.

Jung, Y.S., Bang, S., Choi, K., Kim, E., Kim, Y., Kim, J., Park, J., Koo, H., Moon, R.T., Song, K. & Lee, I. (2006). TC1 (C8orf4) enhances the Wnt/beta-catenin pathway by relieving antagonistic activity of Chibby. *Cancer Research*, 66: 723-728.

Koesters, R. & Doeberitz, M.V. (2003). The Wnt signalling pathway in solid childhood tumours. *Cancer Letters*, 198: 123-138.

Kong, X.T., Choi, S.H., Inoue, A., Takita, J., Yokota, J., Kanada, R., Yamamoto, K., Bessho, F., Yanagisawa, M. & Hayashi, Y. (1997). Alterations of the tumour suppressor gene DCC in neuroblastoma. *European Journal of Cancer*, 33: 1962-1965.

Koppen, A., Ait-Aissa, R., Koster, J., Ora, I., Bras, J., van Sluis, P.G., Caron, H., Versteeg, R. & Valentijn, L.J. (2008). Dickkopf-3 expression is a marker for neuroblastic tumour maturation and is down-regulated by MYCN. *International Journal of Cancer*, 122: 1455-1464.

Lastowska, M., Cotterill, S., Bown, N., Cullinane, C., Variend, S., Lunec, J., Strachan, T., Pearson, A.D. & Jackson, M.S. (2002). Breakpoint position on 17q identifies the most aggressive neuroblastoma tumours. *Genes, Chromosomes and Cancer*, 34: 428-436.

Laureys, G., Speleman, F., Opdenakker, G., Benoit, Y. & Leroy, J. (1990). Constitutional translocation t(1;17)(p36;q12-21) in a patient with neuroblastoma. *Genes, Chromosomes and Cancer*, 2: 252-254.

Laureys, G., Speleman, F., Versteeg, R., van der Drift, P., Chan, A., Leroy, J., Francke, U., Opdenakker, G. & Van Roy, N. (1995). Constitutional translocation t(1;17)(p36.31-p36.13;q11.2-q12.1) in a neuroblastoma patient. Establishment of somatic cell hybrids and identification of PND/A12M2 on chromosome 1 and NF1/SCYA7 on chromosome 17 as breakpoint flanking single copy markers. *Oncogene*, 10: 1087-1093.

Leskov, K.S., Klokov, D.Y., Li, J., Kinsella, T.J. & Boothman, D.A. (2003). Synthesis and functional analyses of nuclear clusterin, a cell death protein. *Journal of Biological Chemistry*, 278: 11590-11600.

Li, F.Q., Mofunanya, A., Harris, K. & Takemaru, K. (2008). Chibby cooperates with 14-3-3 to regulate beta-catenin subcellular distribution and signalling activity. *Journal of Cell Biology*, 181: 1141-1154.

Li, F.Q., Singh, A.M., Mofunanya, A., Love, D., Terada, N., Moon, R.T. & Takemaru, K. (2007). Chibby promotes adipocyte differentiation through inhibition of beta-catenin signalling. *Molecular Cell Biology*, 27: 4347-4354.

Linguegia, E., de Weille, J.R., Bassilana, F., Heurteaux, C., Sakai, H., Waldmann, R. & Lazdunski, M. (1997). A modulatory subunit of acid sensing ion channels in brain and dorsal root ganglion cells. *The Journal of Biological Chemistry*, 272: 29778-29783.

Liu, T., Liu, P.Y., Tee, A.E., Haber, M., Norris, M.D., Gleave, M.E. & Marshall, G.M. (2009). Over-expression of clusterin is a resistance factor to the anti-cancer effect of histone deacetylase inhibitors. *European Journal of Cancer*, 45: 1846-1854.

Liu, X., Mazanek, P., Dam, V., Wang, Q., Zhao, H., Guo, R., Jagannathan, J., Cnaan, A., Maris, J.M. & Hogarty, M.D. (2008). Deregulated Wnt/beta-catenin program in high-risk neuroblastomas without MYCN amplification. *Oncogene*, 27: 1478-1488.

Lourda, M., Trougakos, I.P. & Gonos, E.S. (2006). Development of resistance to chemotherapeutic drugs in human osteosarcoma cell lines largely depends on up-regulation of clusterin/apolipoprotein J. *International Journal of Cancer*, 120: 611-622.

Love, D., Li, F.Q., Burke, M.C., Cyge, B., Ohmitsu, M., Cabello, J., Larson, J.E., Brody, S.L., Cohen, J.C. & Takemaru, K. (2010). Altered lung morphogenesis, epithelial cell differentiation and mechanics in mice deficient in the Wnt/beta-catenin antagonist Chibby. *PLoS One*, 5: 13600.

Lupski, J.R. (2007) Genomic rearrangements and sporadic disease. *Nature Genetics*, 39: 43-47.

Maris, J.M. & Matthay, K.K. (1999). Molecular biology of neuroblastoma. *Journal of Clinical Oncology*, 17: 2264-2279.

Marques-Bonet, T. & Eichler, E.E. (2009). The evolution of human segmental duplications and the core duplicon hypothesis. *Cold Spring Harbor Symposium on Quantitative Biology*, 74: 355-362.

Marques-Bonet, T., Kidd, J.M., Ventura, M., Graves, T.A., Cheng, Z., Hillier, L.W., Jiang, Z.S., Baker, C., Malfavon-Borja, R., Fulton, L.A., Nazareth, L.V., Muzny, D.M., Alkan, C., Aksay, G., Girirajan, S., Siswara, P., Chen, L., Cardone, M.F., Navarro, A., Gibbs, R.A., Mardis, E.R., Wilson, R.K. & Eichler, E.E. (2009a). A burst of segmental duplications in the genome of the African great ape ancestor. *Nature*, 458: 877-881.

Marques-Bonet, T., Ryder, O.A. & Eichler, E.E. (2009b). Sequencing primate genomes: what have we learned? *Annual Reviews of Genomics and Human Genetics*, 10: 355-386.

McLaughlin, L., Zhu, G., Mistry, M., Ley-Ebert, C., Stuart, W.D., Florio, C.J., Groen, P.A., Witt, S.A., Kimball, T.R., Witte, D.P., Harmony, J.A. & Aronow, B.J. (2000). Apolipoprotein J/clusterin limits the severity of murine autoimmune myocarditis. *Journal of Clinical Investigation*, 106: 1105-1113.

Mefford, H.C., Sharp, A.J., Baker, C., Itsara, A., Jiang, Z.S., Buysse, K., Huang, S.W., Maloney, V.K., Crolla, J.A., Baralle, D., Collins, A., Mercer, C., Norga, K., de Ravel, T., Devriendt, K., Bongers, E.M.H.F., de Leeuw, N., Reardon, W., Gimelli, S., Bena, F., Hennekam, R.C., Male, A., Gaunt, L., Clayton-Smith, J., Simonic, I., Park, S.M., Mehta, S.G., Nik-Zainal, S., Woods, C.G., Firth, H.V., Parkin, G., Fichera, M., Reitano, S., Lo Giudice, M., Li, K.E., Casuga, I., Broomer, A., Conrad, B., Schwerzmann, M., Raber, L., Gallati, S., Striano, P., Coppola, A., Tolmie, J.L., Tobias, E.S., Lilley, C., Armengol, L., Spysschaert, Y., Verloo, P., De Coene, A., Goossens, L., Mortier, G., Speleman, F., van Binsbergen, E., Nelen, M.R., Hochstenbach, R., Poot, M., Gallagher, L., Gill, M., McClellan, J., King, M.C., Regan, R., Skinner, C., Stevenson, R.E., Antonarakis, S.E., Chen, C.F., Estivill, X., Menten, B., Gimelli, G., Gribble, S., Schwartz, S., Sutcliffe, J.S., Walsh, T., Knight, S.J.L., Sebat, J., Romano, C., Schwartz, C.E., Veltman, J.A., de Vries, B.B.A., Vermeesch, J.R., Barber, J.C.K., Willatt, L., Tassabehji, M. & Eichler, E.E. (2008). Recurrent rearrangements of chromosome 1q21.1 and variable pediatric phenotypes. *New England Journal of Medicine*, 359: 1685-1699.

Mekel-Bobrov, N., Posthuma, D., Gilbert, S.L., Lind, P., Gosso, M.F., Luciano, M., Harris, S.E., Bates, T.C., Polderman, T.J., Whalley, L.J., Fox, H., Starr, J.M., Evans, P.D., Montgomery, G.W., Fernandes, C., Heutink, P., Martin, N.G., Boomsma, D.I., Deary, I.J., Wright, M.J., de Geus, E.J. & Lahn, B.T. (2007). The ongoing adaptive evolution of ASPM and Microcephalin is not explained by increased intelligence. *Human Molecular Genetics*, 16: 600-608.

Mestdagh, P., Bostrom, A.K., Impens, F., Fredlund, E., Van Peer, G., De Antonellis, P., von Stedingk, K., Ghesquiere, B., Schulte, S., Dews, M., Thomas-Tikhonenko, A.,

Schulte, J.H., Zollo, M., Schramm, A., Gevaert, K., Axelson, H., Speleman, F. & Vandesompele, J. (2010a). The miR-17-92 microRNA cluster regulates multiple components of the TGF-beta pathway in neuroblastoma. *Molecular Cell*, 40: 762-773.

Mestdagh, P., Fredlund, E., Pattyn, F., Schulte, J.H., Muth, D., Vermeulen, J., Kumps, C., Schlierf, S., De Preter, K., Van Roy, N., Noguera, R., Laureys, G., Schramm, A., Eggert, A., Westermann, F., Speleman, F. & Vandesompele, J. (2010b). MYCN/c-MYC-induced microRNAs repress coding gene networks associated with poor outcome in MYCN/c-MYC-activated tumours. *Oncogene*, 29: 1394-1404.

Miyake, H., Chi, K.N. & Gleave, M.E. (2000a). Antisense TRPM-2 oligodeoxynucleotides chemosensitize human androgen-independent PC-3 prostate cancer cells both in vitro and in vivo. *Clinical Cancer Research*, 6: 1655-1663.

Miyake, H., Nelson, C., Rennie, P.S. & Gleave, M.E. (2000b). Acquisition of chemoresistant phenotype by overexpression of the antiapoptotic gene testosterone-repressed prostate message-2 in prostate cancer xenograft models. *Cancer research*, 60: 2547-2554.

Miyake, H., Nelson, C., Rennie, P.S. & Gleave, M.E. (2000c). Testosterone-repressed prostate message-2 is an antiapoptotic gene involved in progression to androgen independence in prostate cancer. *Cancer research*, 60: 170-176.

Moretti, R.M., Marelli, M.M., Mai, S., Cariboni, A., Scaltriti, M., Bettuzzi, S. & Limonta, P. (2007). Clusterin isoforms differentially affect growth and motility of prostate cells: possible implications in prostate tumourigenesis. *Cancer Res*, 67: 10325-10333.

Ohno, S. (1970). *Evolution by gene duplication*. New York:Springer-Verlag.

Paar, V., Gluncic, M., Rosandic, M., Basar, I. & Vlahovic, I. (2011). Intra-gene higher order repeats in Neuroblastoma BreakPoint Family (NBPF) genes distinguish humans from chimpanzees. *Molecular Biology and Evolution*, 28: 1877-1892.

Popesco, M.C., Maclaren, E.J., Hopkins, J., Dumas, L., Cox, M., Meltesen, L., McGavran, L., Wyckoff, G.J. & Sikela, J.M. (2006). Human lineage-specific amplification, selection, and neuronal expression of DUF1220 domains. *Science*, 313: 1304-1307.

Ramos, C. & Robert, B. (2005). msh/Msx gene family in neural development. *Trends in Genetics*, 21: 624-632.

Redon, R., Ishikawa, S., Fitch, K.R., Feuk, L., Perry, G.H., Andrews, T.D., Fiegler, H., Shapero, M.H., Carson, A.R., Chen, W.W., Cho, E.K., Dallaire, S., Freeman, J.L., Gonzalez, J.R., Gratacos, M., Huang, J., Kalaitzopoulos, D., Komura, D., MacDonald, J.R., Marshall, C.R., Mei, R., Montgomery, L., Nishimura, K., Okamura, K., Shen, F., Somerville, M.J., Tchinda, J., Valsesia, A., Woodwark, C., Yang, F.T., Zhang, J.J., Zerjal, T., Zhang, J., Armengol, L., Conrad, D.F., Estivill, X., Tyler-Smith, C., Carter, N.P., Aburatani, H., Lee, C., Jones, K.W., Scherer, S.W. & Hurles, M.E. (2006). Global variation in copy number in the human genome. *Nature*, 444: 444-454.

Revet, I., Huizenga, G., Koster, J., Volckmann, R., van Sluis, P., Versteeg, R. & Geerts, D. (2010). MSX1 induces the Wnt pathway antagonist genes DKK1, DKK2, DKK3, and SFRP1 in neuroblastoma cells, but does not block Wnt3 and Wnt5A signalling to DVL3. *Cancer Letters*, 289: 195-207.

Reyes-Mugica, M., Lin, P., Yokota, J. & Reale, M.A. (1998). Status of deleted in colorectal cancer gene expression correlates with neuroblastoma metastasis. *Laboratory Investigation*, 78: 669-675.

Rhodes, D.R., Kalyana-Sundaram, S., Mahavisno, V., Varambally, R., Yu, J., Briggs, B.B., Barrette, T.R., Anstet, M.J., Kincead-Beal, C., Kulkarni, P., Varambally, S., Ghosh, D. & Chinnaiyan, A.M. (2007). Oncomine 3.0: genes, pathways, and networks in a collection of 18,000 cancer gene expression profiles. *Neoplasia*, 9: 166-180.

Rizzi, F. & Bettuzzi, S. (2010). The clusterin paradigm in prostate and breast carcinogenesis. *Endocrine- Related Cancer*, 17: 1-17.

Roberts, T., Chernova, O. & Cowell, J.K. (1998). NB4S, a member of the TBC1 domain family of genes, is truncated as a result of a constitutional t(1;10)(p22;q21) chromosome translocation in a patient with stage 4S neuroblastoma. *Human Molecular Genetics*, 7: 1169-1178.

Santilli, G., Aronow, B.J. & Sala, A. (2003). Essential requirement of apolipoprotein J (clusterin) signalling for IkappaB expression and regulation of NF-kappaB activity. *The Journal of Biological Chemistry*, 278: 38214-38219.

Sauka-Spengler, T. & Bronner-Fraser, M. (2008). A gene regulatory network orchestrates neural crest formation. *Nature Reviews Molecular Cell Biology*, 9: 557-568.

Savelyeva, L., Corvi, R. & Schwab, M. (1994). Translocation involving 1p and 17q is a recurrent genetic alteration of human neuroblastoma cells. *The American Journal of Human Genetics*, 55: 334-340.

Schwab, M., Praml, C. & Amler, L.C. (1996). Genomic instability in Ip and human malignancies. *Genes, Chromosomes and Cancer*, 16: 211-229.

Sharp, A.J., Hansen, S., Selzer, R.R., Cheng, Z., Regan, R., Hurst, J.A., Stewart, H., Price, S.M., Blair, E., Hennekam, R.C., Fitzpatrick, C.A., Segraves, R., Richmond, T.A., Guiver, C., Albertson, D.G., Pinkel, D., Eis, P.S., Schwartz, S., Knight, S.J. & Eichler, E.E. (2006). Discovery of previously unidentified genomic disorders from the duplication architecture of the human genome. *Nature Genetics*, 38: 1038-1042.

She, X., Cheng, Z., Zollner, S., Church, D.M. & Eichler, E.E. (2008). Mouse segmental duplication and copy number variation. *Nature Genetics*, 40: 909-914.

Singh, A.M., Li, F.Q., Hamazaki, T., Kasahara, H., Takemaru, K.I. & Terada, N. (2007). Chibby, an antagonist of the Wnt/beta-catenin pathway, facilitates cardiomyocyte differentiation of murine embryonic stem cells. *Circulation*, 115: 617-626.

Stefansson, H., Rujescu, D., Cichon, S., Pietilainen, O.P.H., Ingason, A., Steinberg, S., Fossdal, R., Sigurdsson, E., Sigmundsson, T., Buizer-Voskamp, J.E., Hansen, T., Jakobsen, K.D., Muglia, P., Francks, C., Matthews, P.M., Gylfason, A., Halldorsson, B.V., Gudbjartsson, D., Thorgeirsson, T.E., Sigurdsson, A., Jonasdottir, A., Jonasdottir, A., Bjornsson, A., Mattiasdottir, S., Blondal, T., Haraldsson, M., Magnusdottir, B.B., Giegling, I., Moller, H.J., Hartmann, A., Shianna, K.V., Ge, D.L., Need, A.C., Crombie, C., Fraser, G., Walker, N., Lonnqvist, J., Suvisaari, J., Tuulio-Henriksson, A., Paunio, T., Toulopoulou, T., Bramon, E., Di Forti, M., Murray, R., Ruggeri, M., Vassos, E., Tosato, S., Walshe, M., Li, T., Vasilescu, C., Muhleisen, T.W., Wang, A.G., Ullum, H., Djurovic, S., Melle, I., Olesen, J., Kiemeney, L.A., Franke, B., Sabatti, C., Freimer, N.B., Gulcher, J.R., Thorsteinsdottir, U., Kong, A., Andreassen, O.A., Ophoff, R.A.,

Georgi, A., Rietschel, M., Werge, T., Petursson, H., Goldstein, D.B., Nothen, M.M., Peltonen, L., Collier, D.A., St Clair, D. & Stefansson, K. (2008). Large recurrent microdeletions associated with schizophrenia. *Nature*, 455: 232-261.

Subramanian, C., Jarzembowski, J.A., Halsey, S.M., Kuick, R., Opipari, A.W., Jr., Castle, V.P. & Kwok, R.P. (2011). CLU blocks HDACI-mediated killing of neuroblastoma. *Tumour Biology*, 32: 285-294.

Sudmant, P.H., Kitzman, J.O., Antonacci, F., Alkan, C., Malig, M., Tsalenko, A., Sampas, N., Bruhn, L., Shendure, J. & Eichler, E.E. (2010). Diversity of human copy number variation and multicopy genes. *Science*, 330: 641-646.

Szatmari, P., Paterson, A.D., Zwaigenbaum, L., Roberts, W., Brian, J., Liu, X.Q., Vincent, J.B., Skaug, J.L., Thompson, A.P., Senman, L., Feuk, L., Qian, C., Bryson, S.E., Jones, M.B., Marshall, C.R., Scherer, S.W., Vieland, V.J., Bartlett, C., Mangin, L.V., Goedken, R., Segre, A., Pericak-Vance, M.A., Cuccaro, M.L., Gilbert, J.R., Wright, H.H., Abramson, R.K., Betancur, C., Bourgeron, T., Gillberg, C., Leboyer, M., Buxbaum, J.D., Davis, K.L., Hollander, E., Silverman, J.M., Hallmayer, J., Lotspeich, L., Sutcliffe, J.S., Haines, J.L., Folstein, S.E., Piven, J., Wassink, T.H., Sheffield, V., Geschwind, D.H., Bucan, M., Brown, W.T., Cantor, R.M., Constantino, J.N., Gilliam, T.C., Herbert, M., Lajonchere, C., Ledbetter, D.H., Lese-Martin, C., Miller, J., Nelson, S., Samango-Sprouse, C.A., Spence, S., State, M., Tanzi, R.E., Coon, H., Dawson, G., Devlin, B., Estes, A., Flodman, P., Klei, L., McMahon, W.M., Minshew, N., Munson, J., Korvatska, E., Rodier, P.M., Schellenberg, G.D., Smith, M., Spence, M.A., Stodgell, C., Tepper, P.G., Wijsman, E.M., Yu, C.E., Roge, B., Mantoulan, C., Wittemeyer, K., Poustka, A., Felder, B., Klauck, S.M., Schuster, C., Poustka, F., Bolte, S., Feineis-Matthews, S., Herbrecht, E., Schmotzer, G., Tsiantis, J., Papanikolaou, K., Maestrini, E., Bacchelli, E., Blasi, F., Carone, S., Toma, C., Van Engeland, H., de Jonge, M., Kemner, C., Koop, F., Langemeijer, M., Hijmans, C., Staal, W.G., Baird, G., Bolton, P.F., Rutter, M.L., Weisblatt, E., Green, J., Aldred, C., Wilkinson, J.A., Pickles, A., Le Couteur, A., Berney, T., McConachie, H., Bailey, A.J., Francis, K., Honeyman, G., Hutchinson, A., Parr, J.R., Wallace, S., Monaco, A.P., Barnby, G., Kobayashi, K., Lamb, J.A., Sousa, I., Sykes, N., Cook, E.H., Guter, S.J., Leventhal, B.L., Salt, J., Lord, C., Corsello, C., Hus, V., Weeks, D.E., Volkmar, F., Tauber, M., Fombonne, E., Shih, A. & Meyer, K.J. (2007). Mapping autism risk loci using genetic linkage and chromosomal rearrangements. *Nature Genetics*, 39: 319-328.

Takemaru, K.I., Yamaguchi, S., Lee, Y.S., Zhang, Y., Carthew, R.W. & Moon, R.T. (2003). Chibby, a nuclear beta-catenin-associated antagonist of the Wnt/Wingless pathway. *Nature*, 422: 905-909.

Trougakos, I.P. & Gonos, E.S. (2002). Clusterin/apolipoprotein J in human aging and cancer. *The International Journal of Biochemistry and Cell Biology*, 34: 1430-1448.

Trougakos, I.P., Lourda, M., Antonelou, M.H., Kletsas, D., Gorgoulis, V.G., Papassideri, I.S., Zou, Y., Margaritis, L.H., Boothman, D.A. & Gonos, E.S. (2009). Intracellular clusterin inhibits mitochondrial apoptosis by suppressing p53-activating stress signals and stabilizing the cytosolic Ku70-Bax protein complex. *Clinical Cancer Research*, 15: 48-59.

Usakin, L.A., Kogan, G.L., Kalmykova, A.I. & Gvozdev, V.A. (2005). An alien promoter capture as a primary step of the evolution of testes-expressed repeats in the Drosophila melanogaster genome. *Molecular Biology and Evolution*, 22: 1555-1560.

Van Roy, N., De Preter, K., Hoebeeck, J., Van Maerken, T., Pattyn, F., Mestdagh, P., Vermeulen, J., Vandesompele, J. & Speleman, F. (2009). The emerging molecular pathogenesis of neuroblastoma: implications for improved risk assessment and targeted therapy. *Genome Medicine*, 1: 74.

Vandepoele, K., Andries, V. & Van Roy, F. (2009). The NBPF promoter has been recruited from the unrelated EVI5 gene before simian radiation. *Molecular Biology and Evolution*, 26: 1321-1332.

Vandepoele, K., Andries, V., Van Roy, N., Staes, K., Vandesompele, J., Laureys, G., De Smet, E., Berx, G., Speleman, F. & van Roy, F. (2008). A constitutional translocation t(1;17)(p36.2;q11.2) in a neuroblastoma patient disrupts the human *NBPF1* and *ACCN1* genes. *PLoS One*, 3: 1-12.

Vandepoele, K., Staes, K., Andries, V. & van Roy, F. (2010). Chibby interacts with NBPF1 and clusterin, two candidate tumour suppressors linked to neuroblastoma. *Experimental Cell Research*, 316: 1225-1233.

Vandepoele, K., Van Roy, N., Staes, K., Speleman, F. & van Roy, F. (2005). A novel gene family NBPF: Intricate structure generated by gene duplications during primate evolution. *Molecular Biology and Evolution*, 22: 2265-2274.

Varga, A.C. & Wrana, J.L. (2005). The disparate role of BMP in stem cell biology. *Oncogene*, 24: 5713-5721.

Verde, I., Pahlke, G., Salanova, M., Zhang, G., Wang, S., Coletti, D., Onuffer, J., Jin, S.L. & Conti, M. (2001). Myomegalin is a novel protein of the golgi/centrosome that interacts with a cyclic nucleotide phosphodiesterase. *Journal of Biological Chemistry*, 276: 11189-11198.

Vila-Carriles, W.H., Kovacs, G.G., Jovov, B., Zhou, Z.H., Pahwa, A.K., Colby, G., Esimai, O., Gillespie, G.Y., Mapstone, T.B., Markert, J.M., Fuller, C.M., Bubien, J.K. & Benos, D.J. (2006). Surface expression of ASIC2 inhibits the amiloride-sensitive current and migration of glioma cells. *Journal of Biological Chemistry*, 281: 19220-19232.

Vinogradova, T.V., Zhulidov, P.A., Illarionova, A.E. & Sverdlov, E.D. (2002). A new family of KIAA1245 genes with and without HERV-K LTRs in their introns. *Russian Journal of Bioorganic Chemistry*, 28: 312-315.

Voronina, V.A., Takemaru, K., Treuting, P., Love, D., Grubb, B.R., Hajjar, A.M., Adams, A., Li, F.Q. & Moon, R.T. (2009). Inactivation of Chibby affects function of motile airway cilia. *Journal of Cell Biology*, 185: 225-233.

Waldmann, R., Champigny, G., Bassilana, F., Heurteaux, C. & Lazdunski, M. (1997). A proton-gated cation channel involved in acid-sensing. *Nature*, 386: 173-177.

Waldmann, R., Voilley, N., Mattei, M.G. & Lazdunski, M. (1996). The human degenerin MDEG, an amiloride-sensitive neuronal cation channel, is localised on chromosome 17q11.2-17q12 close to the microsatellite D17S798. *Genomics*, 37: 269-270.

White, P.S., Thompson, P.M., Gotoh, T., Okawa, E.R., Igarashi, J., Kok, M., Winter, C., Gregory, S.G., Hogarty, M.D., Maris, J.M. & Brodeur, G.M. (2005). Definition and characterisation of a region of 1p36.3 consistently deleted in neuroblastoma. *Oncogene*, 24: 2684-2694.

Willett-Brozick, J.E., Savul, S.A., Richey, L.E. & Baysal, B.E. (2001). Germ line insertion of mtDNA at the breakpoint junction of a reciprocal constitutional translocation. *Human Genetics*, 109: 216-223.

Yang, C.R., Leskov, K., Hosley-Eberlein, K., Criswell, T., Pink, J.J., Kinsella, T.J. & Boothman, D.A. (2000). Nuclear clusterin/XIP8, an x-ray-induced Ku70-binding protein that signals cell death. *Proceedings of the National Academy of Sciences of the United States of America*, 97: 5907-5912.

Zhang, H., Kim, J.K., Edwards, C.A., Xu, Z., Taichman, R. & Wang, C.Y. (2005). Clusterin inhibits apoptosis by interacting with activated Bax. *Nature Cell Biology*, 7: 909-915.

9

Sympathetic Neurotransmitters in Neuroblastoma – Between Physiology and Pathology

Magdalena Czarnecka, Jason Tilan and Joanna Kitlinska
Georgetown University
USA

1. Introduction

Neuroblastomas arise from precursors of sympathetic neurons due to defects in their normal development (Edsjo et al., 2007). Consequently, the tumors exhibit various degrees of neuronal differentiation manifested by expression of markers characteristic for sympathetic neurons and release of their physiological neurotransmitters (Bourdeaut et al., 2009). Since the levels of neuroblastoma cell differentiation determines clinical phenotype of the disease and its outcome, the factors regulating this process have been extensively studied and recently introduced to the clinic (Edsjo et al., 2007; Maris, 2010). Surprisingly, however, little attention has been paid to the role the sympathetic neurotransmitters excessively released from neuroblastoma cells play in this pathological condition. Despite their known role in the regulation of proliferation and survival of other cell types, in the neuroblastoma field those factors have been treated merely as markers of neuronal differentiation. Very often, even if studies on functional effects of neurotransmitters on neuroblastoma cells have been performed, these cells have been considered purely as a neuronal model (Laifenfeld et al., 2002; Lopes et al., 2010). Therefore, the results of such studies have been interpreted in the context of other neurological disorders, but not assessed in terms of their implications for neuroblastoma biology and therapy. Research conducted in our laboratory focuses on growth-promoting functions of one of such neurotransmitters, neuropeptide Y (NPY). We were able to show that this physiological peptide acts as a crucial mitogenic and angiogenic factor for neuroblastomas and significantly contributes to their progression (Kitlinska et al., 2005; Lu et al., 2010). However, the role of other sympathetic neurotransmitters in biology of these tumors remains understudied. This chapter summarizes our current knowledge on the role these molecules play in the regulation of neuroblastoma growth, and identifies problems which thus far have not been addressed.

2. Sympathetic neuron differentiation

The sympathetic nervous system consists of two major components - sympathetic neurons organized in ganglia and neuroendocrine chromaffin cells, which form the adrenal gland (Huber, 2006). Even though neuroblastomas often develop in adrenals, they are believed to arise from precursors of sympathetic neurons, which are also present in immature adrenal glands (Edsjo et al., 2007; Hoehner et al., 1996).

The sympathetic nervous system is the major derivative of the neural crest and develops in a process tightly controlled by local microenvironments encountered by neural crest cells during their migration within an embryo (Huber, 2006). The essential factors involved in this process are bone morphogenic proteins (BMPs) released from dorsal aorta, which initiate the differentiation of neural crest cells toward sympathoadrenal lineage (Huber, 2006) (Fig. 1). The subsequent development of sympathoneural phenotype is triggered by induction of multiple transcription factors, such as Phox2B, MASH-1, GATA3, Hand2 and MYCN (Huber, 2006). During this process, immature sympathetic neurons acquire expression of TrkA receptor and become dependent on its ligand, nerve growth factor (NGF), for their survival (Glebova & Ginty, 2005). The mature sympathetic neurons attain the adrenergic phenotype associated with the ability to synthesize and release in a controllable manner their main neurotransmitter - norepinephrine (Huber, 2006). Consequently, the enzymes involved in the synthesis of this catecholamine, tyrosine hydroxylase (TH) and dopamine β-hydroxylase (DBH), are considered as the most characteristic sympathetic markers (Fig. 1, 2) (Glebova & Ginty, 2005; Huber, 2006). However, other neurotransmitters released from sympathetic neurons, such as NPY, are also frequently used for their identification (Bowden & Gibbins, 1992; Damon, 2008; Pahlman et al., 1991).

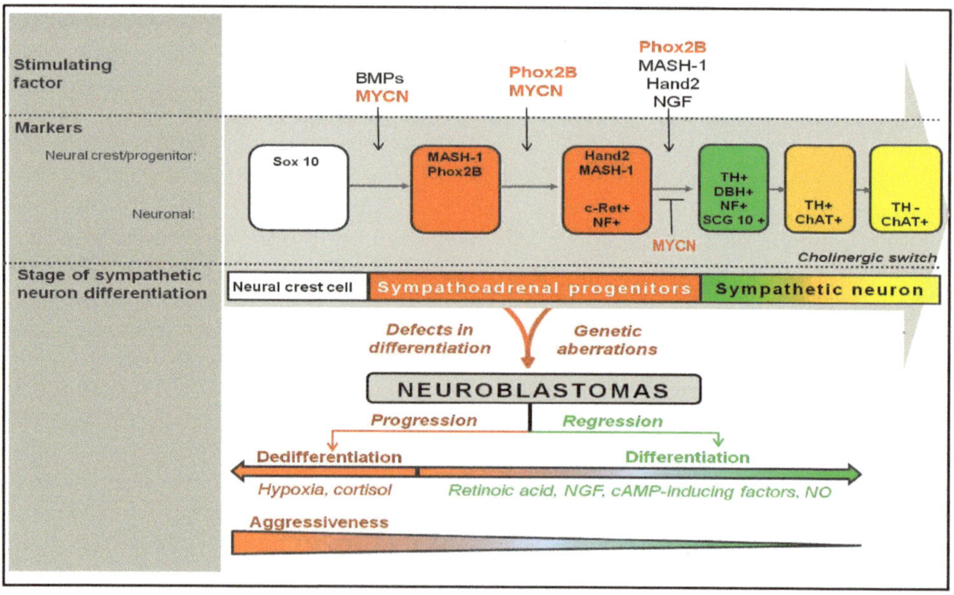

Fig. 1. Sympathetic neuron differentation and neuroblastoma development.

Even though development of the adrenergic phenotype is considered as the end stage of sympathetic neuron differentiation, in their small subset innervating sweat glands, periosteum and skeletal muscle vasculature, this process proceeds further and the neurons undergo a "cholinergic switch" (Glebova & Ginty, 2005). In this process, the adrenergic neurons acquire additional cholinergic features, such as expression of the enzyme involved in acetylcholine synthesis, choline acetyltransferase (ChAT), and the ability to release this neurotransmitter (Fig. 1) (Glebova & Ginty, 2005). In this transient stage, the neurons have both adrenergic and cholinergic characteristics. Subsequently, however, their adrenergic properties are lost and the neurons become purely cholinergic (Glebova & Ginty, 2005). Interestingly, all these stages of sympathetic differentiation are reflected in various phenotypes of neuroblastomas (Bourdeaut et al., 2009).

3. Neuroblastoma as a disorder of neuronal differentiation

Neuroblastoma is an extremely heterogeneous disease with phenotypes ranging from spontaneously regressing to highly metastatic, aggressive tumors (Janoueix-Lerosey et al., 2010). This phenotypical diversity is attributed to the fact that neuroblastomas arise at different stages of sympathetic neuron development. Consequently, the diverse clinical features of the disease are strongly associated with different levels of neuronal differentiation observed within tumor tissue (Fig. 1) (Bourdeaut et al., 2009). The undifferentiated neuroblastomas, which represent the most aggressive tumors, lack morphological features of mature neurons and do not exhibit adrenergic properties, such as expression of enzymes involved in catecholamine synthesis - TH and DBH. Instead, they are characterized by high expression of genes normally active in sympathetic precursors, such as Phox2B (Bourdeaut et al., 2009). In contrast, poorly differentiated neuroblastomas preserve some neuronal morphology and in the vast majority are highly adrenergic, with elevated expression of TH, DBH and with catecholamine synthesis. In some, however, the adrenergic properties are accompanied by expression of cholinergic markers, which corresponds to the transient state of dual adrenergic and cholinergic properties observed in sympathetic neurons undergoing the "cholinergic switch" (Bourdeaut et al., 2009). In line with this, the differentiating tumors with the least malignant clinical features are characterized by down-regulation of adrenergic properties and enhanced cholinergic phenotype (Bourdeaut et al., 2009).

Neuroblastoma tumorigenesis is associated with genetic aberrations targeting crucial factors involved in the regulation of normal sympathetic differentiation. The most aggressive neuroblastomas are often associated with amplification of MYCN, while the hereditary form of the disease is driven by mutations in the genes encoding transcription factor, Phox2B or the direct target of its transcriptional regulation, anaplastic lymphoma kinase (ALK) (Bachetti et al. 2010; Bourdeaut et al., 2005; Janoueix-Lerosey et al., ; Mosse et al., 2008). ALK mutations are also present in sporadic neuroblastomas (Chen et al., 2008; George et al., 2008). Interestingly, despite the genetic nature of the disease, differentiating factors are able to inhibit growth of already existing neuroblastomas and induce their maturation even in the presence of oncogenic mutations (Edsjo et al., 2007). Such a differentiation is also believed to contribute to spontaneous regression observed in stage 4S neuroblastomas and incomplete penetrance of the familial disease. Thus, the deregulation of normal sympathetic differentiation is indispensible for neuroblastoma development and may be, at least partially, independent of genetic aberrations (Edsjo et al., 2007; Prasad et al., 2003).

Neuroblastoma cell differentiation, manifested by morphological changes, up-regulation of neuronal markers and down-regulation of oncogenes, can be triggered in vitro by a variety of factors (Fig. 1) (Edsjo et al., 2007). The most extensively studied is retinoic acid and its derivatives, which have been recently introduced to the clinic as a routine treatment following chemotherapy (Handler et al., 2000; Maris, 2010; Sidell, 1982). Similar effects, however, can also be achieved with other factors, such as NGF in neuroblastoma cells with induced TrkA receptor expression, nitric oxide and cyclic AMP (cAMP) -stimulating factors, such as prostaglandins and pituitary adenylate cyclase activating polypeptide (PACAP), as well as a stable analog of cAMP, dibutyryl cAMP (Kume et al., 2008; Matsushima & Bogenmann, 1990; Monaghan et al., 2008; Prasad et al., 2003; Revoltella & Butler, 1980; Reynolds & Perez-Polo, 1981; Rodriguez-Martin et al., 2000) (Fig. 1). Depending on the type of differentiation factor and cell line used, such a morphological differentiation is associated with augmenting the adrenergic features of the cells manifested by increase in norepinephrine synthesis or, conversely, in down-regulation of adrenergic markers and enhancement of cholinergic properties (Handler et al., 2000; Kume et al., 2008; Pahlman et al., 1981). In some cases, stimulation of the mixed adrenergic and cholinergic phenotype has been observed (Monaghan et al., 2008). Thus, the differentiation factors shift the neuroblastoma cells toward more mature phenotype, with the cholinergic phenotype representing the most mature cells, mimicking the final stage of differentiation observed in sympathetic neurons and human neuroblastomas. In contrast, there are several factors, such as glucocorticoids and hypoxia, known to induce dedifferentiation of neuroblastoma cells associated with down-regulation of neuronal markers (Fig. 1) (Jogi et al., 2003; Yaniv et al., 2008).

4. Catecholamines – The physiological neurotransmitters in pathological condition

Due to their origin, sympathetic neurotransmitters are an integral part of neuroblastoma biology. The levels of catecholamines and/or their metabolites are elevated in over 90% of neuroblastoma patients and their plasma and urinary levels are utilized as a diagnostic tool (Monsaingeon et al., 2003) (Fig. 2). The pattern of catecholamine secretion reflects the level of neuroblastoma differentiation. The differentiating tumors release a relatively high amount of actual sympathetic neurotransmitters, norepinephrine and epinephrine (Zambrano & Reyes-Mugica, 2002). Paradoxically, however, systemic levels of these catecholamines are rarely elevated in neuroblastoma patients, while concentrations of their metabolites - free normetanephrine and vanillylmandelic acid - are significantly higher than normal (Davidson et al., 2011). This phenomenon is attributed to the fact that poorly differentiated neuroblastomas lack catecholamine storing mechanisms, which leads to an uncontrolled release of norepinephrine and its rapid metabolism (Itoh & Omori, 1973).
In contrast, patients with undifferentiated neuroblastomas are characterized by relatively high levels of dopamine and its metabolite, homovanilic acid (Zambrano & Reyes-Mugica, 2002). These dopaminergic features of aggressive tumors result from their immature adrenergic phenotype manifested by a decreased ability to convert dopamine to norepinephrine. Consequently, the high ratio of dopamine to norepinephrine and/or its metabolites has been postulated as an unfavorable prognostic factor (Strenger et al., 2007; Zambrano & Reyes-Mugica, 2002). Thus, measurement of multiple catecholamines and their metabolites appear to be necessary for proper diagnosis and stratification of neuroblastoma (Fig. 2) (Monsaingeon et al., 2003).

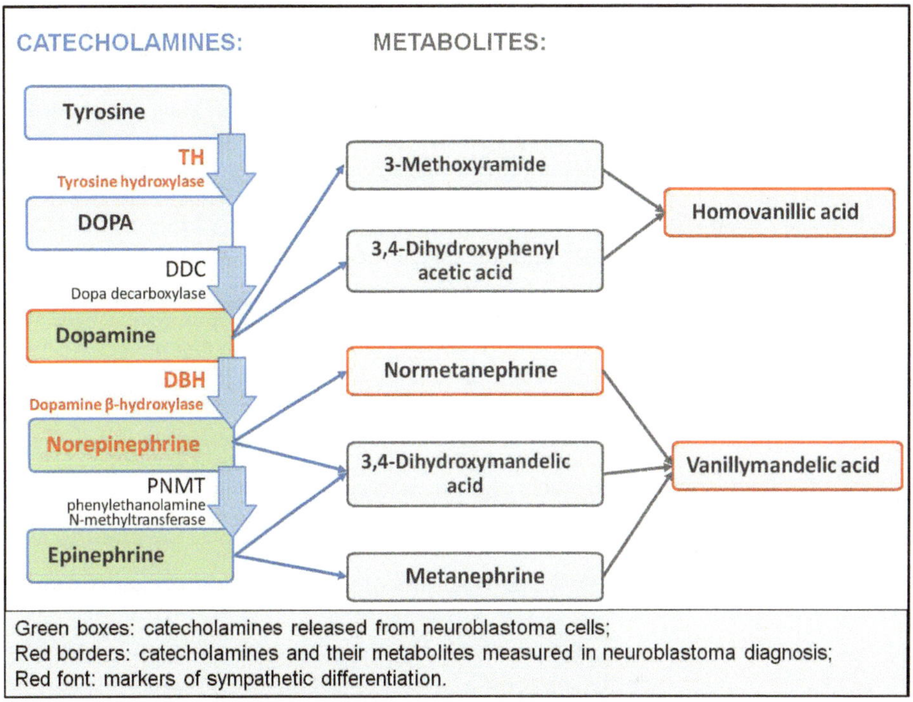

Fig. 2. Catecholamines and their metabolites in neuroblastoma

4.1 Functions of norepinephrine and epinephrine

Aside from releasing catecholamines, neuroblastoma cells also express their receptors – most often α2-adrenergic receptors (AR), but in some cell lines additionally β2-AR (Bawa-Khalfe et al., 2007; Parsley et al., 1999). Consequently, norepinephrine has been found to exert significant effects on neuroblastoma cell physiology. Treatment with exogenous norepinephrine inhibited neuroblastoma cell proliferation, while promoting their survival and inducing morphological differentiation manifested by neurite outgrowth comparable to this observed upon retinoic acid stimulation (Fig. 3) (Laifenfeld et al., 2002; Yaniv et al., 2008). These changes were accompanied by the decrease in expression of a marker of pluripotency, Oct4 and up-regulation of neuronal markers, such as growth-associated protein 43 (GAP-43). The norepinephrine-induced neuronal differentiation of neuroblastoma cells was mediated by α2-AR and p44/42 mitogen-activated protein kinase (MAPK) pathway (Yaniv et al., 2008; Yaniv et al., 2010). However, in the studies described above, neuroblastoma cells have been used solely as models of neuronal cells and the data interpreted in the context of neuronal plasticity. Thus, the role of endogenous norepinephrine in regulation of neuroblastoma cell proliferation and differentiation, as well its effect on neuroblastoma tumor growth have never been explored.

As sympathetic neurotransmitters, norepinephrine and epinephrine are highly released during stress. Therefore, their stimulatory effect on the growth of various tumor types has been proposed as a mechanism of stress-induced augmentation of cancer progression. Further studies revealed that these catecholamines act mainly by increasing tumor vascularization. This effect is driven by β-ARs present on cancer cells, the stimulation of which results in an increased release of angiogenic factors - vascular endothelial growth factor (VEGF) and interleukins 6 and 8 (IL-6 and IL-8) (Fig. 3) (Nilsson et al., 2007; Thaker et al., 2006; Wong et al., 2007; Yang et al., 2009; Yang et al., 2006; Yang & Chou, 2004). Adrenergic stimulation has also been shown to increase the secretion of metalloproteases, MMP-2 and MMP-9, which further augments angiogenic and metastatic processes (Yang et al., 2006). In addition to those indirect activities, catecholamines can also exert direct effects on endothelial cells through α-ARs (Fig. 3). Phenylepinephrine, a non-vasoconstrictive α-AR agonist, has been shown to induce endothelial cell proliferation and migration, as well as promote capillary formation. These effects were potentiated by hypoxia (Vinci et al., 2007), which is also a known stimulator of norepinephrine release from the sympathetic nerves (Borovsky et al., 1998). Thus, the direct angiogenic effect of norepinhephrine can be particularly pronounced in hypoxic areas of tumors. However, as mentioned before, all of the above studies on the angiogenic effects of norepinephrine and epinephrine have been performed on tumors developing in adults, in the context of the stress response. The role of their angiogenic effects in the growth of catecholamine-rich neuroblastomas has never been directly tested.

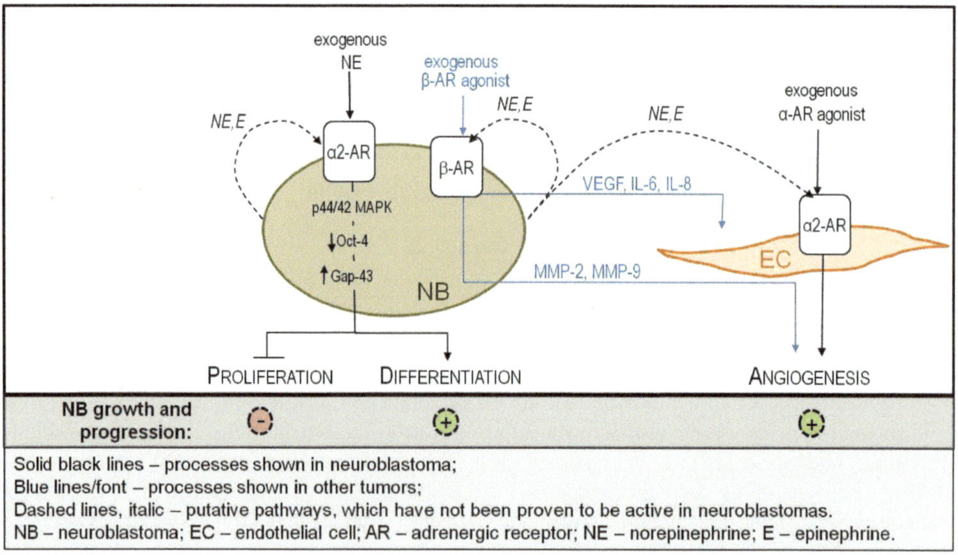

Fig. 3. Potential effects of norepinephrine and epinephrine on neuroblastoma growth and progression

4.2 Dopamine

Another catecholamine which is highly released from neuroblastomas is dopamine. Under physiological conditions, this catecholamine serves mainly as a brain neurotransmitter. However, it can also be released form peripheral sympathetic neurons and chromaffin cells, despite the fact that in these cells most of it is converted to norepinephrine or epinephrine (Fig. 2) (Goldstein, 2003). A similar phenomenon is observed with neuroblastomas, particularly the undifferentiated tumors that are characterized by an "immature adrenergic system" and low levels of enzymes converting dopamine to norepinephrine (Zambrano & Reyes-Mugica, 2002). As in case of other catecholamines, the role of the endogenous dopamine in the regulation of neuroblastoma growth has not been explored. However, the studies designed to test the potential role of dopamine in the development of neurodegenerative diseases have shown that this catecholamine, if given at high concentrations (100-500μM), becomes toxic for neuroblastoma cells (Fig. 4). This effect is driven by intracellular dopamine, the oxidation of which creates reactive oxygen species (ROS) and triggers apoptosis and autophagy (Bisaglia et al., 2010; Gimenez-Xavier et al., 2009; Junn & Mouradian, 2001). Whether or not endogenous dopamine is present in neuroblastoma cells at these toxic concentrations and, if not, what are its effects at the levels present locally in the tumor tissue remains to be elucidated.

As previously shown for other catecholamines, dopamine is also involved in the regulation of tumor angiogenesis. However, in contrast to norepinephrine and epinephrine, dopamine decreases vascularization in a variety of tumor types and animal models (Fig. 4) (Asada et al., 2008; Chakroborty et al., 2004; Sarkar et al., 2008). The mechanism underlying this effect involves blocking VEGF-induced proliferation and migration of mature endothelial cells and their progenitors (Chakroborty et al., 2008). This effect is mediated by endothelial D2 receptors, which upon dopamine stimulation enhance endocytosis of VEGF receptor 2 (VEGF-R2) and decrease its membrane expression. This, in turn, interferes with VEGF signaling by reducing VEGF-induced phosphorylation of VEGF-R2 and preventing the activation of downstream kinases - focal adhesion kinase (FAK) and p42/44 MAPK (Basu et al., 2001; Sarkar et al., 2004).

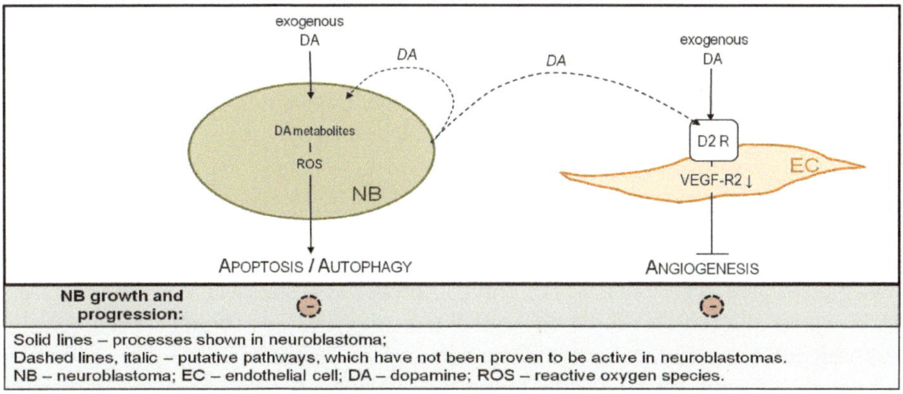

Fig. 4. Potential functions of dopamine in neuroblastoma.

In contrast to D2 receptor-mediated anti-angiogenic effects, stimulation of D1 dopamine receptors has been shown to increase endothelial cell proliferation and angiogenesis (Lindgren et al., 2009). This effect, however, has been shown mainly for brain microvascular endothelial cells stimulated by selective D1 receptor agonists (Bacic et al., 1991; Lindgren et al., 2009; Lu et al., 2008). On the contrary, in cancer models, the inhibitory effect of D2 receptor-preferring dopamine prevails, reducing tumor vascularization and growth (Asada et al., 2008; Chakroborty et al., 2004; Sarkar et al., 2008). The specific effects of endogenous dopamine on neuroblastoma vascularization, as well as their biological and clinical relevance, have yet to be determined.

5. Neuropeptide Y – neuronal marker or growth factor?

Neuropetide Y (NPY) is a 36-amino acid peptide, which is normally co-released with norepinephrine from mature sympathetic nerves. Consequently, as shown for catecholamines, the elevated plasma levels of NPY have been reported in neuroblastoma patients (Grouzmann et al., 1989). However, early attempts to use it as a general diagnostic marker failed due to high variability of the peptide's concentrations. More detailed analyses revealed that release of NPY is elevated in stage 3/4 and stage 4s neuroblastomas, but not in stage 1/2 (Dotsch et al., 1998; Kogner et al., 1994). Also, among patients with advanced disease, the NPY levels were diverse, with many cases comparable to healthy controls. However, the increased plasma concentrations of NPY in patients from this group strongly correlated with poor clinical outcome of the disease (death and relapse) and MYCN amplification (Dotsch et al., 1998; Kogner et al., 1994). Interestingly, in advanced neuroblastomas, the elevated levels of NPY in a patient's plasma did not correlate with its high mRNA levels in the tumor tissue (Cohen et al., 1990; Dotsch et al., 1998). Similarly, based on the data from the Oncogenomics data base, high mRNA levels of NPY in tumor tissues correlated with better survival (Wei et al., 2004). This observation is in agreement with NPY being a sympathetic marker up-regulated by numerous differentiation factors (Bowden & Gibbins, 1992; Damon, 2008; Edsjo et al., 2007; Pahlman et al., 1991). The discrepancies between NPY mRNA levels and its release can be explained by a defect in neurotransmitter storage mechanisms observed in neuroblastoma (Itoh & Omori, 1973). It is plausible that despite high expression of NPY in differentiating tumors, the release of the peptide is tightly controlled and needs certain stimulation to occur, as observed in mature sympathetic neurons. In contrast, undifferentiated tumors synthesize less NPY, but release it in an uncontrolled manner, which leads to elevated systemic levels of the peptide in neuroblastoma patients, as well as further depletion of the peptide in neuroblastoma tissue. Such an uncontrolled secretion has been already described for catecholamines (Davidson et al., 2011; Itoh & Omori, 1973).

The clinical reports associating elevated plasma NPY levels with poor prognosis of neuroblastoma suggested that the peptide can be a growth factor for these tumors. Indeed, neuroblastoma cells express not only NPY, but also its G protein-coupled receptors - mainly Y2 receptors (Y2Rs), with low levels of Y5R co-expression in some cell lines (Kitlinska et al., 2005; Korner et al., 2004). We have shown that this autocrine loop stimulates neuroblastoma cell proliferation via p44/42 MAPK pathway (Fig. 5) (Kitlinska et al., 2005). More importantly, blocking the NPY/Y2R mitogenic signaling reduces basal levels of p44/42 MAPK activity in neuroblastoma cells and significantly inhibits their proliferation (Lu et al., 2010). This effect is associated with an increase in neuroblastoma cell apoptosis mediated by the Bim pathway, known to be activated upon growth factor withdrawal (Lu et al., 2010). Altogether, these observations suggest that the NPY/Y2R autocrine loop is essential to maintain neuroblastoma in their proliferative state

Aside from being a mitogenic factor for neuroblastomas, NPY is also known to stimulate angiogenesis via its direct proliferative and pro-migratory effect on endothelial cells (Lee et al., 2003b; Movafagh et al., 2006; Zukowska-Grojec et al., 1998). Strikingly, the angiogenic effect of NPY is also mediated by Y2Rs, which are expressed in activated endothelial cells (Lee et al., 2003a; Movafagh et al., 2006). Therefore, in vivo, NPY stimulates neuroblastoma tumor growth via two independent mechanisms - a direct proliferative effect on nuroblastoma cells and indirectly, via increasing tumor vascularization (Fig. 5). Since both of these actions are mediated by Y2Rs, blocking Y2Rs in neuroblastoma xenografts leads to substantial inhibition in tumor growth associated with reduced proliferation levels, increased apoptosis, decreased tumor vascularization and marked focal fibrosis (Lu et al., 2010). Thus, the above data gathered in our laboratory indicate that NPY and its Y2Rs are promising new targets in neuroblastoma therapy. However, further studies are required to increase the efficiency of Y2R blockage, as well as to elucidate the role of NPY in other processes involved in regulation of tumor progression, such as chemoresistance and metastases.

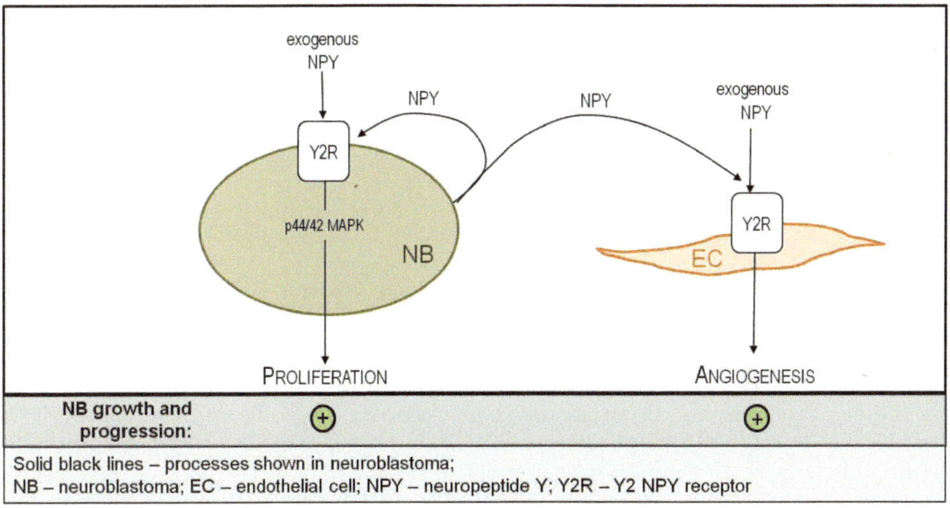

Fig. 5. Growth-promoting actions of NPY in neuroblastoma

6. Acetylcholine – the end stage of neuroblastoma differentiation

As described above, the most differentiated neuroblastomas exhibit cholinergic properties manifested by the expression of the proteins involved in synthesis and release of acetylcholine (Bourdeaut et al., 2009). Similar cholinergic features are acquired by neuroblastoma cells differentiated with retinoic acid (Handler et al., 2000). Neuroblastoma cells have also been shown to express functional muscarinic receptors of acetylcholine (M_1-M_5) (Baumgartner et al., 1993). Stimulation of serum-starved neuroblastoma cells with a non-specific muscarinic agonist, carbochol, resulted in an increase in their survival. This effect was mediated by M_3 muscarinic receptors and the p44/42 MAPK pathway (Fig. 6) (Greenwood & Dragunow, 2010). The pro-survival activity of muscarinic receptors can be further augmented by their ligand-dependent cross-talk with VEGFR2, which augments PI3K/Akt/mTOR pathway activation (Fig. 6) (Edelstein et al., 2011). Again, whether or not endogenous acetylcholine also serves as a survival factor for differentiating neuroblastomas and the role of other muscarinic receptors present in neuroblastoma cells, remains to be elucidated.

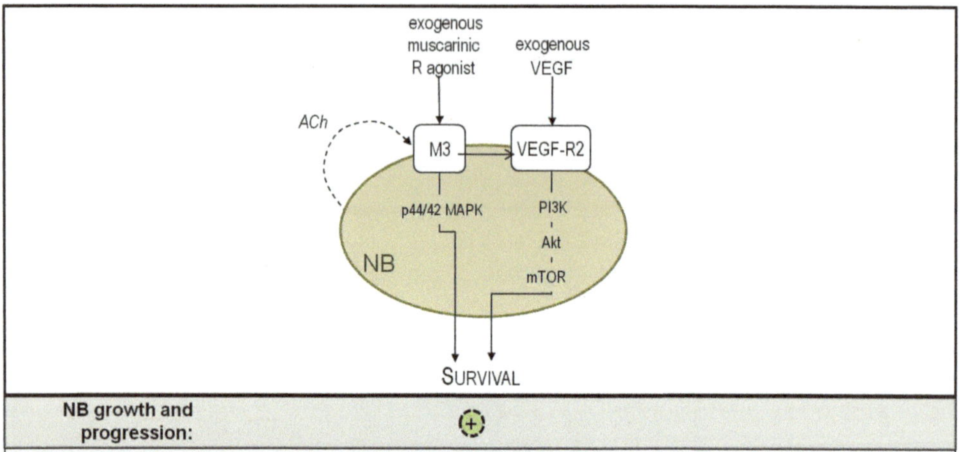

Solid black lines – processes shown in neuroblastoma;
Dashed lines, italic – putative pathways, which have not been proven to be active in neuroblastomas.
NB – neuroblastoma; EC – endothelial cell; ACh – acetylcholine.

Fig. 6. Potential effects of cholinergic stimulation on neuroblastoma growth

7. Conclusions

Neuroblastomas, along with pheochromocytomas, sympathetic nervous system-derived tumors of adulthood, are extremely rich in sympathetic neurotransmitters (Bourdeaut et al., 2009; Cohen et al., 1990; Dotsch et al., 1998; Grouzmann et al., 1989). They are also known to express their receptors, which creates functional autocrine loops (Baumgartner et al., 1993; Bawa-Khalfe et al., 2007; Kitlinska et al., 2005; Parsley et al., 1999). Sympathetic neurotransmitters, in turn, are known to be potent regulators of many processes involved in the regulation of tumor growth, such as cell proliferation, survival, migration and angiogenesis (Greenwood & Dragunow, 2010; Kitlinska et al., 2005; Laifenfeld et al., 2002; Lee et al., 2003b; Tilan & Kitlinska, 2010; Yaniv et al., 2008). Their involvement in the pathogenesis of neurological disorders and stress-induced exacerbation of various diseases has been well characterized (Thaker & Sood, 2008). Surprisingly, however, despite highly elevated levels of these neurotransmitters in sympathetic tumors, their functions in these malignancies have been underappreciated. Our recent studies on NPY and its growth-promoting effects brought the first definitive data proving the crucial role of endogenous sympathetic neurotransmitters in neuroblastoma biology and their potential value as targets in its therapy (Lu et al., 2010). Nevertheless, many seemingly obvious connections, such as the potential role of angiogenic activity of norepinephrine in neuroblastoma progression, have not been made.

8. References

Asada, M., Ebihara, S., Numachi, Y., Okazaki, T., Yamanda, S., Ikeda, K., Yasuda, H., Sora, I. & Arai, H. (2008). Reduced tumor growth in a mouse model of schizophrenia, lacking the dopamine transporter. Int J Cancer, 123, 3, (Aug 1), pp. 511-8

Bachetti, T., Di Paolo, D., Di Lascio, S., Mirisola, V., Brignole, C., Bellotti, M., Caffa, I., Ferraris, C., Fiore, M., Fornasari, D., Chiarle, R., Borghini, S., Pfeffer, U., Ponzoni,

M., Ceccherini, I. & Perri, P. (2010). PHOX2B-mediated regulation of ALK expression: in vitro identification of a functional relationship between two genes involved in neuroblastoma. PLoS One, 5, 10, pp. 13108

Bacic, F., Uematsu, S., McCarron, R.M. & Spatz, M. (1991). Dopaminergic receptors linked to adenylate cyclase in human cerebromicrovascular endothelium. J Neurochem, 57, 5, (Nov), pp. 1774-80

Basu, S., Nagy, J.A., Pal, S., Vasile, E., Eckelhoefer, I.A., Bliss, V.S., Manseau, E.J., Dasgupta, P.S., Dvorak, H.F. & Mukhopadhyay, D. (2001). The neurotransmitter dopamine inhibits angiogenesis induced by vascular permeability factor/vascular endothelial growth factor. Nat Med, 7, 5, (May), pp. 569-74

Baumgartner, M.K., Wei, J. & Aronstam, R.S. (1993). Retinoic acid-induced differentiation of a human neuroblastoma cell line alters muscarinic receptor expression. Brain Res Dev Brain Res, 72, 2, (Apr 16), pp. 305-8

Bawa-Khalfe, T., Altememi, G.F., Mandyam, C.D., Schwarz, L.A., Eikenburg, D.C. & Standifer, K.M. (2007). The presence of beta2-adrenoceptors sensitizes alpha2A-adrenoceptors to desensitization after chronic epinephrine treatment. BMC Pharmacol, 7, pp. 16

Bisaglia, M., Greggio, E., Maric, D., Miller, D.W., Cookson, M.R. & Bubacco, L. (2010). Alpha-synuclein overexpression increases dopamine toxicity in BE2-M17 cells. BMC Neurosci, 11, pp. 41

Borovsky, V., Herman, M., Dunphy, G., Caplea, A. & Ely, D. (1998). CO2 asphyxia increases plasma norepinephrine in rats via sympathetic nerves. Am J Physiol, 274, 1 Pt 2, (Jan), pp. R19-22

Bourdeaut, F., Janoueix-Lerosey, I., Lucchesi, C., Paris, R., Ribeiro, A., de Pontual, L., Amiel, J., Lyonnet, S., Pierron, G., Michon, J., Peuchmaur, M. & Delattre, O. (2009). Cholinergic switch associated with morphological differentiation in neuroblastoma. J Pathol, 219, 4, (Dec), pp. 463-72

Bourdeaut, F., Trochet, D., Janoueix-Lerosey, I., Ribeiro, A., Deville, A., Coz, C., Michiels, J.F., Lyonnet, S., Amiel, J. & Delattre, O. (2005). Germline mutations of the paired-like homeobox 2B (PHOX2B) gene in neuroblastoma. Cancer Lett, 228, 1-2, (Oct 18), pp. 51-8

Bowden, J.J. & Gibbins, I.L. (1992). Vasoactive intestinal peptide and neuropeptide Y coexist in non-noradrenergic sympathetic neurons to guinea pig trachea. J Auton Nerv Syst, 38, 1, (Apr), pp. 1-19

Chakroborty, D., Chowdhury, U.R., Sarkar, C., Baral, R., Dasgupta, P.S. & Basu, S. (2008). Dopamine regulates endothelial progenitor cell mobilization from mouse bone marrow in tumor vascularization. J Clin Invest, 118, 4, (Apr), pp. 1380-9

Chakroborty, D., Sarkar, C., Mitra, R.B., Banerjee, S., Dasgupta, P.S. & Basu, S. (2004). Depleted dopamine in gastric cancer tissues: dopamine treatment retards growth of gastric cancer by inhibiting angiogenesis. Clin Cancer Res, 10, 13, (Jul 1), pp. 4349-56

Chen, Y., Takita, J., Choi, Y.L., Kato, M., Ohira, M., Sanada, M., Wang, L., Soda, M., Kikuchi, A., Igarashi, T., Nakagawara, A., Hayashi, Y., Mano, H. & Ogawa, S. (2008). Oncogenic mutations of ALK kinase in neuroblastoma. Nature, 455, 7215, (Oct 16), pp. 971-4

Cohen, P.S., Cooper, M.J., Helman, L.J., Thiele, C.J., Seeger, R.C. & Israel, M.A. (1990). Neuropeptide Y expression in the developing adrenal gland and in childhood neuroblastoma tumors. Cancer Res, 50, 18, (Sep 15), pp. 6055-61

Damon, D.H. (2008). TH and NPY in sympathetic neurovascular cultures: role of LIF and NT-3. Am J Physiol Cell Physiol, 294, 1, (Jan), pp. C306-12

Davidson, D.F., Hammond, P.J., Murphy, D. & Carachi, R. (2011). Age-related medical decision limits for urinary free (unconjugated) metadrenalines, catecholamines and metabolites in random urine specimens from children. Ann Clin Biochem, 48, Pt 4, (Jul), pp. 358-66

Dotsch, J., Christiansen, H., Hanze, J., Lampert, F. & Rascher, W. (1998). Plasma neuropeptide Y of children with neuroblastoma in relation to stage, age and prognosis, and tissue neuropeptide Y. Regul Pept, 75-76, (Sep 25), pp. 185-90

Edelstein, J., Hao, T., Cao, Q., Morales, L. & Rockwell, P. (2011). Crosstalk between VEGFR2 and muscarinic receptors regulates the mTOR pathway in serum starved SK-N-SH human neuroblastoma cells. Cell Signal, 23, 1, (Jan), pp. 239-48

Edsjo, A., Holmquist, L. & Pahlman, S. (2007). Neuroblastoma as an experimental model for neuronal differentiation and hypoxia-induced tumor cell dedifferentiation. Semin Cancer Biol, 17, 3, (Jun), pp. 248-56

George, R.E., Sanda, T., Hanna, M., Frohling, S., Luther, W., 2nd, Zhang, J., Ahn, Y., Zhou, W., London, W.B., McGrady, P., Xue, L., Zozulya, S., Gregor, V.E., Webb, T.R., Gray, N.S., Gilliland, D.G., Diller, L., Greulich, H., Morris, S.W., Meyerson, M. & Look, A.T. (2008). Activating mutations in ALK provide a therapeutic target in neuroblastoma. Nature, 455, 7215, (Oct 16), pp. 975-8

Gimenez-Xavier, P., Francisco, R., Santidrian, A.F., Gil, J. & Ambrosio, S. (2009). Effects of dopamine on LC3-II activation as a marker of autophagy in a neuroblastoma cell model. Neurotoxicology, 30, 4, (Jul), pp. 658-65

Glebova, N.O. & Ginty, D.D. (2005). Growth and survival signals controlling sympathetic nervous system development. Annu Rev Neurosci, 28, pp. 191-222

Goldstein, D.S. (2003). Catecholamines and stress. Endocr Regul, 37, 2, (Jun), pp. 69-80

Greenwood, J.M. & Dragunow, M. (2010). M3 muscarinic receptors promote cell survival through activation of the extracellular regulated kinase (ERK1/2) pathway. Eur J Pharmacol, 640, 1-3, (Aug 25), pp. 38-45

Grouzmann, E., Comoy, E. & Bohuon, C. (1989). Plasma neuropeptide Y concentrations in patients with neuroendocrine tumors. J Clin Endocrinol Metab, 68, 4, (Apr), pp. 808-13

Handler, A., Lobo, M.D., Alonso, F.J., Paino, C.L. & Mena, M.A. (2000). Functional implications of the noradrenergic-cholinergic switch induced by retinoic acid in NB69 neuroblastoma cells. J Neurosci Res, 60, 3, (May 1), pp. 311-20

Hoehner, J.C., Gestblom, C., Hedborg, F., Sandstedt, B., Olsen, L. & Pahlman, S. (1996). A developmental model of neuroblastoma: differentiating stroma-poor tumors' progress along an extra-adrenal chromaffin lineage. Lab Invest, 75, 5, (Nov), pp. 659-75

Huber, K. (2006). The sympathoadrenal cell lineage: specification, diversification, and new perspectives. Dev Biol, 298, 2, (Oct 15), pp. 335-43

Itoh, T. & Omori, K. (1973). Biosynthesis and storage of catecholamines in pheochromocytoma and neuroblastoma cells. J Lab Clin Med, 81, 6, (Jun), pp. 889-96

Janoueix-Lerosey, I., Schleiermacher, G. & Delattre, O. (2010). Molecular pathogenesis of peripheral neuroblastic tumors. Oncogene, 29, 11, (Mar 18), pp. 1566-79

Jogi, A., Ora, I., Nilsson, H., Poellinger, L., Axelson, H. & Pahlman, S. (2003). Hypoxia-induced dedifferentiation in neuroblastoma cells. Cancer Lett, 197, 1-2, (Jul 18), pp. 145-50

Junn, E. & Mouradian, M.M. (2001). Apoptotic signaling in dopamine-induced cell death: the role of oxidative stress, p38 mitogen-activated protein kinase, cytochrome c and caspases. J Neurochem, 78, 2, (Jul), pp. 374-83

Kitlinska, J., Abe, K., Kuo, L., Pons, J., Yu, M., Li, L., Tilan, J., Everhart, L., Lee, E.W., Zukowska, Z. & Toretsky, J.A. (2005). Differential effects of neuropeptide Y on the growth and vascularization of neural crest-derived tumors. Cancer Res, 65, 5, (Mar 1), pp. 1719-28

Kogner, P., Bjork, O. & Theodorsson, E. (1994). Plasma neuropeptide Y in healthy children: influence of age, anaesthesia and the establishment of an age-adjusted reference interval. Acta Paediatr, 83, 4, (Apr), pp. 423-7

Korner, M., Waser, B. & Reubi, J.C. (2004). High expression of neuropeptide y receptors in tumors of the human adrenal gland and extra-adrenal paraganglia. Clin Cancer Res, 10, 24, (Dec 15), pp. 8426-33

Kume, T., Kawato, Y., Osakada, F., Izumi, Y., Katsuki, H., Nakagawa, T., Kaneko, S., Niidome, T., Takada-Takatori, Y. & Akaike, A. (2008). Dibutyryl cyclic AMP induces differentiation of human neuroblastoma SH-SY5Y cells into a noradrenergic phenotype. Neurosci Lett, 443, 3, (Oct 10), pp. 199-203

Laifenfeld, D., Klein, E. & Ben-Shachar, D. (2002). Norepinephrine alters the expression of genes involved in neuronal sprouting and differentiation: relevance for major depression and antidepressant mechanisms. J Neurochem, 83, 5, (Dec), pp. 1054-64

Lee, E.W., Grant, D.S., Movafagh, S. & Zukowska, Z. (2003a). Impaired angiogenesis in neuropeptide Y (NPY)-Y2 receptor knockout mice. Peptides, 24, 1, (Jan), pp. 99-106

Lee, E.W., Michalkiewicz, M., Kitlinska, J., Kalezic, I., Switalska, H., Yoo, P., Sangkharat, A., Ji, H., Li, L., Michalkiewicz, T., Ljubisavljevic, M., Johansson, H., Grant, D.S. & Zukowska, Z. (2003b). Neuropeptide Y induces ischemic angiogenesis and restores function of ischemic skeletal muscles. J Clin Invest, 111, 12, (Jun), pp. 1853-62

Lindgren, H.S., Ohlin, K.E. & Cenci, M.A. (2009). Differential involvement of D1 and D2 dopamine receptors in L-DOPA-induced angiogenic activity in a rat model of Parkinson's disease. Neuropsychopharmacology, 34, 12, (Nov), pp. 2477-88

Lopes, F.M., Schroder, R., da Frota, M.L., Jr., Zanotto-Filho, A., Muller, C.B., Pires, A.S., Meurer, R.T., Colpo, G.D., Gelain, D.P., Kapczinski, F., Moreira, J.C., Fernandes Mda, C. & Klamt, F. (2010). Comparison between proliferative and neuron-like SH-SY5Y cells as an in vitro model for Parkinson disease studies. Brain Res, 1337, (Jun 14), pp. 85-94

Lu, C., Everhart, L., Tilan, J., Kuo, L., Sun, C.C., Munivenkatappa, R.B., Jonsson-Rylander, A.C., Sun, J., Kuan-Celarier, A., Li, L., Abe, K., Zukowska, Z., Toretsky, J.A. & Kitlinska, J. (2010). Neuropeptide Y and its Y2 receptor: potential targets in neuroblastoma therapy. Oncogene, 29, 41, (Oct 14), pp. 5630-42

Lu, C., Pelech, S., Zhang, H., Bond, J., Spach, K., Noubade, R., Blankenhorn, E.P. & Teuscher, C. (2008). Pertussis toxin induces angiogenesis in brain microvascular endothelial cells. J Neurosci Res, 86, 12, (Sep), pp. 2624-40

Maris, J.M. (2010). Recent advances in neuroblastoma. N Engl J Med, 362, 23, (Jun 10), pp. 2202-11

Matsushima, H. & Bogenmann, E. (1990). Nerve growth factor (NGF) induces neuronal differentiation in neuroblastoma cells transfected with the NGF receptor cDNA. Mol Cell Biol, 10, 9, (Sep), pp. 5015-20

Monaghan, T.K., Mackenzie, C.J., Plevin, R. & Lutz, E.M. (2008). PACAP-38 induces neuronal differentiation of human SH-SY5Y neuroblastoma cells via cAMP-mediated activation of ERK and p38 MAP kinases. J Neurochem, 104, 1, (Jan), pp. 74-88

Monsaingeon, M., Perel, Y., Simonnet, G. & Corcuff, J.B. (2003). Comparative values of catecholamines and metabolites for the diagnosis of neuroblastoma. Eur J Pediatr, 162, 6, (Jun), pp. 397-402

Mosse, Y.P., Laudenslager, M., Longo, L., Cole, K.A., Wood, A., Attiyeh, E.F., Laquaglia, M.J., Sennett, R., Lynch, J.E., Perri, P., Laureys, G., Speleman, F., Kim, C., Hou, C., Hakonarson, H., Torkamani, A., Schork, N.J., Brodeur, G.M., Tonini, G.P., Rappaport, E., Devoto, M. & Maris, J.M. (2008). Identification of ALK as a major familial neuroblastoma predisposition gene. Nature, 455, 7215, (Oct 16), pp. 930-5

Movafagh, S., Hobson, J.P., Spiegel, S., Kleinman, H.K. & Zukowska, Z. (2006). Neuropeptide Y induces migration, proliferation, and tube formation of endothelial cells bimodally via Y1, Y2, and Y5 receptors. Faseb J, 20, 11, (Sep), pp. 1924-6

Nilsson, M.B., Armaiz-Pena, G., Takahashi, R., Lin, Y.G., Trevino, J., Li, Y., Jennings, N., Arevalo, J., Lutgendorf, S.K., Gallick, G.E., Sanguino, A.M., Lopez-Berestein, G., Cole, S.W. & Sood, A.K. (2007). Stress hormones regulate interleukin-6 expression by human ovarian carcinoma cells through a Src-dependent mechanism. J Biol Chem, 282, 41, (Oct 12), pp. 29919-26

Pahlman, S., Meyerson, G., Lindgren, E., Schalling, M. & Johansson, I. (1991). Insulin-like growth factor I shifts from promoting cell division to potentiating maturation during neuronal differentiation. Proc Natl Acad Sci U S A, 88, 22, (Nov 15), pp. 9994-8

Pahlman, S., Odelstad, L., Larsson, E., Grotte, G. & Nilsson, K. (1981). Phenotypic changes of human neuroblastoma cells in culture induced by 12-O-tetradecanoyl-phorbol-13-acetate. Int J Cancer, 28, 5, (Nov 15), pp. 583-9

Parsley, S., Gazi, L., Bobirnac, I., Loetscher, E. & Schoeffter, P. (1999). Functional alpha2C-adrenoceptors in human neuroblastoma SH-SY5Y cells. Eur J Pharmacol, 372, 1, (May 7), pp. 109-15

Prasad, K.N., Cole, W.C., Yan, X.D., Nahreini, P., Kumar, B., Hanson, A. & Prasad, J.E. (2003). Defects in cAMP-pathway may initiate carcinogenesis in dividing nerve cells: a review. Apoptosis, 8, 6, (Dec), pp. 579-86

Revoltella, R.P. & Butler, R.H. (1980). Nerve growth factor may stimulate either division or differentiation of cloned C1300 neuroblastoma cells in serum-free cultures. J Cell Physiol, 104, 1, (Jul), pp. 27-33

Reynolds, C.P. & Perez-Polo, J.R. (1981). Induction of neurite outgrowth in the IMR-32 human neuroblastoma cell line by nerve growth factor. J Neurosci Res, 6, 3, pp. 319-25

Rodriguez-Martin, E., Casarejos, M.J., Bazan, E., Canals, S., Herranz, A.S. & Mena, M.A. (2000). Nitric oxide induces differentiation in the NB69 human catecholamine-rich cell line. Neuropharmacology, 39, 11, (Aug 23), pp. 2090-100

Sarkar, C., Chakroborty, D., Chowdhury, U.R., Dasgupta, P.S. & Basu, S. (2008). Dopamine increases the efficacy of anticancer drugs in breast and colon cancer preclinical models. Clin Cancer Res, 14, 8, (Apr 15), pp. 2502-10

Sarkar, C., Chakroborty, D., Mitra, R.B., Banerjee, S., Dasgupta, P.S. & Basu, S. (2004). Dopamine in vivo inhibits VEGF-induced phosphorylation of VEGFR-2, MAPK, and focal adhesion kinase in endothelial cells. Am J Physiol Heart Circ Physiol, 287, 4, (Oct), pp. H1554-60

Sidell, N. (1982). Retinoic acid-induced growth inhibition and morphologic differentiation of human neuroblastoma cells in vitro. J Natl Cancer Inst, 68, 4, (Apr), pp. 589-96

Strenger, V., Kerbl, R., Dornbusch, H.J., Ladenstein, R., Ambros, P.F., Ambros, I.M. & Urban, C. (2007). Diagnostic and prognostic impact of urinary catecholamines in neuroblastoma patients. Pediatr Blood Cancer, 48, 5, (May), pp. 504-9

Thaker, P.H., Han, L.Y., Kamat, A.A., Arevalo, J.M., Takahashi, R., Lu, C., Jennings, N.B., Armaiz-Pena, G., Bankson, J.A., Ravoori, M., Merritt, W.M., Lin, Y.G., Mangala, L.S., Kim, T.J., Coleman, R.L., Landen, C.N., Li, Y., Felix, E., Sanguino, A.M., Newman, R.A., Lloyd, M., Gershenson, D.M., Kundra, V., Lopez-Berestein, G., Lutgendorf, S.K., Cole, S.W. & Sood, A.K. (2006). Chronic stress promotes tumor growth and angiogenesis in a mouse model of ovarian carcinoma. Nat Med, 12, 8, (Aug), pp. 939-44

Thaker, P.H. & Sood, A.K. (2008). Neuroendocrine influences on cancer biology. Semin Cancer Biol, 18, 3, (Jun), pp. 164-70

Tilan, J. & Kitlinska, J. (2010). Sympathetic Neurotransmitters and Tumor Angiogenesis-Link between Stress and Cancer Progression. J Oncol, 2010, pp. 539706

Vinci, M.C., Bellik, L., Filippi, S., Ledda, F. & Parenti, A. (2007). Trophic effects induced by alpha1D-adrenoceptors on endothelial cells are potentiated by hypoxia. Am J Physiol Heart Circ Physiol, 293, 4, (Oct), pp. H2140-7

Wei, J.S., Greer, B.T., Westermann, F., Steinberg, S.M., Son, C.G., Chen, Q.R., Whiteford, C.C., Bilke, S., Krasnoselsky, A.L., Cenacchi, N., Catchpoole, D., Berthold, F., Schwab, M. & Khan, J. (2004). Prediction of clinical outcome using gene expression profiling and artificial neural networks for patients with neuroblastoma. Cancer Res, 64, 19, (Oct 1), pp. 6883-91

Wong, H.P., Yu, L., Lam, E.K., Tai, E.K., Wu, W.K. & Cho, C.H. (2007). Nicotine promotes colon tumor growth and angiogenesis through beta-adrenergic activation. Toxicol Sci, 97, 2, (Jun), pp. 279-87

Yang, E.V., Kim, S.J., Donovan, E.L., Chen, M., Gross, A.C., Webster Marketon, J.I., Barsky, S.H. & Glaser, R. (2009). Norepinephrine upregulates VEGF, IL-8, and IL-6 expression in human melanoma tumor cell lines: implications for stress-related enhancement of tumor progression. Brain Behav Immun, 23, 2, (Feb), pp. 267-75

Yang, E.V., Sood, A.K., Chen, M., Li, Y., Eubank, T.D., Marsh, C.B., Jewell, S., Flavahan, N.A., Morrison, C., Yeh, P.E., Lemeshow, S. & Glaser, R. (2006). Norepinephrine up-regulates the expression of vascular endothelial growth factor, matrix metalloproteinase (MMP)-2, and MMP-9 in nasopharyngeal carcinoma tumor cells. Cancer Res, 66, 21, (Nov 1), pp. 10357-64

Yang, Z.R. & Chou, K.C. (2004). Bio-support vector machines for computational proteomics. Bioinformatics, 20, 5, (Mar 22), pp. 735-41

Yaniv, S.P., Ben-Shachar, D. & Klein, E. (2008). Norepinephrine-glucocorticoids interaction does not annul the opposite effects of the individual treatments on cellular plasticity in neuroblastoma cells. Eur J Pharmacol, 596, 1-3, (Oct 31), pp. 14-24

Yaniv, S.P., Lucki, A., Klein, E. & Ben-Shachar, D. (2010). Dexamethasone enhances the norepinephrine-induced ERK/MAPK intracellular pathway possibly via dysregulation of the alpha2-adrenergic receptor: implications for antidepressant drug mechanism of action. Eur J Cell Biol, 89, 9, (Sep), pp. 712-22

Zambrano, E. & Reyes-Mugica, M. (2002). Hormonal activity may predict aggressive behavior in neuroblastoma. Pediatr Dev Pathol, 5, 2, (Mar-Apr), pp. 190-9

Zukowska-Grojec, Z., Karwatowska-Prokopczuk, E., Rose, W., Rone, J., Movafagh, S., Ji, H., Yeh, Y., Chen, W.T., Kleinman, H.K., Grouzmann, E. & Grant, D.S. (1998). Neuropeptide Y: a novel angiogenic factor from the sympathetic nerves and endothelium. Circ Res, 83, 2, (Jul 27), pp. 187-95

Part 3

Neuroblastoma,
Therapeutic Targets - Present and Future

10

The Different Faces of Angiogenesis in Neuroblastoma

Pietro Luigi Poliani[1] and Domenico Ribatti[2]
[1]*Department of Pathology, University of Brescia, Brescia*
[2]*Department of Human Anatomy, University of Bari, Bari*
Italy

1. Introduction

Neuroblastoma represents one of the most frequent solid tumour of childhood, arising along the sympathetic nervous system, most frequently in the adrenal gland. Clinically, neuroblastoma is an heterogeneous entity and prognosis vary widely according to different biological variables (such as DNA ploidy and MYCN amplification), patient age, anatomical location and tumour stage at diagnosis (Maris et al., 2002; Schwab et al., 2003). Unfortunately, the majority of patients show systemic disease at the time of diagnosis, with rapid tumour progression and fatal outcome. According to this clinical heterogeneity, the International Pathology Classification System has identified a broad spectrum of different histological features, ranging from undifferentiated/poorly differentiated to differentiating/fully differentiated lesions, with progressive increase in the Schwannian component and differentiation of neuroblastic cells towards a mature ganglionic phenotype (Shimada et al., 1999; Cohn et al., 2009). Of note, as others paediatric tumours, neuroblastoma displays the capacity to undergo spontaneous regression and/or differentiation into benign fully mature lesions, with increase of Schwannian stroma and differentiating/differentiated neuroblasts, that biologically resemble ganglion cells, directly correlated with tumour maturation and better prognosis (Ambros et al., 2002; Haas et al., 1988). Indeed, differentiating and well-differentiated neuroblastic lesions with low mitosis/karyorrhexis index are classified by International Neuroblastoma Pathology Classification consensus as tumours associated with a better prognosis and a higher rate of cure (Peuchmaur et al., 2003; Shimada et al., 1999).

The role of angiogenesis in tumour growth and progression represents a major subject in modern oncology. It is generally accepted that angiogenesis promotes tumour growth and is essential for invasion of surrounding tissues and metastasis. Angiogenesis is tidily regulated by the balance of numerous pro-angiogenic and anti-angiogenic factors. Tumours that fail to recruit new blood vessels remain dormant while tumours characterized by prominent neo-angiogenesis growth faster and display an aggressive behaviour (Carmeliet et al., 2003; Ribatti et al., 1999). A large variety of pro-angiogenic factors have been identified so far to play an important role in the induction of angiogenesis in neuroblastic lesions, including vascular endothelial growth factor (VEGF), interleukin-8 (IL-8), fibroblast growth factor-2 (FGF-2), and angiopoietins (Eggert et al., 2000; Ribatti et al., 1998). High vascular index in neuroblastoma have been demonstrated to correlate with poor prognosis, suggesting a tide correlation between aggressive tumour behaviour and active angiogenesis (Katzenstein et al., 2000). These observations point out to an important role of promising emerging anti-angiogenic strategies for the treatment of neuroblastoma, a lesion characterized by a high degree of vascularity (Pastorino et al., 2009; Marimpietri et al., 2007; Ribatti et al., 2005; Rossler et al., 2008). In this review the recent findings in neuroblastoma angiogenesis as well as the most recent advances in the development of novel anti-angiogenetic approaches in the treatment of neuroblastoma will be discussed.

However, although it has been well established that angiogenesis in neuroblastoma correlates with tumour progression, advanced stages and worst prognosis (Carmeliet et al., 2003), little is known about the role of angiogenesis in the maturation phase of undifferentiated neuroblastomas towards a more differentiated phenotype. As previously described, neuroblastic lesions show a wide spectrum of histological variability that reflects different steps of tumour maturation, whose molecular mechanisms are not still fully understood. Recent findings have suggested that the same molecular pathways driving the development of normal neuroectodermal-derived tissues might also be involved in neuroblastoma maturation (Christiansen et al., 2000; Hoehner et al., 1998). Between these, angiogenesis plays a key role during neural differentiation, exerting a trophic activity (Ribatti et al., 2007; Kitlinska et al., 2005). In line with these observations, recent findings have shown that specific angiogenetic pathways play a crucial role during the maturation phase of neuroblastic tumours and contribute to neuroblast maturation (Poliani et al., 2007).

Finally, it has been suggested that cross-talk between Schwann cells and neuroblasts influences the biology and clinical behaviour of neuroblastic tumours (Kwiatkowski et al., 1998). Schwannian stroma rich tumours have been shown to have low vascularity, suggesting that Schwann cells may influence neuroblast biology by producing soluble factors capable of inducing neuroblast differentiation and inhibiting tumour neo-angiogenesis (Ambros et al., 1996).

These observations indicate a different role of different angiogenetic pathways in neuroblastoma, with some of them mimicking physiological steps leading to maturation of vasculature in developing normal neuroectodermal-derived tissues, thus contributing to the maturation stage of neuroblastic tumours, and others that sustain tumour neo-angiogenesis and contribute to tumour aggressiveness and progression.

In conclusions, this review will focus on the most recent advances in the field of angiogenesis in neuroblastic lesions keeping in mind that understanding the mechanisms of angiogenesis will provide the basis for a rational and targeted approach to the development of specific treatments targeting tumour angiogenesis or promoting neuroblastic maturation in patients affected by neuroblastoma.

2. Role of angiogenesis in tumour growth and progression

During solid tumour development, an avascular phase precede the fully active vascular phase. Assuming that tumour development is dependent on angiogenesis and that this depends on the release of angiogenic factors, the acquisition of an angiogenic ability can be considered as an expression of progression from neoplastic transformation to tumour growth and metastasis (Ribatti et al., 1999). The avascular phase appears to correspond to a small colony of neoplastic cells that reaches a steady state before proliferation and acquisition of an invasive behaviour. In fact, dormant tumours can been found during autopsies of individuals who died of causes other than cancer (Black & Welch, 1993). Moreover, in situ carcinomas are a frequent finding in individuals aged 50 to 70 years who died of trauma, but are diagnosed in only 0.1% of patients during life. Malignant tumours can grow beyond the critical size of 2 mm at their site of origin by exploiting the host's pre-existing vessels. These finding support the notion that only a very small subset of dormant tumours enters the vascular phase and rapidly progress.

The role of angiogenesis in tumour growth has become evident thanks to a series of studies demonstrating that tumour progression is clearly related to the degree of angiogenesis, as seen in different types of tumours, including neuroblastoma. In fact, high vascular density and active angiogenesis in neuroblastoma have been shown to correlate with poor prognosis and tumour progression (Ribatti et al., 2004).

Tumour angiogenesis is strictly linked to the switch in the balance between positive and negative regulators, and mainly depends on the release by neoplastic cells of specific growth factors for endothelial cells, that stimulate the growth of the host's blood vessels or the down-regulation of natural angiogenic inhibitors. In normal tissues, vascular quiescence is maintained by the dominant influence of endogenous angiogenic inhibitors over angiogenic stimuli. This switch depends on increased production of one or more positive regulators of angiogenesis, such as vascular endothelial growth factor (VEGF), fibroblast growth factor-2 (FGF-2), IL-8, placental growth factor (PlGF), transforming growth factor-β (TGF-β), platelet derived growth factor (PDGF), pleiotrophins and others. These factors can be directly produced by tumour cells, mobilized from the extracellular matrix, or released from host cells recruited to the tumour. The switch clearly involves more than a simple up-regulation of angiogenic activity and has thus been regarded as the result of the net balance between positive and negative regulators (Ribatti et al., 2007).

Considerable differences exist between normal and tumour vasculature. Tumour endothelial cells may divide up to 50 times more frequently than normal endothelial cells and are qualified by peculiar molecular and morphological features, mostly related to an immature phenotype. This immaturity of tumour vessels led H. Dvorak to define a tumour as "a wound that never heals" (Dvorak, 1986).

Moreover, although the tumour vasculature originates from the host vessels engaging similar angiogenetic mechanisms, the organization may differ dramatically depending on the tumour type and location and tumour-associated blood vessels display many structural and functional abnormalities (Ribatti et al., 2006). Their unusual leakage, rapid growth and remodelling capacity, along with the expression of distinctive surface molecules, mediate the dissemination of neoplastic cells into the bloodstream and contribute to maintain the tumour microenvironment. Similar to normal blood vessels, tumour vasculature consists of endothelial cells, pericytes and their enveloping basement membrane. Common features, regardless of their origin, size and growth pattern, include the absence of an hierarchy, the formation of large-caliber sinusoidal vessels and a markedly heterogeneous density.

A complex interrelationship has also been described between tumour hypoxia and tumour angiogenesis. Hypoxia in tumours develops both as chronic hypoxia, resulting from long diffusion distances between tumour vessels, and/or acute hypoxia, resulting from a transient collapse of tumour vessels. Most of the solid tumours contain a hypoxic microenvironment, a condition that is associated with poor prognosis and resistance to treatment. Of note, the production of important angiogenic factors, such as FGF-2, VEGF, TGF-β , TNF- β and IL-8, is regulated by hypoxia. Accordingly, VEGF-mRNA expression is rapidly and reversibly induced by exposure of cultured endothelial cells to low PO_2 (Levy et al., 1995).

There are also increasing evidences that stromal cells as well as inflammatory cells within the tumour, such as lymphocytes, neutrophils, macrophages and mast cells, cooperate with endothelial and cancer cells in promoting angiogenesis, by mean of the production of different growth factors and proteases (Parket et al., 2000).

Finally, it is increasingly recognized that oncogenes, such as mutated RAS or SRC, may also contribute to tumour angiogenesis by enhancing the production of pro-angiogenic factors, such as VEGF and inhibitors of angiogenesis such as thrombospondin-1 (TSP-1) (Rak et al., 1995; Ellis et al., 1998). In line with these observations it has been demonstrated that down-regulation of RAS-oncogene in a melanoma driven by doxycycline-inducible ras led to tumour regression within 12 days (Tang et al., 2005) and that cells expressing low levels of RAS remain dormant and non-angiogenic, whereas cells expressing high levels of RAS produce a full-blown tumours with marked up-regulation of TSP-1 levels (Watnick et al., 2003).

3. Role of angiogenesis in the maturation phase of neuroblastic lesions

As described previously a correlation between angiogenesis and poor outcome in human neuroblastomas have been demonstrated (Eggert et al., 2000; Ribatti et al., 2001; Ribatti et al., 2002; Ribatti et al., 2004). However, little is known about the role of angiogenesis in the maturation of undifferentiated neuroblasts towards a mature ganglionic phenotype. In fact, as others paediatric tumours, neuroblastoma displays the capacity to undergo spontaneous regression in infants and/or differentiation into benign ganglioneuroma in older patients (Pritchard et al., 1994; Maris et al., 2002). This peculiarity reflects the wide spectrum of histological variability within the neuroblastic tumours, ranging from undifferentiated to differentiating or fully differentiated lesions (Figure 1, Panel A). Moreover, along with young age (<18 months) and localized disease, differentiation has been strongly correlated to a better prognosis (Ambros et al., 1996). Spontaneous or treatment-induced maturation characterizes a subgroup of neuroblastomas and constitutes the basis for maturation targeting therapies, such as retinoic acid treatment (Ferrari-Toninelli et al., 2010; Matthay et al., 1999; Mora et al., 2004; Giannini et al., 2000). Nevertheless, the molecular mechanisms that drive maturation of neuroblastic lesions are still poorly understood. Schwannian stroma cells have been claimed to be implicated in differentiation of neuroblastomas (Coco et al., 2005; Ambros et al., 1996) as well as a large variety of transcriptional factors and different genes involved in neural development and differentiation of normal neuroectodermal-derived tissues (Hoehner et al. 1998; Kitlinska et al., 2005; Ferrari-Toninelli et al., 2010; Christiansen et al., 2000; Koppen et al., 2008). Gene expression profiles studies recently allowed to identify genes differentially expressed between undifferentiated and differentiated neuroblastic lesions. These studies led to the identification of different molecular patterns of differentiation, ranging from undifferentiated pre-adrenergic/adrenergic neuroblastomas with frequent MYCN amplification to cholinergic-committed or fully cholinergic neuroblastomas that may reflect a fully differentiated phenotype (Bourdeaut et al., 2009).

Angiogenesis has been described to plays a key role during neural differentiation, exerting a trophic activity and promoting the maturation of vasculature in developing normal neuronal tissue (Kitlinska et al., 2005). We have recently described that the human carcinoembryonic antigen-related cell adhesion molecule 1 (CEACAM1), a transmembrane glycoprotein that belongs to the carcinoembryonic antigen (CEA) gene family, is peculiarly expressed in the microvessels among differentiating neuroblastic/ganglion cells and is related to the tumour maturation (Poliani et al., 2007). CEACAM1 exerts a large variety of biological functions, including a strong pro-angiogenic role during the activation phase of angiogenesis, being expressed in the developing immature blood vessels of both in newly normal formed vessels and in different tumours (Wagener et al., 2000; Volpert et al., 2002). Microvascular endothelial cells over-expressing CEACAM1 show up-regulation of various angiogenic factors, including VEGF, angiopoietins and IL-8, indicating that CEACAM1 expression in endothelial cells switches them to an angiogenic phenotype, a mechanism active during the formation of new vessels in physiological conditions such as wound healing and embryonic development, but silent in endothelial cells of large mature quiescent vessels (Wagener et al., 2000). Accordingly, CEACAM1 has been found to be expressed transiently in the microvessels of the developing central nervous system (Sawa et al., 1994), suggesting a role in the induction of capillary formation during tissue development rather than in the maintenance of mature vasculature. Interestingly, CEACAM1 have been also found to be expressed in microvessels of the normal adrenal gland, particularly during fetal development (Figure 1, Panel B). We have investigated the role of CEACAM1/VEGF-mediated angiogenesis in neuroblastic tumours at different stages of maturation, demonstrating that CEACAM1 is transiently expressed in microvessels among differentiating neuroblast/ganglion cells whereas it is completely absent in poorly differentiated/undifferentiated tumours as well as in fully mature ganglioneuromas. Interestingly, strong VEGF expression was observed in differentiating neuroblast/ganglion cells adjacent to CEACAM1 positive microvessels (Figure 1, Panel C). In contrast, CEACAM1 is not expressed in poorly differentiated/undifferentiated neuroblastomas, characterized by high levels of VEGF and VEGFR (FLK-1), in keeping with several studies reporting the association of VEGF expression with tumour aggressiveness and a poor prognosis (Backman et al., 2002; Eggert et al., 2000) and suggesting that in poorly differentiated/undifferentiated lesions VEGF expression is independent from CEACAM1 and may follow different molecular pathways. Accordingly, we have also demonstrated that conditioned medium from human neuroblastoma SH-SY5Y cell lines collected at different stages of differentiation caused a progressive in vitro up-regulation of CEACAM1 expression in human umbilical vein endothelial cells (Poliani et al., 2007).

Overall, our data indicate a crucial role of CEACAM1/VEGF mediated angiogenesis during the maturation phase of neuroblastic tumours, mimicking physiologic events leading to maturation of vasculature in developing neuroectodermal-derived tissues. Endothelial up-regulation of CEACAM-1 activate angiogenesis via increased expression of VEGF in neuroblastic cells triggering an angiogenic cascade that promote and maintain VEGF induced angiogenesis. This feature could be involved in the complex mechanism driving the switch from immature to differentiating forms of neuroblastomas. Conversely, in poorly differentiated/undifferentiated neuroblastomas the VEGF sustained angiogenesis does not reproduce physiological steps, it is associated with tumour aggressiveness and may involve other molecular pathways.

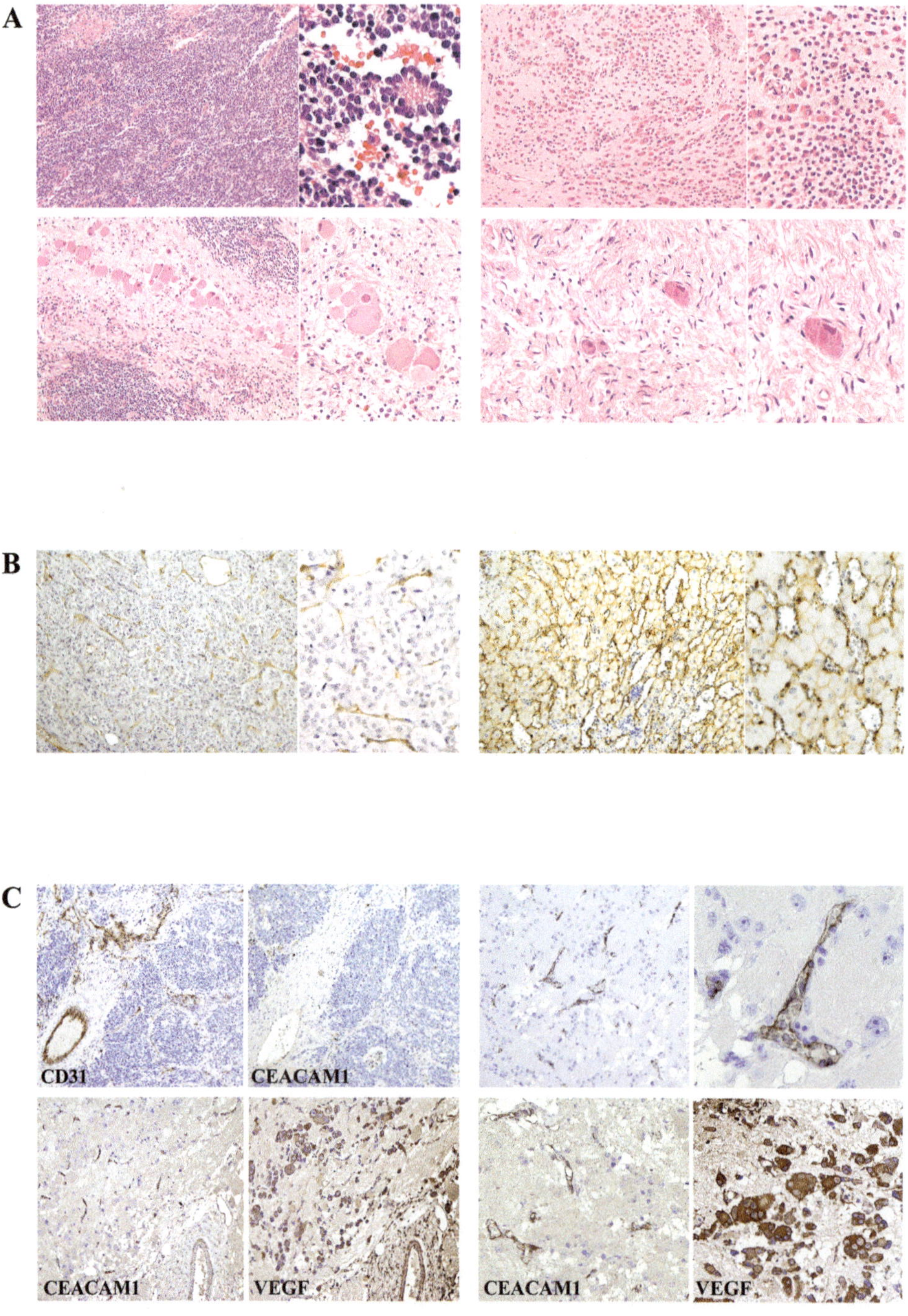

Fig. 1. Histological variants of neuroblastic tumours and CEACAM1/VEGF expression.

Panel A: neuroblastic lesions show a wide spectrum of different histological variants reflecting different maturation phases, ranging from undifferentiated/poorly differentiated neuroblastomas with neuronal rosettes (upper left images), differentiating lesions with larger cells acquiring a ganglionic phenotype (upper right images), mixed lesions (ganglioneuroblastomas) with both immature and fully mature ganglionic cells (lower left panels) and fully differentiated lesions with mature ganglion cells and progressive increase in the Schwannian component (lower right panels). *Panel B:* CEACAM1 is only weakly expressed in the microvessels of normal adult adrenal gland (left images) while strong and diffuse expression is present in the developing microvessels of normal fetal adrenal gland (right images). *Panel C:* Serial sections from a representative case of undifferentiated neuroblastoma showing no expression of CEACAM1 in the tumour vessels that stain positive for CD31 (upper left images). On the contrary, differentiating neuroblastomas show CEACAM1-positive microvessels adjacent to differentiating neuroblastic/ganglion cells (upper right images). Serial tissue sections from a representative case of differentiating neuroblastoma show CEACAM1-positive microvessels adjacent to VEGF-positive differentiating neuroblastic cells (lower images, on the right a detail at higher magnification).

4. Role of Schwann cells in angiogenesis

As previously described, neuroblastic lesions exhibits a large variety of histological features reflecting the different steps of tumour maturation, ranging from immature neuroblastoma, with small undifferentiated neuroblasts with scarce Schwannian stroma, to progressively maturing neuroblastomas composed of larger neuroblastic/ganglion-like cells with abundant Schwannian stroma. Diagnostic categories of Schwannian stroma-rich/dominant tumours include mature and maturing ganglioneuroma and ganglioneuroblastoma of intermixed and nodular type. Categories of Schwannian stroma-poor neuroblastoma tumours include differentiating, poorly differentiated and undifferentiated (Shimada et al., 1999). Importantly, the increasing presence of Schwannian stroma and differentiating/differentiated neuroblasts, that biologically resemble ganglion cells, directly correlates with tumour maturation and better prognosis, with the exception of nodular ganglioneuroblastoma, (Peuchmaur et al., 2003; Nagoshi et al., 1992).

Interestingly, in addition to a more differentiated phenotype, Schwannian stroma rich tumours also display low vascularity (Meitar et al., 1996). A correlation between low vascular density and absence of microvascular proliferation in Schwannian stroma-rich tumours have been demonstrated (Peddinti et al., 2007). On the contrary, high vascular index and abnormal blood vessels have been associated to clinical aggressiveness in Schwannian stroma-poor neuroblastoma tumours (Meitar et al., 1996; Peddinti et al., 2007).

This association between abundant Schwannian stroma, neuronal differentiation and decrease vascularity had led to the hypothesis that Schwann cells may secrete soluble factors capable of inducing neuroblast differentiation and inhibit angiogenesis (Huang et al., 2000). In fact, Schwann cells have been shown to secrete potent angiogenesis inhibitors, such as secreted protein acid rich in cysteine (SPARC) and pigment epithelium-derived factor

(PEDF) (Chlenski et al., 2002; Crawford et al., 2001). Moreover, angiogenesis is inhibited in neuroblastoma xenograft model in which mouse Schwann cells were induced to infiltrate the tumour by engrafting neuroblastoma cells in the sciatic nerve of nude mice (Liu et al., 2005). Moreover, significantly higher number of cancer-associated fibroblasts have been demonstrated in Schwannian stroma-poor tumours compared to Schwannian stroma rich/dominant ganglioneuroblastomas/ganglioneuromas, consistent with the established pro-angiogenic function of cancer-associated fibroblasts (Zeine et al., 2009).

5. Novel treatments targeting angiogenesis

It has been already discussed in the previous paragraphs that high vascularity is a peculiar feature of neuroblastoma and promote tumour growth and aggressiveness. A large spectrum of angiogenic factors, including VEGF, have been reported to be expressed in neuroblastomas. Understanding the key mechanisms promoting angiogenesis in neuroblastoma represent a clue step in the development of effective anti-angiogenic strategies. The following paragraphs will aid to summarize the state of the art of the most current and experimental anti-angiogenic strategies in the treatment of neuroblastoma.

5.1 Retinoids

Retinoic acid has been shown to induce neuroblastoma maturation throughout different molecular pathways (Ferrari-Toninelli, 2010). In patients after autologous stem cell transplantation retinoic acid has been introduced as a maintenance treatment (Matthay et al., 1999). The synthetic retinoid N-(4-hydroxyphenyl) retinamide (fenretinide, HPR) inhibits human neuroblastoma cell growth through the induction of programmed cell death (Ponzoni et al., 1995). The contribution of retinoic acid in the control of tumour angiogenesis has been recently demonstrated. HPR inhibits angiogenesis induced by neuroblastoma specimens implanted onto the chorioallantoic membrane (CAM) (Ribatti et al., 2001). Moreover, retinoic acid have been also shown to induce expression of the endogenous angiogenesis inhibitor TSP-1 (Castle et al., 1992).

5.2 TNP-470

TNP-470 treatment have been shown to induce a reduction of tumour growth and microvascular density in mouse model xenograft of poorly differentiated human neuroblastoma cell line SHSY5Y. Moreover, TNP 470 treatment improved animal survival and reduced tumour growth of primary and metastatic murine neuroblastoma (Nagabuchi et al., 1997). Interestingly, TNP-470 also effectively inhibits neuroblastoma growth in animals with minimal disease treated before tumour were clinically apparent after subcutaneous injection of neuroblastoma cells. Furthermore, when TNP-470 is administered to animals with small tumours, the rate of growth is reduced, while does not significantly altered the tumour growth rate when it is administered to animals with large tumours. Moreover, TNP-470-treated tumours exhibited striking chromaffin differentiation, suggesting that by inhibiting angiogenesis, TNP-470 induces metabolic stress resulting in chromaffin differentiation (Katzenstein et al., 1999). A further study, confirmed that TNP-470 effectively inhibits neuroblastoma xenograft growth when administered as a single agent or in association with other chemotherapic agents (Shusterman et al., 2001), indicating that TNP-470 may be useful as adjuvant therapy for high-risk neuroblastoma.

5.3 Thalidomide

Kaicker et al. (2003) investigated the anti-angiogenic and anti-tumour properties of thalidomide in a xenograft model of human neuroblastoma. Indeed, thalidomide treatment did not significantly alter tumour growth as compared with control mice injected with neuroblastoma cells. However, thalidomide suppressed angiogenesis, as demonstrated both by fluorescent angiography and immunohistochemical staining, and induces apoptosis of endothelial cells in neuroblastoma xenografts (Kaicker et al., 2003).

5.4 Endostatin

Davidoff et al. (2001) developed a gene therapy approach in which the genes encoding for endostatin were delivered to murine neuroblastoma cells prior to inoculation of tumour cells into syngenic immunocompetent mice. Although the effect of either angiogenesis inhibition or immunomodulation alone resulted in only a modest delay in tumour growth, when these approaches were used in combination, prevention of the formation of appreciable tumours was effected in 63% mice (Davidoff et al., 2001). Interestingly, continuous administration of recombinant endostatin resulted even in a more significant tumour regression as compared to intermittent administration in neuroblastoma xenografts (Kuroiwa et al., 2003). Streck et al. (2004) evaluated the influence of a pre-existing primary neuroblastoma xenografts on the growth of a new second subcutaneously injected tumour, hypothesizing that an existing primary tumour could inhibit the growth of a secondary tumour, in part mediated by tumour release of endostatin. Decreased angiogenesis and increased apoptosis were seen in the secondary tumours, along with decrease of the weight of liver metastases. Although no difference in microvessel density was seen between groups, apoptosis was seen to significantly increase when the primary tumour was retained (Streck et al., 2004).

5.5 Angiostatin

Pre-clinical use of angiostatin in neuroblastoma has been studied in a gene therapy approach using a recombinant adenovirus encoding the human angiostatin kringle 1-3 directly fused to human serum albumin HSA (Adk3-HSA). However, in human neuroblastoma xenograft models, intravenous injection of this vector showed no delay in tumour growth when compared to tumours treated with the control viral vector (Joseph et al., 2003).

5.6 Thrombospondin

ABT-510, a peptide derivative of TSP-1, significantly suppressed the growth of neuroblastoma xenografts established from two different MYCN-amplified cell lines. In combination with the histone deacetylase inhibitor valproic acid, ABT-510 inhibited more effectively the growth of xenografts compared to single-agent treatment (Yang et al., 2007).

5.7 Bortezomib

Bortezomib is a selective and reversible inhibitor of proteasome that shows a potent antitumor activity and that has been shown to inhibit proliferation and colony formation of neuroblastoma cell lines in a time- and dose-dependent manner. Moreover, bortezomib has been also shown to inhibit angiogenesis in CAMs stimulated by conditioned medium from either neuroblastoma cell lines, xenografts and primary biopsy specimens. (Brignole et al., 2006)

5.8 Combined therapies

Combined vinblastine and rapamycin therapy displayed synergistic inhibition of human neuroblastoma-related angiogenesis (Marimpietri et al., 2007). A significant inhibition of tumour growth and microvessel density was obtained in neuroblastoma-bearing mice when treated with vinblastine or rapamycin throughout the down-modulation of both VEGF and VEGFR-2 expression, as shown also by human neuroblastoma biopsy specimens in the CAM assay. (Brignole et al., 2006). The antitumor activity of bortezomib in combination with fenretinide has also been considered. The single compounds were able to induce a dose-dependent inhibition of cell proliferation, but significant enhanced of the anti-proliferative effects has been demonstrated for the drugs used in combination. Bortezomib and fenretinide in association triggered increased apoptosis and significantly increase survival. Histologic examination and CAM assay of the primary tumours showed that combined therapeutic activity was strictly associated to anti-angiogenic mechanisms (Pagnan et al., 2009).

5.9 Anti-VEGF and anti-VEGF receptor-2 antibodies

In a murine model of human neuroblastoma the monoclonal antibody against VEGF partially suppresses tumour growth (Kim et al., 2001). In a further study, topotecan, either in association with anti-VEGF treatment or alone, have been shown to significantly suppress neuroblastoma xenograft growth in comparison with controls or anti-VEGF treated mice (Kim et al., 2002b). Combined topotecan and anti-VEGF treatment significantly inhibited rebound tumour growth. Moreover, high-affinity blockade of VEGF, using the VEGF-TRAP, a composite decoy receptor based on VEGFR-1 and VEGFR-2 fused to an Fc segment of IgG1, dramatically decreases tumour vasculature in a xenograft model of neuroblastoma (Kim et al., 2002b). Pre-clinical studies using bevacizumab, an inhibitor of VEGF, in neuroblastoma demonstrated a significant reduction in tumour growth without major toxicity (Segerstrom et al., 2006). A further study demonstrated that bevacizumab induces alterations in tumour vessels that, in turn, allows improved delivery and efficacy of chemotherapy (Dickson et al., 2007). Continuous treatment with low dose of vinblastine, a novel monoclonal anti-VEGFR-2 antibody (DC101) or both agents together have also been investigated(Klement et al., 2000). Both DC101 and low-dose vinblastine treatment individually resulted in significant, but ultimately transient, xenograft regression and decrease of tumour vascularity. Remarkably, the combination therapy resulted in a full and sustained regression of large established tumours, without any consequent increase in host toxicity or any signs of acquired drug resistance during the course of treatment which lasted more than 6 months. Activity of DC101 was also shown in a neuroblastoma cell line over-expressing MYCN, in which tumour growth delay was increased by simultaneous irradiation (Gong et al., 2003).

5.10 Inhibitors of the tyrosine kinase of VEGFRs

SU5416, a specific inhibitor of VEGFR-1 and VEGFR-2, has been investigated as angiogenesis inhibitor strategy in neuroblastoma. Efficacy was increased when SU5416 was administered in combination with irradiation or chemotherapy (Backman et al., 2002).

5.11 Novel vascular targeting

Tumour vascular targeting strategies that target and disrupt the existent vessel network of growing tumours have been actively perused (Sieman et al., 2004). Between them, vascular disrupting agents (VDAs), such as ligand-targeted and/or drug-conjugated liposomes have been recently introduced (Thorpe, 2004). Pastorino et al. have described a novel strategy of achieving an anti-neuroblastoma response using a peptide-targeted formulation of liposomal doxorubicin (Pastorino et al., 2003; Pastorino et al., 2006). This approach was active against both established primary tumours and early-phase metastases and induced a selective apoptosis of tumour endothelial cells and destruction of tumour vasculature. This novel strategy markedly enhanced the therapeutic use of doxorubicin and enabled metronomic administration. A dual mechanism of action has been proposed: indirect tumour cell killing via the destruction of tumour endothelium by NGR-targeted liposomes and direct tumour cell killing via localization of liposomal doxorubicin to the tumour interstitial space. This approach has been validated by evaluating tumour vasculature in several murine xenografts of doxorubicin-resistant human cancers, including lung, ovarian and neuroblastoma (Pastorino et al., 2008). The TVT-DOX used in this study was manufactured as large-scale Good Manufacturing Practice (GMP) preparation suited to human clinical trials. Opposing to the untargeted formulation of DOXIL®/CAELYX®, which has been approved for clinical use for the treatment of ovarian cancer and other solid tumours (Northfelt et al., 1997; Gordon et al., 2000), the GMP preparation of TVT-DOX has been demonstrated to effectively target the angiogenic tumour blood vessels and thus, indirectly, kill the tumour cells. Whereas tumour endothelial cell is well accepted as a valid target for cancer therapies, pericytes have been only recently recognized as a novel target for cancer treatment. The membrane associated protease APA is expressed in pericytes associated with tumour blood vessels and its expression has been correlated with tumour progression (Schlingemann et al., 1996; Marchio et al., 2004). Recently, Loi et al (2010) have developed a novel liposomal formulation targeting APA that displays anti-tumour effects and prolongs survival in human neuroblastoma-bearing mice with a significant increase in the level of apoptosis in tumours cells and a pronounced destruction of the tumour vasculature(Loi et al., 2010).

6. Conclusion

Angiogenesis in neuroblastoma has been thoroughly studied. As other solid tumours, the major role of angiogenesis resides in tumour development, maintenance and progression. These observations have led to the development of several different therapeutic strategies aimed to disrupt tumour vascularity. However, in designing novel therapeutic approaches a role of angiogenesis in promoting the mechanisms of maturation of neuroblastic cells has also to be considered. In fact, different angiogenetic pathways are involved in neuroblastoma, some of them sustaining tumour neo-angiogenesis and contributing to tumour aggressiveness and others contributing to the maturation of neuroblastic tumours.

7. Acknowledgments

A kind acknowledgement goes to Dr. M. Cominelli and Dr. V. Vielmi for their assistance in the manuscript preparation and to Dr. M. Ravanini for her assistance in the preparation of the histopathological staining. This work was supported by University of Brescia research fund (ex 60%) and Fondazione G Berlucchi to P.L.P. The authors confirm that there are no conflicts of interest.

8. References

Ambros IM, Zellner A, Roald B, Amann G, Ladenstein R, Printz D et al. (1996). Tyrrole of ploidy, chromosome 1p, and Schwann cells in the maturation of neuroblastoma. *New Engl J Med,* 334:1505–11.

Ambros IM, Hata J, Joshi VV, Roald B, Dehner LP, Tuchler H, et al. (2002) Morphologic features of neuroblastoma (Schwannian stromapoor tumors) in clinically favorable and unfavorable groups. *Cancer,* 94(5):1574–1583.

Backman U, Svensson A & Christofferson R. (2002) Importance of vascular endothelial growth factor A in the progression of experimental neuroblastoma. *Angiogenesis,* 5:267–274.

Black WC & Welch HG. (1993). Advances in diagnostic imaging and overestimations of disease prevalence and the benefits of therapy. *N Engl J Med,* 328: 1237-1243.

Brignole C, Marimpietri D, Pastorino F, Nico B, Di Paolo D, Cioni M et al. (2006). Effects of bortezomib on human neuroblastoma cell growth, apoptosis, and angiogenesis. *J Natl Cancer Inst,* 98:1142-1157.

Carmeliet P. Angiogenesis in health and disease. (2003) *Nat Med,* 9: 653-60.

Castke VP, Ou X, O'Shea S & Dixit VM (1992). Induction of thrombospondin 1 by retinoic acid is importants during differentiation of neuroblastoma cells. *J Clin Invest,* 90:1857-1863.

Chlenski A, Liu S, Crawford SE, Volpert OV, De Vries GH, Evangelista A, Yang Q et al. (2002) SPARC is a key schwannian-derived inhibitor controlling neuroblastoma tumor angiogenesis. *Cancer Res,* 62:7357–7363.

Christiansen JH, Coles EG & Wilkinson DG. (2000). Molecular control of neural crest formation, migration and differentiation. *Curr Opin Cell Biol,* 12:719–724.

Coco S, Defferrari R, Scaruffi P, Cavazzana A, Di Cristofano C, Longo L et al. (2005) Genome analysis and gene expression profiling of neuroblastoma and ganglioneuroblastoma reveal differences between neuroblastic and Schwannian stromal cells. *J Pathol,* 207(3): 346–357.

Cohn SL, Pearson AD, London WB, Monclair T, Ambros PF, Brodeur GM et al. (2009) The International Neuroblastoma Risk Group (INRG) classification system: an INRG Task Force report. *J Clin Oncol,* Jan 10; 27(2): 289-97.

Crawford SE, Stellmach V, Ranalli M, Huang X, Huang L, Volpert O et al. (2001) Pigment epithelium-derived factor (PEDF) in neuroblastoma: a multifunctional mediator of Schwann cell antitumor activity. *J Cell Science,* 114: 4421–4428.

Davidoff AM, Leary MA, Ng CY, Spurbeck WW, Frare P, Vanhove M et al. (2001) Autocrine expression of both endostatin and green fluorescent protein provides a synergistic antitumor effect in a murine neuroblastoma model, *Cancer Gene Ther,* 8: 537-545.

Dickson PV, Hamner JB, Sims TL, Fraga CH, Ng CY, Rajasekeran S et al. (2007) Bevacizumab-induced transient remodeling of the vasculature in neuroblastoma xenografts results in improved delivery and efficacy of systemically administered chemotherapy. *Clin Cancer Res,* 13: 3942-3950.

Dvorak H (1986) Tumors: wounds that not heal. Similarities between tumor stroma generation and wound healing, *New Engl J Med,* 315: 1650-1659.

Ebrahimnejad A, Flayeh R, Unteregger G, Wagener C & Brummer J (2000) Cell adhesion molecule CEACAM1 associates with paxillin in granulocytes and epithelial and endothelial cells. *Exp Cell Res,* 260:365–373.

Eggert A, Ikegaki N, Kwiatkowski J, Zhao H, Brodeur GM & Himelstein BP (2000) High-level expression of angiogenic factors is associated with advanced tumor stage in human neuroblastomas. *Clin Cancer Res,* 6: 1900-8.

Ellis LM, Staley CA, Liu W, Fleming RY, Parikh NU, Bucana CD et al. (1998) Downregulation of vascular endothelial growth factor in a human colon carcinoma cell line transfected with an antisense expression vector specific for c-src. *J Biol Chem,* 273: 1052-1057.

Ferrari-Toninelli G, Bonini SA, Uberti D, Buizza L, Bettinsoli P, Poliani PL et al. (2010) Targeting Notch pathway induces growth inhibition and differentiation of neuroblastoma cells. *Neuro Oncol,* Dec; 12(12): 1231-43.

Giannini G, Kim CJ, Di Marcotullio L, Manfioletti G, Cardinali B, Cerignoli F et al. (2000) Expression of the HMGI(Y) gene products in human neuroblastic tumours correlates with differentiation status. *Br J Cancer,* 83: 1503–9.

Gong H, Pottgen C, Stuben G, Havers W, Stuschke M & Schweigerer L (2003) Arginine deiminase and other antiangiogenic agents inhibit unfavorable neuroblastoma growth: potentiation by irradiation, *Int J Cancer,* 106: 723-728.

Gordon AN, Granai CO, Rose PG, Hainsworth J, Lopez A, Weissman C et al. (2000) Phase II study of liposomal doxorubicin in platinum- and paclitaxel-refractory epithelial ovarian cancer. *J Clin Oncol,* 18: 3093-3100.

Haas D, Ablin AR, Miller C, Zoger S & Matthay KK (1988). Complete pathologic maturation and regression of stage IVS neuroblastoma without treatment. *Cancer,* 62(4): 818–825.

Hoehner JC, Hedborg F, Eriksson L, Sandstedt B, Grimelius L, Olsen L et al. (1988). Developmental gene expression of sympathetic nervous system tumours reflects their histogenesis. *Lab Invest,* 78:29–45.

Huang D, Rutkowski JL, Brodeur GM, Chou PM, Kwiatkowsji JL, Babbo A et al. (2000). Schwann cell-conditioned medium inhibits angiogenesis. *Cancer Res,* 60: 5966-5971.

Joseph JM, Bouquet C, Opolon P, Morizet J, Aubert G, Rössler J et al. (2003). High level of stabilized angiostatin mediated by adenovirus dekivery does not impair the growth of human neuroblastoma xenografts. *Cancer Gene Ther,* 10: 859-866.

Kaicker S, McCrudden KM, Beck L, New T, Huang J, Frischer JS et al. (2003). Thalidomide is anti-angiogenic in a xenograft model of neuroblastoma, *Int J Oncol,* 23: 1651-1655.

Katzenstein HM, Rademaker AW, Senger C, Salwen HR, Nguyen NN, Thorner PS et al. (1999). Effectiveness of the angiogenesis inhibitor TNP-470 in reducing the growth of human neuroblastoma in nude mice inversely correlates with the tumor burden. *Clin Cancer Res,* 5: 4273-4278

Katzenstein HM, Cohn SL, Crawford S & Meitar D (2000). Angiogenesis in neuroblastoma. *J. Clin. Oncol.*, 18; 2789–2791.

Kim E, Moore J, Huang J, Soffer S, Manley CA, O'Toole K et al. (2001). All angiogenesis is not the same: distinct patterns of response to antiangiogenic therapy in experimental neuroblastoma and Wilms tumor. *J Pediatr Surg*, 36: 287-290.

Kim ES, Soffer SZ, Huang J, Mc Crudden KW, Yokoi A, Manley CA et al. (2002a). Distinct response of experimental neuroblastoma to combination antiangiogenic strategies. *J Pediatr Surg*, 37: 518-522.

Kim ES, Seru A, Huang J, Manley CA, Mc Crudden KW, Frischer JS et al. (2002b). Potent VEGF blockade causes regression of coopted vessels in a model of neuroblastoma. *Proc Natl Acad Sci USA*, 99: 11399-11404.

Kitlinska J, Abe K, Kuo L, Pons J, Yu M, Li L et al. (2005). Differential effects of neuropeptide Y on the growth and vascularization of neural crest-derived tumours. *Cancer Res*, 65:1719–1728.

Klement G, Baruchel S, Rak J, Man S, Clark K, Hicklin DJ et al. (2000). Continuous low-dose therapy with vinblastine and VEGF receptor-2 antibody induces sustained tumor regression without overt toxicity. *J Clin Invest*, 105: 1049-1058.

Koppen A, Ait-Aissa R, Koster J, Ora I, Bras J, van Sluis PG, et al. (2008). Dickkopf-3 expression is a marker for neuroblastic tumor maturation and is down-regulated by MYCN. *Int J Cancer*, 122(7):1455–1464.

Kuroiwa M, Takeuchi T, Lee JH, Yoshizawa J, Hirato J, Kaneko S et al. (2003). Contnuous versus intermittent administration of human endostatin in xenografted human neuroblastoma. *J Pediatr Surg*, 38: 1499-1505.

Kwiatkowski JL, Rutkowski JL, Yamashiro DJ, Tennekoon GI & Brodeur GM. (1988). Schwann cell-conditioned medium promotes neuroblastoma survival and differentiation. *Cancer Res*, 58:4602–4606.

Levy AP, Levy NS, Wegner S & Goldberg MA (1995). Transcriptional regulation of the rat vascular endothelial growth factor gene by hypoxia. *J Biol Chem*, 270:13333-13340.

Liu S, Tian Y, Chlenski A, Yang Q, Zage P, Salwen HR et al. (2005). Cross-talk between Schwann cells and neuroblastss influences the biology of neuroblastoma xenografts. *Am J Pathol*, 166: 891-900.

Loi M, Marchiò S, Becherini P, Di Paolo D, Soster M, Curnis F et al. (2010). Combined targeting of perivascular and endothelial tumor cells enhances anti-tumor efficacy of liposomal chemotherapy in neuroblastoma. *J Control Rel*, 145: 66-73.

Marimpietri D, Brignole C, Nico B, Pastorino F, Pezzolo A, Piccardi F et al. (2007). Combined therapeutic effects of vinblastine and rapamycin on human neuroblastoma growth, apoptosis, and angiogenesis. *Clin Cancer Res*, Jul 1;13(13):3977-88.

Maris JM & Denny CT (2002). Focus on embryonal malignancies. *Cancer Cell*, 2:447–450.

Matthay KK, Villablanca JG, Seeger RC, Stram DO, Harris RE, Ramsay NK et al. (1999). Treatment of high-risk neuroblastoma with intensive chemotherapy, radiotherapy, autologous bone marrow transplantation, and 13-cis-retinoic acid. *N Engl J Med*, 341(16):1165–1173.

Meitar D, Crawford SE, Rademaker AW & Cohn SL (1996). Tumor angiogenesis correlates with metastatic disease, N-myc amplification, and poor outcome in human meuroblastoma. *J Clin Oncol*, 14: 405-414.

Mora J & Gerald WL (2004). Origin of neuroblastic tumors: clues for future therapeutics. *Expert Rev Mol Diagn*, 4:293–302.

Nagabuchi E, Vanderkolk WE, Une Y & Ziegler MM (1997). TNP-470 antiangiogenic therapy for advanced murine neuroblastoma. *J Pediatric Surg*, 32: 287-293.

Nagoshi M, Tsuneyoshi M & Enjoii M (1992). S-100 positive undifferentiated neuroblastomas with a special reference to the tumor stroma related to favovable prognosis. *Pathol Res Pract*, 188: 273-283.

Northfelt DW, Dezube BJ, Thommes JA, Levine R, Von Roenn JH, Dosik GM, Rios A et al. (1997). Efficacy of pegylated-liposomal doxorubicin in the treatment of AIDS-related Kaposi's sarcoma after failure of standard chemotherapy. *J Clin Oncol*, 15: 653-659.

Pagnan G, Di Paolo D, Carosio R, Pastorino F, Marimpietri D, Brignole C et al. (2009). The combined therapeutic effects of bortezomib and fenretinide on neuroblastoma cells involve endoplasmic reticulum stress response. *Clin Cancer Res*, 15: 1199-209.

Park CC, Bissell MJ & Barcellos-Hoff MH (2000). The influence of the microenvironment on the malignant phenotype. *Mol Med Today*, 6: 324-329.

Pastorino F, Brignole C, Marimpietri D, Cilli M, Gambini C, Ribatti D et al. (2003). Vascular damage and anti-angiogenic effects of tumor vessel-targeted liposomal chemotherapy. *Cancer Res*, 63: 7400-7409.

Pastorino F, Brignole C, Di Paolo D, Nico B, Pezzolo A, Marimpietri D et al. (2006). Targeting liposomal chemotherapy via both tumor cell-specific and tumor vasculature-specific ligands potentiates therapeutic efficacy. *Cancer Res*, 66: 10073-10082.

Pastorino F, Di Paolo D, Piccardi F, Nico B, Ribatti D, Daga A (2008). Enhanced antitumor efficacy of clinical-grade vasculature-targeted liposomal doxorubicin. *Clin Cancer Res*, 14: 7320-7329.

Pastorino F, Di Paolo D, Loi M, Becherini P, Caffa I, Zorzoli A et al. (2009). Recent advances in targeted anti-vasculature therapy: the neuroblastoma model. *Curr Drug Targets*, Oct;10(10):1021-7.

Peddinti R, Zeine R, Luca D, Seshadri R, Chlenski A, Cole K et al. (2007). Prominent microvascular proliferation in clinically aggressive neuroblastoma. *Clin Cancer Res*, 13: 3499-3506.

Peuchmaur M, d'Amore ES, Joshi VV, Hata J, Roald B, Dehner LP, et al. (2003). Revision of the International Neuroblastoma Pathology Classification: confirmation of favorable and unfavourable prognostic subsets in ganglioneuroblastoma, nodular. *Cancer*, 98:2274–2281.

Poliani PL, Mitola S, Ravanini M, Ferrari-Toninelli G, D'Ippolito C, Notarangelo LD et al. (2007). CEACAM1/VEGF cross-talk during neuroblastic tumour differentiation. *J Pathol*, Apr; 211(5): 541-9.

Ponzoni M, Bocca P, Chiesa V, Decensi A, Pistoia V, Raffaghello L et al. (1995). Differential effects of N-(4-Hydroxyphenyl) retinamide and retinoic acid on neuroblastoma cells: apoptosis versus differentiation. *Cancer Res,* 55: 853-861.

Prall F, Nollau P, Neumaier M, Haubeck HD, Drzeniek Z, Helmchen U, et al. (1996). CD66a (BGP), an adhesion molecule of the carcinoembryonic antigen family, is expressed in epithelium, endothelium, and myeloid cells in a wide range of normal human tissues. *J Histochem Cytochem,* 44:35–41.

Pritchard J & Hickman JA. Why does stage 4s neuroblastoma regress spontaneously? (1994). *Lancet,* 344:869–870.

Rak J, Mitsuhashi Y, Bayko L, Filmus J, Shirasawa S, Sasazuki T et al. (1995). Mutant ras oncogenes upregulate VEGF/VPF expression: implications for induction and inhibition of tumor angiogenesis. *Cancer Res,* 55: 4575-4580.

Ribatti D, Alessandri G, Vacca A, Iurlaro M & Ponzoni M (1998). Human neuroblastoma cells produce extracellular matrix-degrading enzymes, induce endothelial cell proliferation and are angiogenic in vivo. *Int J Cancer,* 77: 449-54.

Ribatti D, Vacca A & Dammacco F. (1999). The role of the vascular phase in solid tumor growth: a historical review. *Neoplasia,* 1: 293-302.

Ribatti D, Surico G, Vacca A, De Leonardis F, Lastilla G, Montaldo PG, et al. (2001). Angiogenesis extent and expression of matrix metalloproteinase-2 and -9 correlate with progression in human neuroblastoma. *Life Sci,* 68: 1161-8.

Ribatti D, Alessandri G, Baronio M, Raffaghello L, Cosimo E, Marimpetri D et al. (2001). Inhibition of neuroblastoma-induced angiogenesis by fenretinide. *Int J Cancer,* 94: 314-321.

Ribatti D, Raffaghello L, Pastorino F, Nico B, Brignole C, Vacca A, et al. (2002). In vivo angiogenic activity of neuroblastoma correlates with MYCN oncogene overexpression. *Int J Cancer,* 102:351-4.

Ribatti D, Marimpietri D, Pastorino F, Brignole C, Nico B, Vacca A et al. (2004). Angiogenesis in neuroblastoma. *Ann N Y Acad Sci,* Dec; 1028: 133-42.

Ribatti D & Ponzoni M (2005). Antiangiogenic strategies in neuroblastoma. *Cancer Treat Rev,* Feb; 31(1): 27-34.

Ribatti D, Poliani PL, Longo V, Mangieri D, Nico B & Vacca A. (2007). Erythropoietin/erythropoietin receptor system is involved in angiogenesis in human neuroblastoma. *Histopathology,* Apr;50(5):636-41.

Ribatti D, Marzullo A, Longo V & Poliani L. (2007). Schwann cells in neuroblastoma express erythropoietin. *J Neurooncol,* May; 82(3): 327-8.

Ribatti D, Nico B, Crivellato E & Vacca A. (2007). The structure of the vascular networks of tumors. *Cancer Letters,* 248: 18-23.

Ribatti D, Nico B, Crivellato E, Roccaro AM & Vacca A. (2007). The history of the angiogenic switch concept. *Leukemia,* 21: 44-52.

Rössler J, Taylor M, Geoerger B, Farace F, Lagodny J, Peschka-Süss R et al. (2008). Angiogenesis as a target in neuroblastoma. *Eur J Cancer,* Aug;44(12):1645-56.

Sawa H, Kamada K, Sato H, Sendo S, Kondo A, Saito I, et al. (1994). CCAM expression in the developing rat central nervous system. *Brain Res Dev Brain Res,* 78:35–43.

Schlingemann RO, Oosterwijk E, Wesseling P, Rietveld FJ & Ruiter DJ. (1996). Aminopeptidase ais a constituent of activated pericytes in angiogenesis. *J Pathol,* 179: 436-442.

Schwab M, Westermann F, Hero B & Berthold F. (2003). Neuroblastoma: biology and molecular and chromosomal pathology. *Lancet Oncol,* 4:472–480.

Segerstrom L, Fuchs D, Backman U, Holmquist K, Chistofferson R & Azarbayiani E. (2006). The anti-VEGF antibody bevacizumab potently reduces the growth rate of high-risk neuroblastoma xenografts. *Padiatr Res,* 60: 576-581.

Shimada H, Ambros IM, Dehner LP, Hata J, Joshi VV & Roald B. (1999). Terminology and morphologic criteria of neuroblastic tumors: recommendations by the International Neuroblastoma Pathology Committee. *Cancer,* 86(2):349–363.

Shimada H. The International Neuroblastoma Pathology Classification (2003). *Pathologica,* 95(5): 240–241.

Shusterman S, Grupp SA, Barr R, Carpentieri D, Zhao H & Maris JM. (2001). The angiogenesis inhibitor TNP-470 effectively inhibits human neuroblastoma xenografts growth, especially in the setting of subclinical disease. *Clin Cancer Res,* 7: 977-984.

Siemann DW, Chaplin DJ & Horsman MR (2004). Vascular-targeting therapies for treatment of malignant diseases. *Cancer,* 100: 2491-2499.

Streck C, Zhang Y, Zhou J, Ng CYG & Davidoff A (2004). Endostatin-mediated concomitant resistance in neuroblastoma. *J Pediatr Surg,* 405-411.

Tang Y, Kim M, Carrasco D, Kung AL, Chin L & Weissleder R (2005). In vivo assessment of RAS-dependent maintenance of tumor angiogenesis by real-time magnetic resonance imaging. *Cancer Res,* 65: 8324-8330.

Thorpe PE (2004). Vascular targeting agents as cancer therapeutics. *Clin Cancer Res,* 10: 415-427.

Vacca A & Ribatti D (2006). Bone marrow angiogenesis in multiple myeloma. *Leukemia,* 20: 193-199.

Volpert O, Luo W, Liu TJ, Estrera VT, Logothetis C & Lin SH. (2002). Inhibition of prostate tumour angiogenesis by the tumour suppressor CEACAM1. *J Biol Chem,* 277:35696–35702.

Wagener C & Ergun S. (2000). Angiogenic properties of the carcinoembryonic antigen-related cell adhesion molecule 1. *Exp Cell Res,* 261:19–24.

Wassberg E, Hedborg F, Skoldenberge E, Stridsberg M & Christofferson R (1999). Inhibition of angiogenesis induced chromaffin differentiation and apoptosis in neuroblastoma. *Am J Pathol,* 154: 395-400.

Watnick RS, Cheng YN, Rangarajan A & Weinberg RA (2003). Ras modulates Myc activity to repress thrombospondin-1 expression and increase tumor angiogenesis. *Cancer Cell,* 3: 219-231.

Yang Q, Tian Y, Liu S, Chlenski A, Salwen HR, Henkin J et al. (2007). Thrombospondin-1 peptide ABT-510 combined with valproic acid is an effective antiangiogenesis strategy in neuroblastoma. *Cancer Res,* 67: 1716-1724.

Zeine R, Salwen HR, Peddinti R, Tian Y, Guerrero L, Yang Q et al. (2009). Presence of cancer-associated fibroblasts inversely correlates with Schwannian stroma in neuroblastoma tumors. *Mod Pathol,* 22: 950-958.

11

MicroRNA Target Signatures in Advanced Stage Neuroblastoma

Victoria R. Chu and Inhan Lee
miRcore
U.S.A.

1. Introduction

Neuroblastoma is a solid cancer that arises from precursor cells of the sympathetic nervous system. It is known for its extreme heterogeneity, ranging from spontaneous regression to rapid progression to metastasis. Prognostic factors include age and genetic abnormalities, with greater likelihood of survival in infants, suggesting that neuroblastoma is a developmental disorder (Jiang et al., 2011). Considering that neuroblastoma accounts for 15% of all cancer deaths among children, novel therapeutic targets are clearly needed. Furthermore, early differentiation of children who will not develop advanced-stage neuroblastoma would reduce long-term side effects due to treatment, improving quality of life of survivors. Since neuroblastoma arises from precursor cells, understanding the mechanism by which it becomes advanced-stage cancer might also provide insight into how normal stem cells transform into cancer stem cells. This chapter examines factors differentiating advanced, metastatic neuroblastoma from low-risk, localized neuroblastoma.

Common genetic abnormalities in neuroblastoma include the genetic amplification (multiple DNA copies) of MYCN, chromosome 1p36 and 11q23 deletion, and the gain of chromosome 17q22 (review in Jiang et al., 2011). Since all of these genetic abnormalities correlate with poor clinical outcome, they have been investigated as potential driving factors in advanced stage neuroblastoma. However, as advanced neuroblastoma also occurs without such genetic abnormalities, the signatures of advanced neuroblastoma must be determined to understand the mechanism of its progression. For example, though amplification of transcription factor MYCN was linked early on with a poor outcome (Bordow et al., 1998), MYCN status cannot fully account for all advanced-stage cases. In addition to DNA-level abnormalities, expression level changes of transcripts in advanced stage have been studied to accurately predict the disease outcome (Asgharzadeh et al., 2006; Oberthuer et al., 2006). However, MYCN transcript levels could not dependably identify advanced stage neuroblastoma either. It is clear that multiple gene regulation should be considered in deciphering neuroblastoma progression (De Preter et al., 2010; Overthuer et al., 2010). To differentiate the underlying mechanism of progression, several studies have assessed DNA abnormality and transcription level changes together, comparing, for example, all transcription levels of advanced-stage neuroblastoma with and without MYCN amplification. Recent research on transcript-level changes has incorporated microRNA expression changes (Lin et al., 2010).

MicroRNAs (miRNAs) are endogenous regulatory RNAs ranging in size from 16 to 25 nucleotides that are processed from hairpin-structured precursors by the enzyme Dicer (Kim, 2005). Once a mature single strand miRNA becomes part of a miRNA-RiboNucleoProtein complex (miRNP), it mostly functions as a negative regulator of other genes' protein production by directly interacting with the target genes' mRNAs in sequence-complementary fashion. Though originally identified in terms of its translational repression function in animal, it also helps degrade target mRNAs themselves. So far, more than a thousand miRNAs have been identified in human (http://mirbase.org) (Kozomara & Griffiths-Jones, 2010), some of them potentially regulating about 200 genes (Lim et al., 2005). As with transcription factors and other endogenous genes with regulatory roles, expression of each miRNA is strictly controlled and exhibits characteristic patterns based on biological context, such as tissue type or developmental stages. In line with the critical roles of miRNAs in biological processes, their deregulation is frequently observed in many diseases, including neuroblastoma.

Neuroblastoma-related miRNAs have been researched mainly in regard to two biological processes, anti-apoptosis (tumorigenesis), and epithelial mesenchymal transition (EMT: metastasis related). TP53 is a well-known transcription factor that induces apoptosis and miR-34 family transcription (He et al., 2007). In neuroblastoma, TP53 mutation is uncommon, whereas deletion on chromosome 1p36 (where mir-34a is located) frequently occurs. Another frequent deletion site of 11q23 coincides with mir-34b and mir-34c chromomal positions, implying the importance of the mir-34 family in neuroblastoma. On the other hand, MYCN amplification is frequent in neuroblastoma and several miRNAs are induced by MYCN, including the mir-17-92 cluster, which has been shown to be significantly upregulated in MYCN-amplified cells (Schulte et al., 2008) and has been identified with a direct anti-proliferation function (Matsubara et al., 2007). In neuroblastoma, upregulation of the mir-17-92 cluster is correlated with the obstruction of the TGF-beta signaling pathway, thereby preventing apoptosis (Mestdagh et al., 2010a). MYCN also achieves anti-apoptotic function by downregulating other miRNAs which prevent cell proliferation. Low levels of MYCN allow for the over-expression of miR-184, which has been shown to reduce neuroblastoma tumor growth (Foley et al., 2010; Tivnan et al., 2010). While MYCN affects transcripton of certain miRNAs, some miRNAs can down-regulate MYCN translation, such as miR-34 (Christoffersen et al., 2010). let-7 and miR-101 are also found to target MYCN and inhibit proliferation of MYCN-amplified neuroblastoma cells (Buechner et al., 2011). Similarly, Foley et al. demonstrate that miR-10a and miR-10b indirectly downregulate MYCN by targeting NCOR2, though the intermediate processes between NCOR2 and MYCN need further study (Foley et al., 2011). Therefore, miR-34 family deletion and MYCN amplification in neuroblastoma together respond to tumorigenesis through anti-apoptotic process.

Metastasis may also be brought on by altered levels of miRNA. Guo et al. show that 54 different miRNAs are significantly altered in metastatic as opposed to primary neuroblastoma tumors (Guo et al., 2010). A more specific study showed that overexpression of miR-524-5p decreases the invasive potential of neuroblastoma cells (Bray et al., 2011).

Recently, the miR-34 family has been identified as blocking EMT by downregulating SNAI1 (Kim et al., 2011), showing its dual function of blocking tumorigenesis and metastasis. Haug et al. found that miR-92 downregulates tumor suppressor DKK3 (Haug et al, 2011), which normally inhibits the Wnt signaling pathway. The canonical Wnt signaling can induce EMT mostly by degrading E-cadherin (Heuberger & Birchmeier, 2010). All this implies that a large network stretching across miR-34, MYCN, and the miR-17-92 cluster is responsible for both tumorogenesis and metastasis in neuroblastoma (Fig. 1). Hence, miRNAs hold promise as biomarkers for diagnostic and therapeutic purposes.

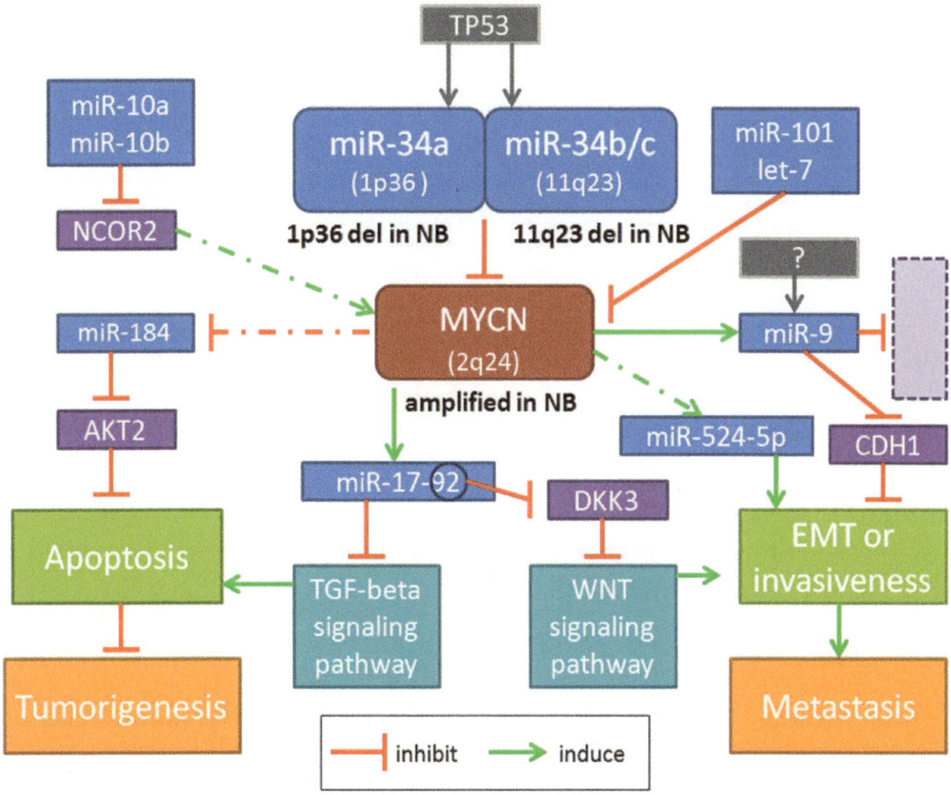

Fig. 1. Schematic diagram of miRNA network in neuroblastoma tumorigenesis and metastasis, including miR-9 from this study. The dotted box represents our six predicted targets in this study.

The problem remains that miRNAs' small size and similar sequences often make their global expression data noisier than mRNA data. Given that miRNAs regulate the expression of target mRNAs, correlating miRNA with mRNA expression could increase biomarker signals, leading to biomarkers with superior resolution and potentially revealing master regulators. To realize this potential, we need accurate miRNA target identification. While other areas of miRNA research have undergone continuous development, target prediction has lagged behind, partly due to the imperfect miRNA-mRNA bindings found in animals. As experimental and evolutionary evidence indicates that the 5′-end of miRNAs (the nucleotide position 1-8 at the 5′-end, also called the seed sequence) is important for recognition of target sequences in 3′-UTRs (untranslated regions) of mRNA, many computational algorithms utilize only 6-8 nucleotides (nt) of the ~22 mer miRNA to predict target mRNAs. However, there exist many genome-wide sequences matching this short stretch of 6-8 nt, resulting in a large number of false positives among the predicted targets and thus invalidating miRNA-mRNA correlations. Although a database of miRNAs and their experimentally verified targets exists (Papadopoulos et al., 2009), the list therein is still far from comprehensive.

We have identified a new class of miRNA targets, called miBridge, in which the 5′- and 3′-end of a miRNA can simultaneously interact with the 3′-UTR and 5′-UTR of a single mRNA (Lee et al., 2009). We will use the terms "3UTR:5emiR" (a miRNA seed sequence and its target site on the 3′-UTR: conventional knowledge) and "5UTR:3emiR" (the 3′-end of a miRNA—the other side of the seed region—and its recognition site in the 5′-UTR: our finding). Whereas other studies have not found global miRNA interactions with the 5′-UTR due to searching against the seed region (5UTR:5emiR), we have found significant 5UTR:3emiR interactions (Ajay, et al., 2010; Lee et al., 2009). This sequence-specific miRNA function through 5UTR:3emiR has been experimentally validated (Lee et al., 2009). In addition to these previous reports establishing the validity and utility of miBridge, we have recently generated a list of genome-wide miBridge targets using version 1 (v.1) prediction parameters. Interestingly, most known miRNA and mRNA (both 5′-UTR and 3′-UTR annotated) have miBridge interactions. Considering both ends of miRNA in the target prediction, miBridge targets are usually fewer in number (about 1/2 to 1/10 of other predictions), while having specific functions which align well with previous expresimental data.

In this chapter, we introduce a new approach to identifying miRNAs which differentiates high-risk (advanced) from low-risk neuroblastoma based on expression data and miBridge target predictions. When we applied the method to neuroblastoma patient datasets of mRNA and miRNA expression levels obtained from the Vandesompele group (Mestdagh et al., 2010b), we found miR-9 to be a consistent biomarker, all six predicted targets being downregulated and their expressions negatively correlated with miR-9 expression. This is interesting since MYCN is one of miR-9's transcription factors, though our analysis did not consider MYCN-amplification status in the advanced stage patient data group. Previous research has shown that miR-9 upregulation correlates with breast cancer metastasis (Ma et al., 2010), supporting our finding of miR-9 as a new biomarker for advanced neuroblastoma. Furthermore, we also found miR-9 to be significantly upregulated in short-term survival patients within the advanced stage neuroblastoma group in other publicly available data (Scaruffi et al., 2009), confirming the validity of our finding. To increase the specificity of differentiating high-risk and short-term survival groups, further research is needed to identify additional miR-9 activating factors besides MYCN as well as the common biological pathways of miR-9 target genes in neuroblasts (Fig. 1).

2. MicroRNA and target gene signature in advanced neuroblastoma

Expression levels of mRNA depend on various factors including DNA copy number, DNA methylation, histone acetylation, active transcription factors, splicing factors, and regulating miRNAs. Here we analyze mRNA expression in a miRNA-centric manner, comparing it with miRNA expression data to increase the specificity of advanced neuroblastoma signatures. This is based on our hypothesis that if a miRNA's function is important and causal to progress neuroblastoma and the expression of the miRNA is up (down)-regulated in the advanced stage, its targets will be preferentially down (up)-regulated in the advanced neuroblastoma. Therefore, we will define a miRNA and its targets as important to the advanced neuroblastoma if such cases are found. Note that this method proceeds without bias of previous knowledge and simply searches for consistent expression data across different datasets (mRNA and miRNA expression), thus allowing novel findings.

The Vandesompele group, which has recently identified correlations between MYCN-induced miRNAs and poor outcome in MYCN-activated tumors (Mestdagh et al., 2010b), kindly provided us matching mRNA and miRNA expression patterns with an annotation file. We also downloaded the mRNA data, disease state, and MYCN amplification status from the Gene Express Omnibus (Series accession number GSE21713). The disease states followed the International Neuroblastoma Staging System's four stages. Stages 1 and 2 indicating the cancer is still localized, while stages 3 and 4 indicate metastasis of the original tumor. To understand global genetic differences in advanced neuroblastoma, we defined two groups for comparison: stage 4 as one group and stage 1 and 2 as another, regardless of MYCN amplification status. Stage 3 data were excluded in order to obtain maximal contrast between the non-metastatic stages and metastatic stage 4. By comparing miRNA and mRNA expression of these two groups, we expected to obtain a more specific advanced neuroblastoma signature, which might not be apparent through mRNA or miRNA analysis alone.

2.1 mRNA expression analysis

2.1.1 Differently expressed mRNAs in advanced neuroblastoma

In total, there are 30 primary tumor sample data from 14 stage 4 patients and 16 stage 1 and 2 patients. Briefly, the Vandesomepele group derived the expression data as follows: after each sample expression dataset was obtained using GeneChip Human Exon 1.0 ST Arrays (Affymetrix), all exon data were combined to transcript clusters (hg18/core exons), to obtain expression information per gene after normalization according to the RMA-sketch algorithm using Affymetrix Power Tools. We used these RMA normalized data calculated by the Vandesomepele group to obtain differentially expressed genes between the two groups. Student t-tests were performed using Microsoft Excel functions and mRNA lists with p-values less than 0.05 were prepared as up- and down-regulated mRNAs using HUGO Gene Nomenclature Committe (HGNC) gene symbol annotation. We ignored transcripts without gene symbol annotation or empty data points among patient samples. If more than two probe sets corresponded to one gene symbol, we chose the probe set with lower p-values. Among a total 372 up-regulated and 689 down-regulated mRNAs with gene symbols having $p < 0.05$, the top 50 genes with the greatest fold changes are shown in Table 1.

Down-Regulated Gene	p-value	Log2 (Fold Change)	Up-Regulated Gene	p-value	Log2(Fold Change)
ALCAM	0.012519	-1.1404	ACTA2	0.017706	0.84008
APBA1	0.000975	-1.00703	BIRC5	0.007473	0.88797
ATP2B4	0.008721	-1.02324	CCNA2	0.009386	0.79357
CADM3	0.002402	-1.24665	CDC45L	0.007403	0.75931
CDH6	0.049003	-1.01205	CDCA5	0.008474	0.77314
DOC2B	0.013732	-1.02395	CMBL	0.004642	0.72441
DRD2	0.001234	-1.08816	DDX1	0.046072	1.22142
ECEL1	0.003074	-1.10837	E2F3	0.000912	0.74161
EPB41L3	0.008477	-1.37384	FN1	0.008058	1.03848
HIST1H1A	0.016193	-1.34667	FOXM1	0.008946	0.9346
HS6ST3	0.000384	-1.10939	GJC1	0.002895	0.82971
LRRTM4	0.040988	-1.31354	HIST1H2BM	0.037272	0.85818
NRCAM	0.031584	-1.04967	HMGB2	0.006813	0.883
NTRK1	0.001072	-1.79752	MAD2L1	0.012955	0.92231
PGM2L1	0.010537	-1.14954	MYBL2	0.019576	0.82346
PLXNC1	0.000939	-1.08949	MYCN	0.019589	1.23078
PMP22	0.003898	-1.62031	NAG	0.020134	1.26792
PRKCA	0.011104	-1.04588	ODC1	0.001326	1.3045
PRPH	0.003777	-1.41955	PAICS	0.000609	0.74121
PTN	0.00069	-1.19001	PHGDH	0.026183	0.88181
RAB3C	0.025466	-1.00737	RRM2	0.00773	1.46016
REEP1	0.002232	-1.00576	SLC16A1	0.000721	0.93447
SCG2	0.009003	-1.21159	TYMS	0.016238	0.95479
SCN9A	0.0207	-1.02774	VCAN	0.019634	0.99934
SYN3	0.006658	-1.04893			
TMEM176A	0.006741	-1.11877			

Table 1. Top 50 genes with the greatest fold changes among differently expressed mRNAs in advanced neuroblastoma ($p < 0.05$).

2.1.2 Mapping differentiated mRNAs to regulating miRNAs

For all mRNAs identified as differentially regulated, their regulating miRNAs were predicted using the miBridge miRNA target prediction method (v.1).We then calculated enrichment scores for miRNAs based on their target enrichment tests among the differentially regulated mRNAs. Score over 0 means that the predicted miRNA is significant in the system, 1 being optimal. Table 2 shows the predicted regulating miRNAs (within the miRNA list in the array measured) with target enrichment score over 0. Within the mir-17-92 cluster, hsa-miR-18* targets are enriched in the down-regulated mRNAs, supporting our hypothesis and miRNA target predictions (though miR-92a is not included in this $p < 0.05$ list, inclusion of genes with less than 15 empty values in patient samples yields a miR-92a score of 0.04 and the prediction that it is up-regulated in advanced neuroblastoma

Regulating miRNA	Enrichment score	Predicted as
hsa-miR-9	0.03642	up
hsa-miR-18a*	0.3787	up
hsa-miR-136	0.3765	up
hsa-miR-152	0.03642	up
hsa-miR-185	0.7552	up
hsa-miR-205	0.49874	up
hsa-miR-214	0.46397	up
hsa-miR-221	0.73754	up
hsa-miR-324-3p	0.49392	up
hsa-miR-326	0.97012	up
hsa-miR-328	0.86602	up
hsa-miR-346	0.51208	up
hsa-miR-500	0.03642	up
hsa-miR-610	0.08688	up
hsa-miR-650	0.81604	up
hsa-miR-489	0.64438	down

Table 2. Predicted miRNAs as potential regulators of advanced neuroblastoma (enrichment score > 0).

2.2 miRNA expression analysis

The miRNA expression data were obtained from the same patient samples analyzed in the mRNA expression: total 14 stage 4 patients and 16 stage 1 and 2 patients. We used the RMA normalized data with 312 mature miRNA annotations as provided by the Vandesomepele group. Student t-test was performed using Microsoft Excel functions; miRNA lists of score > 0 are shown in Table 3.

up-regulated miRNA	p-value	Log2 (fold change)	down-regulated miRNA	p-value	Log2 (fold change)
hsa-miR-9	0.037541	1.173707	hsa-miR-15a	0.044916	-0.49254
hsa-miR-9*	0.018107	1.235894	hsa-miR-24	0.030286	-0.44341
hsa-miR-18a	0.02853	0.570961	hsa-miR-26a	0.007846	-0.53493
hsa-miR-18a*	0.001933	0.58714	hsa-miR-26b	0.011224	-0.44942
hsa-miR-19a	0.038493	0.588543	hsa-miR-30a-3p	0.023514	-0.68173
hsa-mir-92	0.006916	0.782683	hsa-miR-30b	0.00698	-0.50628
hsa-miR-105	0.036113	1.681312	hsa-miR-30e-3p	0.023054	-0.77332
hsa-miR-320	0.023005	0.362074	hsa-miR-95	0.012503	-0.91388
hsa-miR-375	0.03906	1.901862	hsa-miR-103	0.0395	-0.35021
hsa-miR-517a	0.045293	1.423221	hsa-miR-125b	0.00271	-0.89665
hsa-miR-520g	0.024751	1.757529	hsa-miR-128a	0.016545	-0.73381
hsa-miR-526b*	0.049281	0.601139	hsa-miR-137	0.000167	-1.78508
hsa-miR-645	0.014262	0.758181	hsa-miR-140	0.010729	-0.3409
			hsa-miR-148b	0.009921	-0.56818
			hsa-miR-149	0.002849	-1.13549
			hsa-miR-190	0.048211	-1.23233
			hsa-miR-204	0.008341	-2.21371
			hsa-miR-215	0.005819	-1.68041
			hsa-miR-216	0.042686	-1.38497
			hsa-miR-218	0.045402	-0.86703
			hsa-miR-324-3p	0.034135	-0.52073
			hsa-miR-324-5p	0.028667	-0.74833
			hsa-miR-326	0.048664	-0.71389
			hsa-miR-330	0.010354	-0.98399
			hsa-miR-331	0.004691	-0.73239
			hsa-miR-340	0.010086	-0.77428
			hsa-miR-488	0.01028	-1.08969
			hsa-miR-491	0.042597	-0.68084
			hsa-miR-628	0.000553	-1.00498

Table 3. Differentially expressed miRNAs in the advanced neuroblastoma (student t-test $p < 0.05$)

We found that two miRNAs predicted as up-regulated with enrichment score > 0, miR-9 and miR-18a*, are actually up-regulated in microarray experiments with student t-test $p < 0.05$. Since miR-18a* is a minor strand (less present than miR-18a) within the mir-17-92 cluster, we conclude that miR-9 is the most consistent miRNA in terms of its expression and its targets' expression in our analysis. Fig. 2 shows the box plots of miR-9 expressions in advanced and low-risk stage patient samples together with five other miRNAs whose expression values are most significantly changed in up- and down-regulated miRNAs.

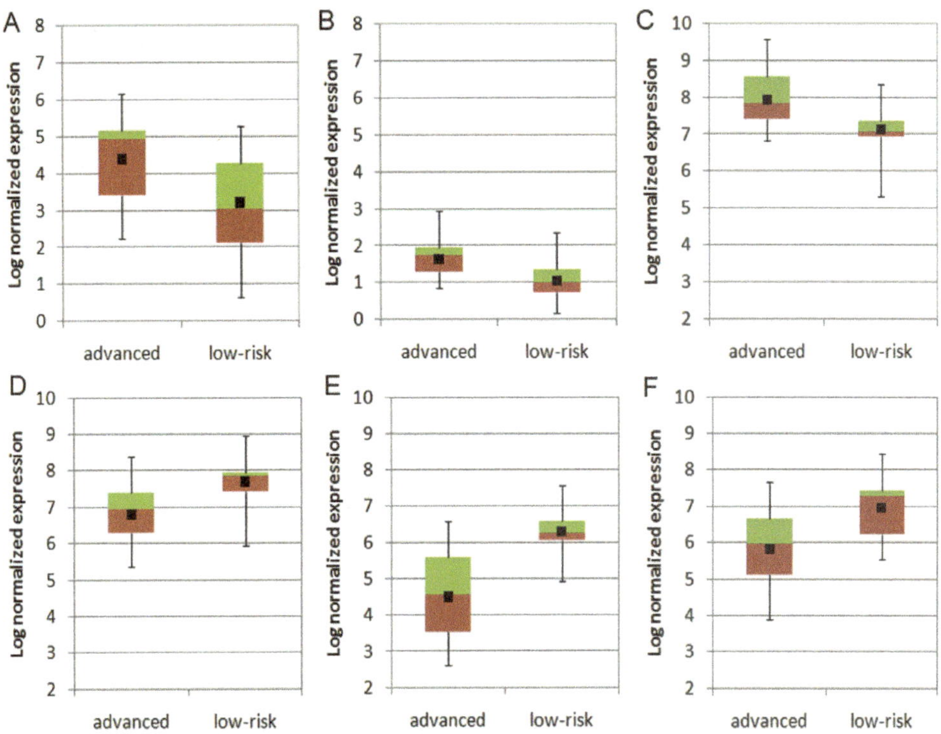

Fig. 2. Box plots of miR-9 (A), miR-18a* (B), miR-92 (C), miR-125b (D), miR-137 (E), and miR-149 (F) expression between advanced and low-risk stage neuroblastoma patient samples.

2.3 Correlation of mRNA and miRNA expression data

We found miR-9 to have the most consistent signal in terms of miRNA and mRNA expression level changes in advanced neuroblastoma. Note that miRNA expression pattern alone does not justify further in-depth analyses of miR-9 since other miRNAs have higher fold changes or lower p-value. Our approach thus provides a new way to prioritize important miRNAs. Interestingly, miR-9's seven predicted targets genes are found only in the down-regulated genes. However, this does not mean that expressions of miR-9 and its target genes are negatively correlated across entire samples. Fig. 3 shows the Pearson product moment correlation coefficient of miR-9 and its seven target genes across the 30 patient samples. For context, correlations between miR-9 and all mRNA expression are also shown. The correlations of miR-9 and target genes stand out from all other correlations, six of the seven targets being negatively correlated with miR-9. The six negatively correlated predicted targets are AGPAT4, BTBD9, GABBR1, KCNK10, LRRTM4, and S100PBP. Among them, LRRTM4 is in Table 1, containing top 50 greatest fold change genes. Fig. 4 shows the scatter plots of the two most negatively correlated miR-9 target genes.

Though miR-9 can target multiple genes at the same time, the expression of each target gene varies from person to person, so that its function on each target gene might vary among patients. In our analysis, six genes are predicted as functional targets in the neuroblastoma, potentially responsible for disease progression. As an example, some outliers shown in the circle in Fig. 4B are no longer outliers in the S100PBP case in Fig. 4A. Therefore, rather than one miRNA or one miRNA and its target, collective miR-9 targets and miR-9 might allow more accurate prediction of whether a neuroblastoma will progress to advanced stage.

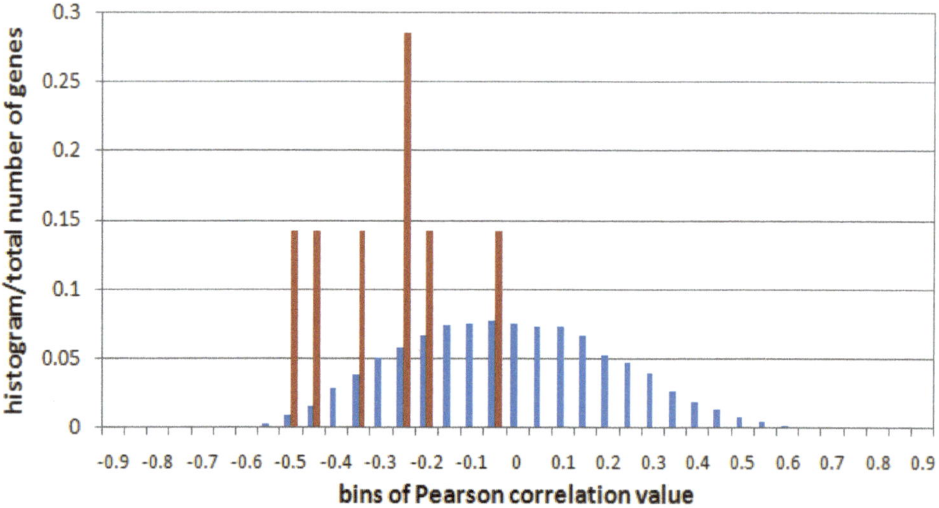

Fig. 3. Histogram of Pearson correlation values between miR-9 and gene expressions. The red bars show miR-9 target genes found in the down-regulated genes; blue bars represent all genes measured in the microarray experiments (total 1,4159 genes excluding ones with blank data > 5 among samples).

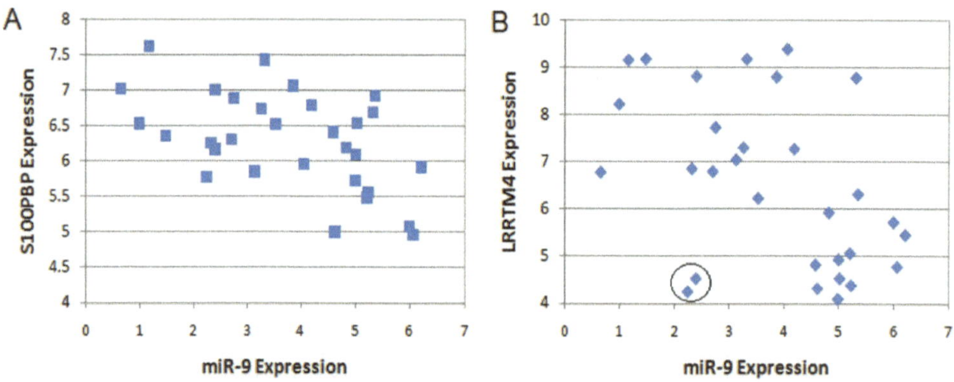

Fig. 4. Scatter plots showing miR-9 and target gene expressions for 30 patient samples. Pearson correlation coefficient of miR-9 and S100PBP is -0.53 (A) and that of miR-9 and LRRTM4 is -0.48 (B).

3. miR-9 signature in short - and long - lived patients

Scaruffi et al. published research on non-coding RNA expressions with regard to outcome in high-risk neuroblastoma (Scaruffi et al., 2009). Among 31 high-risk, stage 4 neuroblastoma samples, miRNA expressions came from 17 short-term survivors (dead within 36 months from diagnosis) and 14 long-term survivors (alive with an overall survival time > 36 months) were deposited in GEO (Series accession number GSE16444). We downloaded the data, which were log_2-transformed and quantile normalized, after obtaining the raw data using miRNA microarray System protocol v. 1.5 (Agilent Tenchnologies). Since they removed probes with less than 50% of detected slops across all arrays, many low signals were not present. We used the downloaded data to identify differential miRNAs between short- and long-term survivor groups. Significance was calculated with a student's t-test (unpaired, two-tailed, unequal variance); miRNAs up- and down-regulated in short-term survivors with p-values less than 0.05 are shown in Table 4.

up-regulated miRNA	p-value	Log_2 (fold change)	down-regulated miRNA	p-value	Log_2 (fold change)
hsa-miR-9	0.0377472	0.68625181	hsa-miR-22	0.040065	-0.990610191
hsa-miR-210	0.0284823	1.147684424	hsa-miR-139-3p	0.0478034	-0.803202819
hsa-miR-425	0.0127439	0.62221312	hsa-miR-181c*	0.0497988	-1.015817709
hsa-miR-758	0.0080157	1.01630988	hsa-miR-302a	0.0338064	-0.915468934
hsa-miR-885-5p	0.0117879	1.125425787	hsa-miR-502-3p	0.0481067	-0.69939469
hsa-miR-885-3p	0.0118758	0.669348934	hsa-miR-886-3p	0.0424204	-1.691328238
hsa-miR-877	0.0276158	0.571214174			
hsa-miR-936	0.0388439	0.656436824			

Table 4. Differentially expressed miRNAs in short-term survivors compared with long-term survivors. All patients had advanced neuroblastoma.

Due to the distinct difference between diseased and healthy status, the overall number of differentially expressed miRNAs with a certain p-value cutoff may be much greater than that within the disease group. Within the disease group, though neuroblastoma has diverse outcomes, differentiating stages within the neuroblastoma is more difficult than differentiating disease from normal. To increase differentiating power, we did not include stage 3 neuroblastoma data in our section 2 analysis. Here, we further differentiate a narrower range within stage 4. Therefore, it is not surprising that fewer miRNAs were differentiated here than between advanced and low-risk neuroblastoma. Also, it is common for different research groups to produce differing lists of significantly changed genes.

However, if underlying causes exist for advanced neuroblastoma which further lead to short-term survival, we might identify them from a persistent signal in various contexts. We find miR-9, the only miRNA common between Table 3 and 4, to be such a consistent signal. We want to emphasize that miR-9 must be evaluated in connection with target gene expressions. It was found to be the most consistent miRNA in terms of down-regulating target mRNAs when induced. Moreover, its expression differs between short- and long-term survivors. When it comes to identifying miRNA signature from expression data, it is therefore crucial to compare a miRNA's target expression patterns with its own expression. While many studies focus on global correlations between miRNA and mRNA expressions without a clear regulating matrix, our method of assessing consistency clearly helps pinpoint the signature miRNA in the disease progression.

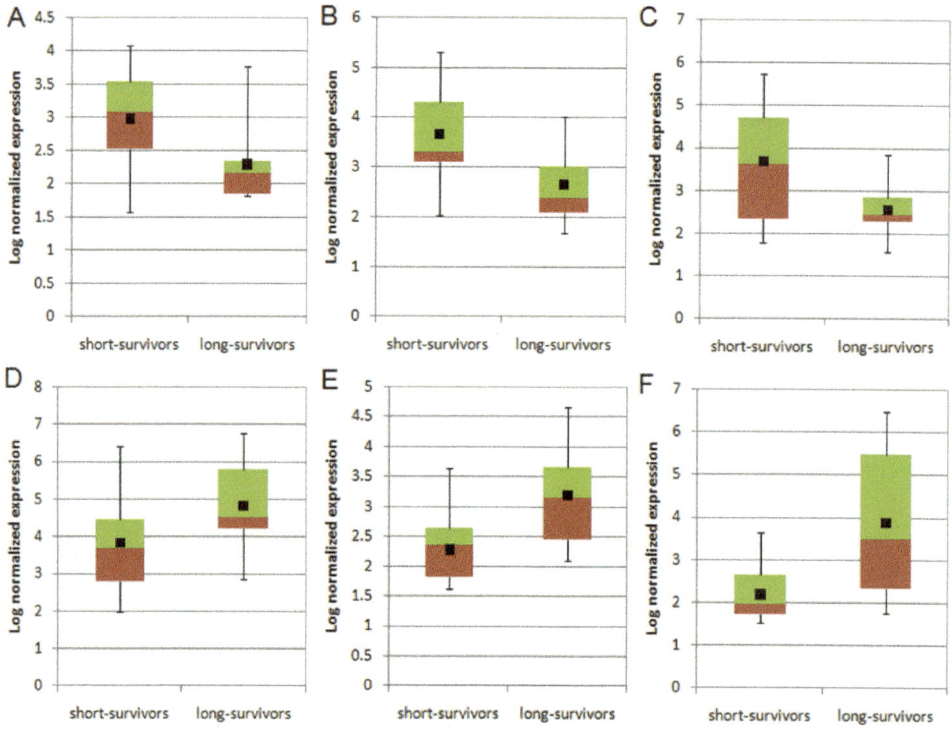

Fig. 5. Box plots of miR-9 (A), miR-758 (B), miR-885-5p (C), miR-22 (D), miR-302a (E), and miR-886-3p (F) expressions of neuroblastoma between short- and long-term survivors in advanced stage patients.

Fig. 5 shows the box plot of miR-9 and five other miRNA expressions (chosen in order of smaller p-values) of samples from short- and long-term survivors in the Table 4. Though the p-value of miR-9 is not as low as others, its differentiating power is close to that of miR-758. In Fig. 2, the miR-9 level itself may not be powerful enough to differentiate advanced stage from low-risk neuroblastoma. Here, the data suggest that the broader range of miR-9 expression in advanced stage is due to its differentiating power between two sub-groups of advanced stage patients (absolute number of normalized data in each dataset is not meaningful). In terms of early prognostic power, miR-9 and its targets hold high promise. Further investigation using larger samples is needed.

4. miR-9 functional model in advanced neuroblastoma

Recently, Ma et al. reported that miR-9 directly targets E-cadherin (CDH1), leading to increased cell motility and invasiveness in breast cancer (Ma et al., 2010). Though in a different cell type, since the function of CDH1 in solid tumors is the same, we expect miR-9 to function similarly in the neuroblastoma. Moreover, as a MYCN-activated miRNA, miR-9 fits well within the neuroblastoma miRNA networks (Fig. 1) as a function of developing advanced metastasized neuroblastoma. Our identification of miR-9 and its targets thus makes sense functionally as an early prognostic marker for developing high mortality neuroblastoma. Fig. 1 includes miR-9 and CDH1 as a functional model of developing advanced stage neuroblastoma.

5. Conclusion

We have used our new method to analyze mRNA and miRNA expression data to identify signature miRNA and target genes in stage 4 neuroblastoma. To obtain maximal contrast between the non-metastatic stages and metastatic stage 4, we excluded stage 3 data and combined stage 1 and 2 as low-risk. When we compared advanced and low-risk stage neuroblastoma, miR-9 related expressions had the most consistent data between mRNA and miRNA expression. We also confirmed that six out of the seven predicted targets were negatively correlated with miR-9 expression across entire samples. Furthermore, miR-9 expression was significantly up-regulated in samples from short-term survivors compared with those from long-term survivors within the same advanced-stage neuroblastoma group. In addition to these data-driven analyses, note that miR-9 has been identified as inducing metastasis in breast cancer by targeting E-cadherin. Therefore, our claim of expressions of miR-9 and its targets as a signature of advancing neuroblastoma fits well with previous studies. Further investigation with a larger number of samples is needed.

6. Acknowledgment

We thank the Vandesompele group for providing paired mRNA and miRNA expression data of samples from neuroblastoma patients.

7. References

Ajay, S. S., Athey, B. D., & Lee, I. (2010). Unified translation repression mechanism for microRNAs and upstream AUGs. *BMC Genomics*, Vol. 11, pp. (155)

Asgharzadeh, S., Pique-Regi, R., Sposto, R., Wang, H., et al. (2006). Prognostic significance of gene expression profiles of metastatic neuroblastomas lacking MYCN gene amplification. *J Natl Cancer Inst*, Vol. 98, No. 17, pp. (1193-203)

Bordow, S. B., Norris, M. D., Haber, P. S., Marshall, G. M., et al. (1998). Prognostic significance of MYCN oncogene expression in childhood neuroblastoma. *J Clin Oncol*, Vol. 16, No. 10, pp. (3286-94)

Bray, I., Tivnan, A., Bryan, K., Foley, N. H., et al. (2011). MicroRNA-542-5p as a novel tumor suppressor in neuroblastoma. *Cancer Lett*, Vol. 303, No. 1, pp. (56-64)

Buechner, J., Tomte, E., Haug, B. H., Henriksen, J. R., et al. (2011). Tumour-suppressor microRNAs let-7 and mir-101 target the proto-oncogene MYCN and inhibit cell proliferation in MYCN-amplified neuroblastoma. *Br J Cancer*, Vol. 105, No. 2, pp. (296-303)

Chen, Y., & Stallings, R. L. (2007). Differential patterns of microRNA expression in neuroblastoma are correlated with prognosis, differentiation, and apoptosis. *Cancer Res*, Vol. 67, No. 3, pp. (976-83)

Christoffersen, N. R., Shalgi, R., Frankel, L. B., Leucci, E., et al. (2010). p53-independent upregulation of miR-34a during oncogene-induced senescence represses MYC. *Cell Death Differ*, Vol. 17, No. 2, pp. (236-45)

De Preter, K., Vermeulen, J., Brors, B., Delattre, O., et al. (2010). Accurate outcome prediction in neuroblastoma across independent data sets using a multigene signature. *Clin Cancer Res*, Vol. 16, No. 5, pp. (1532-41)

Foley, N. H., Bray, I., Watters, K. M., Das, S., et al. (2011). MicroRNAs 10a and 10b are potent inducers of neuroblastoma cell differentiation through targeting of nuclear receptor corepressor 2. *Cell Death Differ*, Vol. 18, No. 7, pp. (1089-98)

Foley, N. H., Bray, I. M., Tivnan, A., Bryan, K., et al. (2010). MicroRNA-184 inhibits neuroblastoma cell survival through targeting the serine/threonine kinase AKT2. *Mol Cancer*, Vol. 9, pp. (83)

Guo, J., Dong, Q., Fang, Z., Chen, X., et al. (2010). Identification of miRNAs that are associated with tumor metastasis in neuroblastoma. *Cancer Biol Ther*, Vol. 9, No. 6, pp. (446-52)

Haug, B. H., Henriksen, J. R., Buechner, J., Geerts, D., et al. (2011). MYCN-regulated miRNA-92 inhibits secretion of the tumor suppressor DICKKOPF-3 (DKK3) in neuroblastoma. *Carcinogenesis*, Vol. 32, No. 7, pp. (1005-12)

He, L., He, X., Lim, L. P., de Stanchina, E., et al. (2007). A microRNA component of the p53 tumour suppressor network. *Nature*, Vol. 447, No. 7148, pp. (1130-4)

He, L., Thomson, J. M., Hemann, M. T., Hernando-Monge, E., et al. (2005). A microRNA polycistron as a potential human oncogene. *Nature*, Vol. 435, No. 7043, pp. (828-33)

Heuberger, J., & Birchmeier, W. (2010). Interplay of cadherin-mediated cell adhesion and canonical Wnt signaling. *Cold Spring Harb Perspect Biol*, Vol. 2, No. 2, pp. (a002915)

Jiang, M., Stanke, J., & Lahti, J. M. (2011). The connections between neural crest development and neuroblastoma. *Curr Top Dev Biol*, Vol. 94, pp. (77-127)

Kim, N. H., Kim, H. S., Li, X.-Y., Lee, I., et al. (2011). A p53/miRNA-34 Axis Regulates Snail1-Dependent Cancer Cell Epithelial-Mesenchymal Transition. *J Cell Biol*, Vol. 195, No. 3, pp. (417-433)

Kim, V. N. (2005). MicroRNA biogenesis: coordinated cropping and dicing. *Nat Rev Mol Cell Biol*, Vol. 6, No. 5, pp. (376-85)

Kozomara, A., & Griffiths-Jones, S. (2010). miRBase: integrating microRNA annotation and deep-sequencing data. *Nucleic Acids Res*, Vol. 39, No. Database issue, pp. (D152-7)

Lee, I., Ajay, S. S., Yook, J. I., Kim, H. S., et al. (2009). New class of microRNA targets containing simultaneous 5'-UTR and 3'-UTR interaction sites. *Genome Res*, Vol. 19, No. 7, pp. (1175-83)

Lim, L. P., Lau, N. C., Garrett-Engele, P., Grimson, A., et al. (2005). Microarray analysis shows that some microRNAs downregulate large numbers of target mRNAs. *Nature*, Vol. 433, No. 7027, pp. (769-73)

Lin, R. J., Lin, Y. C., Chen, J., Kuo, H. H., et al. (2010). microRNA signature and expression of Dicer and Drosha can predict prognosis and delineate risk groups in neuroblastoma. *Cancer Res*, Vol. 70, No. 20, pp. (7841-50)

Ma, L., Young, J., Prabhala, H., Pan, E., et al. (2010). miR-9, a MYC/MYCN-activated microRNA, regulates E-cadherin and cancer metastasis. *Nat Cell Biol*, Vol. 12, No. 3, pp. (247-56)

Matsubara, H., Takeuchi, T., Nishikawa, E., Yanagisawa, K., et al. (2007). Apoptosis induction by antisense oligonucleotides against miR-17-5p and miR-20a in lung cancers overexpressing miR-17-92. *Oncogene*, Vol. 26, No. 41, pp. (6099-105)

Mestdagh, P., Bostrom, A. K., Impens, F., Fredlund, E., et al. (2010a). The miR-17-92 microRNA cluster regulates multiple components of the TGF-beta pathway in neuroblastoma. *Mol Cell*, Vol. 40, No. 5, pp. (762-73)

Mestdagh, P., Fredlund, E., Pattyn, F., Schulte, J. H., et al. (2010b). MYCN/c-MYC-induced microRNAs repress coding gene networks associated with poor outcome in MYCN/c-MYC-activated tumors. *Oncogene*, Vol. 29, No. 9, pp. (1394-404)

Oberthuer, A., Berthold, F., Warnat, P., Hero, B., et al. (2006). Customized oligonucleotide microarray gene expression-based classification of neuroblastoma patients outperforms current clinical risk stratification. *J Clin Oncol*, Vol. 24, No. 31, pp. (5070-8)

Oberthuer, A., Hero, B., Berthold, F., Juraeva, D., et al. (2010). Prognostic impact of gene expression-based classification for neuroblastoma. *J Clin Oncol*, Vol. 28, No. 21, pp. (3506-15)

Papadopoulos, G. L., Reczko, M., Simossis, V. A., Sethupathy, P., et al. (2009). The database of experimentally supported targets: a functional update of TarBase. *Nucleic Acids Res*, Vol. 37, No. Database issue, pp. (D155-8)

Scaruffi, P., Stigliani, S., Moretti, S., Coco, S., et al. (2009). Transcribed-Ultra Conserved Region expression is associated with outcome in high-risk neuroblastoma. *BMC Cancer*, Vol. 9, pp. (441)

Schulte, J. H., Horn, S., Otto, T., Samans, B., et al. (2008). MYCN regulates oncogenic MicroRNAs in neuroblastoma. *Int J Cancer*, Vol. 122, No. 3, pp. (699-704)

Tivnan, A., Foley, N. H., Tracey, L., Davidoff, A. M., et al. (2010). MicroRNA-184-mediated inhibition of tumour growth in an orthotopic murine model of neuroblastoma. *Anticancer Res*, Vol. 30, No. 11, pp. (4391-5)

Tivnan, A., Tracey, L., Buckley, P. G., Alcock, L. C., et al. (2011). MicroRNA-34a is a potent tumor suppressor molecule in vivo in neuroblastoma. *BMC Cancer*, Vol. 11, pp. (33)

12

Retinoic-Acid-Induced Downregulation of the 67 KDa Laminin Receptor Correlates with Reduced Biological Aggressiveness of Human Neuroblastoma Cells

Juan M. Escamilla[1], Christine Bäuerl[1], Carlos M. R. López[1], Satu P. Pekkala[1], Samuel Navarro[2] and Domingo Barettino[1]
[1]Instituto de Biomedicina de Valencia, Consejo Superior de Investigaciones Científicas, Valencia, [2]Dept. of Pathology, School of Medicine, University of Valencia, Valencia Spain

1. Introduction

Neuroblastoma is a common tumor of the childhood arising from embryonal sympathetic neural cell precursors. Despite of the improved therapeutic strategies, the survival rate of high-risk neuroblastoma patients is poor. Although complete clinical remissions can be achieved, relapse is relatively frequent, indicating a role for the persistence of the minimal residual disease (for review, Maris, 2010). Treatments with derivatives of retinoic acid (RA), the biologically active form of vitamin A, produce significant improvements on the therapy of high-risk neuroblastoma patients, when used together with intensive multimodal therapies (Reynolds et al., 2003, for review). Despite some controversy on dosage and treatment schedules (Matthay & Reynolds, 2000; Reynolds et al., 2003), treatment with 13-*cis*-RA (isotretinoin) has been reported to produce a modest but significant increase in the event-free survival of high-risk neuroblastoma patients (Matthay et al., 2009; Matthay et al., 1999). RA and its derivatives, the retinoids, are differentiating agents that induce growth arrest, differentiation and/or apoptosis of neuroblastoma cells *in vitro* (Lovat et al., 1997; Pahlman et al., 1984; Sidell, 1982; Thiele et al., 1985). However the molecular bases of RA therapeutic actions in neuroblastoma have not been established yet.

With the aim of identifying possible molecular targets for RA treatment, we have analyzed RA-induced gene expression changes in SH-SY5Y cultured human neuroblastoma cells (Lopez-Carballo et al., 2002), by means of Ordered Differential Display RT-PCR (Matz et al., 1997). Among more than 60 genes identified, we could found *LAMR1* (also called *RPSA*), encoding the precursor for the 67-KDa Laminin Receptor (67LR) (Wewer et al., 1986; Yow et al., 1988), whose mRNA levels were remarkably reduced after RA treatment. The 67LR is a multifunctional protein which is involved in cell adhesion, required for maintaining of cell viability (Scheiman et al., 2010; Susantad & Smith, 2008), acts as receptor for infectious agents like viruses and prions (Vana et al., 2009) and mediates the actions of the green tea polyphenol epigallocatechin-3-gallate (Umeda et al., 2008). Expression of 67LR has been correlated with the biological aggressiveness, and the invasive and metastatic capacities of tumors from diverse origin. Many examples in which the expression of 67LR is increased in a tumor in respect to the corresponding normal tissue have been reported, and elevated expression of 67LR correlates with tumor progression and has been considered as adverse prognostic factor in several human cancers (Castronovo, 1993; Menard et al., 1997; Menard et al., 1998; Viacava et al., 1997, for review). *LAMR1* encodes a 37 KDa precursor protein (Wewer et al., 1986; Yow et al., 1988), that is acylated and glycosylated to generate the mature 67LR (Buto et al., 1998; Katagiri et al., 2005; Landowski et al., 1995) A role of 67LR in stabilizing the binding of integrins to laminin has been postulated (Magnifico et al., 1996), and it has been proposed that binding of 67LR contributes to laminin remodeling, thereby facilitating laminin degradation by proteolytic enzymes and increasing the release of motility fragments (Ardini et al., 2002; Berno et al., 2005; Vande Broek et al., 2001). Therefore, 67LR could play a role in the degradation of basal membrane whose major component is laminin, a critical step of the metastasis process and a prerequisite for tumor vascularization, involving the invasion of tumor mass by endothelial cells.

We report here that RA treatment of human neuroblastoma cells induces a reduction on the mRNA and protein levels of 67LR. In parallel, RA treatment impaired neuroblastoma cell migration towards laminin in haptotaxis assays *in vitro* and reduced invasiveness through *Matrigel* in *in vitro* invasion assays, processes in which 67LR played a major role. In addition, we show by immunohistochemical methods that more than two thirds of the human high-risk neuroblastic tumors assayed expressed 67LR to certain extent. The results showed here support an important role for 67LR in migration towards and invasion through the basement membrane, critical steps on the metastasis process. RA-induced downregulation of 67LR correlates with a reduction in the biological aggressiveness *in vitro* of neuroblastoma cells, and supports the idea of 67LR as an important molecular target for the therapeutic actions of RA in neuroblastoma.

2. Experimental procedures

2.1 Cell culture and treatments

SH-SY5Y cells (ATCC no. CRL-2266) were cultured in DMEM containing 10% heat-inactivated FBS, 100 U/ml penicillin and 100 μg/ml streptomycin. LA-N-1 cells (ECACC no. 06041201) were grown in a 1:1 mixture of EMEM and Ham's F-12 medium containing 10% heat-inactivated FBS, 100 U/ml penicillin, 100 μg/ml streptomycin and 1% non-essential amino acids. Cell cultures were kept in a humidified incubator at 37°C with 5% CO_2. The medium was replaced every 2 days and the cells were split before they reached confluence. Cycloheximide (CHX), all-*trans*-retinoic acid (RA), and LY294002 (LY) were purchased from Sigma. The different compounds were dissolved in Dimethyl-sulfoxide and added to the culture medium at the indicated concentrations. Peptide P11 (Ac-CDPGYIGSR-NH_2, (Graf et al., 1987b) and its Scrambled control (Ac-YCIPGDRGS-NH_2) were synthesized and purified by HPLC to >90%. Peptides were dissolved in serum-free culture medium at 60 μg/ml (60 μM).

2.2 RNA analysis

Northern Blot analysis of total RNA from SH-SY5Y cells with [^{32}P]-labeled probes were performed as previously described (Lopez-Carballo et al., 2002). *LAMR1* probe consisted of a 1 Kb fragment obtained from the EST clone IMAGE 1271323. Probes for Cyclophilin A (*PPIA)* and beta-actin (*ACTB*) consisted in cDNA fragments generated by RT-PCR. For quantification of the *LAMR1* expression levels, duplicate Northern Blots were exposed to Fuji IP capture plates, measured using a Fuji FLA-5000 laser scanner and analyzed using Fuji ImageQuant software. *LAMR1* absolute values were normalized to the values obtained for *ACTB*.

2.3 Western blot

Whole cell extracts were obtained by lysis of the cells in RIPA buffer (50 mM Hepes pH 7.4, 150 mM NaCl, 1.5 mM $MgCl_2$, 1 mM EGTA, 10% Glycerol) containing 0.5% Nonidet P-40, 0.1% SDS, protease inhibitors (1 mM PMSF, 40 μg/ml aprotinin and 40 μg/ml leupeptin) and phosphatase inhibitors (1 mM sodium ortovanadate, 1 mM NaF). After 10 min incubation on ice, the lysate was cleared by centrifugation (16,100xg, 10 min, 4°C), and protein concentration determined. Extracts were diluted with 2x sample buffer containing freshly added 50 mM Dithiothreitol. Western blot analysis of proteins from whole cell extracts was performed as described (Lopez-Carballo et al., 2002). Antibodies against the 67-KDa Laminin Receptor (Wewer et al., 1987), were obtained from Abcam. Monoclonal antibodies against the 37-KDa Laminin Receptor precursor (MPLR, Buto et al., 1997) were a generous gift of Dr. S. Menard (Istituto Nazionale Tumori, Milan, Italy). Antibodies against beta-actin were purchased from Sigma. Horseradish-peroxidase-conjugated secondary antibodies were obtained from GE Healthcare, and Jackson ImmunoResearch. Chemiluminiscent signals were developed with ECL (GE Healthcare).

2.4 Immunofluorescence

SH-SY5Y neuroblastoma cells were treated with RA or vehicle for 96 h, scraped from the plate and washed in PBS. A drop of the cell suspension was applied onto poly-lysine-coated slides and let to settle for 10 min at room temperature. The slides were fixed with 4% paraformaldehyde in PBS for 20 min, and washed three times with PBS. After blocking with 3% Bovine Serum Albumin in Phosphate Buffered Saline (PBS) for 40 min, slides were sequentially incubated with Anti-67-KDa Laminin Receptor (Abcam, diluted 1:50 in the same buffer) and Fluorescein-isothiocyanate (FITC)-conjugated anti-rabbit IgG (Jackson ImmunoResearch, diluted 1:100 in the same buffer). After washing with PBS, the slides were counter-stained with Hoechst 33258 (Scharlab, 50 mg/ml) for 5 min, rinsed with PBS and mounted with anti-fade mounting medium (Dako-Cytomation). Slides were sequentially photographed in a Leica fluorescence microscope equipped with FITC- and UV-specific excitation filters.

2.5 Migration and invasion assays

The effects of RA treatments, and Laminin β1-derived peptide P11 on the migration and invasion capacities of SH-SY5Y neuroblastoma cells were tested according to published protocols (Albini et al., 1987; McCarthy et al., 1983), with slight modifications. A modified, light-opaque Boyden chamber (Falcon HTS FluoroBlok, 8 μm pore size; Becton-Dickinson) was used in both migration and invasion assays. Cells were treated with 1 μM RA or vehicle in culture medium during the indicated times, and labeled in the plate with Calcein AM (5 μM; Molecular Probes-Invitrogen), during 30 min at 37°C. Labeled cells were detached from the plate by scraping and counted. Migration/haptotaxis assays (see Fig. 3A) were used to measure cell movement toward an immobilized laminin-rich extracellular matrix protein gradient. For that purpose, the lower chamber of the plate was coated with BD *Matrigel*

Matrix (10 μg/cm^2; Becton Dickinson) as attractant and filled with serum-free medium. 50,000 labeled cells in serum-free medium were added onto the upper chamber. As control, equivalent experiments in which coating with *Matrigel* was omitted were set. After 6h of incubation at 37°C, the fluorescent light emitted by the cells that migrated through the opaque filter was measured with a Victor^2 multilabel counter (PerkinElmer Life and Analytical Sciences). The assays were performed at least in triplicate. For invasion assays (see Fig. 3C) the porous membrane of the Boyden chamber was covered with BD *Matrigel* matrix (5 μg/cm^2 in serum-free medium; Becton Dickinson) and allowed to gel for 30 min. 50,000 calcein-labeled cells were carefully layered on top of the *Matrigel* layer and culture medium containing 10% FBS as chemoattractant to promote cell invasion was placed into the lower well. The fluorescent light emitted by cells in the lower chamber after 6 h incubation at 37°C was measured in triplicate assays as above. Peptide blocking of 67LR was performed by incubating 50,000 labeled cells in 500 μl of serum-free medium with P11 peptide or Scrambled control peptide (60 μg/ml; 60μM) for 30 min at 37°C and added to the upper chamber of migration/haptotaxis or invasion assays prepared as described above. For statistical analysis, one-way ANOVA together with Tukey post-hoc test were employed.

2.6 Immunocytochemistry

Immunohistochemical study was performed following streptavidin-biotin method with antigen retrieval using citrate buffer 0.1M, pH 6.0 and heating with autoclave at 1.5 atm during 3 minutes. Primary antibody (Anti-67-KDa Laminin Receptor, Abcam) was diluted 1:100. Positive controls include internal epithelial tissues as well as one case of invasive breast carcinoma. Negative controls consisted in substitution of the primary antibody by mouse ascites and/or PBS. Immunohistochemistry was performed on a tissue microarray composed of cylinders of 1.5 mm in diameter of 49 cases of Neuroblastoma that was assembled using a manual tissue arrayer (MTA , Beecher Inc, USA) (Noguera et al., 2009).

3. Results

3.1 RA treatment of SH-SY5Y neuroblastoma cells results in downregulation of the expression of the metastasis-associated 67-KDa Laminin receptor

To identify differentially expressed genes during RA treatment of human neuroblastoma cells we have used the Ordered Differential Display RT-PCR technique (Matz et al., 1997). One of the displayed fragments, showing strong downregulation after 24 h of RA treatment, was amplified and sequenced. The sequence obtained (data not shown) corresponded to the *LAMR1* gene (also called *RPSA*), encoding the 67 KDa Laminin Receptor (67LR; Wewer et al., 1986; Yow et al., 1988). Because 67LR has been described as a metastasis-associated gene, whose expression levels are related to tumoral progression (Menard et al., 1997; Menard et al., 1998; Sobel, 1993) we decided to study the regulation of *LAMR1* transcription by RA with some detail. As shown on the Northern Blot in Fig. 1a, *LAMR1* expression levels were significantly reduced after a 24 h RA treatment. This delayed downregulation profile resembled that reported for the coordinate repression of the *ID1*, *ID2* and *ID3* HLH genes (Lopez-Carballo et al., 2002).

As was the case for the ID genes, the mechanism by which RA downregulates *LAMR1* expression appears to be complex. The reduction on the levels of *LAMR1* mRNA observed after 24 h of RA treatment did not occur when cells were pre-treated with the protein synthesis inhibitor Cycloheximide (CHX), indicating an indirect regulation that requires newly synthesized proteins (Fig. 1b). RA activates the PI3K/Akt signaling pathway through a non-genomic mechanism (Lopez-Carballo et al., 2002; Masiá et al., 2007). Such activation is also required for the downregulation of the expression of *LAMR1,* since it did not occur in cells treated with RA in the presence of the PI3K inhibitor LY290004 (Fig. 1b).

3.2 RA treatment reduces the presence of the 67-KDa Laminin receptor at the cell surface

67LR is synthesized as a 37-KD precursor (37LRP) subunit, which is processed to the mature form of the protein on the cell surface (Buto et al., 1998; Landowski et al., 1995). Using antibodies recognizing the mature form of this protein in Western Blots (Wewer et al., 1987), we have detected that RA treatment results in a decrease on the levels of 67LR in cellular extracts of SH-SY5Y cells(Fig. 2A). By means of a monoclonal antibody specific for the 37LRP (Buto et al., 1997), we observed a parallel reduction on the expression of the precursor protein (Fig. 2B). A similar RA-induced decrease in 67LR protein expression could be observed in another neuroblastoma cell line, LA-N-1 (Fig.2C). Immunofluorescent

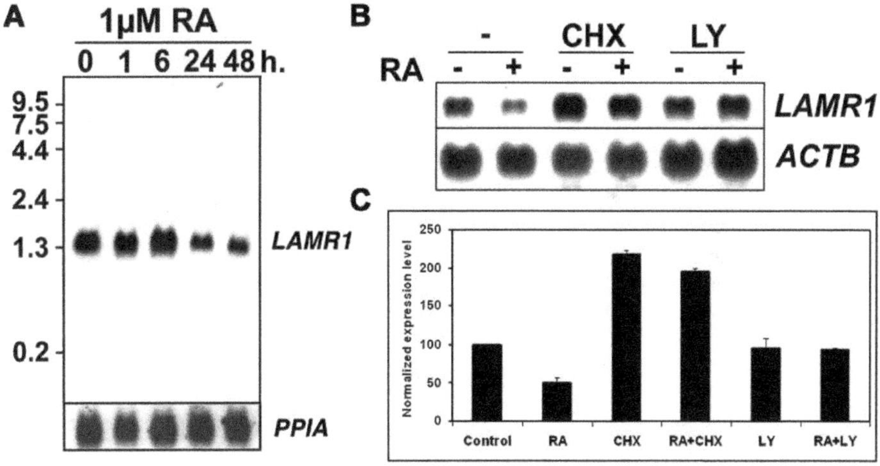

Fig. 1. (A-C) RA-induced downregulation of the expression of *LAMR1.*

A. Northern Blot. Each lane contains 15 µg of total RNA from SH-SY5Y neuroblastoma cells treated with 1 µM RA for the times indicated in the figure. The blot was sequentially hybridized with [^{32}P]-labeled DNA probes specific for the mRNAs of 67LR (*LAMR1,* 1.3 kb), and cyclophilin A (peptidyl- prolyl-isomerase A, *PPIA,* 1 Kb) as internal loading control.
B. Northern Blot. Each lane contains 15 µg of total RNA from SH-SY5Y neuroblastoma cells pre-treated during 30 min with vehicle (-), Cycloheximide (CHX) or 10 µM LY294002 (LY), and then treated with 1 µM RA (+) or vehicle (-) during 24 h in the presence of the inhibitor. The blot was sequentially hybridized with [^{32}P]-labeled DNA probes specific for the mRNAs of the 67LR (*LAMR1,* 1.4 Kb), and Actin-β (*ACTB,* 2 Kb) as internal control.
C. Quantitative analysis of the experiment shown in (B). The radioactivity present in each band on the blot was determined with a Fuji FLA5000 phosphorimager. The values obtained for *LAMR1* probe were normalized with the corresponding *ACTB* values. The graph shows the average (bars) and standard deviation (error bars) of a duplicate experiments.

staining with the same antibody used on fig 2A, showed that 67LR is less abundant on the membranes of RA treated SH-SY5Ycells, as compared with untreated cells (Fig. 2D).

3.3 RA treatment of neuroblastoma cells reduces migration towards and invasion through Matrigel

Laminin is a basal membrane specific glycoprotein. Apart from its structural function, this protein presents a biological activity linked to adhesion, migration, growth and differentiation of certain cell types. Laminin is the major component of the commercial basal membrane preparation *Matrigel* (Kleinman & Martin, 2005, for review), that was used in the following experiments as source of laminin-rich matrix. RA has been reported to reduce the migratory, invasive and metastatic capacity of neuroblastoma cells in *in vitro* assays

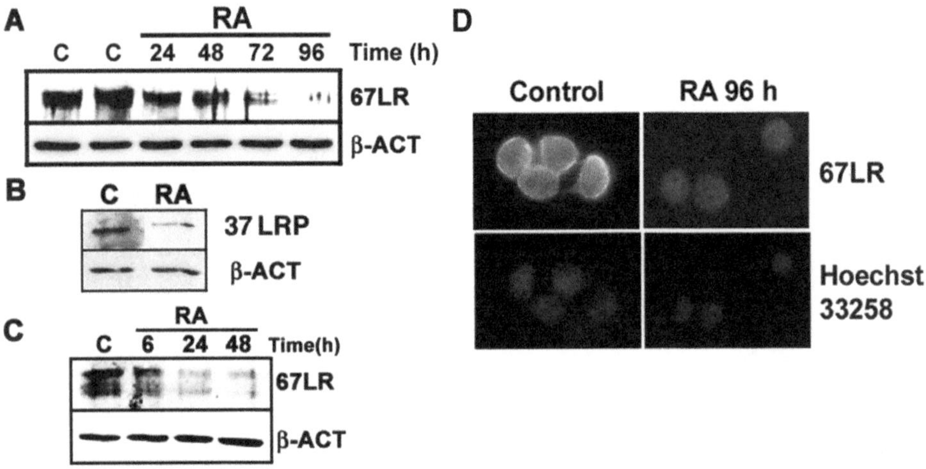

Fig. 2. (A-D) RA-induced reduction on the levels of the 67LR protein.

A. Western Blot. Each lane contains 20 µg of protein extract from SH-SY5Y neuroblastoma cells treated with 1 µM RA for the times indicated in the figure. The blot was sequentially incubated with specific antibodies raised against 67LR protein, and with β-actin antibodies (β-ACT), as loading control. B. Western Blot. Each lane contains 20 µg of protein extract from SH-SY5Y neuroblastoma cells treated with 1 µM RA or vehicle for 72 h. The blot was sequentially incubated with a monoclonal antibody against the 37 KDa Laminin Receptor Precursor protein (37LRP), and with β-actin antibodies (β-ACT), as loading control. C. Western Blot. Each lane contains 20 µg of protein extract from LA-N-1 neuroblastoma cells treated with 1 µM RA for the times indicated in the figure. The blot was sequentially incubated with specific antibodies raised against 67LR protein, and with β-actin antibodies (β-ACT), as loading control. D. Immunofluorescence Microscopy. SH-SY5Y cells were treated during 96 h with 1 µM RA or vehicle, scraped from the plate, and applied onto Poly-lysine-coated slides. The slides were fixed with 4% paraformaldehyde in PBS, and sequentially incubated with rabbit Anti-67LR and FITC-conjugated anti-rabbit IgG. After washing with PBS, the slides were counter-stained with Hoechst 33258 and sequentially photographed in a Leica fluorescence microscope equipped with FITC- and UV-specific excitation filters.

(Joshi et al., 2006; Joshi et al., 2007; Meseguer et al., 2011; Voigt & Zintl, 2003). To look for RA-induced biological effects in neuroblastoma cells that could be related to the observed downregulation of the 67LR, we used assays for migration/haptotaxis towards *Matrigel* and for invasion through *Matrigel*. Migration and invasion assays described here were based on published methods (Albini et al., 1987; McCarthy et al., 1983), and conducted measuring the proportion of calcein-labeled migrating cells in modified Boyden chamber assays, using FluoroBlok light-opaque transwell inserts. Calcein-labeled SH-SY5Y cells (50,000 cells/well) were seeded onto the upper chamber of a FluoroBlok Insert in serum-free DMEM. For migration/haptotaxis assays, the lower chamber was coated with *Matrigel* (10 µg/cm^2) and contained serum-free DMEM. (Fig. 3A). Similar experiments without *Matrigel* coating were set as negative controls for these experiments. Haptotaxis assays with neuroblastoma cells have shown increased migration when *Matrigel* is used as attractant. Surprisingly, short treatments with RA (24 h) resulted in a transient increase on cell migration that however occurred independently of the presence of chemoattractant. Treatment of SH-SY5Y cells

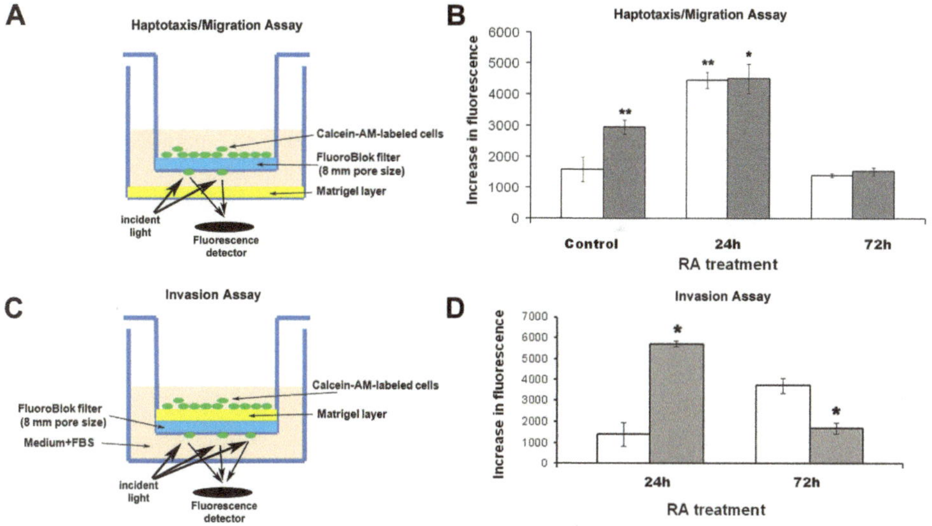

Fig. 3. (A-D) RA treatment reduces migration towards and invasion through *Matrigel*.

A. Schematic representation of the Haptotaxis/migration towards *Matrigel* assay. B. Effect of RA on cell migration towards *Matrigel*. Cells treated with 1 µM RA as indicated or untreated controls were assayed in the absence (empty bars) or in the presence (grey bars) of *Matrigel* as chemoattractant, and the increase in fluorescence was measured. The graph shows the average +/- SD of triplicate experiments. The asterisks indicate a statistically significative difference between the corresponding sample and the untreated control without chemoattractant (ANOVA test; * $p<0.05$; ** $p<0.01$). C. Schematic representation of the invasion assay. D. Effect of RA on cell invasion through *Matrigel*. Cells treated with RA as indicated (grey bars) and their corresponding untreated controls (empty bars) were assayed, and the increase in fluorescence was measured. The graph shows the average +/- SD of triplicate experiments. The asterisks indicate a statistically significative difference between the sample and its untreated control. (ANOVA test; * $p<0.05$).

with RA for 72 h reduced their migration rate and ablated the haptotactic attractive effect of *Matrigel* (Fig. 3B). For *in vitro* invasion assays the porous membrane separating both

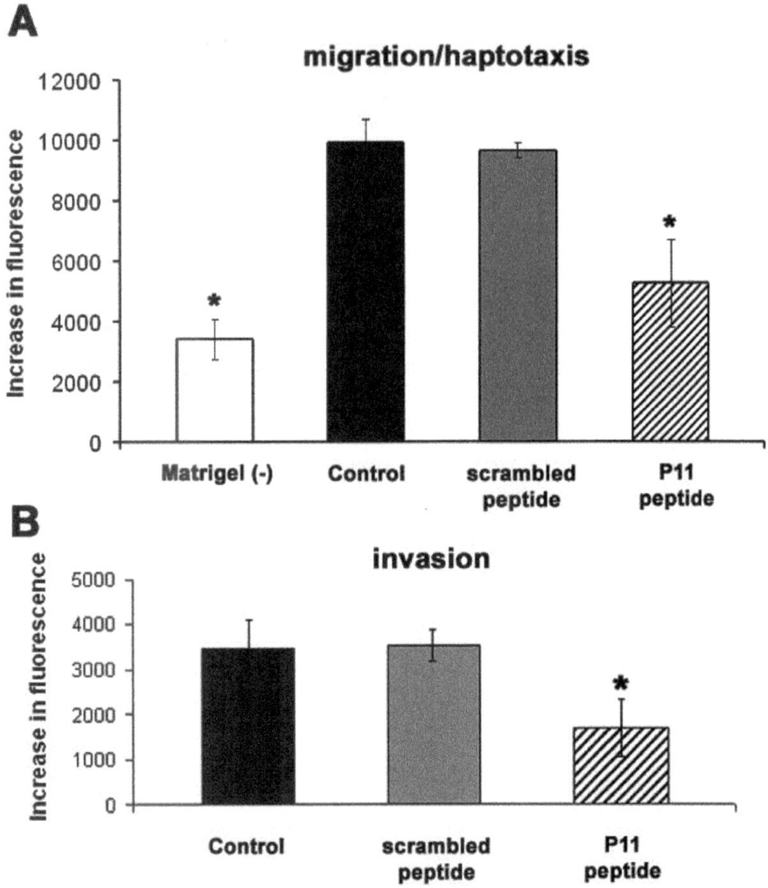

Fig. 4. (A-B) The 67-KDa laminin receptor is involved in migration towards and invasion through *Matrigel*.

A. Effect of Laminin peptide P11 on cell migration towards Matrigel. Untreated cells (black bar), as well as cells treated with scrambled peptide (grey bar) or P11 peptide (hatched bar) were assayed for migration using *Matrigel* as chemoattractant, together with a negative control experiment where the attractant was omitted (empty bar). The graph shows the average +/- SD of triplicate experiments. The asterisks indicate a statistically significative difference between the sample and its control. (ANOVA test; * $p<0.05$).
B. Effect of laminin peptide P11 on cell invasion through Matrigel. Untreated cells (black bar), as well as cells treated with scrambled peptide (grey bar) or P11 peptide (hatched bar) were used for *in vitro Matrigel* invasion assays. The graphs show the average +/- SD of triplicate experiments. The asterisks indicate a statistically significative difference between the sample and its control. (ANOVA test; * $p<0.05$).

chambers of a FluoroBlok transwell was covered with *Matrigel* (5μg/cm^2), simulating the basal membrane and 5% FBS was added to the lower chamber as chemoattractant (Fig. 3C). Similarly to what occurred with the migration assay, a transient increase on the invasive capacity of neuroblastoma cells was detected on *Matrigel* invasion assays after 24 h of RA treatment. Nevertheless, treatment with RA for 72 h resulted in strong reduction on the invasiveness of SH-SY5Y neuroblastoma cells (Fig. 3D). In the human neuroblastoma cell line LA-N-1 the effects of RA on migration/haptotaxis and in *in vitro* invasion were equivalent to those reported for SH-SY5Y cells (data not shown).

3.4 The 67-KDa Laminin receptor is involved in migration towards and invasion through Matrigel

The 67LR binds to the sequence CDPGYIGSR from the Laminin β1 chain (Graf et al., 1987b), and a peptide with that sequence (P11 peptide) impaired the activity of 67LR *in vitro* in laminin-mediated cell attachment and haptotaxis experiments (Graf et al., 1987a) and reduced the formation of experimental metastases *in vivo* (Iwamoto et al., 1987), probably by blocking the Laminin binding sites on 67LR. To assess the involvement of 67LR on the haptotaxis and invasiveness capacities of neuroblastoma cells, we have used P11 peptide to specifically block 67LR. Neuroblastoma cells were incubated with P11 peptide (60 μg/ml), or a scrambled peptide of the same chemical composition but different amino acid sequence. Afterwards the cells were used either on migration/haptotaxis experiments or in *in vitro* invasion assays as above. The results obtained showed that incubation of SH-SY5Y cells with P11 peptide significatively reduced migration towards *Matrigel*, whereas addition of the scrambled control peptide had no relevant effect. (Fig. 4A).

Similarly, addition of peptide P11 also reduced the invasion of neuroblastoma cells through *Matrigel*, whereas incubation with the control peptide had no remarkable effect on invasion (Fig. 4B). These results indicate the involvement of 67LR on laminin-induced migration/haptotaxis and in invasion through *Matrigel*-coated filters. Taken together, our results strongly support that RA-induced downregulation of 67LR contributes to the observed reduction of the biological aggressiveness of neuroblastoma cells after RA treatment.

3.5 Expression of the 67-KDa Laminin receptor in human neuroblastoma tumors

The expression of 67LR in human neuroblastoma primary tumors was tested by immunocytochemistry with the same 67LR antibody used for Western Blots and Expression of 67LR in neuroblastoma tumor samples was analyzed by immunohistochemistry with anti-67LR antibodies. The graph shows the percentage of the analyzed neuroblastoma samples (n=60) showing weak or no signal (empty sector), moderate intensity signal (hatched sector) or strong signal (black sector).

immunofluorescence. The antibody provided good results with paraffin sections, showing specific staining on epithelial tissues and invasive carcinomas used as positive controls (data not shown). Paraffin sections of a tissue microarray including 49 high-risk primary neuroblastoma tumor samples, including40 cases with *MYCN* amplification (100 to 500 copies per haploid genome) and 9 cases with *MYCN* gain (2 to 4 copies per haploid genome), and complete sections from 11 additional poorly differentiated neuroblastoma tumors were analyzed. From these 60 different human primary neuroblastoma samples 17 showed no or weak signal (28.33%), 22 showed positive staining with moderate intensity signal (36.67%), and 21 (35%) showed strong signal (Fig. 5).

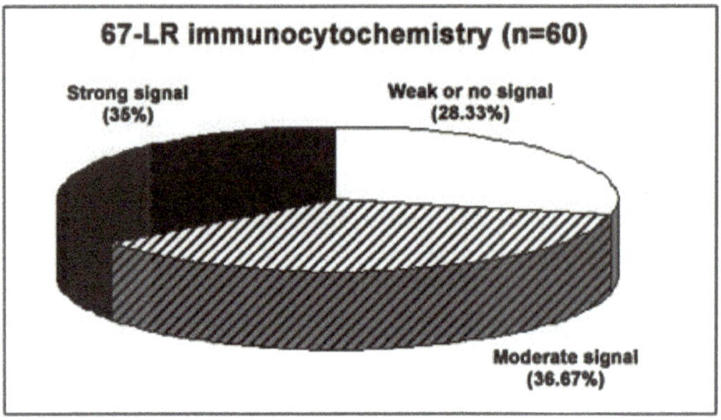

Fig. 5. Expression of 67LR in neuroblastoma tumor samples.

Photomicrographs of representative neuroblastoma tumor sections stained for 67LR are shown in Figure 6, including sections showing no signal (Fig. 6A), weak signal (Fig 6B), moderate intensity signal (Fig. 6 C and D), and strong signal (Fig. 6 E and F). Nuclear staining was detected in these strongly labeled tumor sections, which is an unexpected location for 67LR. Nevertheless, it has to be noted that shedding of 67LR by tumor cells has been reported (Berno et al., 2005; Karpatova et al., 1996; Moss et al., 2006), and it appears

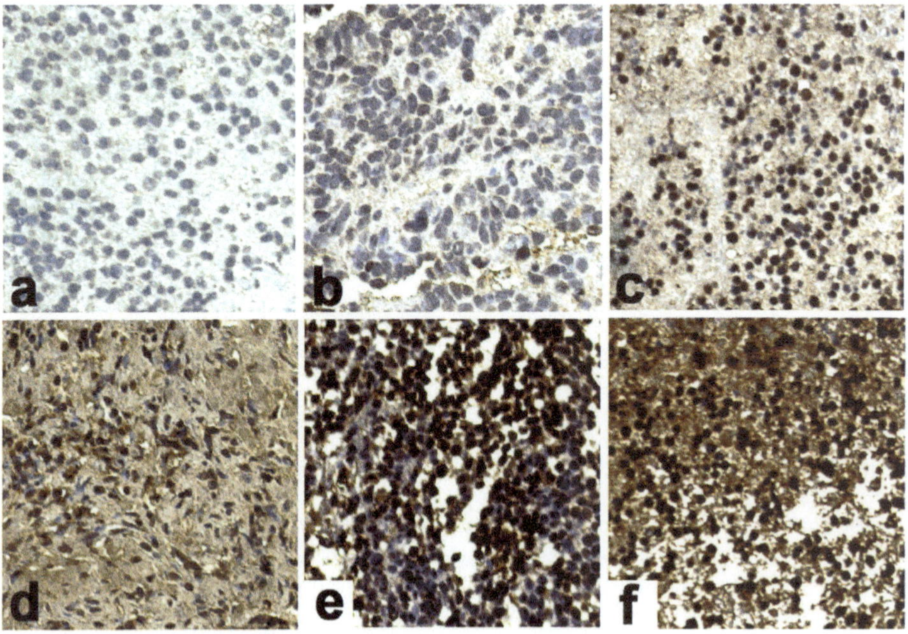

Fig. 6. (a-f) Immunohistochemical detection of 67LR in neuroblastoma tumor samples.

Photomicrographs of representative neuroblastoma tumor paraffin sections stained for 67LR antibody and counterstained with hematoxylin, including sections showing no signal (A), weak signal (B), moderate intensity signal (C and D), and strong signal (E and F).\

conceivable that artefactual location of shed 67LR molecules could occur during the fixation and inclusion procedures. In summary, over 71% of the assayed neuroblastoma samples showed expression of 67LR by immunocytochemistry, with a full range of expression levels.

4. Discussion

The 67LR has been involved in the biological aggressiveness of tumor cells, by helping to laminin remodeling and favoring its degradation by proteolytic enzymes (Ardini et al., 2002; Berno et al., 2005; Vande Broek et al., 2001). Remodeling of the tumor microenvironment and degradation of basement membrane components are two crucial steps in the development of metastases (Wang et al., 2005b). Here we show that RA treatment of neuroblastoma cells results in a reduction of the expression of 67LR. Concomitant to the downregulation of 67LR, RA treatments result in a reduction in cell migration towards *Matrigel* and an impairment in neuroblastoma cells invasiveness in *in vitro* assays. Finally, the involvement of 67LR in migration and invasion of neuroblastoma cells is supported by experiments in which impairment of the 67LR activity by laminin-derived P11 peptide results in reduced migration and invasion capacities for neuroblastoma cells. Taken together all these results support the idea that RA-induced downregulation of 67LR would account for the observed reductions of the migration capacity and invasiveness *in vitro*, and therefore would contribute of a marked reduction of the biological aggressiveness of neuroblastoma cells. RA treatments have been shown to be effective for the therapy of human neuroblastoma, especially in avoiding relapse when applied in a context of minimal residual disease after intensive therapies (Matthay & Reynolds, 2000; Reynolds et al., 2003) The reduction of the ability of migrating towards the basement membrane and degrading it would fit into the range of actions that would lead to effective therapeutic effects in that context.

Several lines of evidence suggest that the 67LR could be a useful therapeutic target for cancer treatment. The anti-cancer cytokines TNFα and IFNγ downregulate the expression of 67LR in transformed keratinocytes (Clausse et al., 1998). Blocking of 67LR with specific antibodies or laminin peptides, or downregulating its expression by anti-sense RNA leads to decreased migration and invasiveness *in vitro* to reduced metastatic and angiogenic potentials in different experimental metastasis models (Iwamoto et al., 1987; Narumi et al., 1999; Satoh et al., 1999; Tanaka et al., 2000)

Remarkably, short term RA treatments induce a transient increase in neuroblastoma cell migration and invasion *in vitro*. The increase in migration appears to be nonspecific, since also occurs in the absence of laminin chemoattractant. Similar RA-induced rapid transient increases in migration and invasion in neuroblastoma cells have been reported (Joshi et al., 2006; Meseguer et al., 2011), and correlated to the expression of tissue transglutaminase (Joshi et al., 2006). Blocking of RA signaling *in vivo* also impaired neuroblast migration from the subventricular zone of the brain to the olfactory bulb (Wang et al., 2005a), suggesting that short term RA-induced increases in migration probably reflects a physiological feature of RA action on the regulation of neurogenesis. Coupling of differentiation with migration has been described for mouse cortical neurons and the involvement of proneural bHLHs transcription factors in migration has been proposed (Ge et al., 2006). Remarkably, RA treatment of neuroblastoma cells results in changes in the expression patterns of bHLH factors including induction of proneural bHLH factors like *NEUROD6* and *NEUROD1* (Jogi et al., 2002; Lopez-Carballo et al., 2002).

Another important aspect is the mechanism through which RA induces the downregulation of *LAMR1* gene, which appears to be complex. It has reported that *LAMR1* is downregulated by p53, through an AP-2 binding element located in its first intron (Modugno et al., 2002). It

is noteworthy that RA treatment of N1E-115 neuroblastoma cells results in the induction of p73, a protein structurally and functionally related to p53 (De Laurenzi et al., 2000).In addition, accumulation of transactivation-deficient DeltaN-p73α in undifferentiated neuroblastic tumors has been reported (Douc-Rasy et al., 2002). Recently it has been reported that 67LR is a hypoxia-inducible factor target gene in gastric cancer (Liu et al., 2010). In neuroblastoma the hypoxia-inducible factors play an important role in maintaining an undifferentiated stem cell-like phenotype, that correlates with poor outcome (Holmquist-Mengelbier et al., 2006; Noguera et al., 2009; Pietras et al., 2009; Pietras et al., 2010).
Finally, we show that more than 71% of the high-grade primary neuroblastoma samples expressed 67LR as revealed by immunocytochemical analysis. The striking differences found in the expression levels of 67LR among the samples open the possibility that these differences could reflect diversity in biological aggressiveness of the tumor cells that may contribute to the differences in the clinical outcome and the heterogeneity of the therapeutic response.

5. Conclusion

RA-induced downregulation of 67LR correlates with a reduction in the biological aggressiveness *in vitro* of neuroblastoma cells, and supports the idea of 67LR as an important molecular target for the therapeutic actions of RA in neuroblastoma.

6. Acknowledgment

The authors are indebted to Dr. S. Menard (Milan, Italy) for the gift of the antibody against 37LRP. C. M. R. L. was supported by *Programa de Personal Técnico de Apoyo* (PTA-2003-02-00207; Ministry of Education and Science, Spain). This work was supported by grants from the Spanish former Ministry of Education and Science and Ministry of Science and Innovation (SAF2003-00311, SAF2006–00647 and SAF2007–60780) and Generalitat Valenciana (GRUPOS 03/15 and ACOMP 09/212) (to D. B.) , and Instituto de Salud Carlos III (RD20-102 to S. N.).

7. References

Albini, A., Iwamoto, Y., Kleinman, H. K., Martin, G. R., Aaronson, S. A., Kozlowski, J. M. & McEwan, R. N. (1987). A rapid in vitro assay for quantitating the invasive potential of tumor cells. *Cancer Res*, Vol. 47, No. 12, pp. 3239-3245.

Ardini, E., Sporchia, B., Pollegioni, L., Modugno, M., Ghirelli, C., Castiglioni, F., Tagliabue, E. & Menard, S. (2002). Identification of a novel function for 67-kDa laminin receptor: increase in laminin degradation rate and release of motility fragments. *Cancer Res*, Vol. 62, No. 5, pp. 1321-1325.

Berno, V., Porrini, D., Castiglioni, F., Campiglio, M., Casalini, P., Pupa, S. M., Balsari, A., Menard, S. & Tagliabue, E. (2005). The 67 kDa laminin receptor increases tumor aggressiveness by remodeling laminin-1. *Endocr Relat Cancer*, Vol. 12, No. 2, pp. 393-406.

Buto, S., Ghirelli, C., Aiello, P., Tagliabue, E., Ardini, E., Magnifico, A., Montuori, N., Sobel, M. E., Colnaghi, M. I. & Menard, S. (1997). Production and characterization of monoclonal antibodies directed against the laminin receptor precursor. *Int J Biol Markers*, Vol. 12, No. 1, pp. 1-5.

Buto, S., Tagliabue, E., Ardini, E., Magnifico, A., Ghirelli, C., van den Brule, F., Castronovo, V., Colnaghi, M. I., Sobel, M. E. & Menard, S. (1998). Formation of the 67-kDa laminin receptor by acylation of the precursor. *J Cell Biochem*, Vol. 69, No. 3, pp. 244-251.

Castronovo, V. (1993). Laminin receptors and laminin-binding proteins during tumor invasion and metastasis. *Invasion Metastasis*, Vol. 13, No. 1, pp. 1-30.

Clausse, N., van den Brule, F., Delvenne, P., Jacobs, N., Franzen-Detrooz, E., Jackers, P. & Castronovo, V. (1998). TNF-alpha and IFN-gamma down-regulate the expression of the metastasis-associated bi-functional 37LRP/p40 gene and protein in transformed keratinocytes. *Biochem Biophys Res Commun*, Vol. 251, No. 2, pp. 564-569.

De Laurenzi, V., Raschella, G., Barcaroli, D., Annicchiarico-Petruzzelli, M., Ranalli, M., Catani, M. V., Tanno, B., Costanzo, A., Levrero, M. & Melino, G. (2000). Induction of neuronal differentiation by p73 in a neuroblastoma cell line. *J Biol Chem*, Vol. 275, No. 20, pp. 15226-15231.

Douc-Rasy, S., Barrois, M., Echeynne, M., Kaghad, M., Blanc, E., Raguenez, G., Goldschneider, D., Terrier-Lacombe, M. J., Hartmann, O., Moll, U., Caput, D. & Benard, J. (2002). DeltaN-p73alpha accumulates in human neuroblastic tumors. *Am J Pathol*, Vol. 160, No. 2, pp. 631-639.

Ge, W., He, F., Kim, K. J., Blanchi, B., Coskun, V., Nguyen, L., Wu, X., Zhao, J., Heng, J. I., Martinowich, K., Tao, J., Wu, H., Castro, D., Sobeih, M. M., Corfas, G., Gleeson, J. G., Greenberg, M. E., Guillemot, F. & Sun, Y. E. (2006). Coupling of cell migration with neurogenesis by proneural bHLH factors. *Proc Natl Acad Sci U S A*, Vol. 103, No. 5, pp. 1319-1324.

Graf, J., Iwamoto, Y., Sasaki, M., Martin, G. R., Kleinman, H. K., Robey, F. A. & Yamada, Y. (1987a). Identification of an amino acid sequence in laminin mediating cell attachment, chemotaxis, and receptor binding. *Cell*, Vol. 48, No. 6, pp. 989-996.

Graf, J., Ogle, R. C., Robey, F. A., Sasaki, M., Martin, G. R., Yamada, Y. & Kleinman, H. K. (1987b). A pentapeptide from the laminin B1 chain mediates cell adhesion and binds the 67,000 laminin receptor. *Biochemistry*, Vol. 26, No. 22, pp. 6896-6900.

Holmquist-Mengelbier, L., Fredlund, E., Lofstedt, T., Noguera, R., Navarro, S., Nilsson, H., Pietras, A., Vallon-Christersson, J., Borg, A., Gradin, K., Poellinger, L. & Pahlman, S. (2006). Recruitment of HIF-1alpha and HIF-2alpha to common target genes is differentially regulated in neuroblastoma: HIF-2alpha promotes an aggressive phenotype. *Cancer Cell*, Vol. 10, No. 5, pp. 413-423.

Iwamoto, Y., Robey, F. A., Graf, J., Sasaki, M., Kleinman, H. K., Yamada, Y. & Martin, G. R. (1987). YIGSR, a synthetic laminin pentapeptide, inhibits experimental metastasis formation. *Science*, Vol. 238, No. 4830, pp. 1132-1134.

Jogi, A., Persson, P., Grynfeld, A., Pahlman, S. & Axelson, H. (2002). Modulation of basic helix-loop-helix transcription complex formation by Id proteins during neuronal differentiation. *J Biol Chem*, Vol. 277, No. 11, pp. 9118-9126.

Joshi, S., Guleria, R., Pan, J., DiPette, D. & Singh, U. S. (2006). Retinoic acid receptors and tissue-transglutaminase mediate short-term effect of retinoic acid on migration and invasion of neuroblastoma SH-SY5Y cells. *Oncogene*, Vol. 25, No. 2, pp. 240-247.

Joshi, S., Guleria, R. S., Pan, J., Dipette, D. & Singh, U. S. (2007). Heterogeneity in retinoic acid signaling in neuroblastomas: Role of matrix metalloproteinases in retinoic acid-induced differentiation. *Biochim Biophys Acta*, Vol. 1772, No. 9, pp. 1093-1102.

Karpatova, M., Tagliabue, E., Castronovo, V., Magnifico, A., Ardini, E., Morelli, D., Belotti, D., Colnaghi, M. I. & Menard, S. (1996). Shedding of the 67-kD laminin receptor by human cancer cells. *J Cell Biochem*, Vol. 60, No. 2, pp. 226-234.

Katagiri, Y. U., Kiyokawa, N., Nakamura, K., Takenouchi, H., Taguchi, T., Okita, H., Umezawa, A. & Fujimoto, J. (2005). Laminin binding protein, 34/67 laminin receptor, carries stage-specific embryonic antigen-4 epitope defined by monoclonal antibody Raft.2. *Biochem Biophys Res Commun*, Vol. 332, No. 4, pp. 1004-1011.

Kleinman, H. K. & Martin, G. R. (2005). Matrigel: basement membrane matrix with biological activity. *Semin Cancer Biol*, Vol. 15, No. 5, pp. 378-386.

Landowski, T. H., Dratz, E. A. & Starkey, J. R. (1995). Studies of the structure of the metastasis-associated 67 kDa laminin binding protein: fatty acid acylation and evidence supporting dimerization of the 32 kDa gene product to form the mature protein. *Biochemistry*, Vol. 34, No. 35, pp. 11276-11287.

Liu, L., Sun, L., Zhao, P., Yao, L., Jin, H., Liang, S., Wang, Y., Zhang, D., Pang, Y., Shi, Y., Chai, N. & Zhang, H. (2010). Hypoxia promotes metastasis in human gastric cancer by up-regulating the 67-kDa laminin receptor. *Cancer Sci*, Vol. 101, No. 7, pp. 1653-1660.

Lopez-Carballo, G., Moreno, L., Masia, S., Perez, P. & Barettino, D. (2002). Activation of the phosphatidylinositol 3-kinase/Akt signaling pathway by retinoic acid is required for neural differentiation of SH-SY5Y human neuroblastoma cells. *J Biol Chem*, Vol. 277, No. 28, pp. 25297-25304.

Lovat, P. E., Irving, H., Annicchiarico-Petruzzelli, M., Bernassola, F., Malcolm, A. J., Pearson, A. D., Melino, G. & Redfern, C. P. (1997). Retinoids in neuroblastoma therapy: distinct biological properties of 9- cis- and all-trans-retinoic acid. *Eur J Cancer*, Vol. 33, No. 12, pp. 2075-2080.

Magnifico, A., Tagliabue, E., Buto, S., Ardini, E., Castronovo, V., Colnaghi, M. I. & Menard, S. (1996). Peptide G, containing the binding site of the 67-kDa laminin receptor, increases and stabilizes laminin binding to cancer cells. *J Biol Chem*, Vol. 271, No. 49, pp. 31179-31184.

Maris, J. M. (2010). Recent advances in neuroblastoma. *N Engl J Med*, Vol. 362, No. 23, pp. 2202-2211.

Masia, S., Alvarez, S., de Lera, A. R. & Barettino, D. (2007). Rapid, nongenomic actions of retinoic acid on phosphatidylinositol-3-kinase signaling pathway mediated by the retinoic acid receptor. *Mol Endocrinol*, Vol. 21, No. 10, pp. 2391-2402.

Matthay, K. & Reynolds, C. (2000). Is there a role for retinoids to treat minimal residual disease in neuroblastoma? *Br J Cancer*, Vol. 83, No. 9, pp. 1121-1123.

Matthay, K. K., Reynolds, C. P., Seeger, R. C., Shimada, H., Adkins, E. S., Haas-Kogan, D., Gerbing, R. B., London, W. B. & Villablanca, J. G. (2009). Long-term results for children with high-risk neuroblastoma treated on a randomized trial of myeloablative therapy followed by 13-cis-retinoic acid: a children's oncology group study. *J Clin Oncol*, Vol. 27, No. 7, pp. 1007-1013.

Matthay, K. K., Villablanca, J. G., Seeger, R. C., Stram, D. O., Harris, R. E., Ramsay, N. K., Swift, P., Shimada, H., Black, C. T., Brodeur, G. M., Gerbing, R. B. & Reynolds, C. P. (1999). Treatment of high-risk neuroblastoma with intensive chemotherapy, radiotherapy, autologous bone marrow transplantation, and 13-cis- retinoic acid. Children's Cancer Group. *N Engl J Med*, Vol. 341, No. 16, pp. 1165-1173.

Matz, M., Usman, N., Shagin, D., Bogdanova, E. & Lukyanov, S. (1997). Ordered differential display: a simple method for systematic comparison of gene expression profiles. *Nucleic Acids Res*, Vol. 25, No. 12, pp. 2541-2542.

McCarthy, J. B., Palm, S. L. & Furcht, L. T. (1983). Migration by haptotaxis of a Schwann cell tumor line to the basement membrane glycoprotein laminin. *J Cell Biol*, Vol. 97, No. 3, pp. 772-777.

Menard, S., Castronovo, V., Tagliabue, E. & Sobel, M. E. (1997). New insights into the metastasis-associated 67 kD laminin receptor. *J Cell Biochem*, Vol. 67, No. 2, pp. 155-165.

Menard, S., Tagliabue, E. & Colnaghi, M. I. (1998). The 67 kDa laminin receptor as a prognostic factor in human cancer. *Breast Cancer Res Treat*, Vol. 52, No. 1-3, pp. 137-145.

Meseguer, S., Mudduluru, G., Escamilla, J. M., Allgayer, H. & Barettino, D. (2011). MicroRNAs-10a and -10b Contribute to Retinoic Acid-induced Differentiation of Neuroblastoma Cells and Target the Alternative Splicing Regulatory Factor SFRS1 (SF2/ASF). *J Biol Chem*, Vol. 286, No. 6, pp. 4150-4164.

Modugno, M., Tagliabue, E., Ardini, E., Berno, V., Galmozzi, E., De Bortoli, M., Castronovo, V. & Menard, S. (2002). p53-dependent downregulation of metastasis-associated laminin receptor. *Oncogene*, Vol. 21, No. 49, pp. 7478-7487.

Moss, B. L., Taubner, L., Sample, Y. K., Kazmin, D. A., Copie, V. & Starkey, J. R. (2006). Tumor shedding of laminin binding protein modulates angiostatin production in vitro and interferes with plasmin-derived inhibition of angiogenesis in aortic ring cultures. *Int J Cancer*, Vol. 118, No. 10, pp. 2421-2432.

Narumi, K., Inoue, A., Tanaka, M., Isemura, M., Shimo-Oka, T., Abe, T., Nukiwa, T. & Satoh, K. (1999). Inhibition of experimental metastasis of human fibrosarcoma cells by anti-recombinant 37-kDa laminin binding protein antibody. *Jpn J Cancer Res*, Vol. 90, No. 4, pp. 425-431.

Noguera, R., Fredlund, E., Piqueras, M., Pietras, A., Beckman, S., Navarro, S. & Pahlman, S. (2009). HIF-1alpha and HIF-2alpha are differentially regulated in vivo in neuroblastoma: high HIF-1alpha correlates negatively to advanced clinical stage and tumor vascularization. *Clin Cancer Res*, Vol. 15, No. 23, pp. 7130-7136.

Pahlman, S., Ruusala, A. I., Abrahamsson, L., Mattsson, M. E. & Esscher, T. (1984). Retinoic acid-induced differentiation of cultured human neuroblastoma cells: a comparison with phorbolester-induced differentiation. *Cell Differ*, Vol. 14, No. 2, pp. 135-144.

Pietras, A., Hansford, L. M., Johnsson, A. S., Bridges, E., Sjolund, J., Gisselsson, D., Rehn, M., Beckman, S., Noguera, R., Navarro, S., Cammenga, J., Fredlund, E., Kaplan, D. R. & Pahlman, S. (2009). HIF-2alpha maintains an undifferentiated state in neural crest-like human neuroblastoma tumor-initiating cells. *Proc Natl Acad Sci U S A*, Vol. 106, No. 39, pp. 16805-16810.

Pietras, A., Johnsson, A. S. & Pahlman, S. (2010). The HIF-2alpha-driven pseudo-hypoxic phenotype in tumor aggressiveness, differentiation, and vascularization. *Curr Top Microbiol Immunol*, Vol. 345, No., pp. 1-20.

Reynolds, C. P., Matthay, K. K., Villablanca, J. G. & Maurer, B. J. (2003). Retinoid therapy of high-risk neuroblastoma. *Cancer Lett*, Vol. 197, No. 1-2, pp. 185-192.

Satoh, K., Narumi, K., Abe, T., Sakai, T., Kikuchi, T., Tanaka, M., Shimo-Oka, T., Uchida, M., Tezuka, F., Isemura, M. & Nukiwa, T. (1999). Diminution of 37-kDa laminin binding protein expression reduces tumour formation of murine lung cancer cells. *Br J Cancer*, Vol. 80, No. 8, pp. 1115-1122.

Scheiman, J., Jamieson, K. V., Ziello, J., Tseng, J. C. & Meruelo, D. (2010). Extraribosomal functions associated with the C terminus of the 37/67 kDa laminin receptor are required for maintaining cell viability. *Cell Death Dis*, Vol. 1, No. 5, pp. e42.

Sidell, N. (1982). Retinoic acid-induced growth inhibition and morphologic differentiation of human neuroblastoma cells in vitro. *J Natl Cancer Inst*, Vol. 68, No. 4, pp. 589-596.

Sobel, M. E. (1993). Differential expression of the 67 kDa laminin receptor in cancer. *Semin Cancer Biol*, Vol. 4, No. 5, pp. 311-317.

Susantad, T. & Smith, D. R. (2008). siRNA-mediated silencing of the 37/67-kDa high affinity laminin receptor in Hep3B cells induces apoptosis. *Cell Mol Biol Lett*, Vol. 13, No. 3, pp. 452-464.

Tanaka, M., Narumi, K., Isemura, M., Abe, M., Sato, Y., Abe, T., Saijo, Y., Nukiwa, T. & Satoh, K. (2000). Expression of the 37-kDa laminin binding protein in murine lung tumor cell correlates with tumor angiogenesis. *Cancer Lett*, Vol. 153, No. 1-2, pp. 161-168.

Thiele, C. J., Reynolds, C. P. & Israel, M. A. (1985). Decreased expression of N-myc precedes retinoic acid-induced morphological differentiation of human neuroblastoma. *Nature*, Vol. 313, No. 6001, pp. 404-406.

Umeda, D., Yano, S., Yamada, K. & Tachibana, H. (2008). Green tea polyphenol epigallocatechin-3-gallate signaling pathway through 67-kDa laminin receptor. *J Biol Chem*, Vol. 283, No. 6, pp. 3050-3058.

Vana, K., Zuber, C., Pflanz, H., Kolodziejczak, D., Zemora, G., Bergmann, A. K. & Weiss, S. (2009). LRP/LR as an alternative promising target in therapy of prion diseases, Alzheimer's disease and cancer. *Infect Disord Drug Targets*, Vol. 9, No. 1, pp. 69-80.

Vande Broek, I., Vanderkerken, K., De Greef, C., Asosingh, K., Straetmans, N., Van Camp, B. & Van Riet, I. (2001). Laminin-1-induced migration of multiple myeloma cells involves the high-affinity 67 kD laminin receptor. *Br J Cancer*, Vol. 85, No. 9, pp. 1387-1395.

Viacava, P., Naccarato, A. G., Collecchi, P., Menard, S., Castronovo, V. & Bevilacqua, G. (1997). The spectrum of 67-kD laminin receptor expression in breast carcinoma progression. *J Pathol*, Vol. 182, No. 1, pp. 36-44.

Voigt, A. & Zintl, F. (2003). Effects of retinoic acid on proliferation, apoptosis, cytotoxicity, migration, and invasion of neuroblastoma cells. *Med Pediatr Oncol*, Vol. 40, No. 4, pp. 205-213.

Wang, T. W., Zhang, H. & Parent, J. M. (2005a). Retinoic acid regulates postnatal neurogenesis in the murine subventricular zone-olfactory bulb pathway. *Development*, Vol. 132, No. 12, pp. 2721-2732.

Wang, W., Goswami, S., Sahai, E., Wyckoff, J. B., Segall, J. E. & Condeelis, J. S. (2005b). Tumor cells caught in the act of invading: their strategy for enhanced cell motility. *Trends Cell Biol*, Vol. 15, No. 3, pp. 138-145.

Wewer, U. M., Liotta, L. A., Jaye, M., Ricca, G. A., Drohan, W. N., Claysmith, A. P., Rao, C. N., Wirth, P., Coligan, J. E., Albrechtsen, R. & et al. (1986). Altered levels of laminin receptor mRNA in various human carcinoma cells that have different abilities to bind laminin. *Proc Natl Acad Sci U S A*, Vol. 83, No. 19, pp. 7137-7141.

Wewer, U. M., Taraboletti, G., Sobel, M. E., Albrechtsen, R. & Liotta, L. A. (1987). Role of laminin receptor in tumor cell migration. *Cancer Res*, Vol. 47, No. 21, pp. 5691-5698.

Yow, H. K., Wong, J. M., Chen, H. S., Lee, C. G., Davis, S., Steele, G. D., Jr. & Chen, L. B. (1988). Increased mRNA expression of a laminin-binding protein in human colon carcinoma: complete sequence of a full-length cDNA encoding the protein. *Proc Natl Acad Sci U S A*, Vol. 85, No. 17, pp. 6394-6398.

13

Application of Molecular Mimicry to Target GD2 Ganglioside

Irena Horwacik and Hanna Rokita
The Jagiellonian University, Faculty of Biochemistry, Biophysics and Biotechnology, Laboratory of Molecular Genetics and Virology
Poland

1. Introduction

GD2 ganglioside is an important example of tumour-associated carbohydrate antigens. Over expression of the GD2 ganglioside is a hallmark of neuroblastoma, while its expression on normal cells is restricted. The antigen is stably expressed on cells of the tumour, and retained during a therapy of the disease (Kramer et al., 2001). The facts allow to use its presence to diagnose neuroblastoma, monitor response to treatment, and target the tumour cells (Navid et al., 2010; Reuland et al., 2001; Swerts et al., 2005).

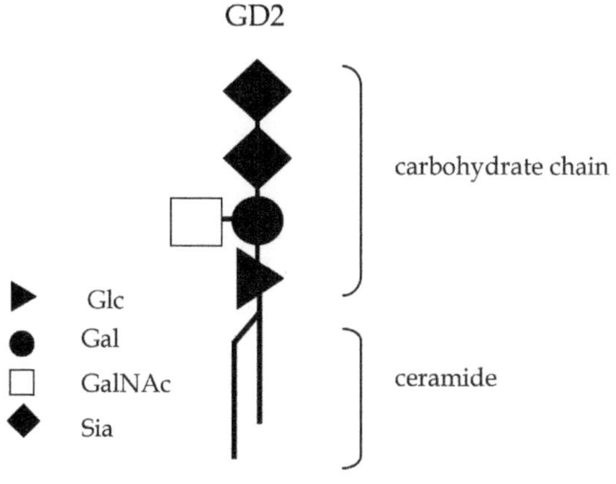

Fig. 1. A schematic representation of the GD2 ganglioside structure (abbreviations: Glc, glucose; Gal, galactose; GalNAc,, N-acetylgalactosamine; Sia, sialic acid).

The GD2 ganglioside is a member of glycolipids, compounds that are commonly present in outer plasma membrane of animal cells. The GD2 ganglioside is a polar molecule. The hydrophilic part is made from a carbohydrate chain, charged due to the presence of two sialic acid residues, and exposed to cell outside. The second part of the molecule is hydrophobic in nature, functions as a membrane anchor, and it is formed by a ceramide, fatty acid sphingosine (Fig. 1). Gangliosides were shown to be involved in many aspects of cancer biology. Changes in their expression may influence cell signalling pathways, morphology, proliferation, invasiveness, and tumour progression, as shown in cell cultures and *in vivo* (Ruan et al., 1999; Yoshida et al., 2001). The gangliosides are shed from cell membranes, and are present in sera of cancer patients (Czaplicki et al., 2009). Immunomodulating activities of the GD2 ganglioside were also described (Ladish et al., 1994). The GD2 ganglioside allows for successful targeting of neuroblastoma with monoclonal antibodies binding the tumour-associated carbohydrate antigen (Kushner et al., 2011; Yu et al., 2011). Novel active approaches targeting the GD2 ganglioside are under development to improve weak-immunogenicity of the self antigen, including GD2 ganglioside-KLH conjugates, anti-idiotypes, and peptide mimetics (Foon et al., 2000; Chapman et al., 2000,). In the chapter we review approaches to improve immunogencity of the GD2 ganglioside, with emphasis on application of peptide mimetics.

2. Molecular mimicry phenomenon

A molecular mimicry phenomenon relies on similarities between chemically diverse molecules, *i.e.*, a surrogate and an original antigen (epitope) in the context of their ability to bind to a given target. Numerous data highlight that peptides, which are small molecules, consisting of amino acids linked with the peptide bond in a linear order, can be carbohydrate mimetics, inhibitors of carbohydrate-protein interactions, but also immunogens. Such peptides can be isolated from phage-displayed peptide libraries, synthetic libraries constructed with combinatorial chemistry, or rationally designed (Aina et al., 2007; Johnson & Pinto, 2008; Pande et al., 2010).

Antigenicity of peptide mimetics relies on their ability to bind to receptors, such as antibodies, enzymes, or lectins. Their reactivity can be measured with several assays (ELISA, Western blot). Additional competition tests for binding between mimicking peptides and the natural ligand can prove, if the peptides can bind at or near the antigen binding site. Further studies often include evaluation of residues critical for binding, their replacement, shortening or extension of the peptide length. All of these can help to characterise the binding. Moreover, structures of free and the receptor-bound mimetics can be compared experimentally, or with application of computational docking (Huang et al., 2011). As a result, lead compounds can be identified, and further developed to replace natural antigens in diagnostic assays, and in therapy (Deroo & Muller, 2001).

The nature of the peptide-carbohydrate mimicry is extensively studied, as more examples are reported (Jonson & Pinto, 2008). On the molecular level, structural mimicry can be distinguished, if a peptide can replicate three-dimensional (3D) interactions made by the carbohydrate with the target binding site. The contacts are mediated due to a certain arrangement of functional groups. The interaction does not require for such a peptide to have a similar 3D shape, as the mimicked carbohydrate. Instead, it may be facilitated by a high degree of flexibility that characterises peptides. This can allow for an arrangement of peptide functional groups within the target binding site that is critical for the structural mimicry to occur. Another type of interactions, namely functional mimicry, takes place, when a peptide does not interact with the binding site of the target in the same way, as the mimicked carbohydrate. Here, the peptide binds engaging different set of residues at the binding site of the target. A peptide can also made contacts at a distinct site, as compared to the carbohydrate. Based on the extensive data published, one can conclude that there is no consistent or preferred mechanism by which peptides mimic carbohydrates. Moreover,

mixed types of the above described binding modes are often observed (Agostino et al., 2011, see also examples in the paragraph 4.3).
Immunological mimicry may be desired, if the use of an original antigen in vaccine formulation is not the best suited. Immunologically functional mimetics (mimotopes) induce antibodies that cross react with the original antigen. Mimotopes can be useful, if a natural antigen is unknown, hard to purify, or synthesise, or weakly immunogenic (Popkov et al., 2000; Tai et al., 1985). This also applies in general to carbohydrates that due to chirality are costly, and uneasy in their synthesis. Here, application of carbohydrate mimicking peptides as surrogates is justified, and often possible (Fleuridor et al., 2001; Kieber-Emmons et al., 2000). However, discrepancies between antigenicity and immunogenicity of mimicking peptides are often observed (El Kasmi et al., 1999; Willers et al., 1999). Many antigenic peptides isolated with antibodies are not immunogenic, because they do not bind the same paratope, as the natural epitope. Based on the published data, it is still unclear to what extent antibody bound conformation of a peptide, or conformation of the peptide in solution is related to immunogenicity (Theillet et al., 2009). It is known, that biologically functional mimicry can be affected for example by the sequence, flexibility of free peptides, a phage environment, conjugation to carrier protein, expression on a protein scaffold, a fit induced during interactions between the selecting antibody and the mimic.
Many features of peptides can justify their use in place of carbohydrates. The methodology of their synthesis is well established, and can be automatic. The peptide structure can be modified in order to delay their degradation *in vivo*. Although, peptides in general are highly flexible, there are approaches to restrain their conformation through introduction of structure constrains, or their presentation as a part of a larger protein scaffold. More importantly, peptides are thymus dependent antigens, and therefore attractive surrogates of generally weakly immunogenic carbohydrates. Furthermore, peptides can be conjugated to carrier proteins, and even transferred to a DNA sequence, depending on the delivery schedule, and types of the immune response desired. The molecular mimicry lays a basis for application of anti-idiotypic antibodies, and peptide mimetics of the GD2 ganglioside isolated from phage displayed-libraries, as novel candidates to induce immune responses against neuroblastoma.

3. Anti-idiotypic antibodies to target the GD2 ganglioside

Monoclonal antibodies are effective means to fight cancer. The molecules can affect signalling pathways critical for malignancy, trigger, or enhance anti-tumour immune responses (Weiner et al., 2009). Monoclonal antibodies binding the GD2 ganglioside, *e.g.*, the 14.G2a (mouse monoclonal antibody, IgG2a), the 3F8 (mouse monoclonal antibody, IgG3), the ch14.18 (chimeric antibody consisting of variable regions of the murine monoclonal antibody 14.18, and the constant regions of human IgG-K) were tested in clinical trials (Modak & Cheung, 2010). Recently, treatment with the ch14.18 was shown to significantly improve event-free survival, and overall survival in a phase III clinical trial in patients with high risk neuroblastoma (Yu et al., 2011). Moreover, approaches to reduce the treatment-associated pain are being developed (Kushner et al., 2011; Sorkin et al., 2010). On the one side, HAMA (human anti-mouse antibody), and HACA (human anti-chimeric antibody) responses can be induced in patients after administration of antibodies, and if acute unable the further treatment. On the other side, induction of idiotypic network measured by presence of anti-anti-idiotypic antibodies and binding the GD2 ganglioside antibodies, 6 and 11 months after the 3F8 administration, was associated with long-term survival of patients with stage 4 neuroblastoma (Cheung et al., 2000).

Three major types of anti-Ig molecules can be induced, based on which part of the antibody they will recognize, *i.e.*, anti-isotypic, anti-allotypic, anti-idiotypic antibodies. Isotypic determinants consist of epitopes specific to one of five heavy chains (H), or one of two light chains (L) of antibodies. Allotypic determinants reflect allelic polymorphism existing in various regions of Ig constant genes. Thus, a particular isotype of an antibody common to members of a species may exist in several allogenic forms. Additionally, each Ig molecule has a unique (not-shared by any other member of the species) relatively minor differences that are defined by the hypervariable sequences in the variable region (*i.e.*, antigen binding region). The collection of such unique determinants on a given Ig defines its idiotypes. It is suggested that network of anti-idiotypic antibodies may have a physiological function by regulating immune responses (Mak & Saunders, 2006).

Anti-idiotypic antibodies binding specific paratopes can be induced with anti-GD2 ganglioside antibodies (termed Ab1). Some anti-idiotypic antibodies can be used as surrogate antigens in immunizations to target the GD2 ganglioside. Variable regions of such anti-idiotypic antibodies (Ab2β) may "immunologically resemble" the GD2 ganglioside, yet are not identical with the glycolipid. They react with the Ab1 antibody, and upon administration induce anti-anti-idiotypic antibodies (Ab3), also specific toward the GD2 ganglioside (Ab1') (Bhattacharya-Chatterjee et al., 2000; Saleh et al., 1993).

The first anti-idiotypic antibody for neuroblastoma, used in clinical trials, was the monoclonal anti-idiotypic antibody for the 3F8, A1G4. In the phase I study in relapsed or high risk patients, administration of the anti-idiotype intravenously (i.v.) at 0.1, 0.3, 1 mg/kg for a total of 10 doses, induced anti-GD2 ganglioside antibody responses at all doses tested. No dose limiting toxicities (DLTs) were observed (Modak & Cheung, 2007 as cited in Modak & Cheung, 2010). 1A7 is yet another anti-idiotypic antibody. It was raised against the 14.G2a antibody. The 1A7 was tested in melanoma patients. 47 advanced melanoma patients received 1, 2, 4, 8-mg doses of the 1A7 mixed with QS-21 adjuvant (100 μg), subcutaneously (s.c.), weekly for 4 weeks and then monthly until disease progression. In 40 out of 47 patients that continued on study beyond 3 months, anti-GD2 ganglioside antibody responses were detected. In 20 patients the antibody concentrations ranged from 34-240 μg/ml. The responses were predominately IgG. There was no additional toxicity, such as abdominal pain. Authors concluded that although objective responses had been minimal, the approach should be tested in prospective randomised trials to further investigate possible favourable impact on disease progression (Foon et al., 2000).

Zeytin et al. constructed DNA vaccine (pc1A7VHLnVL) encoding secreted form of the single chain variable fragment of the 1A7 (1A7scFV). Intramuscular injection of the DNA vaccine to mice induced both antibodies against the 1A7 antibody, and against the GD2 ganglioside. However, no cellular immune responses were observed (Zeytin et al., 2000). On the contrary, GD2 ganglioside specific delayed-type hypersensitivity reactions (DTH) to the challenge with syngeneic GD2-positive melanoma cells D142.34 were induced by s.c. injection of mouse anti-idiotypic antibody TA412G Cl1 with complete Freund adjuvant in C57BL/6 mice, but not in in C57BL/6 $CD4^{-/-}$ mice. This suggested involvement of $CD4^{+}$ T cells in the observed DTH reactions. Additionally, 3 out of 6 of anti-idiotypic antibodies (TA17A Cl2, TA412G Cl1, TB310B Cl1), precipitated by alum and administered to rabbits, induced IgG antibodies binding GD2 ganglioside positive melanoma WM115, and glioma 251 MG cells (Basak at al., 2003).

4. Generation of peptide mimetics of the GD2 ganglioside

Peptide displayed on bacteriophages, plasmids, polysomes, and various types of synthetic peptide libraries are invaluable sources of new ligands. They can be further tested as therapeutic leads, and therefore have a potential commercial value. In the following chapters, the technology of screening of peptide libraries based on filamentous bacteriophage display will be characterised. This will be followed by review of currently undertaken approaches to generate peptides mimicking the GD2 ganglioside.

4.1 The filamentous bacteriophage life cycle

The phage display is a powerful and challenging method to study interactions of proteins with other molecules including peptides, nucleic acids, and carbohydrates. Generally, the technique applies filamentous bacteriophages of the genus *Inovirus* (M13, fd, f1) infecting *Escherichia coli,* although other viral species, *i.e.*, T4, λ could be employed for peptide display.

The wild filamentous viruses are rod-like structures, 930 nm in length, and 6.5 nm in diameter. Their protein capsid is mainly build of a small protein, the major coat protein p8, which is present in 2700 copies, and covers like a cylinder a circular single-stranded DNA genome. The DNA is build of 6400 bases, and encodes for eleven genes. At one end of the virion, there are five copies of each of p3 and p6 proteins, and the other end contains five copies of each of p7 and p9 proteins. The filamentous phages infect male *E. coli* bacteria that have F pilus, made of subunits of pilin protein. The structure interacts with the p3 protein in the first step of infection. The further steps of the life cycle involve amplification of viral ssDNA, which is mediated by viral proteins p2, p5, p10 and host bacterium proteins. A double stranded circular DNA called a replicative form (RF) arises as an intermediate in the process. The minus strand of the RF form is used for transcription. Numerous copies of the viral ssDNA, covered with dimers of the p5 protein are produced as a result of the replication. This induces collapse of the DNA to a rod, leaving only the packaging signal exposed.

The viral proteins that build the capsid, as well as proteins p4, p1, p11 are synthesised, and then embedded in bacterial membranes. The p4, p1, p11 proteins form sites (channels) in the bacterial envelope which bring cytoplasmic and outer membranes in a close contact. Here, a process of assembly of new viral particles takes place. The filamentous phages do not kill the infected bacteria, but slow the ratio of bacterial growth by half. The assembly process allows packing of all the capsid protein, integrated to the cytoplasmic membrane, around the DNA extruding from the cytoplasm. The end that leaves first the bacterium contains the p7 and the p9 protein, interacting with the packaging signal. The process of exchange of the p5 to the p8 continues till the end of the DNA is reached. Then, the p3 and the p6 are added, and a newly formed bacteriophage particle is released (Rakonjac et al., 2011).

4.2 Phage display technology

Because of the nature of the membrane-associated assembly, there is virtually no constrains on the size of DNA to be packed in the capsid. Therefore, the bacteriophage vectors are useful for construction of genomic, cDNA libraries, and display of peptides or even whole proteins on the surface of phage particles. The most prominent example of the protein display is construction of libraries of antibody fragments that are proved sources of human fragments of monoclonal antibodies (Rakonjac et al., 2011).

A large number of libraries consisting of variants of peptides are available. They differ by number of clones, length of peptide sequences that can be random, or constrained due to the presence of cysteine residues forming a disulfide bond. Although all protein building the capsid can be used for display, the most common are libraries utilizing the p3; and the p8 proteins for presentation of foreign sequences. The pivotal concept is that the peptides displayed on the bacteriophage surface, and the DNA sequence coding for that peptide are physically linked in one viral particle. This enables easy verification of sequences of peptides isolated from the libraries. The libraries are constructed by cloning of oligonucleotides encoding for peptides in frame with the gene of the protein used for display. Oligonucleotides encoding for peptides can be inserted between sequences encoding the leader sequence and the mature p8 (Fig. 2). Peptides are encoded by NNK or NNS (where N is A, T, C, G; K is G and T; S is G and C). The cloning can result in all copies of the p3 and the p8 expressed as fusion proteins, or only some of the proteins carrying peptides. The later can be achieved by introduction into the viral genome of an additional copy of the recombinant gene, besides the wild-type gene. The recombinant gene can also be delivered to bacteria on a separate genome (a phagemid). Moreover, peptide libraries can be expressed as a part of a larger protein scaffold (Uchiyama et al., 2005).

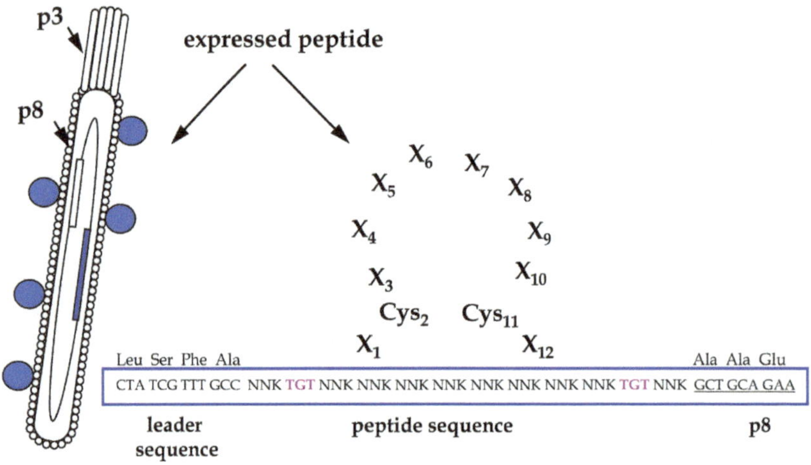

Fig. 2. A schematic representation of the constrained peptide library LX-8. Peptides are expressed as fusion with the p8 protein. Two genes encoding p8 proteins are present in the bacteriophage genome, a wild type (white), and a recombinant one (colour filled). The leader sequence is removed during processing of the p8 (Bonnycastle et al., 1996).

The process of screening of phage-displayed peptide libraries is called a panning. During the purification process a peptide library is allowed to interact with screening molecules such as for examples antibodies, enzymes, receptors, lectins, or hormones. The target receptor can be coated to plastic surfaces, membranes, or used in a solution phase. Affinity interactions are basis for most of the screening protocols. Therefore pre-adsorption steps are necessary to reduce the numbers of phage clones that bind to other than screening molecules, *e.g.*, blocking agents, washing buffer ingredients, and surfaces used for target coating. Phages captured via their displayed peptides by the target screening molecule can be retained during washing steps. Then, they are amplified in bacteria, and the panning is repeated. A resulting pool of phages is enriched in peptides that bind the target molecule used for the screening. From such pools single clones can be isolated. Next, the peptides are decoded through DNA sequencing, and then characterised in the phage-displayed environment, as well as in a free form (Fig. 3). The screening can also be designed and

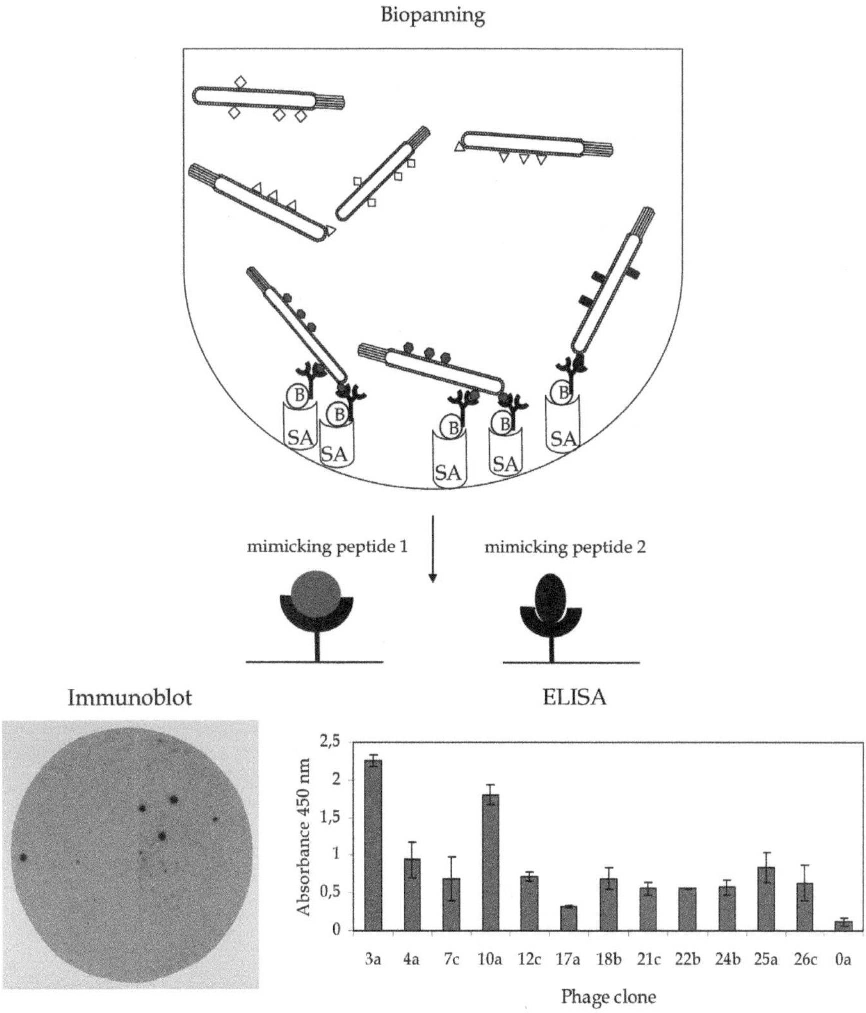

Fig. 3. A schematic representation of a biopanning (top). Biotinylated antibodies are immobilised in streptavidin-coated wells. The pre-adsorbed library of phage-displayed peptides can interact with the immobilised target molecules (see text for more details). Immunoblotting and ELISA can be used to analyse phage clones isolated from peptide libraries (bottom). The examples from the screening of the LX-8 library with the 14.G2a were included (see Horwacik et al., 2007 for more details). Replicas of bacteria infected with phages on nitrocellulose membranes were incubated with the 14.G2a antibody and the secondary HRP-conjugated antibody, and then developed (bottom left). ELISA with immobilised 14.G2a antibody was used to capture specific phage clones. Phage binding was detected with anti-p8 antibodies. The 0a phage is a negative control (bottom right).

conducted on target molecules expressed on the surface of whole cells, or even in mice. Applicability of the technique is enormous, and includes new ligand identification, quest for agonist and antagonists of receptors, elucidation of binding motifs, epitope mapping, analyses of enzymatic activity, new drug and vaccine design (Dudak et al., 2011, Smith & Petrenko, 1997).

4.3 Isolation and optimisation of peptide mimetics of the GD2 ganglioside isolated from phage-displayed libraries

It is a common finding that in addition to binding to original epitopes, antibodies can cross-react with several antigens (Van Regenmortel, 2001). Phage display techniques were used to exploit the molecular mimicry phenomenon to isolate peptide surrogates to tumour-associated carbohydrate antigens, *e.g.*, Lewis Y (Kieber-Emmons et al., 1999), sialylated Lewis a/x (O et al., 1999), and GD3 (Willers et al., 1999). The examples of the peptides mimicking the GD2 ganglioside, the antibodies used for their identification, as well as references were for convenience collected in the Table 1. Following is the description of their antigenic and immunogenic properties, analysed with experimental and computational tools, as well as strategies that were used to improve their mimicry.

Antibody	Peptide name	Peptide sequence	Reference
ME36.1	P9	LDVVLAWRDGLSGAS	Qiu et al., 1999
	P10	GVVWRYTAPVHLGDG	Monzavi-Karbassi et al., 2007
	P10s	WRYTAPVHLGDG	
Ch14.18	MD	CDGGWLSKGSWC	Förster-Waldl et al., 2005
	MA	CGRLKMVPDLEC	Bleeke et al., 2009
	C3	CGRL**HL**VPDLEC	
14.G2a	47	EDPSHSLGLDVALFM	Bolesta et al., 2005
	47-LDA	EDPSHSLGLD**A**ALFM	
14.G2a	94	RCNPNMEPPRCF	Horwacik et al., 2007
	94-12-F/W-AAEGD	RCNPNMEPPRC**WAAEGD**	Horwacik et al., 2011

Table 1. Examples of mimicking peptides isolated with the anti-GD2 ganglioside monoclonal antibodies.

4.3.1 Peptides isolated with the ME36.1 antibody

The ME36.1 monoclonal antibody displays reactivity with the gangliosides GD2 and GD3. The antibody was used to screen the 15-mer library build with the fUSE5 vector. Qiu et al. reported in 1999 results of a panning of the library with the ME36.1 antibody. 16 peptides were isolated. Sequence analysis revealed presence of mainly unique sequences, which indicated that many peptides could mimic the GD2 ganglioside binding to the ME36.1. Interestingly, some similarities between the peptides isolated with the ME36.1 and the BR55-2 (binding Lewis-Y) were found, *i.e.*, presence of WRY and AP sequences in the peptide P10 (GVVWRYTAPVHLGDG), and WRDG in the peptide P9 (LDVVLAWRDGLSGAS) that is similar to YRGD found in a peptide isolated with the BR55-2.

ELISA was applied to compare ganglioside reactivity of IgM in sera samples of non-immunised animals, and animals immunized with the P10. For vaccinations the P10 was presented as multiple antigenic peptides of 8 peptide clusters (MAP), injected intraperitoneally (i.p.) with QS-21 adjuvant. The obtained results suggested that the P10 might induce serum IgM antibodies reactive with multiple gangliosides. The analysis of data comparing dilutions yielding half-maximal binding to different gangliosides showed that the peptide could functionally mimic GD1b, GD1a, GD3, and only to a lesser extent GD2 and GM2. The finding was supported with molecular modelling approach revealing that the P10 interacts with the ME36.1 with only two hydrogen bonds (with Tyr33 and Ser100 from the heavy chain) in common, as compared to the GD2 ganglioside binding network to the antibody (*i.e.*, with Tyr33, His35, Asp50, Asn52, Asn59, and Ser100 from the heavy chain, and Tyr93 from the light chain).
In efforts to improve the immunological mimicry of the GD2 ganglioside, a shorter peptide missing the N-terminal GVV sequence was designed (P10s). It showed a rise in numbers of bonds involved in the ME36.1 interactions (Tyr33, Asp50, Asn59, and Ser100 from the heavy chain, and Tyr93 from the light chain). Additionally, immunisation with the P10s induced IgM in sera with augmented reactivity toward GD2, GD3, GM2 (as compared to the P10). Moreover, the sera collected from mice immunised with the P10s showed higher binding to the GD2 ganglioside positive MCF7 human breast cancer cells, and WM793 melanoma cells, as compared to sera from mice immunised with the P10 (Monzavi-Karbassi et al., 2007).

4.3.2 Peptides isolated with the ch14.18 antibody

Förster-Waldl et al. published in 2005 results from their panning experiments (Förster-Waldl et al., 2005). The group screened a peptide phage-displayed library expressed in the context of the p3, and constrained by presence of additional cysteines at N and C termini of the peptides. The authors reported isolation of 13 different phage-displayed peptides that specifically recognized the ch14.18 antibody, in contrast to wild type phages. An isotype control antibody (cetuximab) was included in the binding assays. In most of the clones R is present in the position 2 of the decamers flanked by cysteines, hydrophobic V, L, or M are in the positions 5 or 6, and acidic D or E occupies the position 10. The antigenicity of the phage-expressed peptides was positively verified with application of a competitive ELISA, to measure their specific binding to the ch14.18 against simultaneously added GD2 ganglioside. Two peptide sequences were chosen for further studies, *i.e.*, the MD peptide (CDGGWLSKGSWC) and the MA peptide (CGRLKMVPDLEC).
In the next step, a computer model of interactions between the ch14.18 and the GD2 ganglioside, or the two peptides was built. The peptide MD was shown not to block the binding site as effectively as the peptide MA. In 2006, additional *in silico* data were published by Fest et al. Eight residues of the ch14.18 were found to interact with both the two peptides and the GD2 ganglioside, *i.e.*, Tyr37, His54, Ser96, Val99, Pro100, Leu102 from the light chain, as well as Gly98 and Gly100 from the heavy chain. Also, dissociation constants were determined with surface plasmion resonance (Fest et al., 2006). Immunogenicity of the both peptides was investigated after their conjugation to KLH. In the sera of mice immunised with both peptide conjugates antibodies of IgM and IgG isotypes recognising the GD2 ganglioside were raised, as detected with ELISA. The sera samples also bound specifically to the GD2 positive M21 melanoma cells (Reimer et al., 2006).
The MA sequence was recently improved, as reported by Bleeke and co-authors. This was achieved after another two rounds of screenings with the ch14.18 of synthetic sub-libraries,

produced on a solid support, and containing systematic alterations based on the MA sequence (Bleeke et al., 2009). The experiments yielded a new mutated sequence C3 CGRL**HL**VPDLEC with significantly improved binding to the ch14.18, as determined with dot blot and surface plasmion resonance measurements using BIACORE.

4.3.3 Peptides isolated with the 14.G2a antibody

Bolesta and co-authors reported screening with the 14.G2a of 15-mer library of linear peptides, fused with the p8 protein (in the f88-4 vector). 6 peptides were isolated, and shown to bind to the 14.G2a antibody by ELISA. Moreover, all the peptides in the free form competed for binding to the 14.G2a with the GD2 ganglioside present on a human neuroblastoma cell line IMR-32 (Bolesta et al., 2005). Importantly, three peptides (47, 9, and 51) cross-reacted with GD2 ganglioside binding antibodies from a serum sample of a neuroblastoma patient. Competition experiments between peptides 47, 9, and 51 showed that they mimic an overlapping epitope of the GD2 ganglioside.

The peptide 47 (EDPSHSLGLDVALFM) with highest score in the competition tests was chosen for further optimisation. Also here, molecular modelling was conducted to build a model of interactions between the 47 peptide, and the antigen binding site of the 14.G2a. Additionally, alanine scanning enabled identification of amino acid residues pivotal for the observed binding. As a result, the LGLDVALFM sequence was found essential for the interactions with the 14.G2a. More importantly, substitution of V with A yielded the 47-LDA (EDPSHSLGLD**A**ALFM) peptide that was 2-fold more effective than the original 47, in the competition assays against the IMR-32 cells.

Based on the findings, the 47-LDA peptide, and two universal T helper epitopes (PADRE, and $P18_{MN}$ epitope from envelope protein of HIV-1 isolate MN) were encoded in a DNA vaccine, constructed in the pNGVL-7 vector that contained the tissue plasminogen activator secretory signal sequence. The vaccine induced anti-GD2 ganglioside IgG antibodies in BALB/c mice. The level of GD2 ganglioside cross-reactive antibodies was further increased with prime-boost strategy that utilised first the 47-LDA construct, and then the GD2 antigen administered in incomplete Freund's adjuvant. The sera samples obtained from immunisations with the DNA construct alone, as well as in combination with the GD2 ganglioside boost, mediated complement dependent lysis of the GD2 positive IMR-32 neuroblastoma, and HT-144 melanoma cells (Bolesta et al., 2005).

Yet another 5 sequences binding to the 14G2a antibodies were isolated, but this time from the constrained library LX-8 (Horwacik et al., 2007). The library displays 12-amino acid peptides. Their structure is constrained by the presence of two cysteines at the positions 2 and 11. Binding motifs were identified through sequence comparisons. LTG or LSG motifs are present in the centre in 3 of 5 isolated peptides. D or N is present in the position 3 of 4 peptides, while P occupies the position 4 in 2 peptides, and L is present in the positions 9 (in 2 peptides), and 10 (in 3 peptides). Finally, S occupies the position 12 in 2 peptides. All five peptides were shown to mimic the GD2 ganglioside, as analysed by ELISA. The peptides presented in the phage-bound form, as well as the free synthetic form competed for binding to the 14.G2a with the GD2 ganglioside present on the IMR-32 cells (Fig. 4). More importantly, the presence of the disulfide bond, formed by the cysteines 2 and 11, is pivotal for the observed mimicry of the GD2 ganglioside for all 5 constrained peptides.

To further characterise antigenic features of the peptides, we analysed reactivity of 3 peptides (65, 85, 94) with other than the 14.G2a mouse monoclonal antibodies that had been raised against gangliosides, *i.e.*, the anti-GD2 antibody 126 (IgM), anti-GD2 antibody ME361-

S2A (IgG2a), and the anti-GD3 antibody ME3.6 (IgG3). But, the peptides did not bind to them, which highlights the fact that peptide-carbohydrate mimicry is observed in the context of a given receptor (the 14.G2a in this case). Additionally, the peptides were shown to occupy overlapping binding sites on the 14.G2a. This finding was supported by *in silico* models of interactions of the peptides with the Fab fragment of the 14.G2a (Horwacik et al., 2011).

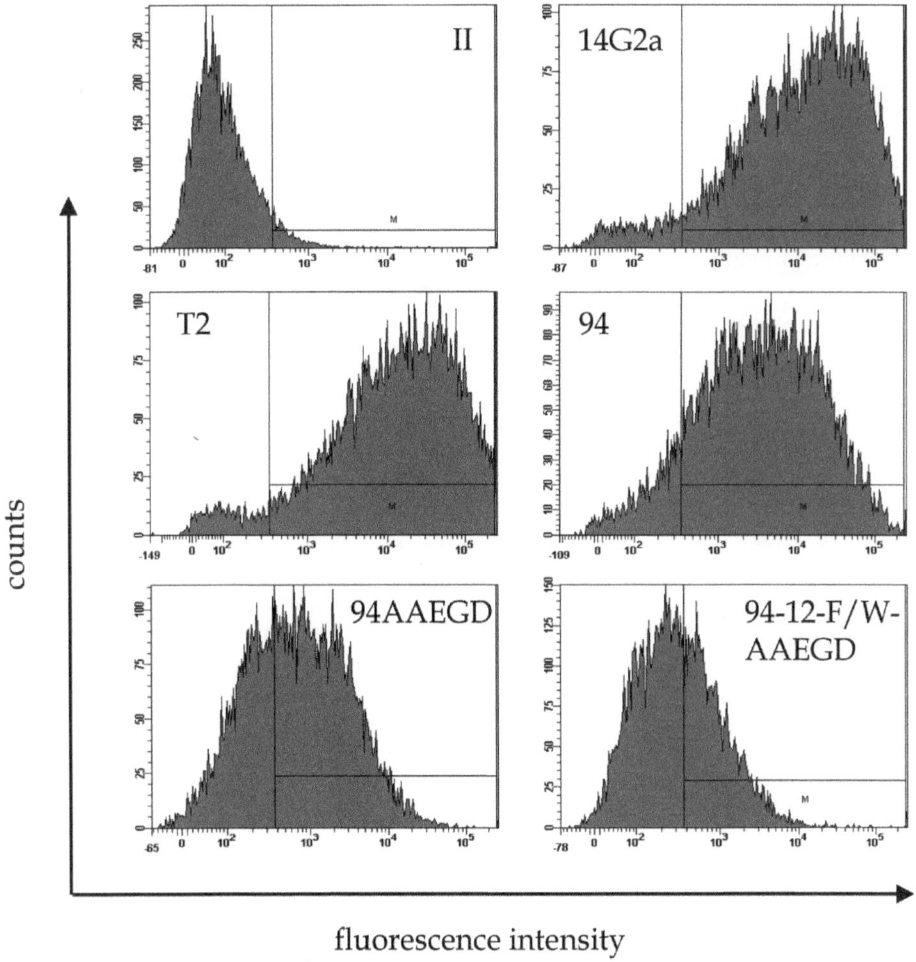

Fig. 4. The peptide 94 can compete with the GD2 ganglioside present on IMR-32 neuroblastoma for biding to the 14.G2a (as analysed by flow cytometry). The inhibitory effect is significantly improved for modified peptides 94-AAEGD and 94-12-F/W-AAEGD. No inhibition was detected with a control peptide T2. The pool of GD2-positive IMR-32 cells was determined by comparison of cells stained with the 14.G2a and the secondary FITC-conjugated (Fab')$_2$ fragments specific to mouse immunoglobulins (14.G2a), and cells stained only with the secondary antibody fragments (II).

The peptide 94 (RCNPNMEPPRCF) was chosen for further analysis and optimisation of the binding to the 14.G2a. Alanine scanning, replacement analysis, and truncation experiments allowed to elucidate structure-activity relationships that are the basis for the observed mimicry of the GD2 ganglioside by the peptide 94. The experiments showed that C2, N3, M6, E7, C11 are indispensable for the observed binding, as their substitution by alanine resulted in a complete loss of the 14.G2a binding. A new peptide with better binding to the antibody was identified by replacement of F at the position 12 with W. The antigenicity was even further improved with extension of the C terminus with the AAEGD sequence, taken from the N terminus of the viral coat protein p8 (Horwacik et al., 2011). The peptide 94-12-F/W-AAEGD (RCNPNMEPPRC**WAAEGD**) was the best in the competition assay against the IMR-32 cells, and showed 18-fold decrease in the measured IC50 values (half maximal inhibition concentration), as compared to the original 94 sequence (Fig. 4). The obtained peptides are currently being further analysed to verify relationships between their antigenicity and immunogenicity.

4.4 Vaccination using the GD2 mimetics in preclinical settings

Many of the isolated peptides mimicking the GD2 ganglioside were tested in pre-clinical experiments, using several modes of delivery (*e.g.*, DNA vaccines, dendritic cell-based vaccines, KLH-conjugated peptides) with application of syngeneic (Bleeke et al., 2009; Gil et al., 2009; Kowalczyk et al., 2007; Wierzbicki et al., 2008; Wondimu et al., 2008), and heterotransplant mouse models (Bolesta et al., 2005).

4.4.1 Tests of GD2 ganglioside mimics in melanoma models

Sera were collected from animals immunised with the 47-LDA DNA vaccine/GD2 ganglioside boost. Therapeutic efficacy of purified fractions of mouse IgG antibodies containing the GD2 ganglioside cross-reactive antibodies was tested in a heterotransplant model, based on s.c. injection of a human MV3 melanoma (10^6 cells). Multiple i.v. injection of the antibodies were conducted, starting 3 days after the tumour challenge. They lead to significant decrease in tumour growth in the group of animals treated with the GD2 antibodies, as compared to control mice treated with murine IgG. However, none of the mice on therapy with the GD2 ganglioside specific antibodies showed a complete resolution of the melanoma tumours (Bolesta et al., 2005).

Similar indications of anti-melanoma efficacy of vaccines based on the GD2 mimicking peptides were gathered on a syngeneic model with s.c. injections of GD2 ganglioside positive melanoma cells D142.34 to C56BL/6 mice. Peptide vaccines containing the P9, or the P10 conjugated to KLH, or in the form of MAP were delivered s.c. with QS-21 adjuvant. GD2 ganglioside specific antibodies were raised by the immunisations with both peptides, as compared to control group injected with an unrelated peptide. In animals that received vaccines with the peptides, DTH reactions were detected 48, and 72 h after administration of irradiated D142.34 cells, in contrast to injections with GD2 ganglioside negative B78.H1 melanoma cells. In a prophylactic setting, the vaccines with the P10 were more effectively inhibiting s.c. growth of the D142.34 cells than the vaccines with the P9, as evidenced by tumour volume and weight measurements. Moreover, P10-KLH vaccinations in a therapeutic setting, starting 10 days after challenge with the D142.34 cells, delayed growth of tumours, as compared to control peptide vaccination. Although, the statistical significance could not be achieved in the therapeutic setting, the data emphasise that induction of protective responses targeting the melanoma cells with active immunisation with the GD2 mimicking peptides was possible (Wondimu et al., 2008).

4.4.2 Tests of GD2 ganglioside mimics in syngenic neuroblastoma models

A syngeneic mouse model based on injections of NXS2 cells that show heterogeneous expression of the GD2 ganglioside to mice of A strain was reported in 1997 (Lode et al., 1997). The model was applied to test DNA constructs bearing Ig κ leader sequence, T helper epitope for HIV-1 envelope protein, and MA, or MD epitopes separated with flexible glycine-serine linkers in the pSA vector. The construct was used for oral mice immunisation after transfection to attenuated *Salmonella typhimurium* SL7207. The regiment used in a prophylactic setting was shown to significantly reduce spontaneous liver metastases, as determined about a month after removal of s.c. NXS2 tumors. This was correlated with induction of anti-GD2 antibodies responses in sera of mice vaccinated with MA or MD, as well as with significant increase in activity of spleen derived NK cells from pSA-MD immunised mice. The later was evidenced by ability of the NK cells to lyse YAC-1 cells, but not NXS2 cells. However, the effect was only observed with the effector cells co-cultured with irradiated NXS2. Additionally, orally delivered *Salmonella typhimurium* SL7207, carrying the empty vector pSA, was shown to be an effective adjuvant to establish GD2 ganglioside specific antibodies, and NXS2 protective immune responses in A mice, with protein vaccines containing the peptides MD and C3 conjugated to KLH, and absorbed on alum. No $CD8^+$ T cell immune responses were observed with the DNA vaccines. No experiments in therapeutic setting were described (Bleeke et al., 2009; Fest et al., 2006).
On the contrary, sequence of the peptide 47-LDA delivered in the form of DNA construct effectively induced antibody and cell mediated immune responses that inhibited growth of s.c. NXS2 tumour in A mice in therapeutic setting. Kowalczyk and co-authors showed that protection against tumour challenge with NXS2 cells required both innate (NK cells), and adoptive cell-mediated immunity ($CD4^+$ and $CD8^+$ T cells). Furthermore, administration of plasmids encoding IL-15, and IL-21 cytokines together with the 47-LD construct markedly enhanced the tumour protective immunity. In the group of animals that were treated with the combined immunisation regiment, delivered from 1 day after s.c. NXS2 challenge, 6 of 8 animals remained tumour-free more than 90 days. The inclusion of the plasmids encoding IL-15, and IL-21 in the vaccination protocol, significantly increased levels of GD2 ganglioside cross-reactive IgG in sera of mice, as well as CDC and ADCC against NXS2 cells. More importantly, re-challenge experiment in the group of 8 animals that remained tumour free, showed that all the animals survived additional 90 days, in contrast to control mice that developed tumours by day 30. Finally, adoptive transfer of $CD8^+$ T cells from 47-LDA vaccinated and cured mice to NXS2-challenged mice, significantly influenced tumour control, as most of the mice survived tumour-free for more than 90 days (Kowalczyk et al., 2007).
The $CD8^+$ T cell responses induced with the 47-LDA construct were further investigated. Interestingly, they were shown to be MHC class I restricted to syngeneic neuroblastoma cells (NXS2, Neuro2a), but independent of the GD2 ganglioside expression. This suggested that than GD2 vaccine induced responses cross-reactive with other the GD2 antigen present on neuroblastoma cells. The hypothesis was confirmed with experiments showing that the 14G2a cross reacts with a 105 kDa protein, ALCAM/CD166 (activated leukocyte cell

adhesion molecule). When the expression of CD166 was silenced using specific shRNA in Neuro2a, the cells were no longer killed by $CD8^+$ T cells from mice immunised with the 47-LDA construct. Additionally, such cells induced progressive growth of s.c. tumours in mice, despite of the combined immunisation with the 47-LDA, IL-15, IL-21 constructs that preceded the challenge. This finding shed new light on application of peptide mimicking the GD2 ganglioside. Here the 47-LDA was shown to induce responses to conformation-dependent epitope of CD166 protein (Wierzbicki et al., 2008).
In the following report in 2009, the 47-LDA mimotope was expressed as a fusion protein with the mouse IgG2a Fc region, and used for vaccination based on dendritic cells (DC). Targeting the mimotope vaccine to activating Fcγ receptors of DC allowed for selective expansion of adoptively transferred $CD8^+$ T in NXS2-tumour bearing syngeneic mice. Anti-tumour responses were also observed with virotherapy, after delivery of recombinant oncolytic vaccinia virus expressing the 47-LDA- Fcγ2a fusion protein (Gil et al., 2009).

5. Conclusion

Tumour associated-carbohydrate antigens are highly over expressed in tumour cells, and therefore are attractive targets for both passive and active immunization approaches. Both, mimicking peptides and anti-idiotypic antibodies can functionally mimic carbohydrates, including the GD2 ganglioside. Furthermore, such surrogate antigens often induce humoral and cellular immune responses, which the carbohydrate itself is usually unable to induce. Peptides are easier to manufacture and modify than carbohydrates. Additionally, they can be used to manipulate immune responses, *i.e.*, to present cryptic epitopes, and to break tolerance by focusing the response on critical epitopes delivered in a different molecular environment. The data on application of the molecular mimicry to target the GD2 ganglioside adds knowledge on structural-activity relationships of such mimicking peptides, and anti-idiotypic antibodies, and correlates of their immunogenicity. This extends our understanding of vaccine design in cancer. Hopefully, this will boost research on future vaccines targeting neuroblastoma.

6. Acknowledgment

We acknowledge financial support: in years 2006-2010 from the research grant no. N302 034 31/3063 from the Polish Ministry of Science and Higher Education (to Irena Horwacik); from the Jagiellonian University Grant no. WBBB 8. The Faculty of Biochemistry, Biophysics and Biotechnology of the Jagiellonian University is a beneficiary of the structural funds from the European Community (POIG.02.01.00-12-064/08).

7. References

Agostino, M.; Sandrin, M.S.; Thompson, P.E.; Farrugia, W.; Ramsland, P.A. & Yuriev, E. (2011). Carbohydrate-Mimetic Peptides: Structural Aspects of Mimicry and Therapeutic Implications. *Expert Opinion on Biological Therapy*, Vol.11, No.2, (February 2011), pp. 211-224, ISSN 1744-7682

Aina, O.H.; Liu, R.; Sutcliffe, J.L.; Marik, J.; Pan, C.X. & Lam, K.S. (2007). From Combinatorial Chemistry to Cancer-Targeting Peptides. *Molecular Pharmacology*, Vol.4, No.5, (September-October 2007), pp. 631-651, ISSN 1521-0111

Basak, S.; Birebent, B.; Purev, E.; Somasundaram, R.; Maruyama, H.; Zaloudik, J.; Swoboda, R.; Strittmatter, W.; Li, W.; Luckenbach, A.; Song, H.; Li, J.; Sproesser, K.; Guerry, D.; Nair, S.; Furukawa, K. & Herlyn, D. (2003). Induction of Cellular Immunity by Anti-Idiotypic Antibodies Mimicking GD2 Ganglioside. *Cancer Immunology and Immunotherapy*, Vol.52, No.3, (March 2003), pp. 145-154, ISSN 0340-7004

Bhattacharya-Chatterjee, M.; Chatterjee, S.K. & Foon, K.A. (2000). Anti-Idiotype Vaccine Against Cancer. *Immunology Letters*, Vol.74, No.1, (September 2000), pp. 51-58, ISSN 0165-2478

Bleeke, M.; Fest, S.; Huebener, N.; Landgraf, C.; Schraven, B.; Gaedicke, G.; Volkmer, R. & Lode, H.N. (2009). Systematic Amino Acid Substitutions Improved Efficiency of GD2-Peptide Mimotope Vaccination Against Neuroblastoma. *The European Journal of Cancer*, Vol.45, No.16, (November 2009), pp. 2915-2921, ISSN 0959-8049

Bolesta, E.; Kowalczyk, A.; Wierzbicki, A.; Rotkiewicz, P.; Bambach, B.; Tsao, C.Y.; Horwacik, I.; Kolinski, A.; Rokita, H.; Brecher, M.; Wang, X.; Ferrone, S. & Kozbor, D. (2005). DNA Vaccine Expressing the Mimotope of GD2 Ganglioside Induces Protective GD2 Cross-Reactive Antibody Responses. *Cancer Research*, Vol.65, No.8, (April 2005), pp. 3410-3418, ISSN 1538-7445

Bonnycastle, L.L.; Mehroke, J.S.; Rashed, M.; Gong, X. & Scott, J.K. (1996). Probing the Basis of Antibody Reactivity with a Panel of Constrained Peptide Libraries Displayed by Filamentous Phage. *Journal of Molecular Biology*, Vol.258, No.5, (May 1996), pp. 747-762, ISSN 0022-2836

Chapman, P.B.; Morrisey, D.; Panageas, K.S.; Williams, L.; Lewis, J.J.; Israel, R.J.; Hamilton, W.B. & Livingston, P.O. (2000). Vaccination with a Bivalent G(M2) and G(D2) Ganglioside Conjugate Vaccine: a Trial Comparing Doses of G(D2)-Keyhole Limpet Hemocyanin. *Clinical Cancer Research*, Vol.6, No.12, (December 2000), pp. 4658-4662, ISSN 1557-3265

Cheung, N.K.; Guo, H.F.; Heller, G. & Cheung, I.Y. (2000). Induction of Ab3 and Ab3' Antibody was Associated with Long-Term Survival after Anti-G(D2) Antibody Therapy of Stage 4 Neuroblastoma. *Clinical Cancer Research*, Vol.6, No.7, (July 2000), pp. 2653-60, ISSN 1557-3265

Czaplicki, D.; Horwacik, I.; Kowalczyk, A.; Wieczorek, A.; Bolek-Marzec, K.; Balwierz, W.; Kozik, A. & Rokita, H. (2009). New Method for Quantitative Analysis of GD2 Ganglioside in Plasma of Neuroblastoma Patients. *Acta Biochimica Polonica*, Vol.56, No.3, (August 2009), pp. 423-431, ISSN 0001-527X

Deroo, S. & Muller, C.P. (2001). Antigenic and Immunogenic Phage Displayed Mimotopes as Substitute Antigens: Applications and Limitations. *Combinatorial Chemistry and High Throughput Screening*, Vol.4, No.1, (February 2001), pp. 75-110, ISSN 1875-5402

Dudak, F.C.; Boyaci, I.H. & Orner, B.P. (2011). The Discovery of Small-Molecule Mimicking Peptides Through Phage Display. *Molecules*, Vol.16, No.1, (January 2011), pp. 774-789, ISSN 1420-3049

El Kasmi, K.C.; Deroo, S.; Theisen, D.M.; Brons, N.H. & Muller, C.P. (1999). Crossreactivity of Mimotopes and Peptide Homologues of a Sequential Epitope with a Monoclonal Antibody does not Predict Crossreactive Immunogenicity. *Vaccine*, Vol.18, No.3-4, (September 1999), pp. 284-290, ISSN 0264-410X

Fest, S.; Huebener, N.; Weixler, S.; Bleeke, M.; Zeng, Y.; Strandsby, A.; Volkmer-Engert, R.; Landgraf, C.; Gaedicke, G.; Riemer, A.B.; Michalsky, E.; Jaeger, I.S.; Preissner, R.; Förster-Wald, E.; Jensen-Jarolim, E. & Lode, H.N. (2006). Characterization of GD2 Peptide Mimotope DNA Vaccines Effective Against Spontaneous Neuroblastoma Metastases. *Cancer Research*, Vol.66, No.21, (November 2006), pp. 10567-10575, ISSN 1538-7445

Fleuridor, R., Lees, A. & Pirofski, L. (2001). A Cryptococcal Capsular Polysaccharide Mimotope Prolongs the Survival of Mice with Cryptococcus Neoformans Infection. *The Journal of Immunology*, Vol.166, No.2, (January 2001), pp. 1087-1096, ISSN 0022-1767

Foon, K.A.; Lutzky, J.; Baral, R.N.; Yannelli, J.R.; Hutchins, L.; Teitelbaum, A.; Kashala, O.L.; Das, R.; Garrison, J.; Reisfeld, R.A. & Bhattacharya-Chatterjee, M. (2000). Clinical and Immune Responses in Advanced Melanoma Patients Immunized with an Anti-Idiotype Antibody Mimicking Disialoganglioside GD2. *Journal of Clinical Oncology*, Vol.18, No.2, (January 2000), pp. 376-384, ISSN 1527-7755

Förster-Waldl, E.; Riemer, A.B.; Dehof, A.K.; Neumann, D.; Brämswig, K.; Boltz-Nitulescu, G.; Pehamberger, H.; Zielinski, C.C.; Scheiner, O.; Pollak, A.; Lode, H. & Jensen-Jarolim, E. (2005). Isolation and Structural Analysis of Peptide Mimotopes for the Disialoganglioside GD2, a Neuroblastoma Tumor Antigen. *Molecular Immunology*, Vol.42, No.3, (February 2005), pp. 319-325, ISSN 0161-5890

Gil, M.; Bieniasz, M.; Wierzbicki, A.; Bambach, B.J.; Rokita, H. & Kozbor, D. (2009). Targeting a Mimotope Vaccine to Activating Fcgamma Receptors Empowers Dendritic Cells to Prime Specific CD8+ T Cell Responses in Tumor-Bearing Mice. *The Journal of Immunology*, Vol.183, No.10, (November 2009), pp. 6808-6818, ISSN 0022-1767

Horwacik, I.; Czaplicki, D.; Talarek, K.; Kowalczyk, A.; Bolesta, E.; Kozbor, D. & Rokita, H. (2007). Selection of Novel Peptide Mimics of the GD2 Ganglioside from a Constrained Phage-Displayed Peptide Library. *International Journal of Molecular Medicine*, Vol.19, No.5, (May 2007), pp. 829-839, ISSN 1791-244X

Horwacik, I.; Kurciński, M.; Bzowska, M.; Kowalczyk, A.K.; Czaplicki, D.; Koliński, A. & Rokita, H. (2011). Analysis and Optimization of Interactions Between Peptides Mimicking GD2 Ganglioside and Monoclonal Antibody 14G2a. *International Journal of Molecular Medicine*, Vol.28, No.1, (July 2011), pp. 47-57, ISSN 1791-244X

Huang, J.; Ru, B. & Dai, P. (2011). Bioinformatics Resources and Tools for Phage Display. *Molecules*, Vol.16, No.1, (January 2011), pp. 694-709, ISSN 1420-3049

Johnson, M.A. & Pinto, B.M. (2008). Structural and Functional Studies of Peptide–Carbohydrate Mimicry. *Topics in Current Chemistry*, Vol.273, (2008), pp. 55-116, ISSN 0340-1022

Kieber-Emmons, T.; Luo, P.; Qiu, J.; Chang, T.Y.; O, I.; Blaszczyk-Thurin, M. & Steplewski, Z. (1999). Vaccination with Carbohydrate Peptide Mimotopes Promotes Anti-Tumor Responses. *Nature Biotechnolology*, Vol.17, No.7, (July 1999), pp. 660-665, ISSN 1087-0156

Kieber-Emmons, T.; Monzavi-Karbassi, B.; Wang, B.; Luo, P. & Weiner, D.B. (2000). Cutting Edge: DNA Immunization with Minigenes of Carbohydrate Mimotopes Induce Functional Anti-Carbohydrate Antibody Response. *The Journal of Immunology*, Vol.165, No.2, (July 2000), pp. 623-627, ISSN 0022-1767

Kowalczyk, A.; Wierzbicki, A.; Gil, M.; Bambach, B.; Kaneko, Y.; Rokita, H.; Repasky, E.; Fenstermaker, R.; Brecher, M.; Ciesielski, M. & Kozbor, D. (2007). Induction of Protective Immune Responses against NXS2 Neuroblastoma Challenge in Mice by Immunotherapy with GD2 Mimotope Vaccine and IL-15 and IL-21 Gene Delivery. *Cancer Immunology and Immunotherapy*, Vol.56, No.9, (September 2007), pp. 1443-1458, ISSN 0340-7004

Kramer, K.; Gerald, W.L.; Kushner, B.H.; Larson, S.M.; Hameed, M. & Cheung, N.K. (2001). Disaloganglioside GD2 Loss Following Monoclonal Antibody Therapy is Rare in Neuroblastoma. *Medical and Pediatric Oncology*, Vol.36, No.1, (January 2001), pp. 194-196, ISSN 0098-1532

Kushner, B.H.; Kramer, K.; Modak, S. & Cheung, N.K. (2011). Successful Multifold Dose Escalation of Anti-GD2 Monoclonal Antibody 3F8 in Patients with Neuroblastoma: a Phase I Study. *Journal of Clinical Oncology*, Vol.29, No.9, (March 2011), pp. 1168-1174, ISSN 1527-7755

Ladisch, S.; Li, R. & Olson, E. (1994). Ceramide Structure Predicts Tumor Ganglioside Immunosuppressive Activity. *Proceedings of the National Academy of Sciences of the United States of America*, Vol.94, No.5, (March 1994), pp. 1974-1978, ISSN 1091-6490

Lode, H.N.; Xiang, R.; Varki, N.M.; Dolman, C.S.; Gillies, S.D. & Reisfeld, R.A. (1997). Targeted Interleukin-2 Therapy for Spontaneous Neuroblastoma Metastases to Bone Marrow. *Journal of the National Cancer Institute*, Vol.89, No.21, (November 1997), pp. 1586-94, ISSN 1460-2105

Mak, T.W. & Saunders, M.E. (2006). The Immune Response: Basic and Clinical Principles, Elsevier Academic Press, ISBN-13 978-0-12-088451-3, San Diego, USA

Modak, S. & Cheung, N.K. (2010). Neuroblastoma: Therapeutic Strategies for a Clinical Enigma. *Cancer Treatment Reviews*, Vol.36, No.4, (June 2010), pp. 307-317, ISSN 0305-7372

Monzavi-Karbassi, B.; Hennings, L.J.; Artaud, C.; Liu, T.; Jousheghany, F.; Pashov, A.; Murali, R.; Hutchins, L.F. & Kieber-Emmons, T. (2007). Preclinical Studies of Carbohydrate Mimetic Peptide Vaccines for Breast Cancer and Melanoma. *Vaccine*, Vol.25, No.16, (April 2007), pp. 3022-3031, ISSN 0264-410X

Navid, F.; Santana, V.M. & Barfield, R.C. (2010). Anti-GD2 Antibody Therapy for GD2-Expressing Tumors. *Current Cancer Drug Targets*, Vol.10, No.2, (March 2010), pp. 200-209, ISSN 1568-0096

O, I.; Kieber-Emmons, T.; Otvos, L. & Blaszczyk-Thurin, M. (1999). Peptides Mimicking Sialyl-Lewis a Isolated From a Random Peptide Library and Peptide Array. *Annals of the New York Academy of Sciences*, Vol.886, (December 1999), pp. 276-279, ISSN 00778923

Pande, J.; Szewczyk, M.M. & Grover, A.K. (2010). Phage Display: Concept, Innovations, Applications and Future. *Biotechnology Advances*, Vol.28, No.6, (November-December 2010), pp. 849-858, ISSN 0734-9750

Popkov, M.; Sidrac-Ghali, S.; Alakhov, V. & Mandeville, R. (2000). Epitope-Specific Antibody Response to HT-1080 Fibrosarcoma Cells by Mimotope Immunization. *Clinical Cancer Research*, Vol.6, No.9, (September 2000), pp. 3629-3635, ISSN 1557-3265

Qiu, J.; Luo, P.; Wasmund, K.; Steplewski, Z. & Kieber-Emmons, T. (1999). Towards the Development of Peptide Mimotopes of Carbohydrate Antigens as Cancer Vaccines. *Hybridoma,* Vol.18, No.1, (February 1999), pp. 103-112, ISSN 1554-0014

Rakonjac, J.; Bennett, N.J.; Spagnuolo, J.; Gagic, D. & Russel, M. (2011). Filamentous Bacteriophage: Biology, Phage Display and Nanotechnology Applications. *Current Issues in Molecular Biology*, Vol.13, No.2, (April 2011), pp. 51-76, ISSN 1467-3037

Reuland, P.; Geiger, L.; Thelen, M.H.; Handgretinger, R.; Haase, B.; Müller-Schauenburg, W.; Niethammer, D. & Bares, R. (2001). Follow-up in Neuroblastoma: Comparison of Metaiodobenzylguanidine and a Chimeric Anti-GD2 Antibody for Detection of Tumor Relapse and Therapy Response. *Journal of Pediatric Hematology/Oncology*, Vol.23, No.7, (October 2001), pp. 437-442, ISSN 1077-4114

Riemer, A.B.; Förster-Waldl, E.; Brämswig, K.H.; Pollak, A.; Zielinski, C.C.; Pehamberger, H.; Lode, H.N.; Scheiner, O. & Jensen-Jarolim, E. (2006). Induction of IgG Antibodies Against the GD2 Carbohydrate Tumor Antigen by Vaccination with Peptide Mimotopes. *European Journal of Immunology*, Vol.36, No.5, (May 2006), pp. 1267-1274, ISSN 1521-4141

Ruan, S.; Raj, B.K. & Lloyd, K.O. (1999). Relationship of Glycosyltransferases and mRNA Levels to Ganglioside Expression in Neuroblastoma and Melanoma Cells. *Journal of Neurochemistry*, Vol.72, No.2, (February 1999), pp. 514-521, ISSN 0022-3042

Saleh, M.N.; Stapleton, J.D.; Khazaeli, M.B. & LoBuglio, A.F. (1993). Generation of a Human Anti-Idiotypic Antibody That Mimics the GD2 Antigen. *The Journal of Immunology*, Vol.151, No.6, (September 1993), pp. 3390-3398, ISSN 0022-1767

Smith, G.P. & Petrenko, V.A. (1997). Phage Display. *Chemical Reviews,* Vol.97, No.2, (April 1997), pp. 391-410, ISSN 0009-2665

Sorkin, L.S.; Otto, M.; Baldwin, W.M.; Vail, E.; Gillies, S.D.; Handgretinger, R.; Barfield, R.C.; Ming Yu, H. & Yu, A.L. (2010). Anti-GD(2) with an FC Point Mutation Reduces Complement Fixation and Decreases Antibody-Induced Allodynia. *Pain*, Vol. 149, No. 1, (April 2010), pp. 135-142, ISSN 0304-3959

Swerts, K.; Ambros, P.F.; Brouzes, C.; Navarro, J.M.; Gross, N.; Rampling, D.; Schumacher-Kuckelkorn, R.; Sementa, A.R.; Ladenstein, R. & Beiske, K. (2005). Standardization of the Immunocytochemical Detection of Neuroblastoma Cells in Bone Marrow. *Journal of Histochemistry and Cytochemistry*, Vol.53, No.12, (December 2005), pp. 1433-1440, ISSN 0022-1554

Tai, T.; Cahan, L.D.; Tsuchida, T.; Saxton, R.E.; Irie, R.F. & Morton, D.L. (1985). Immunogenicity of Melanoma-Associated Gangliosides in Cancer Patients. *International Journal of Cancer*, Vol.35, No.5, (May 1985), pp. 607-612, ISSN 0020-7136

Theillet, F.X.; Saul, F.A.; Vulliez-Le Normand, B.; Hoos, S.; Felici, F.; Weintraub, A.; Mulard, L.A.; Phalipon, A.; Delepierre, M. & Bentley, G.A. (2009). Structural Mimicry of O-Antigen by a Peptide Revealed in a Complex With an Antibody Raised Against Shigella flexneri Serotype 2a. *Journal of Molecular Biology*, Vol.388, No.4, (May 2009), pp. 839-850, ISSN 0022-2836

Uchiyama, F.; Tanaka, Y.; Minari, Y. & Tokui, N. (2005). Designing Scaffolds of Peptides for Phage Display Libraries. *Journal of Biosciences and Bioengineering*, Vol.99, No.5, (May 2005), pp. 448-456, ISSN 1389-1723

Van Regenmortel, M.H. (2001). Antigenicity and Immunogenicity of Synthetic Peptides. *Biologicals*, Vol.29, No.3-4, (September-December 2001), pp. 209-213, ISSN 1045-1056

Weiner, L.M.; Dhodapkar, M.V. & Ferrone, S. (2009). Monoclonal Antibodies for Cancer Immunotherapy. *The Lancet*, Vol.373, No.9668, (March 2009), pp. 1033-1040, ISSN 0140-6736

Wierzbicki, A.; Gil, M.; Ciesielski, M.; Fenstermaker, R.A.; Kaneko, Y.; Rokita, H.; Lau, J.T. & Kozbor, D. (2008). Immunization with a Mimotope of GD2 Ganglioside Induces CD8+ T Cells That Recognize Cell Adhesion Molecules on Tumor Cells. *The Journal of Immunology*, Vol.181, No.9, (November 2008), pp. 6644-6653, ISSN 0022-1767

Willers, J.; Lucchese, A.; Kanduc, D. & Ferrone, S. (1999). Molecular Mimicry of Phage Displayed Peptides Mimicking GD3 Ganglioside. *Peptides*, Vol.20, No.9, (September 1999), pp. 1021-1026, ISSN 0196-9781

Wondimu, A.; Zhang, T.; Kieber-Emmons, T.; Gimotty, P.; Sproesser, K.; Somasundaram, R.; Ferrone, S.; Tsao, C.Y. & Herlyn, D. (2008). Peptides Mimicking GD2 Ganglioside Elicit Cellular, Humoral and Tumor-Protective Immune Responses in Mice. *Cancer Immunology and Immunotherapy*, Vol.57, No.7, (July 2008), pp. 1079-1089, ISSN 0340-7004

Yoshida, S.; Fukumoto, S.; Kawaguchi, H.; Sato, S.; Ueda, R. & Furukawa, K. (2001). Ganglioside G(D2) in Small Cell Lung Cancer Cell Lines: Enhancement of Cell Proliferation and Mediation of Apoptosis. *Cancer Research*, Vol.61, No.10, (May 2001), pp. 4244-4252, ISSN 0008-5472

Yu, A.L.; Gilman, A.L.; Ozkaynak, M.F.; London, W.B.; Kreissman, S.G.; Chen, H.X.; Smith, M.; Anderson, B.; Villablanca, J.G.; Matthay, K.K.; Shimada, H., Grupp, S.A.; Seeger, R.; Reynolds, C.P.; Buxton, A.; Reisfeld, R.A.; Gillies, S.D.; Cohn, S.L.; Maris, J.M.; Sondel, P.M. & Children's Oncology Group. (2011). Anti-GD2

Antibody with GM-CSF, Interleukin-2, and Isotretinoin for Neuroblastoma. *The New England Journal of Medicine*, Vol.363, No.14, (September 2010), pp. 1324-1334, ISSN 1533-4406

Zeytin, H.E.; Tripathi, P.K.; Bhattacharya-Chatterjee, M.; Foon, K.A. & Chatterjee, S.K. (2000). Construction and Characterization of DNA Vaccines Encoding the Single-Chain Variable Fragment of the Anti-Idiotype Antibody 1A7 Mimicking the Tumor-Associated Antigen Disialoganglioside GD2. *Cancer Gene Therapy*, Vol.7, No.11, (November 2000), pp. 1426-1436, ISSN 0929-1903

14

Small Molecule Drugs and Targeted Therapies for Neuroblastoma

Chengyuan Xue[1], Andrei Gudkov[2],
Michelle Haber[1] and Murray D. Norris[1]
[1]*Children's Cancer Institute Australia for Medical Research,
Lowy Cancer Research Centre, UNSW, Sydney,*
[2]*Roswell Park Cancer Institute, Buffalo, New York,*
[1]*Australia*
[2]*USA*

1. Introduction

Neuroblastoma currently accounts for approximately 15% of all childhood cancer related deaths despite intensive multimodal chemotherapy (Maris & Matthay, 1999). Innovative treatment approaches are therefore needed for this disease. Recent advancements in molecular genetics of neuroblastoma have enabled the identification of several prospective molecular targets that provide opportunities for the development of new therapeutic strategies. Targeted therapy is defined as a type of treatment that employs chemical small molecules or other substances, such as monoclonal antibodies, to specifically identify and attack cancer cells. This type of therapy contrasts with traditional chemotherapy that relies on the elimination of rapidly dividing cells, regardless of whether or not they are malignant. Thus, targeted therapies offer a number of potential advantages over conventional chemotherapy including: (1) an increased therapeutic index (i.e. effective cancer treatment with less side effects) due to the targeting of a unique characteristic within the tumour cells, which is usually absent in normal cells of the body (Oeffinger, Mertens et al., 2006); and (2) a decreased likelihood of the development of resistance to the targeted therapy due to the molecular target being essential for the viability of the cancer.

Targeted cancer therapies ultimately interfere with one or more biological pathways within the cancer cell that are critical to its growth or survival. Examples of these pathways include signal transduction, apoptosis, regulation of gene transcription, and tumour angiogenesis. Most targeted therapeutics are either chemical small molecules or monoclonal antibodies. The former can act on targets located inside the cell since they are typically able to diffuse across the lipid bilayer, whereas most monoclonal antibodies usually cannot penetrate the cell's plasma membrane and hence are directed against targets that are either outside cells or on the cell surface. This chapter will review some of the recent findings involving the development of potential small molecule drugs as targeted therapies for childhood neuroblastoma.

2. Cell-based small molecule drug screening

Small molecule drugs or therapeutics are simple organic chemicals with low molecular weights, usually under 1000 Daltons. Compared to larger molecular weight pharmaceuticals such as proteins and peptides, small molecule drugs can be delivered orally or intravenously, and in most instances, more easily penetrate cell membranes and the blood brain barrier. The process of discovery and development of small molecule drugs involves the identification of a target, the discovery of drug candidates that can block or activate the target, product development, pre-clinical research on animals, and finally human clinical trials. The screening of collections or libraries of small molecules has long been used in the pharmaceutical industry as a method of finding drug candidates. The screening process generally falls into one of the two categories: Virtual screening and real screening. Virtual screening is based on computationally inferred or simulated real screening. By using this methodology, huge numbers of chemicals can be screened, and it is also possible to design and investigate compounds that have yet to be synthesized. Real screening on the other hand, is conducted using a variety of readout systems involving either biochemical assays or cell-based assays.

Most *in vitro* screening assays utilize a surrogate readout system that relies on labelled molecules or some type of biochemical reaction, and is often done in so called high-throughput screening (HTS) facilities. HTS can experimentally test the activity of thousands of compounds against a target on a daily basis and provides real information for drug discovery. In addition to biochemical assays, various cell-based assays such as reporter gene assays, secondary messenger assays, cell-based enzyme-linked immunosorbent assay (ELISA), cell-based proximity assays, and pathway screening are also used in current HTS (Digan, Pou et al., 2005). The advantage of a cell-based readout is that one can use a functional assay, thus bringing selection conditions closer to the final application of the compounds. It also allows testing the desired activity of the compounds while filtering out cytotoxic ones in one assay. A cell-based assay normally includes a cell line or a primary cell population, a target molecule that records the cellular response, instruments for conducting and monitoring the assay, and methods of data analyses. The choice of cells for the readout is a compromise between those systems that most adequately reflect the "disease" properties *in vitro*, and the requirements of high throughput screening. For drug discovery screening, a cell-based assay, in certain aspects, is more useful than an *in vitro* assay, as potential liabilities can be assessed earlier, and structure-activity relationships can be explored at reasonable cost in a shorter timeframe. Although cell-based approaches are sometimes less robust due to certain problems with living cells, this technology is proving to be one of the most successful ways in identifying bioactive compounds (Gudkov & Komarova, 2003).

Chemical libraries are available from many vendors and differ in their origin, composition, complexity and purity. They consist of large sets of individual organic molecules usually dissolved in DMSO and formatted to facilitate their transfer to microtitre plates for screening purposes (Gudkov & Komarova, 2003). Following establishment of a read-out system, an initial library screening will yield a number of "hits", with an acceptable hit rate usually below 0.5%. These hits are then subjected to a filtering process to remove those compounds representing false positives. Additional rounds of screening, including screening of focussed libraries generated around the best and most active compounds, is performed with the aim of finding further compounds with increased activity and specificity. After completing the screening process, the chemical structure of particularly promising compounds can be used as a starting point for modifications in order to further improve potency and selectivity, ultimately leading to the selection of "lead compounds". Use of cell-based readout systems, has led to the discovery of small molecule inhibitors, including p53 inhibitors such as pifithrin-α (Komarov, Komarova et al., 1999), P-glycoprotein modulators (Kondratov, Komarov et al., 2001) and the Multidrug Resistance-Associated Protein 1 (MRP1) inhibitor, Reversan (Burkhart, Watt et al., 2009). The methodology of drug screening in cell-based readout systems and its application in the discovery of p53 inhibitors have been comprehensively reviewed previously (Gudkov & Komarova, 2003).

3. MycN targeted inhibition

3.1 Rationale for targeting Myc oncoproteins

Target-based drug discovery begins with the identification of the function of a potential therapeutic drug target and an understanding its role in the disease process. In this regard, amplification of the *MYCN* oncogene in neuroblastoma tumours represents one of the most powerful prognostic markers yet identified for this disease (Maris & Matthay, 1999). *MYCN* belongs to the *MYC* family of proto-oncogenes (including *CMYC* and *MYCL*), and these genes encode a family of basic helix-loop-helix leucine zipper transcription factors. Myc proteins localize to the nucleus and form heterodimers with the basic helix-loop-helix molecule, Max. Myc/Max heterodimers bind to DNA at specific 'E-box' sequences (CAC(G/A)TG) to drive transcription of target genes that are important for proliferation, differentiation and apoptosis. Max also heterodimerizes with Mxd or Mnt proteins to influence the transcription of other downstream genes and often to antagonize the proliferative effects of Myc proteins (Meyer & Penn, 2008). Among Myc proteins, MycN and c-Myc share several regions of homology as well as similar cellular functions. Replacement of the *CMYC* gene with the *MYCN* gene in mice does not affect murine embryonic development, indicating MycN is capable of replacing most of the essential c-Myc functions required for embryonic development and for proliferation of differentiated cells (Malynn, de Alboran et al., 2000). The universal deregulation of *CMYC* gene expression in tumour cells and the high dependency of tumour growth on elevated c-Myc levels suggests that this oncoprotein represents an attractive target for cancer therapy (Prochownik & Vogt, 2010). The same concept applies to the *MYCN* gene in neuroblastoma as the genetic feature most consistently associated with treatment failure is amplification of the *MYCN* gene that strongly correlates with advanced disease (Brodeur, Seeger et al., 1984; Seeger, Brodeur et al., 1985). These notions are supported by numerous experimental data showing that inhibition of c-Myc or MycN significantly halts tumour cell growth and proliferation (Ponzielli, Katz et al., 2005; Gustafson & Weiss, 2010).

3.2 Challenges in targeting Myc by small molecule drugs

Although many efforts have been made to develop anti-Myc therapeutics, to date, no specific Myc modulators have approached clinical trials. The difficulty in identifying drugs that target Myc oncoproteins for the treatment of cancer is multifactorial. Myc is considered a challenging therapeutic target for a number of reasons (Prochownik & Vogt, 2010) that includes (1) Despite its high level of expression in cancer, *MYC* genes are rarely mutated, with the exception of mutations found in primary Burkitt and AIDS-related lymphomas (~30%); (2) Difficulties exist in Myc inhibitor design. For instance, targeting the association between Myc and Max or other essential cofactors involves the disruption of protein–protein interactions. The surfaces at which these interactions occur tend to be large, flat, and relatively featureless, and often lack recognizable motifs or clefts. In addition, disruption of protein–protein interactions must overcome a large free energy of association from the interacting protein moieties.

Ubiquitous expression of c-Myc in normal proliferating cells also raises concerns about potential side effects of such therapeutic agents. Recent findings, however, demonstrated that whole-mouse genetic inhibition of c-Myc resulted in rapid regression of incipient and established tumours, whereas the side effects to normal tissues were well tolerated and completely reversible even over extended periods of time of Myc inhibition (Soucek, Whitfield et al., 2008). Thus, the inhibition of c-Myc, as well as MycN, appears to be a safe and efficient method to eliminate cancer although the actual effects in human context remain to be tested.

3.3 Targeting Myc oncoproteins

3.3.1 Identification of inhibitors of Myc-Max dimerization

Several *in vitro* and cell-based methods have been used in screening for inhibitors of Myc–Max dimerization (Prochownik & Vogt, 2010). The *in vitro* techniques are based on either fluorescence resonance energy transfer (FRET) or fluorescence polarization, while cell-based screening has employed the yeast 2-hybrid approach, in which the interaction between the bHLH-ZIPdomains of c-Myc and Max has been used to isolate inhibitors of Myc–Max dimerization (Yin, Giap et al., 2003). Seven compounds were identified with specificity for Myc–Max inhibition. It was subsequently shown that these compounds work via common mechanisms involving their direct binding to the dimerization domain of the c-Myc monomer. However, their clinical application is likely to be limited due to their relatively low potencies, and rational design of compounds with greater potencies is underway using structure-based computational approaches (Wang, Hammoudeh et al., 2007). In general, an increasing amount of data suggests that inhibition of the protein-protein interactions between c-Myc and Max by small molecules is a feasible approach toward the inhibition of c-Myc functions. More recently, stabilization of Max homodimers to reduce the amount of Max available for activating c-Myc has also been demonstrated to counteract Myc activity (Berg, 2011). It is highly likely that any small molecule inhibitors of c-Myc will also work to inhibit MycN functions due to the high level of structural and functional homology between the two proteins.

3.3.2 Development of stabilizers of the Max homodimer

High levels of Myc protein in cancer cells require an abundance of Max to become functional. Stabilization of the Max–Max homodimer could therefore preferentially affect such overexpressed Myc and attenuate its oncogenic effects. Max–Max stabilizers have been identified by virtual ligand screening, although this type of screening is dependent on structural information being available for the target molecules (Prochownik & Vogt, 2010). One identified compound, NSC13728, which is an effective stabilizer of Max–Max, strongly interferes with Myc-mediated oncogenic transformation in cell culture while not affecting transformation induced by Jun, Src, or PI3K. Transcriptional activity of Myc was also inhibited. Although virtual ligand screening suggests a binding site for this stabilizer, that site has not been experimentally verified.

3.3.3 Development of MycN inhibitors using cell-based screening

Although targeting MycN has been successfully achieved in the laboratory setting using RNA interference technologies, this approach suffers from the lack of an efficient *in vivo* delivery method. The development of small molecule inhibitors to MycN is needed and in this regard, Lu and colleagues have identified five potential MycN inhibitors in a pilot screen of 2800 compounds from the Cancer Research-UK collection (Lu, Pearson et al., 2003). To make this readout system, neuroblastoma cells were stably transfected with a luciferase gene construct under control of the *ornithine decarboxylase* 1 (*ODC1*) gene promoter. Resulting compounds are subject to further characterization. Similarly to this approach, we have created a cell-based MycN readout system (SHR6-17). This cell line was derived from human neuroblastoma SH-EP cells by stable transfection of a luciferase reporter gene under the control of a minimal heat shock protein promoter that contained 6 copies of the E-box sequence for MYC-specific transactivation. Because the SHR6-17 cells express low Myc proteins, the basal reporter activity is low. However, transduction with *MYCN* lentivirus resulted in the controlled induction of luciferase reporter activity (~5-10 fold). A small molecule library containing 34,000 individual compounds was used for primary screening and a number of promising compounds have been identified.

3.4 Targeting MycN upstream pathways

Available evidence suggests that targeting upstream pathways of MycN may also be an efficacious strategy for neuroblastoma therapy. This idea comes from studies showing that active Ras oncoprotein is needed to block MycN degradation, promoting cooperative Ras and MycN-dependent cell cycle progression in LAN-1 cells (Yaari, Jacob-Hirsch et al., 2005). Mutations in the *RAS* genes have rarely been found in neuroblastomas. Treating the *MYCN*-amplified neuroblastoma cell line LAN1 with the Ras inhibitor, farnesylthiosalicylic acid, or a dominant-negative Ras, led to growth inhibition and a decrease in MycN levels. The growth inhibition is attributed to attenuation of the Raf-MEK-ERK and phosphoinositide 3-kinase-Akt-glycogen synthase-3 (GSK-3) pathways, reduction in cyclin D1, phospho-retinoblastoma, and E2F, and an increase in p27Kip1 and retinoblastoma-binding protein-1. The down-regulation of MycN protein resulted from blocking of Akt-mediated inactivation of GSK-3, leading to GSK-3-dependent phosphorylation with consequent proteosomal degradation of MycN. More recent studies have confirmed that MycN phosphorylation and stability are controlled by the PI3K/Akt/mTOR pathway in neuroblastoma cells, and that activation of Akt predicts poor outcome in neuroblastoma patients (Fulda, 2009). Taken together, these data suggest that targeting pathways upstream of MycN may be a feasible strategy for MycN targeted therapy in neuroblastoma.

3.5 Targeting MYCN downstream pathways

Several potential downstream target genes of MycN have been identified as a result of expression profiling studies in neuroblastoma cell lines and tumours. Some of these genes have been confirmed to be direct or indirect transcriptional targets of MycN and their therapeutic potential has been confirmed (Bell, Chen et al.2010; Gustafson & Weiss, 2010). Representative genes include *ODC1, MDM2, Aurora Kinase A, DKK3* and *SKP2*, and for each of them, small molecule inhibitors are available or under development. Inhibition of Odc1, Mdm2 and Aurora Kinase A in neuroblastoma will be reviewed below.

Apart from the above MycN downstream genes, we are particularly interested in another Myc-regulated gene *MRP4/ABCC4. MRP4/ABCC4* is a known c-Myc target gene found in Burkitt's lymphoma cells (Li, Van Calcar et al., 2003) and we have recently provided direct evidence that it is also a MycN target gene (Porro, Haber et al., 2010). In addition to *MRP1/ABCC1, MRP4/ABCC4* is also a powerful independent predictor of neuroblastoma outcome (Norris, Smith et al., 2005). While this study demonstrated that high levels of *MRP4* could protect neuroblastoma cells from the chemotherapeutic drug irinotecan *in vitro*, the patients in the study received neither irinotecan, nor any other drugs known to be ABCC4 substrates, suggesting that the prognostic significance of this gene could also not be explained in terms of MRP4-mediated cytotoxic drug resistance. We are currently investigating in more detail precisely how MRP4 contributes to highly malignant neuroblastoma using a range of experimental approaches. In particularly, we have provided strong evidence using siRNA-mediated silencing of MRP4 that this transporter contributes to neuroblastoma biology independently of its role in chemotherapeutic drug efflux (Henderson, Haber et al., 2011). This finding suggests that therapeutic targeting of MRP4 has potential clinical utility for this disease, as well as for other cancers expressing high MRP4 levels. Therefore we are using high-throughput screening of chemical libraries to generate novel inhibitors of MRP4. Several MRP4 small molecule inhibitor "hits" have been identified by screening a 30,000 compound library, and further characterization of these compounds is underway.

4. MRP1/ABCC1 targeted inhibition

4.1 Rationale for targeting MRP1

Intrinsic or acquired multidrug resistance (MDR) is one of the major causes of treatment failure in human malignancy, including childhood neuroblastoma (Maris & Matthay, 1999). In the laboratory, MDR mediated by multidrug transporters, such as P-glycoprotein and MRP1, results in resistance to a broad spectrum of structurally unrelated drugs. Amongst these transporters, there is strong evidence demonstrating the clinical relevance of MRP1 in aggressive childhood neuroblastoma. MRP1 is encoded by the *ABCC1* gene (ATP-binding cassette, sub- family C member 1) and acts as an ATP-dependent efflux pump for the transport of organic anions, glutathione-, glucuronate- or sulfate-conjugated drugs, or unconjugated drugs in concert with free glutathione (Hipfner, Deeley et al., 1999; Borst, Evers et al., 2000), including the chemotherapeutic agents vincristine, doxorubicin and etoposide. The down-regulation of MRP1 activity in neuroblastoma cells by antisense mRNA (Kuss, Corbo et al., 2002) or by treatment with MRP1 reversal agents (Norris, Gilbert et al., 2001) results in increased sensitivity to cytotoxic drugs. More importantly, high *MRP1* expression in primary neuroblastoma at diagnosis is strongly associated with poor patient outcome (Norris, Bordow et al., 1996; Haber, Smith et al., 2006). To determine the overall contribution of MRP1 to drug resistance in neuroblastoma, we crossed mice lacking the *MRP1* gene (*MRP1*$^{-/-}$) with human *hMYCN* transgenic mice, which develop neuroblastoma characteristic of the human disease. This cross yielded murine neuroblastoma tumours that were either wild-type (*MRP1*$^{+/+}$) or homozygous null (*MRP1*$^{-/-}$) for *MRP1*. Tumour cells of either *MRP1* genotype were isolated and xenografted into nude mice and these mice were treated with clinically used drugs and monitored for tumour growth (Burkhart, Watt et al., 2009). Results showed that loss of MRP1 significantly increased the latency of tumour progression in response to vincristine and etoposide, both of which are known MRP1 substrates. In contrast, the lack of MRP1 had no effect on the efficacy of cisplatin or cyclophosphamide, which are not substrates for MRP1 (Burkhart, Watt et al., 2009). These data suggest that MRP1 is a major determinant of the response of neuroblastoma tumours to chemotherapy, further supporting the development of MRP1 small molecule inhibitors. Although a number of MRP1 inhibitors have been identified, the number of compounds close to or entered into clinical trials is limited (e.g. sulindac (O'Connor, O'Leary et al., 2007)).

4.2 Reversan modulates MRP1 function *in vitro*

Through our screening efforts (Burkhart, Watt et al., 2009), we have identified 6 structural scaffolds that can effectively inhibit MRP1 function with the most active compounds clustered within the pyrazolopyrimidine scaffold. Reversan, one of the most potent pyrazolopyrimidines identified to date, sensitized MRP1 overexpressing breast cancer cells (MCF7/VP) to a panel of drugs including vincristine (14.6 fold), etoposide (11.6 fold) and doxorubicin (3.8 fold), all of which are MRP1 substrates. In contrast, it did not increase sensitivity to two non-MRP1 substrates cisplatin and paclitaxel. The selectivity of Reversan for MRP1 in terms of modulating drug response was further examined by studying its effects on cell lines overexpressing one of several other multidrug transporters, including P-glycoprotein, MRP2, MRP3, MRP4, or MRP5. Reversan did not sensitize MRP2, MRP3, MRP4 or MRP5 overexpressing cell lines to known substrates of each of these transporters, namely vincristine (MRP2), etoposide (MRP3) or 6-mercaptopurine (MRP4 and MRP5). In contrast, this modulator significantly sensitized P-glycoprotein overexpressing neuroblastoma cells (BECHCb (Borst, Evers et al., 2000)) to vincristine, indicating that Reversan is not totally MRP1 specific.

In addition, effects of Reversan on cytotoxic drug response were examined in human neuroblastoma (BE(2)-C), renal cell carcinoma (SK-RC45) and colon (HCT116) tumour cell lines, which represent tumour types that are clinically refractory to cytotoxic drug treatment as well containing high levels of MRP1 protein. Reversan caused increased sensitivity of these cell lines to one or more cytotoxic drugs with the most dramatic effect observed in combination with vincristine (Burkhart, Watt et al., 2009). Furthermore, when compared to a panel of known drug transporter inhibitors, including verapamil, cyclosporin A, difloxacin, probenecid and PAK104P, for the effects on etoposide sensitivity of MCF7/VP cells, Reversan increased the sensitivity of MCF7/VP cells to etoposide to a level similar to the most potent of these modulators, PAK104P (25-fold). More importantly, Reversan was 6–8 times more potent than the rest of the panel of modulators, including the Phase I clinical trial drug, probenecid (Burkhart, Watt et al., 2009).

4.3 *In vivo* efficacy and toxicity of Reversan

The toxicity of Reversan has been tested in BALB/c mice and has been found to be safe and well tolerated (Burkhart, Watt et al., 2009). Furthermore, when used in combination with either vincristine or etoposide to treat neuroblastoma-prone *hMYCN* transgenic mice, 10 mg/kg Reversan increased tumour sensitivity to these conventional drugs with no increased toxicity. The combination of Reversan with vincristine or etoposide significantly increased the survival time of mice compared to those treated with drug alone. While treatment with vincristine alone increased survival of tumour bearing *hMYCN* mice by approximately 10 days, the addition of Reversan to the vincristine treatment regimen increased survival by an additional 20 days (survival: 4.9 ± 0.49 days saline control, 16.2 ± 0.89 days vincristine alone, 36.5 ± 4.4 days vincristine plus Reversan). For treatment with etoposide alone, the duration of survival of tumour bearing *hMYCN* mice doubled compared to vehicle control and tripled when co-administered with Reversan (survival: 4.9 ± 0.49 days saline control, 11 ± 0.67 days etoposide alone, 16 ± 0.56 days etoposide plus Reversan). The combination of Reversan and cyclophosphamide, which is not an MRP1 substrate, had no effect on the duration of time between treatment and progression compared to cyclophosphamide alone. In addition, Reversan also significantly increased the efficacy of vincristine and etoposide against BE(2)-C human neuroblastoma xenografts. It should also be noted that oral administration of Reversan worked equally as well as ip administration for increasing the efficacy of etoposide administered to tumour-bearing *hMYCN* mice (Burkhart, Watt et al., 2009).

Past attempts at modulating MDR have failed mainly due to nonspecific side effects that became apparent when modulators have been combined with conventional drugs (Szakacs, Paterson et al., 2006). We found that Reversan did not significantly alter the toxicity profile of vincristine in BALB/c mice when treated with vincristine in the clinically relevant range for this drug (DeVita, Hellman et al., 1993) in the presence or absence of 10 mg/kg Reversan (Burkhart, Watt et al., 2009). In contrast, vincristine administered in combination with 10 mg/kg cyclosporin A, a first generation multidrug transporter inhibitor that underwent clinical trials in the 1990's, resulted in rapid weight loss and a dramatic shift in the toxicity profile of vincristine. Neither Reversan nor cyclosporin A were toxic when administered as individual drugs. Importantly, there was no toxicity associated with Reversan at clinically relevant doses of vincristine. Similar results for Reversan were obtained for both males and females in a second mouse strain, ICR, which demonstrates that lack of toxicity was not a gender-specific or strain-specific artefact. In addition, we tested BE(2)-C xenograft-bearing nude mice for signs of hematopoietic toxicity following treatment with etoposide alone or in combination with Reversan on Day 15. There was no effect of Reversan on the number of lymphocytes, monocytes, eosinophils, or basophils. In contrast, there was a significant increase (~2 fold, P=0.027) in the number of neutrophils in mice treated with the drug combination compared to mice treated with etoposide alone. Thus, Reversan did not enhance etoposide-induced neutropenia but rather appeared to have a protective effect on the neutrophil population. There was no significant effect of the etoposide/Reversan combination on the platelet population (Burkhart, Watt et al., 2009). Therefore, we have identified a safe small molecule inhibitor of MRP1 that may have clinical potential in the treatment of neuroblastoma and other cancers that overexpress MRP1.

4.4 Mechanism of action and novelty of Reversan

Classical inhibitors of multidrug transporters are substrates of these pumps themselves, reversing resistance by competitive inhibition. Such inhibitors compete with the conventional drugs for metabolism as well as for efflux (Schuetz, Schinkel et al., 1996; Wandel, Kim et al., 1999). Many of the first and second generation P-glycoprotein inhibitors were such classical inhibitors and it is believed that this mechanism of action contributed to their failures (Thomas & Coley 2003). Currently, third generation P-glycoprotein inhibitors (e.g. tariquidar and zosuquidar) have reached various stages of clinical investigation (Thomas & Coley, 2003). These molecules are potent, highly specific Pgp inhibitors that are not themselves substrates of this transporter (Dantzig, Shepard et al., 1999; Roe, Folkes et al., 1999; Mistry, Stewart et al., 2001). Although, early clinical trials demonstrated that tariquidar could reverse drug efflux in patients (Stewart, Steiner et al., 2000; Agrawal, Abraham et al., 2003) and be co-administered with paclitaxel, vinorelbine or doxorubicin without the need for dose reduction of the chemotherapeutic agents (Thomas & Coley 2003). More recent clinical trials have failed to live up to the early promise and have delivered disappointing results (Pusztai L, 2005; Cripe, Uno et al., 2010; Libby & Hromas, 2010). However, in terms of MRP1, we have recently shown that this transporter has a more fundamental role in neuroblastoma, than that of simply effluxing cytotoxic drugs. Thus, using genetic and pharmacologic inhibition, we have provided the first direct evidence that MRP1 can contribute to neuroblastoma biology independently of chemotherapeutic drug efflux, thereby enhancing its potential as a target for therapeutic intervention (Henderson, Haber et al., 2011). Importantly, in this study, treatment of neuroblastoma-prone *hMYCN* transgenic mice with Reversan in the absence of chemotherapeutic agents, led to a significant delay in tumour progression

Although available evidence indicates that Reversan is not a substrate for MRP1, its exact mechanism of action as well as related pyrazolopyrimidines is currently unknown. Since the original P-glycoprotein modulators that were used to generate libraries in which Reversan was discovered, were found not to be ATPase inhibitors (Kondratov, Komarov et al., 2001), it is likely that the pyrazolopyrimidines are also not inhibitors of ATPase but this remains to be tested. It is possible that Reversan does not interact directly with MRP1 or P-glycoprotein but rather alters the physicochemical properties of the membrane surrounding the transporter, which could then alter the structure of the protein(s) within the membrane and affect its ability to transport. Indeed, it appears that the hydrophobic nature of Reversan and the other similarly active pyrazolopyrimidines may be important for their potency since more hydrophilic pyrazolopyrimidine analogs were found to be less effective in reversing drug resistance (Burkhart, Watt et al., 2009).

While some critics of this field have suggested that inhibitors of multidrug transporters should be specific for individual transporters, or toxicity could be increased due to off-target effects, the results of our own study suggest that this is not the case for Reversan. Despite the fact that Reversan inhibits the function of both MRP1 and P-glycoprotein equally well, it does not significantly alter the toxicity profile of conventional chemotherapeutic agents *in vivo* in contrast to cyclosporin A, which exemplifies the earlier generation of toxic multidrug transporter modulators. It is possible that the problem of off-target toxicities is not related to interactions with other transporters but more related to interplay between P-glycoprotein and CYP3A4 in terms of shared substrates (Schuetz, Schinkel et al., 1996; Wandel, B. Kim et al., 1999). The increase in the effectiveness of conventional chemotherapeutic agents observed with Reversan, as well as the ability of Reversan to inhibit neuroblastoma tumorigenesis in the absence of any antineoplastic agents, highlights the potential use of this compound in the clinical setting. In addition, Reversan has an excellent therapeutic index compared to multidrug inhibitors of the past. Therefore, it appears that Reversan represents a new class of "safe" multidrug transporter inhibitor that may be clinically useful in the treatment of neuroblastoma and other cancers associated with aberrant MRP1/P-glycoprotein expression.

5. Polyamine targeted inhibition - targeting Odc1

Amplification of the *MYCN* oncogene is one of the most powerful predictors of poor clinical outcome in this disease. Although the mechanism by which *MYCN* amplification influences the prognosis of neuroblastoma remain largely unknown, it is widely accepted that identification of the requisite biopathways downstream of this oncogene may provide therapeutic opportunities. This concept has been evidenced by recent success in the treatment of neuroblastoma tumours of *hMYCN*-transgenic mice by targeting the polyamine biosynthesis enzyme ODC1 (Hogarty, Norris et al., 2008; Rounbehler, Li et al., 2009).

It has been shown that *MYCN*-amplified neuroblastomas have co-ordinately deregulated a range of polyamine enzymes (including Odc1, Srm, Sms, Amd1, Oaz2, and Smox) to enhance polyamine biosynthesis (Evageliou & Hogarty, 2009). Polyamines are organic cations that enhance transcription, translation, and replication (Pegg, Secrist et al., 1988) and support many cellular processes governed by *MYC* genes. Their maintenance is essential for cell survival as depletion activates growth arrest or apoptotic checkpoints (Bettuzzi, Davalli et al., 1999). Thus, intracellular polyamines are kept under tight control through posttranscriptional as well as transcriptional regulation, with the rate-limiting enzymes Odc1 and Amd1 having among the shortest half-lives of any mammalian enzyme as a result (Shirahata & Pegg, 1985). Odc1 activity is frequently elevated in cancer through deregulation of *MYC*, resulting in higher polyamine content to support rapid tumour cell proliferation (Pegg, Secrist et al., 1988). Overexpression of *ODC1* has been observed in a range of tumour cells, including neuroblastoma, and a number of studies have provided evidence for the oncogenic and transforming abilities of this protein (Gerner & Meyskens, 2004).

We have investigated the role of *ODC1* in neuroblastoma both in tumour samples and in preclinical models of this disease. In a large cohort of primary untreated neuroblastomas, we found that high levels of *ODC1* expression were strongly predictive of both event-free-survival and overall survival (Hogarty, Norris et al., 2008). These data suggest that inhibiting Odc1 activity should have a therapeutic advantage in treating neuroblastoma. To determine the effects of disabling Odc1 on both tumour initiation and progression, we treated neuroblastoma-prone h*MYCN* mice with α-difluoromethylornithine (DFMO), a known Odc1 inhibitor. DFMO treatment extended tumour latency and survival in homozygous mice and prevented oncogenesis in hemizygous mice. In the latter, transient Odc1 ablation permanently prevented tumour onset consistent with a time-limited window for embryonal tumour initiation. Similarly, an independent study showed DFMO treatment, but not Odc1 heterozygosity, impaired MycN-induced neuroblastoma in h*MYCN* mice (Rounbehler, Li et al., 2009). More importantly, our study demonstrated that combining DFMO with cisplatin, either concomitantly or afterward, prolonged tumour-free survival in these mice, compared with cisplatin alone. Similar results were seen when cyclophosphamide was combined with DFMO. There was no overt toxicity that could be attributed to DFMO in the treated mice (Hogarty, Norris et al., 2008). These data implicate polyamine biosynthesis as an arbiter of MycN oncogenesis and showed initial efficacy for polyamine depletion strategies in neuroblastoma. DFMO is considered a very promising drug due to its high specificity, low toxicity and water-soluble properties allowing oral administration. It is currently undergoing Phase I clinical trial for testing its safety for refractory or relapsed neuroblastoma as there are limited data on its use in paediatric patients.

6. Targeting the p53 pathway

6.1 p53 pathway in neuroblastoma

p53 has been regarded as "the guardian of the genome" for it is a key mediator of cell response to a variety of stresses, inducing growth arrest or apoptosis, thereby eliminating damaged and potentially dangerous cells from the organism (Prives, 1999). This tumour suppressor is mutated in approximately 50% of human malignancies and is functionally inactivated in the majority of cancers that retain wild-type p53 by other members of the pathway (Arf) (Sherr, 1998), or by negative p53 regulators of cellular (Mdm2) (Momand, Jung et al., 1998) or viral origin (E6 of human papillomavirus) (Thomas, Pim et al., 1999). Loss of p53 provides tumour cells with a series of important selective advantages, including high tolerance to growth arrest and death-inducing stimuli and genomic instability that promotes tumour progression by rapid acquisition of mutations (Levine, 1997).

In contrast to adult cancer, *p53* mutations are infrequent (2%) in neuroblastomas. However, Most of the few p53 mutations in neuroblastoma tumours reported are in relapsed or progressive tumours (Tweddle, Malcolm et al., 2001). Similarly, the majority of neuroblastoma cell lines with p53 mutations reported have been established from relapsed or progressive tumours, and in most cases the cell lines are more chemoresistant than wild-type cell lines (Tweddle, Pearson et al., 2003). Recently, a higher incidence of p53 mutations was found in a study on 84 neuroblastomas from 41 patients with relapsed disease, including 38 paired neuroblastomas at different stages of therapy. Inactivating missense p53 mutations were identified in 6/41 (15%) cases, 5 following chemotherapy and/or at relapse and only 1 at both diagnosis and relapse (Carr-Wilkinson, O'Toole et al., 2010). Studies on neuroblastoma cell lines demonstrated that loss of p53 function due to mutations of *p53* gene or gene silencing by p53 shRNA can confer multidrug resistance to neuroblastoma cells (Keshelava, Zuo et al., 2000; Keshelava, Zuo et al., 2001; Xue, Haber et al., 2007). These findings highlight the role of p53 inactivation in tumour progression in some high-risk neuroblastoma patients.

In the majority of neuroblastoma tumours maintaining wild-type *p53* gene, an increasing amount of data shows that the p53 pathway may not be functional due to non-mutational mechanisms. For example, a high incidence of abnormalities in the p53/MDM2/$p14^{ARF}$ pathway was found in human neuroblastoma cell lines established at relapse (53%) (Carr, Bell et al., 2006) and patient samples at relapse (49%) (Carr-Wilkinson, O'Toole et al., 2010). MDM2, the essential negative regulator of p53, is transcriptionally regulated by the *MYCN* oncogene in neuroblastoma (Slack, Chen et al., 2005). Targeted inhibition of MycN leads to reduced Mdm2 expression levels, with concomitant stabilization of p53 protein and stimulation of apoptosis in *MYCN* amplified neuroblastoma cell lines. These data suggest that Mdm2 is a key player in MycN-mediated suppression of p53. This notion was supported by a later study involving crossing the h*MYCN* transgenic model of neuroblastoma and the Mdm2 haploinsufficient mouse model (Chen, Barbieri et al., 2009). The $Mdm2^{+/-}MYCN^{+/+}$ transgenics showed marked delay in tumour development and a lower overall tumour incidence compared to $Mdm2^{+/+}MYCN^{+/+}$ genotype, strongly implicating Mdm2-mediated blockade of p53 as an essential step in the pathogenesis of neuroblastoma. Recently, a miRNA (miR-380-5p), has been identified that represses *p53* expression via a conserved sequence in the *p53* 3' untranslated region (Swarbrick, Woods et al., 2010). This miRNA is highly expressed in mouse embryonic stem cells and neuroblastomas, and its expression correlates with poor outcome in *MYCN*-amplified neuroblastoma. *In vivo* delivery of a miR-380-5p antagonist led to a decrease in tumour size in an orthotopic mouse model of neuroblastoma. This new mechanism of p53 deregulation has uncovered a potential novel therapeutic target for neuroblastoma treatment.

6.2 Small molecule approaches to p53 modulators

Frequent inactivation of p53 in cancer and high sensitivity of tumour cells to p53 suggest that the most straightforward p53-based therapeutic approach to cancer treatment involves restoration or imitation of p53 function in p53-deficient tumours, resulting either in a direct (tumour growth inhibition) or indirect (sensitization to treatment) therapeutic benefit. So far the majority of research efforts have been applied to restoration of p53 function in tumours. However, the development of p53-targeting therapeutic approaches also takes advantage of the fact that this important signalling pathway is relatively well studied, making it possible to develop tools affecting individual components or interactors within the pathway. p53 function is inactivated in tumours either by mutations or deletions within the *p53* gene itself, by viral p53-inactivating proteins (i.e., E6 of papilloma virus), or through deregulation of other members of the pathway such as inactivation of positive (Arf) and overexpression of negative (Mdm2) regulators. Thus, modulation of p53 pathway activity may target any of the above factors. This general strategy is being extensively explored through a variety of approaches (reviewed in (Gudkov & Komarova, 2007; Lane, Cheok et al., 2010; Cheok, Verma et al., 2011)).

6.2.1 Mutant p53 as a target for inhibition

The transcriptional regulatory and tumour suppressor activity of p53 is dependent on the ability of the protein to maintain DNA binding conformation. Human p53 protein containing the most common mutations cannot bind significantly to the DNA-binding sequence of p53-responsive genes (Kern, Kinzler et al., 1991). Normal activity of mutant p53 might be restored, at least in part, by application of antibodies and peptides to a negative regulatory domain at the p53 COOH-terminus (Hupp, Sparks et al., 1995; Selivanova, Ryabchenko et al., 1999). Alternatively, restoration of p53 activity might be realized by stabilizing the active conformation of the DNA-binding domain by chemicals. This idea was confirmed by Foster and colleagues (Foster, Coffey et al., 1999). A chemical library (100,000 compounds) was screened in the study and active chemicals, which promoted conformational stability of wild type p53 as judged by binding with mutant-specific antibodies, were found. These compounds were also effective *in vivo* by slowing tumour growth in mice. A number of small molecules with the potential to reactivate mutant p53 are currently under preclinical development (including CP-31398, MIRA-1 and STIMA-1) or Phase I/II clinical trial in patients with haematologic and prostate neoplasms (PRIMA-1MET/APR-246) (reviewed in (Cheok, Verma et al., 2011)). Recently, more novel p53 activating small-molecule compounds have been identified in cell-based screening. Six lead compounds (BMH-7, BMH-9, BMH-15, BMH-21, BMH-22, and BMH-23) were able to activate p53 and repress the growth of human cancer cells. Two tested compounds suppressed *in vivo* tumour growth in an orthotopic mouse model of human B-cell lymphoma. All compounds interacted with DNA, and two activated the p53 pathway in a DNA damage signaling-dependent manner (Peltonen, Colis et al., 2010).

6.2.2 p53 regulatory proteins as targets

In addition to p53, other members of the p53 pathway (i.e., Mdm2, E6, Arf) make attractive targets for screening purposes. The development of small-peptide effectors that can inhibit Mdm2 binding to p53 protein provides a potential drug target for reactivating the p53 pathway in cancers overexpressing Mdm2 (Böttger, Böttger et al., 1997). Similar inhibition of Jnk binding to p53 by small peptides derived from Jnk/p53 interface can also reduce Jnk-dependent ubiquitination and degradation of p53 (Fuchs, Adler et al., 1998). p14Arf blocks the degradation of p53 by MDM2 through the inhibition of its ubiquitin ligase-associated function (Lowe, 1999). The use of small peptides derived from p14Arf, which map at the p14Arf /Mdm2 interface, can activate p53, providing an additional target for modulating the Mdm2-degradation pathway (Midgley, Desterro et al., 2000). A number of small molecules that indirectly activate the p53 response have also reached clinic trial, of which the most advanced are the p53/Mdm2 interaction inhibitors (Nutlin, MI-219/AT-219, RITA, JNJ-26854165; PXN727 and PXN822) (Cheok, Verma et al., 2011).

Nutlins are cis-imidazoline analogs that inhibit the interaction between Mdm2 and p53, and were discovered by screening a chemical library by Vassiliev and colleagues (Vassilev, Vu et al., 2004). Nutlin-1, Nutlin-2 and Nutlin-3 were all identified in the same screening, of which, Nutlin-3 is the one most well studied. Crystallization data have shown that nutlin-3 mimics the three residues of the helical region of the transactivation domain of p53 (Phe19, Trp23 and Leu26) that are conserved across species and critical for binding to Mdm2. Thus, Nutlin-3 displaces p53 by competing for binding to Mdm2.

The effects of Nutlin-3 on p53 reactivation have been extensively studied in a wide range of cancer cell lines and animals, including neuroblastoma (reviewed in (Shangary & Wang 2009)). For example, Nutlin-3 induces cell cycle arrest in both cancer and normal cells, but selective cell death in cancer cells of different origins. *Ex vivo* experiments using AML, B-CLL and multiple myeloma patient specimens have shown that inhibition of Mdm2 by Nutlin-3 effectively triggers apoptosis. Nutlin-3 synergizes with doxorubicin and cytosine arabinoside in killing myeloblasts in AML and with doxorubicin, chlorambucil, and fludarabine in killing leukemic cells in B-CLL patient specimens. Importantly, both the single agent and the combination effect of Nutlin-3 are selective for cancer versus normal cells. In neuroblastoma cell lines with wild type p53, targeted disruption of the p53-Mdm2 interaction by nutlin-3 stabilizes p53 and selectively activates the p53 pathway, resulting in a pronounced antiproliferative and cytotoxic effect regardless of the *MYCN* amplification status (Van Maerken, Speleman et al., 2006). Furthermore, oral administration of nutlin-3 to mice bearing xenografts of chemoresistant neuroblastoma cells with wild type p53, resulted in inhibition of tumour growth and reduction in metastatic disease (Van Maerken, Ferdinande et al., 2009). Thus, targeting p53/Mdm2 by nutlin-3 or other Mdm2 antagonists may be a viable treatment option for neuroblastoma patients with wild type p53, perhaps particularly for high-risk *MYCN*-amplified disease, since a recent study demonstrated that overexpression of MycN sensitizes neuroblastoma cell lines with wild type p53 to Mdm2/p53 antagonists (Gamble, Kees et al., 2011). To date, the most promising small molecule Mdm2 modulators are still in preclinical development or early stage clinical trial.

7. Targeting kinases and the kinase pathway in neuroblastoma

Deregulation of kinase activity is one of the major mechanisms by which tumour cells evade normal physiological constraints on proliferation. One of the advantages of targeting kinases is that inhibition of kinase activity in normal cells can often be tolerated, which favours selective killing of cancer cells. Small-molecule kinase inhibitors have been intensively pursued as new anticancer therapeutics for many years, with approximately 30 distinct kinase targets having been identified. The vast majority of these inhibitors are being investigated for the treatment of cancer (reviewed in (Zhang, Yang et al., 2009)).

7.1 ALK targeted inhibition

Anaplastic lymphoma kinase (ALK), also known as ALK tyrosine kinase receptor or CD246, is an enzyme that in humans is encoded by the *ALK* gene. ALK plays an important role in the development of the brain and exerts its effects on specific neurons in the nervous system. Recent studies have shown that heritable mutations of *ALK* are a major cause of familial neuroblastoma, and that germline or acquired activation of this cell surface kinase is a tractable therapeutic target for this lethal paediatric malignancy (Mosse, Laudenslager et al., 2008). Specific and potent ALK inhibitors have been discovered and described in the literature. One of the promising ALK inhibitor, PF-2341066 (Pfizer), is currently in clinical development both for c-Met and ALK driven cancer indications (Ardini, Magnaghi et al., 2010).

7.2 Trk targeted inhibition

Trk (Tropomyosin receptor kinase) receptors are a family of tyrosine kinases that regulate synaptic strength and plasticity in the mammalian nervous system. Among the three Trk receptors (A, B and C), TrkB is preferentially expressed in aggressive neuroblastoma tumours and the BDNF/TrkB signaling pathway has been shown to form an autocrine loop in these tumours (Schramm, Schulte et al., 2005). TrKB mediates chemoresistance in neuroblastoma by activation of PI3/AKT survival pathway (Ho, Eggert et al., 2002). Given the apparent roles of *Trk* genes in the biological and clinical behaviour of neuroblastomas, inhibiting Trk receptors may be an important adjunct to therapy. Lestaurtinib (CEP-701) is a Trk-selective tyrosine kinase inhibitor that blocks Trk activation by its ligand. It has been shown that precursor compounds to Lestaurtinib have efficacy in treating neuroblastomas in preclinical xenograft models. Lestaurtinib is currently in a phase I clinical trial in neuroblastoma patients. It is presumed that this agent, by blocking an important survival pathway, will render tumour cells more susceptible to cytotoxic drugs, as suggested by preclinical studies (Brodeur, Minturn et al., 2009).

7.3 PLK1 targeted inhibition

The Polo-like kinase 1 (PLK1) is highly expressed in many human cancers and is a target of the novel small-molecule inhibitor BI 2536, which has shown promising anti-cancer activity in adult malignancies. A recent study showed that elevated PLK1 expression is significantly associated with high-risk neuroblastoma and unfavourable prognosis. Inhibition of PLK1 using BI 2536 exhibits strong anti-tumour activity on human neuroblastoma cells *in vitro* and *in vivo* (Ackermann, Goeser et al., 2011). In addition, BI 2536 significantly inhibited tumour growth in a therapeutic xenograft model of tumour initiating cells, both as a single agent and in combination with the therapeutic agent irinotecan (Grinshtein, Datti et al., 2011). BI 2536 has progressed into clinical studies in patients with locally advanced or metastatic cancers in adults.

7.4 Aurora kinase targeted inhibition

Aurora kinases are a family of three highly homologous serine/threonine kinases (Aurora A, B and C) that play a critical role in regulating many of the processes that are pivotal to mitosis. Each isoform has a different function in the control of mitosis. Aurora A, encoded by the *AURKA* gene, appears to be involved in microtubule formation and/or stabilization at the spindle pole during chromosome segregation and has a critical function in regulating turnover of MycN protein. Aurora A interacts with both MycN and the SCFFbxw7 ubiquitin ligase that ubiquitinates MycN and counteracts degradation of this oncoprotein, thereby uncoupling MycN stability from growth factor-dependent signals (Otto, Horn et al., 2009). Overexpression of *AURKA* in neuroblastoma tumours is associated with high risk, late-stage tumours, unfavorable histology, *MYCN* amplification, disease relapse and decreased progression-free survival. knockdown of this gene by siRNA results in growth inhibition and enhanced chemosensitivity in neuroblastoma cell lines. Similarly, treating neuroblastoma cells *in vitro* with MLN8054, a small molecule Aurora A inhibitor, causes dramatic growth inhibition (Shang, Burlingame et al., 2009). Several small molecule Aurora kinase inhibitors have been developed and are currently undergoing preclinical or clinical trials. However, the clinical activity of the aurora kinase inhibitors in patients with solid tumours has been rather disappointing (reviewed in (Gautschi, 2008; Boss, Beijnen et al., 2009)). Currently, a promising Aurora A inhibitor MLN8237 is in phase II clinical trial for treating young patients with recurrent or refractory solid tumours or leukemia (NCT01154816, USA). Future studies with aurora kinase inhibitors should focus on the possibility of combining these agents with radiotherapy, chemotherapy, or other targeted anticancer agents.

7.5 PI3K/Akt/mTOR pathway as therapeutic target

The prognostic value of the phosphatidylinositol 3'-kinase (PI3K)/Akt/mTOR pathway was first investigated through analysis of 116 primary neuroblastoma samples. Akt activation was identified as a novel prognostic indicator of both decreased event-free and overall survival, and this was correlated with a number of well-established prognostic markers, including *MYCN* amplification, 1p36 aberrations, advanced disease stage, age at diagnosis, and unfavourable Histology (Opel, Poremba et al., 2007). *In vitro* studies also demonstrated that activation of Akt by Insulin-like Growth Factor I protected neuroblastoma cells against TRAIL- or cytotoxic drug-induced apoptosis, indicating that activation of this survival cascade can rescue neuroblastoma cells from cell death. In preclinical studies, the bisphosphonate inhibitor of osteoclasts, zoledronic acid, showed anti-neuroblastoma activity in bony metastases by inhibiting osteoclasts and tumour cell proliferation. Its antitumoral activity involves inhibition of the activation of Ras, c-Raf, ERK1/2 and Akt (Peng, Sohara et al., 2007). Inhibitors of PI3-K and mTOR have been shown to be anti-proliferative and pro-apoptotic in neuroblastoma cells *in vitro* and *in vivo* (Chesler, Schlieve et al., 2006; Johnsen, Segerstrom et al., 2007). The importance of the PI3K/Akt pathway in maintaining neuroblastoma cell growth has attracted interest in the design of molecular targeted therapies for this disease (Sartelet, Oligny et al., 2008). Several strategies have been developed to interfere with distinct components of PI3K/Akt/mTOR pathway signalling (LoPiccolo, Blumenthal et al., 2008; Fulda, 2009). To date, few specific inhibitors of AKT have been discovered. The novel Akt inhibitor, Perifosine, has demonstrated both clinical efficacy and safety in several tumour types (LoPiccolo, Blumenthal et al., 2008). It is currently in Phase 1 clinical trial for paediatric tumours, including neuroblastoma. Thus, drugs targeting PI3K/Akt/mTOR pathway may eventually open novel avenues to improve the poor prognosis of patients with advanced stage neuroblastoma.

8. Future perspectives

Recent advancements in targeted therapy for neuroblastoma using small molecule drugs are not limited to the above-mentioned studies. There are a number of other molecular targets and inhibitors that are being intensively investigated in various cancer types, including neuroblastoma. One such example involves inhibitors of histone deacetylases (HDACs), which are currently in early phase clinical trial for neuroblastoma as well as other cancers (Reviewed in (Witt, Deubzer et al., 2009)). We can anticipate that current molecular genetic research in neuroblastoma will enable the identification of more prospective molecular targets that will provide opportunities for the development of new therapeutic strategies. In this regard, new targets that have recently been identified include S-phase kinase-associated protein 2 (SKP2) (Westermann, Henrich et al., 2007), Endosialin (Rouleau, Smale et al., 2011), cycle checkpoint kinase 1 (CHK1) (Cole, Huggins et al., 2011), and c-Met (Crosswell, Dasgupta et al., 2009). By integrating the analysis of MycN binding sites derived from ChIP-chip experiments with mRNA expression microarrays and clinical data, Murphy and colleagues in a recent comprehensive study on the role of MycN in tumorigenesis, have found a large set of clinically relevant cell cycle genes that are critical to neuroblastoma tumorigenesis. Many of these clinically relevant MycN target genes may warrant further functional study as potential neuroblastoma therapeutic targets (Murphy, Buckley et al., 2011).

In recent years, a number of strategies have been developed to identify synthetic lethal interactions between genes for use in anticancer drug discovery, and a few drugs are currently being investigated in preclinical and clinical studies (reviewed in (Chan & Giaccia, 2011)). Synthetic lethality screening involves searching for genetic interactions between two mutations, whereby the presence of either mutation alone has no effect on cell viability, but the combination of the two mutations leads to cell death. The presence of one of these mutations in cancer cells but not in normal cells can therefore create opportunities to selectively kill cancer cells by mimicking the effect of the second genetic mutation with targeted therapy. One such example of this strategy in neuroblastoma involves cyclin dependent kinase 2 (CDK2), which is found to be a synthetically lethal molecule to MycN (Molenaar, Ebus et al., 2009). Inactivation of CDK2 by either siRNA or small molecule drugs induces apoptosis in *MYCN*-amplified neuroblastoma cell lines, but not in *MYCN* single copy cells, and silencing of *MYCN* by siRNA can abrogate this apoptotic response in *MYCN*-amplified cells. Thus, the synthetically lethal relationship between CDK2 and MycN suggests CDK2 is a potential MYCN-selective target in neuroblastoma therapy.

Another research area that warrants exploration for targeted therapy is that aimed at neuroblastoma differentiation. Conventional chemotherapy often results in dramatic reduction in tumour mass after initial treatment, suggesting a strong primary apoptotic response. However, histopathology reveals that, in many cases, neuroblastoma tumours are composed of both pathogenic undifferentiated neuroblasts and neuronal lineage cells at various stages of differentiation. This suggests that neuroblastoma tumours retain the biochemical pathways mediating both programmed cell death as well as multilineage terminal differentiation and this represents the rationale for involvement of differentiating agents such as retinoic acid derivatives in neuroblastoma therapy. Identification of key molecules (apart from MycN) involved in the differentiation of neuroblastoma will be essential for future development of potent differentiating agents.

The rapid screening of collections of compounds for which the majority have already been approved for clinical use as anticancer agents is another area that holds considerable promise for the development compounds with potential therapeutic value in treating paediatric cancers. Virtually all the new anticancer drugs that are currently being tested in clinical trials as targeted therapies, have been developed for specific adult cancers. Given the size of the adult cancer population by comparison with the total number of paediatric cancer patients, the vast majority of these drugs will never be administered to childhood cancer sufferers. However, compound libraries containing marketed drugs are available for purchase and bioavailability and toxicity studies have already been performed for any promising candidates that might be identified. Recently, a number of promising compounds for treatment of children with neuroblastoma were identified using this strategy and further studies are warranted (De Preter, De Brouwer et al., 2009). As previously discussed, the use of DFMO for inhibiting Odc1 in neuroblastoma is a good example of an off patent drug demonstrating renewed clinical promise as both an anticancer drug as well as a cancer chemopreventive agent (Hogarty, Norris et al., 2008; Rounbehler, Li et al., 2009).

In looking towards future clinical application, targeted therapies may be useful in combination with conventional chemotherapeutic agents in order to achieve synergistic effects, or alternatively, the combination of two targeted therapeutics may also prove efficacious. For example, recent studies have shown that DFMO acts synergistically with PI3 kinase inhibitors to increase apoptosis in neuroblastoma cells (Koomoa, Yco et al., 2008). Overall, despite the existing challenges in the discovery of new drugs, an increased understanding of cancer genetics is allowing the development of powerful drug or drug combinations that may increase the selectivity and safety of chemotherapy by selective killing of cancer cells and protecting normal cells. It is hoped that with this increased understanding and the development of new therapeutic strategies, this will ultimately lead to improved outcomes for children with neuroblastoma and other cancers.

9. Acknowledgements

Children's Cancer Institute Australia for Medical Research is affiliated with the University of New South Wales and Sydney Children's Hospital, Randwick, Sydney, Australia. This work was supported by grants from the National Health and Medical Research Council, Australia, and the Cancer Institute New South Wales, Australia.

10. References

Ackermann, S., Goeser, F., Schulte, J. H., Schramm, A., Ehemann, V., Hero, B., Eggert, A., Berthold, F. & Fischer, M. (2011). Polo-Like Kinase 1 Is a Therapeutic Target in High-Risk Neuroblastoma. *Clinical Cancer Research* 17(4): 731-741.

Agrawal, M., Abraham, J., Balis, F. M., Edgerly, M., Stein, W. D., Bates, S., Fojo, T. & Chen, C. C. (2003). Increased 99mtc-Sestamibi Accumulation in Normal Liver and Drug-Resistant Tumors after the Administration of the Glycoprotein Inhibitor, Xr9576. *Clinical Cancer Research* 9(2): 650-656.

Ardini, E., Magnaghi, P., Orsini, P., Galvani, A. & Menichincheri, M. (2010). Anaplastic Lymphoma Kinase: Role in Specific Tumours, and Development of Small Molecule Inhibitors for Cancer Therapy. *Cancer letters* 299(2): 81-94.

Bell, E., Chen, L., Liu, T., Marshall, G. M., Lunec, J. & Tweddle, D. A. (2010) Mycn Oncoprotein Targets and Their Therapeutic Potential. *Cancer letters* 293(2): 144-157.

Berg, T. (2011). Small-Molecule Modulators of C-Myc/Max and Max/Max Interactions *Curr Top Microbiol Immunol* (348): 139-49.

Bettuzzi S, Davalli. P., Astancolle S, Pinna C, Roncaglia R, Boraldi F, Tiozzo R, Sharrard M, Corti A. (1999). Coordinate Changes of Polyamine Metabolism Regulatory Proteins During the Cell Cycle of Normal Human Dermal Fibroblasts. *FEBS Lett* 446(1): 18-22.

Borst, P., Evers, R., Kool, M. & Wijnholds, J. (2000). A Family of Drug Transporters: The Multidrug Resistance-Associated Proteins. *Journal of the National Cancer Institute* 92(16): 1295-1302.

Boss, D. S., Beijnen, J. H. & Schellens, J. H. M. (2009). Clinical Experience with Aurora Kinase Inhibitors: A Review. *The Oncologist* 14(8): 780-793.

Böttger, A., Böttger, V., Garcia-Echeverria, C., Chène, P., Hochkeppel, H.-K., Sampson, W., Ang, K., Howard, S. F., Picksley, S. M. & Lane, D. P. (1997). Molecular Characterization of the Hdm2-P53 Interaction. *Journal of Molecular Biology* 269(5): 744-756.

Brodeur, G. M., Minturn, J. E., Ho, R., Simpson, A. M., Iyer, R., Varela, C. R., Light, J. E., Kolla, V. & Evans, A. E. (2009). Trk Receptor Expression and Inhibition in Neuroblastomas. *Clinical Cancer Research* 15(10): 3244-3250.

Brodeur, G. M., Seeger, R. C., Schwab, M., Varmus, H. E. & Bishop, J. M. (1984). Amplification of N-Myc in Untreated Human Neuroblastomas Correlates with Advanced Disease Stage. *Science* 224(4653): 1121-4.

Burkhart, C. A., Watt, F., Murray, J., Pajic, M., Prokvolit, A., Xue, C., Flemming, C., Smith, J., Purmal, A., Isachenko, N., Komarov, P. G., Gurova, K. V., Sartorelli, A. C., Marshall, G. M., Norris, M. D., Gudkov, A. V. & Haber, M. (2009). Small-Molecule Multidrug Resistance-Associated Protein 1 Inhibitor Reversan Increases the Therapeutic Index of Chemotherapy in Mouse Models of Neuroblastoma. *Cancer Res* 69(16): 6573-80.

Carr-Wilkinson, J., O'Toole, K., Wood, K. M., Challen, C. C., Baker, A. G., Board, J. R., Evans, L., Cole, M., Cheung, N.-K. V., Boos, J., Köhler, G., Leuschner, I., Pearson, A. D. J., Lunec, J. & Tweddle, D. A. (2010). High Frequency of P53/Mdm2/P14arf Pathway Abnormalities in Relapsed Neuroblastoma. *Clinical Cancer Research* 16(4): 1108-1118.

Carr, J., Bell, E., Pearson, A. D. J., Kees, U. R., Beris, H., Lunec, J. & Tweddle, D. A. (2006). Increased Frequency of Aberrations in the P53/Mdm2/P14arf Pathway in Neuroblastoma Cell Lines Established at Relapse. *Cancer Res* 66(4): 2138-2145.

Chan, D. A. & Giaccia, A. J. (2011). Harnessing Synthetic Lethal Interactions in Anticancer Drug Discovery. *Nat Rev Drug Discov* 10(5): 351-364.

Chen Z, L. Y., Barbieri E, Burlingame S, Hicks J, Ludwig A, Shohet JM. (2009). Mdm2 Deficiency Suppresses Mycn-Driven Neuroblastoma Tumorigenesis in Vivo. *Neoplasia.* 11(8): 753-62.

Cheok, C. F., Verma, C. S., Baselga, J. & Lane, D. P. (2011). Translating P53 into the Clinic. *Nat Rev Clin Oncol* 8(1): 25-37.

Chesler, L., Schlieve, C., Goldenberg, D. D., Kenney, A., Kim, G., McMillan, A., Matthay, K. K., Rowitch, D. & Weiss, W. A. (2006). Inhibition of Phosphatidylinositol 3-Kinase Destabilizes Mycn Protein and Blocks Malignant Progression in Neuroblastoma. *Cancer Res* 66(16): 8139-8146.

Cole, K. A., Huggins, J., Laquaglia, M., Hulderman, C. E., Russell, M. R., Bosse, K., Diskin, S. J., Attiyeh, E. F., Sennett, R., Norris, G., Laudenslager, M., Wood, A. C., Mayes, P. A., Jagannathan, J., Winter, C., Mosse, Y. P. & Maris, J. M. (2011). Rnai Screen of the Protein Kinome Identifies Checkpoint Kinase 1 (Chk1) as a Therapeutic Target in Neuroblastoma. *Proceedings of the National Academy of Sciences* 108(8): 3336-3341.

Cripe, L. D., Uno, H., Paietta, E. M., Litzow, M. R., Ketterling, R. P., Bennett, J. M., Rowe, J. M., Lazarus, H. M., Luger, S. & Tallman, M. S. (2010). Zosuquidar, a Novel Modulator of P-Glycoprotein, Does Not Improve the Outcome of Older Patients with Newly Diagnosed Acute Myeloid Leukemia: A Randomized, Placebo-Controlled Trial of the Eastern Cooperative Oncology Group 3999. *Blood* 116(20): 4077-4085.

Crosswell, H., Dasgupta, A., Alvarado, C., Watt, T., Christensen, J., De, P., Durden, D. & Findley, H. (2009). Pha665752, a Small-Molecule Inhibitor of C-Met, Inhibits Hepatocyte Growth Factor-Stimulated Migration and Proliferation of C-Met-Positive Neuroblastoma Cells. *BMC Cancer* 9(1): 411.

Dantzig, A. H., Shepard, R. L., Law, K. L., Tabas, L., Pratt, S., Gillespie, J. S., Binkley, S. N., Kuhfeld, M. T., Starling, J. J. & Wrighton, S. A. (1999). Selectivity of the Multidrug Resistance Modulator, Ly335979, for P-Glycoprotein and Effect on Cytochrome P-450 Activities. *Journal of Pharmacology and Experimental Therapeutics* 290(2): 854-862.

De Preter, K., De Brouwer, S., Van Maerken, T., Pattyn, F., Schramm, A., Eggert, A., Vandesompele, J. & Speleman, F. (2009). Meta-Mining of Neuroblastoma and Neuroblast Gene Expression Profiles Reveals Candidate Therapeutic Compounds. *Clinical Cancer Research* 15(11): 3690-3696.

DeVita VTJ, Hellman. S., Rosenberg SA. (1993). Cancer: Principles and Practice of Oncology. 4. Philadelphia, J.B. Lippincott Co.

Digan, M. E., Pou, C., Niu, H. & Zhang, J.-H. (2005). Evaluation of Division-Arrested Cells for Cell-Based High-Throughput Screening and Profiling. *Journal of Biomolecular Screening* 10(6): 615-623.

Evageliou, N. F. & Hogarty, M. D. (2009). Disrupting Polyamine Homeostasis as a Therapeutic Strategy for Neuroblastoma. *Clinical Cancer Research* 15(19): 5956-5961.

Foster, B.A., Coffey, H.A., Morin, M.J., Rastinejad F. (1999). Pharmacological Rescue of Mutant P53 Conformation and Function. *Science* 286(5449): 2507-10.

Fuchs, S. Y., Adler, V., Buschmann, T., Yin, Z., Wu, X., Jones, S. N. & Ronai, Z. e. (1998). Jnk Targets P53 Ubiquitination and Degradation in Nonstressed Cells. *Genes & Development* 12(17): 2658-2663.

Fulda, S. (2009). The Pi3k/Akt/Mtor Pathway as Therapeutic Target in Neuroblastoma. *Curr Cancer Drug Targets* 9(6): 729-37.

Gamble, L. D., Kees, U. R., Tweddle, D. A. & Lunec, J. (2011). Mycn Sensitizes Neuroblastoma to the Mdm2-P53 Antagonists Nutlin-3 and Mi-63. *Oncogene*.

Gautschi O, H. J., Mack PC, Purnell PR, Lara PN Jr, Gandara DR. (2008). Aurora Kinases as Anticancer Drug Targets. *Clin Cancer Res.* 14(6): 1639-48.

Gerner, E. W. & Meyskens, F. L. (2004). Polyamines and Cancer: Old Molecules, New Understanding. *Nat Rev Cancer* 4(10): 781-792.

Grinshtein, N., Datti, A., Fujitani, M., Uehling, D., Prakesch, M., Isaac, M., Irwin, M. S., Wrana, J. L., Al-awar, R. & Kaplan, D. R. (2011). Small Molecule Kinase Inhibitor Screen Identifies Polo-Like Kinase 1 as a Target for Neuroblastoma Tumor-Initiating Cells. *Cancer Res* 71(4): 1385-1395.

Gudkov, A. & Komarova, E. (2003). Isolation of P53 Inhibitors by Screening Chemical Libraries in Cell-Based Readout System. Methods in Molecular Biology. 223: 635-647.

Gudkov, A. V. & Komarova, E. A. (2007). Dangerous Habits of a Security Guard: The Two Faces of P53 as a Drug Target. *Human Molecular Genetics* 16(R1): R67-R72.

Gustafson, W. C. & Weiss, W. A. (2010). Myc Proteins as Therapeutic Targets. *Oncogene* 29(9): 1249-1259.

Henderson M J., Haber M, Porro A, Munoz M A., Iraci N, Xue C, Murray J, Flemming C L., Smith J, Fletcher J I., Gherardi S, Kwek C, Russell A J, Valli E, London W B., Buxton A B., Ashton L J., Sartorelli A C., Cohn S L., Schwab M, Marshall G M., Perini G & D, N. M. (2011). Abcc Multidrug Transporters in Childhood Neuroblastoma: Influence on Tumor Biology and Clinical Outcome, Independent of Cytotoxic Drug Efflux. *Journal of the National Cancer Institute* 103(16):1236–1251.

Haber, M., Smith, J., Bordow, S. B., Flemming, C., Cohn, S. L., London, W. B., Marshall, G. M. & Norris, M. D. (2006). Association of High-Level Mrp1 Expression with Poor Clinical Outcome in a Large Prospective Study of Primary Neuroblastoma. *J Clin Oncol* 24(10): 1546-53.

Hipfner, D. R., Deeley, R. G. & Cole, S. P. (1999). Structural, Mechanistic and Clinical Aspects of Mrp1. *Biochim Biophys Acta* 1461(2): 359-76.

Ho, R., Eggert, A., Hishiki, T., Minturn, J. E., Ikegaki, N., Foster, P., Camoratto, A. M., Evans, A. E. & Brodeur, G. M. (2002). Resistance to Chemotherapy Mediated by Trkb in Neuroblastomas. *Cancer Res* 62(22): 6462-6466.

Hogarty, M. D., Norris, M. D., Davis, K., Liu, X., Evageliou, N. F., Hayes, C. S., Pawel, B., Guo, R., Zhao, H., Sekyere, E., Keating, J., Thomas, W., Cheng, N. C., Murray, J., Smith, J., Sutton, R., Venn, N., London, W. B., Buxton, A., Gilmour, S. K., Marshall, G. M. & Haber, M. (2008). Odc1 Is a Critical Determinant of Mycn Oncogenesis and a Therapeutic Target in Neuroblastoma. *Cancer Res* 68(23): 9735-9745.

Hupp, T. R., Sparks, A. & Lane, D. P. (1995). Small Peptides Activate the Latent Sequence-Specific DNA Binding Function of P53. *Cell* 83(2): 237-245.

Johnsen, J. I., Segerstrom, L., Orrego, A., Elfman, L., Henriksson, M., Kagedal, B., Eksborg, S., Sveinbjornsson, B. & Kogner, P. (2007). Inhibitors of Mammalian Target of Rapamycin Downregulate Mycn Protein Expression and Inhibit Neuroblastoma Growth in Vitro and in Vivo. *Oncogene* 27(20): 2910-2922.

Kern, S., Kinzler, K., Bruskin, A., Jarosz, D., Friedman, P., Prives, C. & Vogelstein, B. (1991). Identification of P53 as a Sequence-Specific DNA-Binding Protein. *Science* 252(5013): 1708-1711.

Keshelava N , Z. J., Waidyaratne NS, Triche TJ, Reynolds CP. (2000). P53 Mutations and Loss of P53 Function Confer Multidrug Resistance in Neuroblastoma. *Med Pediatr Oncol.* 35(6): 563-8.

Keshelava, N., Zuo, J. J., Chen, P., Waidyaratne, S. N., Luna, M. C., Gomer, C. J., Triche, T. J. & Reynolds, C. P. (2001). Loss of P53 Function Confers High-Level Multidrug Resistance in Neuroblastoma Cell Lines. *Cancer Res* 61(16): 6185-6193.

Komarov, P. G., Komarova, E. A., Kondratov, R. V., Christov-Tselkov, K., Coon, J. S., Chernov, M. V. & Gudkov, A. V. (1999). A Chemical Inhibitor of P53 That Protects Mice from the Side Effects of Cancer Therapy. *Science* 285(5434): 1733-7.

Komarova, E. & Gudkov, A. V. (1998). Could P53 Be a Target for Therapeutic Suppression? *Seminars in Cancer Biology* 8(5): 389-400.

Komarova, E. A., Chernov, M. V., Franks, R., Wang, K., Armin, G., Zelnick, C. R., Chin, D. M., Bacus, S. S., Stark, G. R. & Gudkov, A. V. (1997). Transgenic Mice with P53-Responsive Lacz: P53 Activity Varies Dramatically During Normal Development and Determines Radiation and Drug Sensitivity in Vivo. *EMBO J* 16(6): 1391-1400.

Kondratov, R. V., Komarov, P. G., Becker, Y., Ewenson, A. & Gudkov, A. V. (2001). Small Molecules That Dramatically Alter Multidrug Resistance Phenotype by Modulating the Substrate Specificity of P-Glycoprotein. *Proc Natl Acad Sci U S A* 98(24): 14078-83.

Koomoa, D.-L. T., Yco, L. P., Borsics, T., Wallick, C. J. & Bachmann, A. S. (2008). Ornithine Decarboxylase Inhibition by A-Difluoromethylornithine Activates Opposing Signaling Pathways Via Phosphorylation of Both Akt/Protein Kinase B and P27kip1 in Neuroblastoma. *Cancer Res* 68(23): 9825-9831.

Kuss, B. J., Corbo, M., Lau, W. M., Fennell, D. A., Dean, N. M. & Cotter, F. E. (2002). In Vitro and in Vivo Downregulation of Mrp1 by Antisense Oligonucleotides: A Potential Role in Neuroblastoma Therapy. *Int J Cancer* 98(1): 128-33.

Lane DP, Cheok CF., Lain S. (2010). P53-Based Cancer Therapy. *Cold Spring Harb Perspect Biol.* 2(9): a001222.

Levine, A. J. (1997). P53, the Cellular Gatekeeper for Growth and Division. *Cell* 88(3): 323-331.

Li, Z., Van Calcar, S., Qu, C., Cavenee, W. K., Zhang, M. Q. & Ren, B. (2003). A Global Transcriptional Regulatory Role for C-Myc in Burkitt's Lymphoma Cells. *Proceedings of the National Academy of Sciences* 100(14): 8164-8169.

Libby, E. & Hromas, R. (2010). Dismounting the Mdr Horse. *Blood* 116(20): 4037-4038.

LoPiccolo, J., Blumenthal, G. M., Bernstein, W. B. & Dennis, P. A. (2008). Targeting the Pi3k/Akt/Mtor Pathway: Effective Combinations and Clinical Considerations. *Drug resistance updates : reviews and commentaries in antimicrobial and anticancer chemotherapy* 11(1): 32-50.

Lowe, S. W. (1999). Activation of P53 by Oncogenes. *Endocrine-Related Cancer* 6(1): 45-8.

Lu, X., Pearson, A. & Lunec, J. (2003). The Mycn Oncoprotein as a Drug Development Target. *Cancer letters* 197(1): 125-130.

Malynn, B. A., de Alboran, I. M., O'Hagan, R. C., Bronson, R., Davidson, L., DePinho, R. A. & Alt, F. W. (2000). N-Myc Can Functionally Replace C-Myc in Murine Development, Cellular Growth, and Differentiation. *Genes & Development* 14(11): 1390-1399.

Maris, J. M. & Matthay, K. K. (1999). Molecular Biology of Neuroblastoma. *Journal of Clinical Oncology* 17(7): 2264.

Meyer, N. & Penn, L. Z. (2008). Reflecting on 25 Years with Myc. *Nat Rev Cancer* 8(12): 976-990.

Midgley CA, D. J., Saville MK, Howard S, Sparks A, Hay RT, Lane DP. (2000). An N-Terminal P14arf Peptide Blocks Mdm2-Dependent Ubiquitination in Vitro and Can Activate P53 in Vivo. *Oncogene.* 19(19): 2312-23.

Mistry, P., Stewart, A. J., Dangerfield, W., Okiji, S., Liddle, C., Bootle, D., Plumb, J. A., Templeton, D. & Charlton, P. (2001). In Vitro and in Vivo Reversal of P-Glycoprotein-Mediated Multidrug Resistance by a Novel Potent Modulator, Xr9576. *Cancer Res* 61(2): 749-758.

Molenaar, J. J., Ebus, M. E., Geerts, D., Koster, J., Lamers, F., Valentijn, L. J., Westerhout, E. M., Versteeg, R. & Caron, H. N. (2009). Inactivation of Cdk2 Is Synthetically Lethal to Mycn over-Expressing Cancer Cells. *Proceedings of the National Academy of Sciences* 106(31): 12968-12973.

Momand, J., Jung, D., Wilczynski, S. & Niland, J. (1998). The Mdm2 Gene Amplification Database. *Nucleic Acids Research* 26(15): 3453-3459.

Mosse, Y. P., Laudenslager, M., Longo, L., Cole, K. A., Wood, A., Attiyeh, E. F., Laquaglia, M. J., Sennett, R., Lynch, J. E., Perri, P., Laureys, G., Speleman, F., Kim, C., Hou, C., Hakonarson, H., Torkamani, A., Schork, N. J., Brodeur, G. M., Tonini, G. P., Rappaport, E., Devoto, M. & Maris, J. M. (2008). Identification of Alk as a Major Familial Neuroblastoma Predisposition Gene. *Nature* 455(7215): 930-935.

Murphy D M, Buckley P G, Bryan K, Watters KM, Koster J, van Sluis P, Molenaar J, Versteeg R, Stallings RL. (2011). Dissection of the Oncogenic Mycn Transcriptional Network Reveals a Large Set of Clinically Relevant Cell Cycle Genes as Drivers of Neuroblastoma Tumorigenesis. *Mol Carcinog* 50(6): 403-11.

Norris, M. D., Bordow, S. B., Marshall, G. M., Haber, P. S., Cohn, S. L. & Haber, M. (1996). Expression of the Gene for Multidrug-Resistance–Associated Protein and Outcome in Patients with Neuroblastoma. *New England Journal of Medicine* 334(4): 231-238.

Norris MD, M. J., Gilbert J, Marshall GM, Haber M. (2001). Reversal of Multidrug Resistance-Associated Protein-Mediated Drug Resistance in Cultured Human Neuroblastoma Cells by the Quinolone Antibiotic Difloxacin. *Med Pediatr Oncol* 36(1): 177-80.

Norris, M. D., Smith, J., Tanabe, K., Tobin, P., Flemming, C., Scheffer, G. L., Wielinga, P., Cohn, S. L., London, W. B., Marshall, G. M., Allen, J. D. & Haber, M. (2005). Expression of Multidrug Transporter Mrp4/Abcc4 Is a Marker of Poor Prognosis in Neuroblastoma and Confers Resistance to Irinotecan in Vitro. *Molecular Cancer Therapeutics* 4(4): 547-553.

O'Connor, R., O'Leary, M., Ballot, J., Collins, C. D., Kinsella, P., Mager, D. E., Arnold, R. D., O'Driscoll, L., Larkin, A., Kennedy, S., Fennelly, D., Clynes, M. & Crown, J. (2007). A Phase I Clinical and Pharmacokinetic Study of the Multi-Drug Resistance Protein-1 (Mrp-1) Inhibitor Sulindac, in Combination with Epirubicin in Patients with Advanced Cancer. *Cancer Chemother Pharmacol* 59(1): 79-87.

Oeffinger, K. C., Mertens, A. C., Sklar, C. A., Kawashima, T., Hudson, M. M., Meadows, A. T., Friedman, D. L., Marina, N., Hobbie, W., Kadan-Lottick, N. S., Schwartz, C. L.,

Leisenring, W. & Robison, L. L. (2006). Chronic Health Conditions in Adult Survivors of Childhood Cancer. *New England Journal of Medicine* 355(15): 1572-1582.

Opel, D., Poremba, C., Simon, T., Debatin, K.-M. & Fulda, S. (2007). Activation of Akt Predicts Poor Outcome in Neuroblastoma. *Cancer Res* 67(2): 735-745.

Otto, T., Horn, S., Brockmann, M., Eilers, U., Schüttrumpf, L., Popov, N., Kenney, A. M., Schulte, J. H., Beijersbergen, R., Christiansen, H., Berwanger, B. & Eilers, M. (2009). Stabilization of N-Myc Is a Critical Function of Aurora a in Human Neuroblastoma. *Cancer cell* 15(1): 67-78.

Pegg, A. E., Secrist, J. A. & Madhubala, R. (1988). Properties of L1210 Cells Resistant to A-Difluoromethylornithine. *Cancer Res* 48(10): 2678-2682.

Peltonen K , Colis L., Liu H, Jäämaa S, Moore HM , Enbäck J, Laakkonen P , Vaahtokari A, Jones RJ, af Hällström TM, Laiho M. (2010). Identification of Novel P53 Pathway Activating Small-Molecule Compounds Reveals Unexpected Similarities with Known Therapeutic Agents *PLoS One.* 5(9): e12996.

Peng, H., Sohara, Y., Moats, R. A., Nelson, M. D., Groshen, S. G., Ye, W., Reynolds, C. P. & DeClerck, Y. A. (2007). The Activity of Zoledronic Acid on Neuroblastoma Bone Metastasis Involves Inhibition of Osteoclasts and Tumor Cell Survival and Proliferation. *Cancer Res* 67(19): 9346-9355.

Ponzielli, R., Katz, S., Barsyte-Lovejoy, D. & Penn, L. Z. (2005). Cancer Therapeutics: Targeting the Dark Side of Myc. *European journal of cancer (Oxford, England : 1990)* 41(16): 2485-2501.

Porro, A., Haber, M., Diolaiti, D., Iraci, N., Henderson, M., Gherardi, S., Valli, E., Munoz, M. A., Xue, C., Flemming, C., Schwab, M., Wong, J. H., Marshall, G. M., Della Valle, G., Norris, M. D. & Perini, G. (2010). Direct and Coordinate Regulation of Atp-Binding Cassette Transporter Genes by Myc Factors Generates Specific Transcription Signatures That Significantly Affect the Chemoresistance Phenotype of Cancer Cells. *Journal of Biological Chemistry* 285(25): 19532-19543.

Prives C, H. P. (1999). The P53 Pathway. *J Pathol.* 187((1)): 112-26.

Prochownik, E. V. & Vogt, P. K. (2010). Therapeutic Targeting of Myc. *Genes Cancer* 1(6): 650-659.

Pusztai L, W. P., Ibrahim N, Rivera E, Theriault R, Booser D, Symmans FW, Wong F, Blumenschein G, Fleming DR, Rouzier R, Boniface G, Hortobagyi GN. (2005). Phase Ii Study of Tariquidar, a Selective P-Glycoprotein Inhibitor, in Patients with Chemotherapy-Resistant, Advanced Breast Carcinoma. *Cancer* 104((4)): 682-91.

Roe, M., Folkes, A., Ashworth, P., Brumwell, J., Chima, L., Hunjan, S., Pretswell, I., Dangerfield, W., Ryder, H. & Charlton, P. (1999). Reversal of P-Glycoprotein Mediated Multidrug Resistance by Novel Anthranilamide Derivatives. *Bioorganic & Medicinal Chemistry Letters* 9(4): 595-600.

Rogel, A., Popliker, M., Webb, C. G. & Oren, M. (1985). P53 Cellular Tumor Antigen: Analysis of Mrna Levels in Normal Adult Tissues, Embryos, and Tumors. *Mol. Cell. Biol.* 5(10): 2851-2855.

Rouleau C, S. R., Sancho J, Fu YS, Kurtzberg L, Weber W, Kruger A, Jones C, Roth S, Bormann C, Dunham S, Krumbholz R, Curiel M, Wallar G, Mascarello J, Campos-Rivera J, Horten B, Schmid S, Miller G, Teicher BA. (2011). Endosialin: A Novel

Malignant Cell Therapeutic Target for Neuroblastoma. *Int J Oncol.* doi: 10.3892/ijo.2011.1091. [Epub ahead of print].

Rounbehler, R. J., Li, W., Hall, M. A., Yang, C., Fallahi, M. & Cleveland, J. L. (2009). Targeting Ornithine Decarboxylase Impairs Development of Mycn-Amplified Neuroblastoma. *Cancer Res* 69(2): 547-553.

Sartelet, H., Oligny, L.-L. & Vassal, G. (2008). Akt Pathway in Neuroblastoma and Its Therapeutic Implication. *Expert Review of Anticancer Therapy* 8(5): 757-769.

Schramm, A., Schulte, J. H., Astrahantseff, K., Apostolov, O., Limpt, V. v., Sieverts, H., Kuhfittig-Kulle, S., Pfeiffer, P., Versteeg, R. & Eggert, A. (2005). Biological Effects of Trka and Trkb Receptor Signaling in Neuroblastoma. *Cancer letters* 228(1): 143-153.

Schuetz, E. G., Schinkel, A. H., Relling, M. V. & Schuetz, J. D. (1996). P-Glycoprotein: A Major Determinant of Rifampicin-Inducible Expression of Cytochrome P4503a in Mice and Humans. *Proc Natl Acad Sci U S A* 93(9): 4001-5.

Seeger, R. C., Brodeur, G. M., Sather, H., Dalton, A., Siegel, S. E., Wong, K. Y. & Hammond, D. (1985). Association of Multiple Copies of the N-Myc Oncogene with Rapid Progression of Neuroblastomas. *New England Journal of Medicine* 313(18): 1111-1116.

Selivanova, G., Ryabchenko, L., Jansson, E., Iotsova, V. & Wiman, K. G. (1999). Reactivation of Mutant P53 through Interaction of a C-Terminal Peptide with the Core Domain. *Mol. Cell. Biol.* 19(5): 3395-3402.

Shang, X., Burlingame, S. M., Okcu, M. F., Ge, N., Russell, H. V., Egler, R. A., David, R. D., Vasudevan, S. A., Yang, J. & Nuchtern, J. G. (2009). Aurora a Is a Negative Prognostic Factor and a New Therapeutic Target in Human Neuroblastoma. *Molecular Cancer Therapeutics* 8(8): 2461-2469.

Shangary S, W. S. (2009). Small-Molecule Inhibitors of the Mdm2-P53 Protein-Protein Interaction to Reactivate P53 Function: A Novel Approach for Cancer Therapy. *Annu Rev Pharmacol Toxicol*(49): 223-41.

Sherr, C. J. (1998). Tumor Surveillance Via the Arf–P53 Pathway. *Genes & Development* 12(19): 2984-2991.

Shirahata, A. & Pegg, A. E. (1985). Regulation of S-Adenosylmethionine Decarboxylase Activity in Rat Liver and Prostate. *Journal of Biological Chemistry* 260(17): 9583-8.

Slack, A., Chen, Z., Tonelli, R., Pule, M., Hunt, L., Pession, A. & Shohet, J. M. (2005). The P53 Regulatory Gene Mdm2 Is a Direct Transcriptional Target of Mycn in Neuroblastoma. *Proc Natl Acad Sci U S A* 102(3): 731-736.

Soucek, L., Whitfield, J., Martins, C. P., Finch, A. J., Murphy, D. J., Sodir, N. M., Karnezis, A. N., Swigart, L. B., Nasi, S. & Evan, G. I. (2008). Modelling Myc Inhibition as a Cancer Therapy. *Nature* 455(7213): 679-683.

Stewart, A., Steiner, J., Mellows, G., Laguda, B., Norris, D. & Bevan, P. (2000). Phase I Trial of Xr9576 in Healthy Volunteers Demonstrates Modulation of P-Glycoprotein in Cd56+ Lymphocytes after Oral and Intravenous Administration. *Clinical Cancer Research* 6(11): 4186-4191.

Swarbrick, A., Woods, S. L., Shaw, A., Balakrishnan, A., Phua, Y., Nguyen, A., Chanthery, Y., Lim, L., Ashton, L. J., Judson, R. L., Huskey, N., Blelloch, R., Haber, M., Norris, M. D., Lengyel, P., Hackett, C. S., Preiss, T., Chetcuti, A., Sullivan, C. S., Marcusson, E. G., Weiss, W., L'Etoile, N. & Goga, A. (2010). Mir-380-5p Represses P53 to

Control Cellular Survival and Is Associated with Poor Outcome in Mycn-Amplified Neuroblastoma. *Nat Med* 16(10): 1134-1140.

Szakacs, G., Paterson, J. K., Ludwig, J. A., Booth-Genthe, C. & Gottesman, M. M. (2006). Targeting Multidrug Resistance in Cancer. *Nat Rev Drug Discov* 5(3): 219-34.

Thomas, H. & Coley, HM. (2003). Overcoming Multidrug Resistance in Cancer: An Update on the Clinical Strategy of Inhibiting P-Glycoprotein. *Cancer Control* 10 ((2)): 159-65.

Thomas, M., Pim, D., Banks L. (1999). The Role of the E6-P53 Interaction in the Molecular Pathogenesis of Hpv. *Oncogene.* Volume 18(53): 7690-7700.

Tweddle, D. A., Malcolm, A. J., Bown, N., Pearson, A. D. J. & Lunec, J. (2001). Evidence for the Development of P53 Mutations after Cytotoxic Therapy in a Neuroblastoma Cell Line. *Cancer Res* 61(1): 8-13.

Tweddle, D. A., Pearson, A. D. J., Haber, M., Norris, M. D., Xue, C., Flemming, C. & Lunec, J. (2003). The P53 Pathway and Its Inactivation in Neuroblastoma. *Cancer letters* 197(1): 93-98.

Van Maerken, T., Ferdinande, L., Taildeman, J., Lambertz, I., Yigit, N., Vercruysse, L., Rihani, A., Michaelis, M., Cinatl, J., Cuvelier, C. A., Marine, J.-C., De Paepe, A., Bracke, M., Speleman, F. & Vandesompele, J. (2009). Antitumor Activity of the Selective Mdm2 Antagonist Nutlin-3 against Chemoresistant Neuroblastoma with Wild-Type P53. *Journal of the National Cancer Institute* 101(22): 1562-1574.

Van Maerken, T., Speleman, F., Vermeulen, J., Lambertz, I., De Clercq, S., De Smet, E., Yigit, N., Coppens, V., Philippé, J., De Paepe, A., Marine, J.-C. & Vandesompele, J. (2006). Small-Molecule Mdm2 Antagonists as a New Therapy Concept for Neuroblastoma. *Cancer Res* 66(19): 9646-9655.

Vassilev LT, Vu BT, Graves B, Carvajal D, Podlaski F, Filipovic Z, Kong N, Kammlott U, Lukacs C, Klein C, Fotouhi N, Liu EA. (2004). In Vivo Activation of the P53 Pathway by Small-Molecule Antagonists of Mdm2. *Science* 303(5659): 844-8.

Wandel, C., B. Kim, R., Kajiji, S., Guengerich, F. P., Wilkinson, G. R. & Wood, A. J. J. (1999). P-Glycoprotein and Cytochrome P-450 3a Inhibition: Dissociation of Inhibitory Potencies. *Cancer Res* 59(16): 3944-3948.

Wang, H., Hammoudeh, D. I., Follis, A. V., Reese, B. E., Lazo, J. S., Metallo, S. J. & Prochownik, E. V. (2007). Improved Low Molecular Weight Myc-Max Inhibitors. *Molecular Cancer Therapeutics* 6(9): 2399-2408.

Westermann, F., Henrich, K.-O., Wei, J. S., Lutz, W., Fischer, M., König, R., Wiedemeyer, R., Ehemann, V., Brors, B., Ernestus, K., Leuschner, I., Benner, A., Khan, J. & Schwab, M. (2007). High Skp2 Expression Characterizes High-Risk Neuroblastomas Independent of Mycn Status. *Clinical Cancer Research* 13(16): 4695-4703.

Witt, O., Deubzer, HE., Lodrini M, Milde T, Oehme I. (2009). Targeting Histone Deacetylases in Neuroblastoma *Curr Pharm Des.* 15(4): 436-47.

Xue, C., Haber, M., Flemming, C., Marshall, G. M., Lock, R. B., MacKenzie, K. L., Gurova, K. V., Norris, M. D. & Gudkov, A. V. (2007). P53 Determines Multidrug Sensitivity of Childhood Neuroblastoma. *Cancer Res* 67(21): 10351-10360.

Yaari, S., Jacob-Hirsch, J., Amariglio, N., Haklai, R., Rechavi, G. & Kloog, Y. (2005). Disruption of Cooperation between Ras and Mycn in Human Neuroblastoma Cells Promotes Growth Arrest. *Clinical Cancer Research* 11(12): 4321-4330.

Yin, X., Giap, C., Lazo, J. S. & Prochownik, E. V. (2003). Low Molecular Weight Inhibitors of Myc-Max Interaction and Function. *Oncogene* 22(40): 6151-6159.

Zhang, J., Yang, P. L. & Gray, N. S. (2009). Targeting Cancer with Small Molecule Kinase Inhibitors. *Nat Rev Cancer* 9(1): 28-39.

15

Molecular Chaperones as Prognostic Markers of Neuroblastoma

Yung-Feng Liao et al.*
Institute of Cellular and Organismic Biology, Academia Sinica
Taipei,
Taiwan

1. Introduction

Neuroblastoma (NB) is a childhood tumor derived from sympathoadreanal lineage of the neural crest progenitor cells, and is the most common malignant disease of infancy, accounting for 96% of cases occurred before the age of 10 (Gurney et al., 1995, Maris and Matthay, 1999). The neuroblastoma cells exhibit characteristics of undifferentiated cells and often metastasize to distant organs (Maris and Matthay, 1999, Maris et al., 2007). Approximately, 60% of patients diagnosed with NB display a stage IV disease and a very poor prognosis. The 5-year survival rate of NB patients is no more than 30%, even with aggressive therapy (Nishihira et al., 2000). As a result, 50% of the NB patients die from this disease that continues to be one of the most difficult challenges among pediatric tumors.

NB is quite a heterogeneous tumor and presents a broad clinical and biologic spectrum ranging from highly undifferentiated tumors with very poor outcomes to the most differentiated benign ganglioneuroma or NBs with high probability of spontaneous regression and hence favorable prognosis. The clinical presentation of NB can be categorized into three distinct patterns based on the tumor histology: (i) life-threatening progression; (ii) maturation to ganglioneuroblastoma (GNB) or ganglioneuroma (GN); and (iii) spontaneous regression (Pritchard and Hickman, 1994). Taking other biological variables into account, NBs can be categorized into two groups in terms of prognosis (Brodeur, 2003, Woods et al., 1992). One, the favorable NB, is associated with young age and

*Wen-Ming Hsu[1], Hsinyu Lee[3,4], Ming-Kuan Hu[9], Hsueh-Fen Juan[3,5], Min-Chuan Huang[8], Hsiu-Hao Chang[2], Bo-Jeng Wang[4,6], Yu-Yin Shih[4,6] and Yeou-Guang Tsay[7]
Departments of [1]Surgery and [2]Pediatrics, National Taiwan University Hospital and National Taiwan University College of Medicine, Taipei, Taiwan
[3]Department of Life Science and Institutes of [4]Zoology and [5]Molecular and Cellular Biology, National Taiwan University, Taipei, Taiwan
[6]Institute of Cellular and Organismic Biology, Academia Sinica, Taipei, Taiwan
[7]Institute of Biochemistry and Molecular Biology and Proteomics Research Center, National Yang-Ming University, Taipei, Taiwan
[8]Graduate Institute of Anatomy and Cell Biology, National Taiwan University College of Medicine, Taipei, Taiwan
[9]School of Pharmacy, National Defense Medical Center, Taipei, Taiwan

early stage at diagnosis, triploid karyotypes with whole chromosome gains, and excellent clinical outcome despite minimal or no therapy. The other, the unfavorable NB, is associated with older age and advanced stage, and pseudodiploid karyotypes with structural changes including deletion of 1p or 11q, unbalanced gain of 17q and/or amplification of the MYCN proto-oncogene. Patients with unfavorable NBs usually have a very poor outcome despite multimodality therapies including bone marrow transplantation. Furthermore, we have also previously shown that the biologic characteristics of NB tumors would significantly influence the surgical decision (Hsu et al., 2006). The role of gross total resection of the primary tumor, a high-risk operation, has been controversial in the treatment of NB, especially in advanced NB. We demonstrated that gross total resection of the primary tumor could carry favorable outcome only in a specific group of NB with certain biomarkers (Hsu et al., 2006). These lines of evidence suggest that a more detailed understanding of the clinical and biologic characteristics of NB is imperative for the selection of appropriate therapeutic intervention on these tumors in order to achieve effective treatment without unnecessary complications. In this review, we will briefly overview the molecular mechanisms implicated in the tumorigenesis of NB and discuss the pathological roles of three chaperone proteins in this tumor. A model will then be proposed to illustrate the aberrant functions of chaperone proteins in predisposing neuroblastic cells into the initiation of NB.

2. The tumorigenesis of neuroblastoma

Aberrant embryonic development of sympathetic nervous system has been suggested to underlie the tumorigenesis of NB. The molecular characterization of clinically relevant prognostic markers is likely to shed light on the molecular mechanisms governing the neuroblast development and lead to the identification of novel therapeutic targets of NB. Since NB exhibits great tendency to differentiate, intensive induction therapy of NB has been widely attempted to improve outcomes. Recent evidence suggests that NB cells exhibit capacity of differentiating into mature cells and can be forced to differentiate upon the treatment of retinoic acid, butyric acid, or cisplatin (Ijiri et al., 2000, Tonini, 1993). A number of molecules normally expressed during embryonic development, including HNK-1, neuropeptide Y, tyrosine hydroxylase, TrkA and CD44, are found in NB (Hoehner et al., 1996, Israel, 1993), suggesting that the tumorigenesis of NB could be a divergence of the embryonic development of the sympathetic nervous system. On the other hand, NB cells with better prognosis are often found to express markers indicative of cell differentiation, such as HNK-1 and TrkA (Cooper et al., 1992, Nakagawara et al., 1993). It is thus plausible that the tumorigenesis of NB might result from the defect in the differentiation of embryonic NB cells (Tonini, 1993). Interestingly, NB can regress spontaneously by apoptosis (Ijiri et al., 2000, Pritchard and Hickman, 1994). The expression of pro-apoptotic genes is evident in NB,that correlates with favorable prognosis, and the survival rate of NB patients is proportional to the expression levels of these genes (Hoehner et al., 1997). Inducers of differentiation, including retinoid acid and cisplatin, could promote apoptosis in NB cells (Tonini, 1993), and NB cells expressing TrkA may undergo cell death when deprived of nerve growth factor (NGF) (Nakagawara et al., 1993), suggesting that the deficient apoptosis of embryonic NB cells could lead to the tumorigenesis of NB. However, what factors may contribute to the regulation of NB cell differentiation or apoptosis is still unclear. Accumulated evidence has suggested that apoptosis and differentiation of NB cells might occur simultaneously (Ijiri et al., 2000, Tonini, 1993). Consistently, NB cells expressing TrkA can be induced to differentiate in the presence of NGF, while undergo apoptosis upon withdrawal of NGF (Nakagawara et al., 1993). It is thus conceivable that factors mediating the tumorigenesis of NB would affect the differentiation and apoptosis of the NB cells simultaneously.

NB tumors are highly vascular and autonomously produce a variety of angiogenic factors, such as VEGF, bFGF, Ang-2, TGF-β, and PDGF-A, that are commonly found in advanced-stage tumors (Eggert et al., 2000). Although it is still debatable (Canete et al., 2000), the vascular index, as expressed by numbers of vessels per square millimeter of tissue area, has been shown to correlate with the adverse prognosis of NB patients (Meitar et al., 1996). Furthermore, the obstruction of angiogenesis may induce differentiation and apoptosis in NB (Wassberg et al., 1999), suggesting that the angiogenic factors produced by NB could also play an important role in the differentiation and apoptosis of NB cells.

Together, these data suggest that failure of either differentiation or regression by apoptotic death of NB cells is critical for the development of NB. This notion can be further supported by these findings (i) that the high frequency of spontaneous differentiation and regression can be observed in 4S tumors as well as those detected by mass screening; (ii) that the neuroblastic tumors (NTs) in adrenal glands obtained from non-afflicted infants at autopsy indicates a high incidence of unrecognized spontaneous resolution; (iii) that expression of apoptosis-related genes has been demonstrated in NB; and (iv) that NB patients with higher apoptotic index have better prognosis. Along these lines, we will describe the functions of three chaperone proteins that are implicated in the differentiation of NB. The alteration of their functions, either individually or combinarotially, could result in the propensity for the neuroblastic cells to transform and initiate the tumorigenesis of NB.

Here, we summarize the roles of three newly identified favorable prognostic markers, whose functionality as chaperones are well-established, in the pathogenesis of NB. Although these biomarkers, including calreticulin, glucose-regulated protein 78, and glucose-regulated protein 75, could be localized to different intracellular organelles, our recent studies have provided compelling evidence demonstrating that these biomarkers share an emerging function in actively governing the neuronal differentiation of neuroblastic cells. These new findings thus propose a model in which some chaperone proteins might not simply be a protein guardian in securing the normal folding of cellular proteins but could vigorously engage in crucial cellular functions by themselves.

3. Molecular chaperones of tumorigenesis

The enhanced expression of molecular chaperones have been found in a variety of tumors, and is often associated with an unfavorable prognosis and resistance to therapy (Calderwood et al., 2006). These molecular chaperones at high levels can promote tumorigenesis through facilitating the accumulation of overexpressed and mutated oncogenes and inhibiting apoptosis of tumor cells. According to Hanahan and Weinbeg (Hanahan and Weinberg, 2000), the tumorigenesis can be organized into six phenotypic changes in cellular functions: (i) autonomy in growth signaling; (ii) resistance to growth inhibition; (iii) evasion of apoptosis; (iv) unlimited proliferative potential; (v) persistent angiogenesis; and (vi) tissue invasion and metastasis. The increased expression of molecular chaperones thus could not only allow tumor cells acquire malignant capabilities, but also actively play a role in most stages of tumor development and the acquisition of drug resistance.

3.1 Calreticulin

Calreticulin (CRT) is a molecular chaperone primarily localized to endoplasmic reticulum, and has emerged as an early stage marker of NB. Although CRT is best known for its critical role in securing the correct folding and maturation of nascent proteins (Ellgaard and Helenius, 2003), it also involves in the regulation of Ca^{2+} homeostasis, the modulation of integrin-dependent adhesion, the alteration of Ca^{2+}-elicited signaling, and the inhibition of the transcriptional activities of steroid receptors (Coppolino et al., 1997, Dedhar et al., 1994, Michalak et al., 1999). The expression of CRT can be up-regulated under stress conditions and apoptosis, suggesting CRT as a stress protein (Nakamura et al., 2000). Consistent with these findings, mice deficient of CRT exhibit significant brain defects (Rauch et al., 2000), suggesting an essential role of CRT in the embryonic development of nervous system.

The role of CRT in tumorigenesis has just begun to be elucidated, evidenced by the differential expression and localization of CRT in malignant versus non-malignant tissues. The nuclear localization of CRT in hepatocellular carcinoma and various carcinomas, but not in nonmalignant liver tissue, suggests that the interaction of calreticulin and nuclear matrix could be critical for the uncontrolled proliferation of carcinomas (Yoon et al., 2000). Furthermore, up-regulated expression of CRT can be observed in breast cancers, suggesting that CRT is pivotal for the malignant progression of carcinomas (Bini et al., 1997, Franzen et al., 1997). Interestingly, vasostatin, the N-terminal fragment of CRT, and the full-length CRT have been shown to suppress tumor growth by directly targeting endothelial cells to inhibit angiogenesis (Pike et al., 1998, Pike et al., 1999). A recent report further demonstrates that CRT can serve as a recognition ligand for LDL receptor-related protein (LRP) and signal for the removal of apoptotic cells in a CRT/LRP-dependent manner (Gardai et al., 2005). These findings depict dual functions of intracellular CRT and extracellular CRT in tumorigenesis. The former is likely to promote tumor growth by entering nuclei to alter the function of transcriptional machinery, while the latter could target specific surface receptors to hinder the growth of malignant cells.

The essential role of CRT in the differentiation of NB cells has recently been established. The up-regulated expression of CRT in NB cells, coincident with the alteration of integrin profile on the surface, is particularly prominent upon differentiation (Combaret et al., 1994, Gladson et al., 1997, Rozzo et al., 1993, Coppolino et al., 1997), substantiating an essential function of CRT in mediating integrin-dependent calcium signaling. CRT in differentiating NB cells is localized to plasma membrane and could play an essential role in neurite outgrowth (Xiao et al., 1999a, Xiao et al., 1999b). These results suggest that CRT in NB, unlike in other carcinomas, can be re-distributed to cell surface to antagonize tumor growth upon induced differentiation. To verify this hypothesis, we evaluate the association of clinicopathologic factors and patient survival with the expression of CRT in patients with NB to determine whether CRT could affect the tumor behavior of NB (Hsu et al., 2005a). Our data show that positive CRT expression is strongly correlated with differentiated histologies in sixty-eight NBs. Its expression is also closely associated with known favorable prognostic factors such as detected from mass screening, younger age

(≤1 year) at diagnosis and early clinical stages, but is inversely correlated with MYCN amplification. Overall, NB patients with higher levels of CRT fare significantly better in long-term survival, substantiating CRT as an independent prognostic factor. Moreover, CRT expression also predicted better survival in patients with advanced-stage NB, and its absence predicted poor survival in patients whose tumor had no MYCN amplification. Altogether, CRT could actively play a part in the differentiation, apoptosis and angiogenesis of NB as well as the pathogenesis of NB.

3.2 Glucose-regulated protein 78

Glucose-regulated protein 78 (GRP78) is a member of the family of heat shock protein 70 (HSP70) that is localized at the endoplasmic reticulum (ER) (Gething, 1999). Like other ER-resident chaperones, GRP78 is essential for the correct folding and translocation of newly-synthesized secretory proteins across the ER membrane, and is also required for the retrotranslocation of aberrant and misfolded polypeptides destined for degradation in proteasome (Gething, 1999). In addition to being a constituent of the quality control system in ER, GRP78 also contributes to the maintenance of Ca^{2+} homeostasis (Chevet et al., 1999). GRP78 expression in normal adult organs is generally maintained at low levels and could become escalated in tumors (Dong et al., 2004), suggesting that GRP78 is required for the propagation of cancers. Consistent with this finding, tumor progression in GRP78 heterozygous mice is significantly attenuated, accompanied by a longer latency period, reduced tumor size, and increased tumor apoptosis (Lee, 2007). Accumulated evidence also suggest that GRP78 overexpression could renders various cancers resistance to chemotherapy (Li and Lee, 2006). These findings provide the rationales for targeting GRP78 as an anticancer approach that could be used in conjunction with standard therapeutic agents to improve the prognosis.

Like other HSP70 family members, GRP78 is constitutively expressed at high levels in neuroepithelial cells of the neural tube, suggesting that GRP78 and other HSP70 proteins could play significant roles in the development and differentiation of neural tissue (Barnes and Smoak, 2000, Walsh et al., 1997). By using a rat pheochromocytoma cell line PC12 as a cellular model of neuroblastoma, the levels of GRP78 protein are significantly enhanced in PC12 cells that are induced by nerve growth factor (NGF) to differentiate (Satoh et al., 2000). The overexpression of exogenous GRP78 can further augment the neurite outgrowth induced by NGF, while the down-regulation of GRP78 blocks the NGF-induced neurite outgrowth (Satoh et al., 2000), suggesting a functional synergism between NGF signaling and GRP78 function with respect to neuronal differentiation. Consistently, the inhibition of cell death in NGF-deprived neuronal cells reduces of the levels of GRP78 transcripts, suggesting a functional role of GRP78 in neuronal cell death (Aoki et al., 1997). The possibility thus exists that GRP78 could affect the differentiation and apoptosis of NB and may have a role in the tumor behavior of this cancer. In supporting this view, data from our lab have confirmed the clinical importance of GRP78 in NB. In a cohort of 68 neuroblastic tumors, forty (58.8%) of them display positive GRP78 expression by immunohistochemistry, and the positive GRP78 immunostaining is tightly correlated with differentiation histology of tumor and early clinical stages, but inversely correlated with MYCN amplification (Hsu et al., 2005b). Our findings also suggest that GRP78 expression could be an independent prognostic biomarker for favorable outcome in NB patients. Given that the differential roles of GRP78 in NB and other solid tumors, it would become increasingly critical to assess GRP78 expression level for the proper management of patients with NB versus other types of cancers.

3.3 Glucose-regulated protein 75

Glucose-regulated protein 75 (GRP75) is a member of heat shock protein 70 family and is first cloned from the cytoplasmic fraction of normal mouse fibroblast (Wadhwa et al., 1993). GRP75, also known as mortalin-2, is a member of mitochondrial molecular chaperones, but could also resides in other organelles, such as ER, plasma membrane, cytoplasmic vesicles, and cytosol (Kaul et al., 2002). GRP75 carries multiple cellular functions ranging from stress response, intracellular trafficking, antigen processing, control of cell proliferation, differentiation, and tumorigenesis (Wadhwa et al., 2002b). It has been shown that GRP75 is distributed in a pancytoplasmic pattern in normal cells but could be redistributed into a perinuclear mode in transformed cells (Wadhwa et al., 1995). The versatilities of GRP75's functions can also be exemplified by its interactions with many cellular proteins, including metabolic enzymes (e.g. diphosphomevalonate decarboxylase), mitochondrial proteins (e.g. voltage-dependent anion channel 1), and proteins involved in proliferation and differentiation (e.g. FGF-1, MKK7, and p53) (Wadhwa et al., 2003, Schwarzer et al., 2002, Wadhwa et al., 1998).

The tumorigenic role of GRP75 is shown by its colocalization with p53 in the perinuclear region of various cancers, possibly through taking part in the suppression of p53 expression (Wadhwa et al., 2002a, Wadhwa et al., 1998). GRP75 can thus serve as a functional chelator of p53 by sequestering it in cytoplasm to suppress p53-dependent gene expression. Consistent with these data, overexpression of GRP75 is found to be crucial for the changes from immortal to malignant phenotypes, leading to aggressive proliferative potential (Czarnecka et al., 2006). The expression of GRP75 is evidently up-regulated in a large number of tumorigenic human cell lines, implicating its overexpression as a marker of cell transformation (Wadhwa et al., 2006). In the acute myeloid leukemia HL-60 cells, the level of GRP75 is down-regulated upon differentiation, while overexpression of GRP75 is able to attenuate RA-induced differentiation and prevent apoptosis (Xu et al., 1999). Furthermore, GRP75 has been shown to be critical for the malignancy of breast cancer cells, and cells with higher levels of GRP75 are prone to exhibit an anchorage-independent phenotype and form tumors in nude mice (Wadhwa et al., 2006). Together, GRP75 actively involves in the molecular mechanisms governing the carcinogenesis of various tumors and could represent an ideal candidate for gene therapy.

The exact role of GRP75 in the tumorigenesis of neuroblastoma is still unclear. We have employed two-dimensional differential gel electrophoresis (2-D DIGE) to identify GRP75 as one of the most dramatically up-regulated proteins in differentiated NB cells. Immunohistochemical analyses of NB tissues further reveal that positive GRP75 immunostaining is strongly correlated with differentiated histologies, mass-screened tumors and early clinical stages, but inversely correlated with MYCN amplification. Consistent with these data, univariate and multivariate survival analyses demonstrate that GRP75 expression is an independent favorable prognostic factor. Our data substantiate an essential role of GRP75 in the differentiation of neuroblastoma and establish a novel function of GRP75 in promoting the differentiation of NB cells. Whether GRP75 localized at different intracellular compartments can play distinctive cellular functions is not clear. Nevertheless, our data demonstrate for the first time that the change in the intracellular distribution of GRP75 coincides with the development of neuronal phenotypes of differentiated NB cells, strongly suggesting a functional role of GRP75 in neuronal differentiation.

4. Conclusion

Current data have clearly suggested that the tumorigenesis of NB is controlled by a complex mechanism and is distinct from that of other cancers. This process could be driven by the intricate interactions among many gene products in multiple pathways. The best-known examples of molecular chaperones involved in the regulation of neuronal differentiation, such as CRT, GRP78, and GRP75, also turn out to be favorable prognostic markers of NB, paving the way for us to unveil the functional roles of molecular chaperones in the tumorigenesis of NB. A recent study has shown that GRP75 and GRP78, another favorable prognostic marker of NB (Hsu et al., 2005b), could bind to RHAMM with an associated downregulation of RHAMM in Jurkat cells (Kuwabara et al., 2006). The GRP75/78-RHAMM complex could then bind to the microtubules to stabilize the microtubules in the interphase and prevent the depolymerization of microtubules for the progression of mitosis (Kuwabara et al., 2006). The essential role of RHAMM in neurite extension has been suggested (Nagy et al., 1995), and the expression of RHAMM has been linked to the progression and metastasis of a variety of cancers (Maxwell et al., 2005). The possibility thus exists that the pancytoplasmic GRP75 in differentiating NB cells, along with GRP78, may prevent these cells from engaging into mitosis by binding with and downregulating RHAMM while promoting the neurite formation simultaneously. These findings thus suggest that the non-chepraone effects of these molecular chaperones might play an even bigger role in tumorigenesis of NB and other cancers.

A number of molecular chaperones of ER and mitochondria, such as CRT, GRP78, GRP75, and GRP94, whose expression is affected by tumorigenic pathways could be re-distributed outside their primary resident organelles, such as plasma membrane, neurites, and nuclei, upon differentiation. Data from others and our own labs have clearly demonstrated the "off-site" localization of these molecular chaperones. There may also be other mechanisms for the re-localization of chaperones to the nuclei and neurites that are associated with the cellular transformation. In contrast, molecular chaperones, such as calnexin in ER, that are constitutively expressed despite oncogenic transformation would mostly remain immotile during differentiation of NB. It remains to be determined whether the off-site expression of molecular chaperones is restricted to specific types of cancer and what fractions of these chaperones are presented on different cellular locations in tumor cells. Nonetheless, in certain cancers, the surface-localized GRP78 has been utilized as a beacon to deliver therapeutic agents specifically into cancer cells (Fu and Lee, 2006). Biologic factors that predict a favorable outcome for neuroblastoma patients are usually associated with differentiation or regression of neuroblastoma cells and early clinical stages. It remains to be investigated whether the expression of these differentiation-associated molecular chaperones, including HSP45, GRP78, GRP75, and calreticulin, in neuroblastic tumors would be sufficient to counteract the MYCN-elicited tumorigenesis of NB. In summary, molecular chaperones that are expressed in increased amounts in NB during differentiation could play an essential role in NB by slowing down its autonomous growth through promoting neuronal differentiation. The increased abundance of molecular chaperones in differentiated NB cells also offers tempting targets for the development of gene therapy that can attenuate the malignant phenotype of NB.

5. Acknowledgements

This work was supported by the National Science Council, Taiwan and Academia Sinica.

6. References

Aoki, T., Koike, T., Nakano, T., Shibahara, K., Kondo, S., Kikuchi, H. & Honjo, T. (1997) Induction of Bip mRNA upon programmed cell death of differentiated PC12 cells as well as rat sympathetic neurons. *J Biochem (Tokyo)*, 121, 122-7.

Barnes, J. A. & Smoak, I. W. (2000) Glucose-regulated protein 78 (GRP78) is elevated in embryonic mouse heart and induced following hypoglycemic stress. *Anat Embryol (Berl)*, 202, 67-74.

Bini, L., Magi, B., Marzocchi, B., Arcuri, F., Tripodi, S., Cintorino, M., Sanchez, J. C., Frutiger, S., Hughes, G., Pallini, V., Hochstrasser, D. F. & Tosi, P. (1997) Protein expression profiles in human breast ductal carcinoma and histologically normal tissue. *Electrophoresis*, 18, 2832-41.

Brodeur, G. M. (2003) Neuroblastoma: biological insights into a clinical enigma. *Nat Rev Cancer*, 3, 203-16.

Calderwood, S. K., Khaleque, M. A., Sawyer, D. B. & Ciocca, D. R. (2006) Heat shock proteins in cancer: chaperones of tumorigenesis. *Trends Biochem Sci*, 31, 164-72.

Canete, A., Navarro, S., Bermudez, J., Pellin, A., Castel, V. & Llombart-Bosch, A. (2000) Angiogenesis in neuroblastoma: relationship to survival and other prognostic factors in a cohort of neuroblastoma patients. *J Clin Oncol*, 18, 27-34.

Chevet, E., Jakob, C. A., Thomas, D. Y. & Bergeron, J. J. (1999) Calnexin family members as modulators of genetic diseases. *Semin Cell Dev Biol*, 10, 473-80.

Combaret, V., Coll, J. L. & Favrot, M. C. (1994) Expression of integrin and CD44 adhesion molecules on neuroblastoma: the relation to tumor aggressiveness and embryonic neural-crest differentiation. *Invasion Metastasis*, 14, 156-63.

Cooper, M. J., Steinberg, S. M., Chatten, J., Evans, A. E. & Israel, M. A. (1992) Plasticity of neuroblastoma tumor cells to differentiate along a fetal adrenal ganglionic lineage predicts for improved patient survival. *J Clin Invest*, 90, 2402-8.

Coppolino, M. G., Woodside, M. J., Demaurex, N., Grinstein, S., ST-Arnaud, R. & Dedhar, S. (1997) Calreticulin is essential for integrin-mediated calcium signalling and cell adhesion. *Nature*, 386, 843-7.

Czarnecka, A. M., Campanella, C., Zummo, G. & Cappello, F. (2006) Mitochondrial chaperones in cancer: from molecular biology to clinical diagnostics. *Cancer Biol Ther*, 5, 714-20.

Dedhar, S., Rennie, P. S., Shago, M., Hagesteijn, C. Y., Yang, H., Filmus, J., Hawley, R. G., Bruchovsky, N., Cheng, H., Matusik, R. J. & *et al.* (1994) Inhibition of nuclear hormone receptor activity by calreticulin. *Nature*, 367, 480-3.

Dong, D., Dubeau, L., Bading, J., Nguyen, K., Luna, M., Yu, H., Gazit-Bornstein, G., Gordon, E. M., Gomer, C., Hall, F. L., Gambhir, S. S. & Lee, A. S. (2004) Spontaneous and controllable activation of suicide gene expression driven by the stress-inducible grp78 promoter resulting in eradication of sizable human tumors. *Hum Gene Ther,* 15, 553-61.

Eggert, A., Ikegaki, N., Kwiatkowski, J., Zhao, H., Brodeur, G. M. & Himelstein, B. P. (2000) High-level expression of angiogenic factors is associated with advanced tumor stage in human neuroblastomas. *Clin Cancer Res,* 6, 1900-8.

Ellgaard, L. & Helenius, A. (2003) Quality control in the endoplasmic reticulum. *Nat Rev Mol Cell Biol,* 4, 181-91.

Franzen, B., Linder, S., Alaiya, A. A., Eriksson, E., Fujioka, K., Bergman, A. C., Jornvall, H. & Auer, G. (1997) Analysis of polypeptide expression in benign and malignant human breast lesions. *Electrophoresis,* 18, 582-7.

Fu, Y. & Lee, A. S. (2006) Glucose regulated proteins in cancer progression, drug resistance and immunotherapy. *Cancer Biol Ther,* 5, 741-4.

Gardai, S. J., Mcphillips, K. A., Frasch, S. C., Janssen, W. J., Starefeldt, A., Murphy-Ullrich, J. E., Bratton, D. L., Oldenborg, P. A., Michalak, M. & Henson, P. M. (2005) Cell-Surface Calreticulin Initiates Clearance of Viable or Apoptotic Cells through trans-Activation of LRP on the Phagocyte. *Cell,* 123, 321-334.

Gething, M. J. (1999) Role and regulation of the ER chaperone BiP. *Semin Cell Dev Biol,* 10, 465-72.

Gladson, C. L., Dennis, C., Rotolo, T. C., Kelly, D. R. & Grammer, J. R. (1997) Vitronectin expression in differentiating neuroblastic tumors: integrin alpha v beta 5 mediates vitronectin-dependent adhesion of retinoic-acid-differentiated neuroblastoma cells. *Am J Pathol,* 150, 1631-46.

Gurney, J. G., Severson, R. K., Davis, S. & Robison, L. L. (1995) Incidence of cancer in children in the United States. Sex-, race-, and 1-year age-specific rates by histologic type. *Cancer,* 75, 2186-95.

Hanahan, D. & Weinberg, R. A. (2000) The hallmarks of cancer. *Cell,* 100, 57-70.

Hoehner, J. C., Gestblom, C., Hedborg, F., Sandstedt, B., Olsen, L. & Pahlman, S. (1996) A developmental model of neuroblastoma: differentiating stroma-poor tumors' progress along an extra-adrenal chromaffin lineage. *Lab Invest,* 75, 659-75.

Hoehner, J. C., Gestblom, C., Olsen, L. & Pahlman, S. (1997) Spatial association of apoptosis-related gene expression and cellular death in clinical neuroblastoma. *Br J Cancer,* 75, 1185-94.

Hsu, W. M., Hsieh, F. J., Jeng, Y. M., Kuo, M. L., Chen, C. N., Lai, D. M., Hsieh, L. J., Wang, B. T., Tsao, P. N., Lee, H., Lin, M. T., Lai, H. S. & Chen, W. J. (2005a) Calreticulin expression in neuroblastoma--a novel independent prognostic factor. *Ann Oncol,* 16, 314-21.

Hsu, W. M., Hsieh, F. J., Jeng, Y. M., Kuo, M. L., Tsao, P. N., Lee, H., Lin, M. T., Lai, H. S., Chen, C. N., Lai, D. M. & Chen, W. J. (2005b) GRP78 expression correlates with histologic differentiation and favorable prognosis in neuroblastic tumors. *Int J Cancer,* 113, 920-7.

Hsu, W. M., Jen, Y. M., Lee, H., Kuo, M. L., Tsao, P. N., Chen, C. N., Lai, D. M., Lin, M. T., Lai, H. S., Chen, W. J. & Hsieh, F. J. (2006) The influence of biologic factors on the surgical decision in advanced neuroblastoma. *Ann Surg Oncol,* 13, 238-44.

Ijiri, R., Tanaka, Y., Kato, K., Misugi, K., Nishihira, H., Toyoda, Y., Kigasawa, H., Nishi, T., Takeuchi, M., Aida, N. & Momoi, T. (2000) Clinicopathologic study of mass-screened neuroblastoma with special emphasis on untreated observed cases: a possible histologic clue to tumor regression. *Am J Surg Pathol,* 24, 807-15.

Israel, M. A. (1993) Disordered differentiation as a target for novel approaches to the treatment of neuroblastoma. *Cancer,* 71, 3310-3.

Kaul, S. C., Taira, K., Pereira-Smith, O. M. & Wadhwa, R. (2002) Mortalin: present and prospective. *Exp Gerontol,* 37, 1157-64.

Kuwabara, H., Yoneda, M., Hayasaki, H., Nakamura, T. & Mori, H. (2006) Glucose regulated proteins 78 and 75 bind to the receptor for hyaluronan mediated motility in interphase microtubules. *Biochem Biophys Res Commun,* 339, 971-6.

Lee, A. S. (2007) GRP78 induction in cancer: therapeutic and prognostic implications. *Cancer Res,* 67, 3496-9.

Li, J. & Lee, A. S. (2006) Stress induction of GRP78/BiP and its role in cancer. *Curr Mol Med,* 6, 45-54.

Maris, J. M., Hogarty, M. D., Bagatell, R. & Cohn, S. L. (2007) Neuroblastoma. *Lancet,* 369, 2106-20.

Maris, J. M. & Matthay, K. K. (1999) Molecular biology of neuroblastoma. *J Clin Oncol,* 17, 2264-79.

Maxwell, C. A., Keats, J. J., Belch, A. R., Pilarski, L. M. & Reiman, T. (2005) Receptor for hyaluronan-mediated motility correlates with centrosome abnormalities in multiple myeloma and maintains mitotic integrity. *Cancer Res,* 65, 850-60.

Meitar, D., Crawford, S. E., Rademaker, A. W. & Cohn, S. L. (1996) Tumor angiogenesis correlates with metastatic disease, N-myc amplification, and poor outcome in human neuroblastoma. *J Clin Oncol,* 14, 405-14.

Michalak, M., Corbett, E. F., Mesaeli, N., Nakamura, K. & Opas, M. (1999) Calreticulin: one protein, one gene, many functions. *Biochem J,* 344 Pt 2, 281-92.

Nagy, J. I., Hacking, J., Frankenstein, U. N. & Turley, E. A. (1995) Requirement of the hyaluronan receptor RHAMM in neurite extension and motility as demonstrated in primary neurons and neuronal cell lines. *J Neurosci,* 15, 241-52.

Nakagawara, A., Arima-Nakagawara, M., Scavarda, N. J., Azar, C. G., Cantor, A. B. & Brodeur, G. M. (1993) Association between high levels of expression of the TRK gene and favorable outcome in human neuroblastoma. *N Engl J Med,* 328, 847-54.

Nakamura, K., Bossy-Wetzel, E., Burns, K., Fadel, M. P., Lozyk, M., Goping, I. S., Opas, M., Bleackley, R. C., Green, D. R. & Michalak, M. (2000) Changes in endoplasmic reticulum luminal environment affect cell sensitivity to apoptosis. *J Cell Biol,* 150, 731-40.

Nishihira, H., Toyoda, Y., Tanaka, Y., Ijiri, R., Aida, N., Takeuchi, M., Ohnuma, K., Kigasawa, H., Kato, K. & Nishi, T. (2000) Natural course of neuroblastoma detected by mass screening: s 5-year prospective study at a single institution. *J Clin Oncol,* 18, 3012-7.

Pike, S. E., Yao, L., Jones, K. D., Cherney, B., Appella, E., Sakaguchi, K., Nakhasi, H., Teruya-Feldstein, J., Wirth, P., Gupta, G. & Tosato, G. (1998) Vasostatin, a calreticulin fragment, inhibits angiogenesis and suppresses tumor growth. *J Exp Med,* 188, 2349-56.

Pike, S. E., Yao, L., Setsuda, J., Jones, K. D., Cherney, B., Appella, E., Sakaguchi, K., Nakhasi, H., Atreya, C. D., Teruya-Feldstein, J., Wirth, P., Gupta, G. & Tosato, G. (1999)

Calreticulin and calreticulin fragments are endothelial cell inhibitors that suppress tumor growth. *Blood,* 94, 2461-8.

Pritchard, J. & Hickman, J. A. (1994) Why does stage 4s neuroblastoma regress spontaneously? *Lancet,* 344, 869-70.

Rauch, F., Prud'homme, J., Arabian, A., Dedhar, S. & ST-Arnaud, R. (2000) Heart, brain, and body wall defects in mice lacking calreticulin. *Exp Cell Res,* 256, 105-11.

Rozzo, C., Ratti, P., Ponzoni, M. & Cornaglia-Ferraris, P. (1993) Modulation of alpha 1 beta 1, alpha 2 beta 1 and alpha 3 beta 1 integrin heterodimers during human neuroblastoma cell differentiation. *FEBS Lett,* 332, 263-7.

Satoh, T., Furuta, K., Tomokiyo, K., Nakatsuka, D., Tanikawa, M., Nakanishi, M., Miura, M., Tanaka, S., Koike, T., Hatanaka, H., Ikuta, K., Suzuki, M. & Watanabe, Y. (2000) Facilitatory roles of novel compounds designed from cyclopentenone prostaglandins on neurite outgrowth-promoting activities of nerve growth factor. *J Neurochem,* 75, 1092-102.

Schwarzer, C., Barnikol-Watanabe, S., Thinnes, F. P. & Hilschmann, N. (2002) Voltage-dependent anion-selective channel (VDAC) interacts with the dynein light chain Tctex1 and the heat-shock protein PBP74. *Int J Biochem Cell Biol,* 34, 1059-70.

Tonini, G. P. (1993) Neuroblastoma: the result of multistep transformation? *Stem Cells,* 11, 276-82.

Wadhwa, R., Kaul, S. C., Ikawa, Y. & Sugimoto, Y. (1993) Identification of a novel member of mouse hsp70 family. Its association with cellular mortal phenotype. *J Biol Chem,* 268, 6615-21.

Wadhwa, R., Pereira-Smith, O. M., Reddel, R. R., Sugimoto, Y., Mitsui, Y. & Kaul, S. C. (1995) Correlation between complementation group for immortality and the cellular distribution of mortalin. *Exp Cell Res,* 216, 101-6.

Wadhwa, R., Taira, K. & Kaul, S. C. (2002a) An Hsp70 family chaperone, mortalin/mthsp70/PBP74/Grp75: what, when, and where? *Cell Stress Chaperones,* 7, 309-16.

Wadhwa, R., Taira, K. & Kaul, S. C. (2002b) Mortalin: a potential candidate for biotechnology and biomedicine. *Histol Histopathol,* 17, 1173-7.

Wadhwa, R., Takano, S., Kaur, K., Deocaris, C. C., Pereira-Smith, O. M., Reddel, R. R. & Kaul, S. C. (2006) Upregulation of mortalin/mthsp70/Grp75 contributes to human carcinogenesis. *Int J Cancer,* 118, 2973-80.

Wadhwa, R., Takano, S., Robert, M., Yoshida, A., Nomura, H., Reddel, R. R., Mitsui, Y. & Kaul, S. C. (1998) Inactivation of tumor suppressor p53 by mot-2, a hsp70 family member. *J Biol Chem,* 273, 29586-91.

Wadhwa, R., Yaguchi, T., Hasan, M. K., Taira, K. & Kaul, S. C. (2003) Mortalin-MPD (mevalonate pyrophosphate decarboxylase) interactions and their role in control of cellular proliferation. *Biochem Biophys Res Commun,* 302, 735-42.

Walsh, D., Li, Z., Wu, Y. & Nagata, K. (1997) Heat shock and the role of the HSPs during neural plate induction in early mammalian CNS and brain development. *Cell Mol Life Sci,* 53, 198-211.

Wassberg, E., Hedborg, F., Skoldenberg, E., Stridsberg, M. & Christofferson, R. (1999) Inhibition of angiogenesis induces chromaffin differentiation and apoptosis in neuroblastoma. *Am J Pathol,* 154, 395-403.

Woods, W. G., Lemieux, B. & Tuchman, M. (1992) Neuroblastoma represents distinct clinical-biologic entities: a review and perspective from the Quebec Neuroblastoma Screening Project. *Pediatrics,* 89, 114-8.

Xiao, G., Chung, T. F., Fine, R. E. & Johnson, R. J. (1999a) Calreticulin is transported to the surface of NG108-15 cells where it forms surface patches and is partially degraded in an acidic compartment. *J Neurosci Res,* 58, 652-62.

Xiao, G., Chung, T. F., Pyun, H. Y., Fine, R. E. & Johnson, R. J. (1999b) KDEL proteins are found on the surface of NG108-15 cells. *Brain Res Mol Brain Res,* 72, 121-8.

Xu, J., Xiao, H. H. & Sartorelli, A. C. (1999) Attenuation of the induced differentiation of HL-60 leukemia cells by mitochondrial chaperone HSP70. *Oncol Res,* 11, 429-35.

Yoon, G. S., Lee, H., Jung, Y., Yu, E., Moon, H. B., Song, K. & Lee, I. (2000) Nuclear matrix of calreticulin in hepatocellular carcinoma. *Cancer Res,* 60, 1117-20.

16

FOXO Transcription Factors as Potential Therapeutic Targets in Neuroblastoma

Michael J. Ausserlechner[1,3], Judith Hagenbuchner[2,3], Stefan Fuchs[3], Kathrin Geiger[3] and Petra Obexer[2,3]
Medical University Innsbruck,
[1]Department of Pediatrics II,
[2]Department of Pediatrics IV,
[3]Tyrolean Cancer Research Institute,
Austria

1. Introduction

The hallmark of cancer cells is deregulated growth, inhibition of differentiation, and delay or blockage of programmed cell death. Tumor cells that are independent of extra- and/or intracellular regulatory mechanisms due to mutations in proto-oncogenes and tumor suppressors acquire the ability of uncontrolled proliferation and invasion into other tissues.

FOXO (FOXO1, FOXO3, FOXO4, FOXO6) transcription factors control apoptosis, stress resistance and longevity in mammalian cells. Their activity and subcellular localization is regulated by phosphorylation on conserved serine/threonin residues via protein kinase B (PKB) and stress-induced kinases. Hyperactivation of PKB contributes to the inactivation of FOXO3 and predicts poor outcome for neuroblastoma patients. Depending on their post-translational modifications and cellular context FOXO transcription factors exert diverse functions thereby either inducing cell death but also cell survival and resistance to environmental stress. Although FOXO transcription factors share the same DNA binding motive and seem to have overlapping functions, knock out animals for single FOXO family members show different defects: Whereas FOXO1 knock-out mice die during embryonic development due to defective vasculature, FOXO3 and FOXO4 knock out mice show a mild phenotype. However, conditional triple-knock-out mice provide evidence that FOXO1, FOXO3 and FOXO4 are critically involved in the maintenance of the hematopoietic stem cell population and the regulation of endothelial cell homeostasis. Consistent with their putative role as tumor suppressors, in cultured neuroblastoma cells the activation of FOXO3 triggers the intrinsic death pathway and induces programmed cell death via induction of the pro-apoptotic BH3-only proteins BCL2L11/Bim and PMAIP1/Noxa. Surprisingly, in neuroblastoma cells FOXO3-mediated cell death depends on the accumulation of reactive oxygen species (ROS). Activation of FOXO3 also causes the repression of the apoptosis-inhibitor protein Survivin and determines sensitivity of neuroblastoma cells to DNA-damaging chemotherapeutic agents. More recently it was shown that beside its function as a tumor suppressor FOXO3 might also facilitate cancer cell survival under certain circumstances. In other tumor types FOXO3 also induces detoxification and stress resistance thereby contributing to tumor stem cell renewal and protection of cancer cells from eradication during chemotherapy. In this respect FOXO3 was recently shown to be essential for the maintenance of leukemia initiating cells in chronic myeloid leukemia and to confer therapy resistance in leukemia cells. Active FOXO3 facilitates metastasis through activation of matrix metalloproteinases, leads to lymph node positivity and predicts poor survival in breast carcinoma. In this article we will therefore review the current knowledge of FOXO transcription factors, their "Janus-faced role" in tumor cell survival and drug sensitivity and discuss whether FOXO3 might be an interesting target for therapeutic intervention in neuroblastoma.

2. A general overview on FOXOs

The forkhead transcription factor family consists of more than 100 members, which are important in various processes including development, cellular differentiation, proliferation, cell cycle arrest, cell death, tumor suppression, stress resistance and metabolism (Carlsson and Mahlapuu 2002). In mammals four members of the forkhead transcription factor class O (FOXO) family are known, named FKHR/FOXO1, FKHRL1/FOXO3, AFX/FOXO4 and FOXO6 (Katoh and Katoh 2004). FOXO transcription factors are homologs of the *Caenorhabditis elegans* protein DAF-16 which regulates the life-span of *C. elegans* (Lin et al, 1997) and were first discovered through the cloning of chromosomal breakpoints associated with cancer. Since the chromosomal translocation disrupted the FOXO-DNA-binding domain in the oncogenic fusion protein it was proposed that all three FOXOs act as tumor suppressors. FOXO proteins function primarily as transcription factors in the nucleus and bind as monomers to a consensus DNA sequence with a DNA-binding "winged-helix" domain, also called forkhead box, a 110 amino acid region in the central part of the protein (Weigelt et al, 2001). FOXO factors bind to the DNA-binding motif TTGTTTAC, TT(G/A)TTTC and (C/A)(A/C)AAA(C/T)AA (Obsil and Obsilova 2010; Furuyama et al, 2000). Bioinformatics analyses showed that a large set of genes contain FOXO-binding sites in their promoter region (Xuan and Zhang 2005). FOXO proteins act as potent transcriptional activators, but gene array analyses indicate that FOXOs can also act as transcriptional repressors (Ramaswamy et al, 2002).

To specify the diverse functions of FOXO transcription factors, knock-out mice were generated. These approaches revealed distinct but overlapping roles of FOXO members in mammals. FOXO1 null mice die during embryonic development due to defective vascularization (Hosaka et al, 2004). *In vitro* experiments further suggest that FOXO1 is important for endothelial cells to respond to vascular endothelial growth factor (VEGF). FOXO3 null mice are viable but exhibit an age-dependent female infertility as a consequence of abnormal follicular activation leading to total depletion of ovarian follicles (reviewed in (Arden 2008a)). Furthermore FOXO3 null mice show defects in the glucose uptake (Castrillon et al, 2003). This implies a role of FOXO factors in glucose metabolism. In lymphoid organs, FOXO3 is the predominant FOXO member and its deficiency leads to lymphoproliferation and widespread organ inflammation. FOXO4 null mice are viable and show no overt phenotype (Hosaka et al, 2004). Since all three FOXO transcription factors recognize the same DNA consensus sequence, the three family members seem to have overlapping functions. Since there is possible functional redundancy between the family members, a triple knock-out mouse with conditional deletions of FOXO1, FOXO3 and FOXO4 was developed. These animals show abnormalities in lymphoid development and a defect in the long-term repopulating activity of the bone-marrow stem cells. Additionally, these mice have a significant reduction in their long-term hematopoietic stem cell population and a decrease in a subset of genes, which are involved in detoxification and prevention of oxidative stress (Tothova et al, 2007b). This suggests that FOXOs play a major role in the response to oxidative stress (Arden 2008b). Furthermore the inactivation of all three FOXO transcription factors results in lymphoblastic thymic lymphomas, leukemias and widespread hemangiomas (Paik et al, 2007). Since these animal models support a critical role of FOXOs in the homeostasis of the stem cell population, deregulation of FOXOs might contribute to the development of various malignancies, among them human neuroblastoma.

3. Regulation of FOXOs by survival and stress signaling

FOXO proteins are post-translationally regulated by phosphorylation, acetylation or ubiquitination via different signaling pathways. These modifications determine the cellular localization of FOXO proteins and the interaction with binding partners. In the absence of growth factors, FOXO3 localizes to the nucleus. Binding of growth factors such as insulin, insulin-like-growth factor (IGF) or neurotrophic factors (nerve growth factor (NGF), brain-derived-neurotrophic-factor (BDNF), neurotrophin-3, -4 (NT-3, -4)) to their cognate receptors induce a signaling cascade that leads to the activation of phosphatidylinositol-3-kinase (PI3K) and the production of phosphoinositol-3-phosphate (PIP3). The second messenger PIP3 serves as an adapter molecule for pleckstrin homology (PH)-domain containing proteins at the cytoplasma membrane, such as the protein kinase B (PKB). The molecular interaction of these proteins at the membrane induces their (auto)phosphorylation and activation (reviewed in (Coffer and Burgering 2004)). When activated, PKB phosphorylates FOXO transcription factors on three highly conserved sites (e.g. FOXO3 on threonin-32, serine-253, serine-315), one located in the forkhead domain, one at the N-terminal and one at the C-terminal site. Phosphorylation by PKB masks the nuclear localization sequence (NLS) of FOXO3 and impedes DNA-binding. Furthermore PKB phosphorylation prevents the interaction with the transcriptional co-activator p300/CBP and promotes binding of FOXO proteins to 14-3-3. Following this binding FOXO3 undergoes a conformational change that results in the exposure of a nuclear export sequence (NES) on its C-terminal site and causes the export of FOXO3 into the cytoplasm (Biggs et al, 1999; Brunet et al, 1999). This conformational change allows FOXO3 to interact with Exportin/Crm1 and Ran, which leads to its export into the cytoplasm via the nuclear pore complex, repression of its transcriptional activity and to ubiquitin-mediated proteasomal degradation. Nuclear re-import is prevented due to masking of its NLS by 14-3-3 proteins (Rena et al, 2002). The PI3K-PKB signaling pathway is negatively regulated by phosphatases such as PTEN (Yamada and Araki 2001) that degrade PIP3 and thereby abrogate this signaling cascade. Loss of PTEN is frequently observed in carcinomas (Li et al, 1997) and hematologic malignancies (Sakai et al, 1998). The overexpression of growth factors that activate the PI3K or mutations in its regulatory subunits also result in hyperactivation of the PI3K-PKB pathway. PKB is dysregulated in a variety of cancers such as neuroblastoma (Opel et al, 2007). In addition to PKB, also the serum and glucocorticoid-inducible kinase (SGK) and the cyclin-dependent-kinase-2 (CDK2) phosphorylate FOXOs at distinct sites, which triggers their export from the nucleus (reviewed in (Coffer and Burgering 2004)). Other kinases which phosphorylate FOXO3 are the serine/threonine kinase CK1 (Rena et al,

2002) and the dual tyrosine phosphorylated regulated kinase 1 (DYRK1), which belongs to the MAP kinase family (Woods et al, 2001).

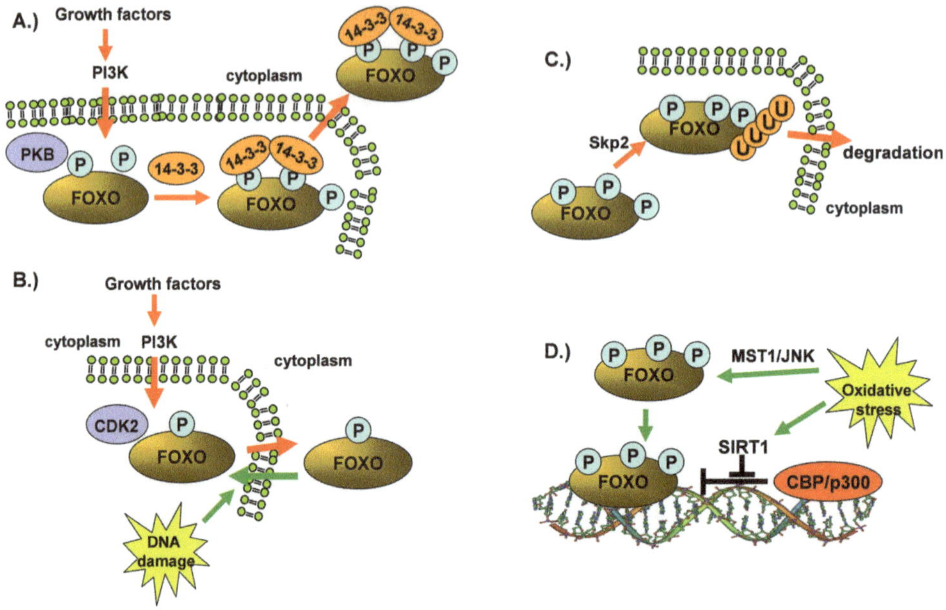

Growth factors such as IGF-1 lead to activation of PKB and CDK2 via PI3K-dependent pathways resulting in phosphorylation of FOXOs at distinct sites. A) PKB-mediated phosphorylation induces the binding of the chaperone protein 14-3-3 and subsequent export into the cytoplasm. B) CDK2-mediated phosphorylation also leads to cytoplasmic localization. Upon DNA-damage the CDK2-triggered phosphorylation activates FOXOs. C) Skp2 of the SCF-E3 ligase complex interacts with and ubiquitylates FOXO1. D) In response to oxidative stress FOXOs translocate into the nucleus as a consequence of direct JNK or MST1 phosphorylation. Acetylation of FOXOs by CBP/p300 inhibits their transcriptional activity. Under conditions of oxidative stress this effect can be overcome by the deacetylase SIRT1. Red arrows indicate negative regulation, whereas green arrows indicate positive regulation.

Fig. 1. Regulation of FOXO proteins in response to external and internal stimuli.

In contrast, oxidative and genotoxic stress results in FOXO3 phosphorylation by c-Jun N-terminal kinase (JNK) and by mammalian sterile 20-like kinase 1 (MST1), which forces translocation of FOXO transcription factors from the cytoplasm to the nucleus even in the presence of growth factor signaling (Sunters et al, 2006; Lehtinen et al, 2006; Essers et al, 2004). Additional posttranslational modifications modify FOXO activity, such as acetylation of lysines in the forkhead domain by CBP/p300 or deacetylation by the protein deacetylase sirtuin-1 (SIRT1). The interaction with SIRT1 modulates the transcriptional function of FOXO3 resulting in the inhibition of FOXO3-induced expression of pro-apoptotic genes and the enhanced expression of genes involved in cell cycle regulation, DNA-repair and stress resistance (Brunet et al, 2004). Deacetylation of FOXO3 preferentially enhances the expression of genes that regulate cell cycle arrest, DNA-repair and stress resistance, which finally induces longevity instead of death inducing factors (Brunet et al, 2004; Furukawa-Hibi et al, 2002). An additional mode of FOXO regulation is its proteasomal degradation, which irreversibly shuts down FOXO activity (Hu et al, 2004). Ubiquitination by ubiquitin-ligase Skp2 or de-ubiquitination by USP7 adds an additional level of control (van der Horst et al, 2006). Poly-ubiquitination depends on phosphorylation of FOXOs by PKB; Skp2 directly interacts with FOXO1 after PKB-specific phosphorylation at serine-253. Deacetylation by SIRT1 and SIRT2 on the lysine residues K242, K259, K290 and K569 facilitates Skp2-mediated FOXO3 ubiquitination and proteasomal degradation (Wang et al, 2011). Furthermore, FOXO proteins have been shown to cooperate with cofactors such as Smad3/4 and the transcription factor p53 as well as with nuclear androgen-, glucocorticoid- and retinoic acid receptors (reviewed in (Calnan and Brunet 2008; van der Vos and Coffer 2008)).

4. Physiological functions of FOXOs

FOXO transcription factors control the expression of various genes which are involved in cell proliferation, cell survival, DNA repair and apoptosis. Cell proliferation is controlled by FOXO3 via inducing the expression of cell cycle breaks such as the Cdk inhibitor (CKI) $p27^{Kip1}$ and the retinoblastoma family member p130. Both proteins are negative regulators of cell cycle progression and induce cell cycle arrest in the G1 phase (Kops et al, 2002b; Dijkers et al, 2000b). Another FOXO3-regulated CKI $p21^{Cip1}$ which is activated in response to tumor-growth factor β (TGFβ) induces cell cycle arrest at G1. FOXO3 can directly bind to the transcription factors Smad3 and Smad4 and the resulting complex further binds to a forkhead and a smad binding element within the $p21^{Cip1}$ promoter leading to increased $p21^{Cip1}$ expression (Seoane et al, 2004). Beside activation of cell cycle inhibitors FOXO3 can also induce cell cycle arrest by repressing the G1 cell cycle activators cyclin D1 and D2 (Schmidt et al, 2002; Fernandez et al, 2004). FOXO transcription factors have also been implicated in the control of G2-M transition and in exit from telophase. In particular FOXO3 regulates the expression and degradation of cyclin B and of Polo-like kinase (Alvarez et al, 2001) and the DNA damage-inducible protein 45 (Gadd45a). Under low stress conditions FOXO3 promotes DNA repair in a Gadd45a dependent mechanism, whereas under high levels of stress FOXO3 induces cell death (Furukawa-Hibi et al, 2002; Tran et al, 2002). Stress stimuli like hypoxia, ionizing radiation, oxidants, UV light or growth factor withdrawal strongly induce Gadd45a. Gadd45a is also involved in cellular mechanisms like G2-M cell cycle progression, genomic stability, nucleotide excision repair, apoptosis and signaling through MAP kinase and JNK (Lal and Gorospe 2006). Similar to PKB activity, the expression level, phosphorylation and subcellular localization of FOXO3 changes during the cell cycle, which is in part regulated by the phosphatase Cdc25A (Leisser et al, 2004). Importantly, FOXOs may also protect cells against reactive oxygen species (ROS) by inducing the two scavenger proteins superoxide dismutase (SOD2/MnSOD) and CAT/Catalase and may even induce therapy resistance by activating the multi-drug resistance gene MDR1 (Hui et al, 2008a; Kops et al, 2002a).

FOXOs not only control proteins involved in cell cycle progression but also regulate pro- and anti-apoptotic genes, particularly in neurons and hematopoietic cells. Two pro-apoptotic proteins whose expression is induced by FOXO3 are the BH3-only proteins PMAIP1/Noxa and BCL2L11/Bim (Dijkers et al, 2000a; Obexer et al, 2007). The Bim promoter contains two conserved forkhead response elements (FHRE). Binding of FOXO3 to these elements results in apoptotic cell death in sympathetic neurons and neuroblastoma cells (Gilley et al, 2003; Obexer et al, 2007). The induction of the BH3-only protein Noxa leads in neuroblastoma cells to apoptosis via the intrinsic death pathway (Obexer et al,

2007). FOXO3 also regulates the transcription of genes which are involved in the extrinsic death pathway, like Fas ligand (FASLG) (Brunet et al, 1999) and tumor necrosis factor-related apoptosis inducing ligand (TRAIL). FOXO3 binds directly three FHRE within the regulatory region of the FASLG promoter and a novel binding site in the sequence of the TRAIL promoter (Modur et al, 2002). Under conditions of oxidative stress FOXO3 strongly induces the expression of the transcriptional repressor B-cell/lymphoma 6 (BCL6). BCL6 represses the anti-apoptotic protein BCL2L1/Bcl-xL which contains a STAT/BCL6 binding site within its promoter (Tang et al, 2002). Via this indirect regulation of Bcl-xL, FOXO3 changes the balance of pro- and anti-apoptotic proteins from survival to cell death induction. Interaction of FOXO factors with other transcription factors influences the transcriptional activity of FOXO proteins and determines the regulation of its target genes. β-catenin directly interacts with FOXO factors and thereby increases the expression of MnSOD. This leads to a shift from apoptosis regulating genes to oxidative stress detoxifying genes, which results in longevity (Essers et al, 2005). Another transcription factor which regulates FOXO3 activity is p53. Binding of p53 to FOXO3 under low stress conditions prevents induction of pro-apoptotic Bim and the transcriptional repressor BCL6, whereas expression of cyclin G2 and $p27^{Kip1}$ are not affected. By modifying the target gene spectrum of FOXO3, the p53/FOXO3 complex induces cell cycle arrest instead of apoptosis (Miyaguchi et al, 2009).

Taken together, FOXO3 is involved in various cell-type specific, cellular functions. Depending on its posttranslational modifications such as phosphorylation, acetylation, ubiquitination or interaction with other transcription factors, FOXO factors regulate even opposite effects, like cell cycle arrest, apoptosis induction or even induction of longevity.

5. Regulation of FOXOs in neural stem cells and neuronal cells

Neural stem cells are the self-renewing population that is important for proper generation of neurons, astrocytes and oligodendrocytes in the developing but also in the adult brain where they play a critical role for learning and for the brain-homeostasis during aging. They participate in memory, behavior, and brain injury repair.

The insulin/IGF1/PI3K/PKB/FOXO signaling controls neural stem cell proliferation. Neural stem cells that overexpress PKB show an enhanced proliferation and a reduced capacity to differentiate (Peltier et al, 2007). In addition to maintaining the replicatory-potential of hematopoietic stem cells (Tothova et al, 2007b) it was recently shown that FOXO3 knockout mice have fewer neural stem cells than wildtype mice and that neural stem cells isolated from $FOXO3^{-/-}$ mice had reduced self-renewal capacity and showed impaired differentiation into different neural lineages. FOXO3 knockout mice and mice with conditional deletion of FOXO3, FOXO4 and FOXO1 in the brain show an increased brain size. Furthermore their neural stem cells have enhanced rates of entry into the cell cycle suggesting that FOXO3 is important to maintain the relative quiescence of neural stem cells and prevents their premature exhaustion (Renault et al, 2009; Paik et al, 2009). One FOXO3 target that might be critical for these neuronal abnormalities is abnormal spindle-like microcephaly-associated (Aspm) which is repressed by FOXO1 and FOXO3. This protein limits neural progenitor expansion during development and prevents early exhaustion of the adult neural stem cell pool (Bond et al, 2002). Adult neurogenesis relies on adult mitotic neural stem cells. Activation of dFOXO in Drosophila causes the elimination of these neural stem cells during the development via Caspase-dependent cell death (Siegrist et al, 2010). In adult neural stem cells that lack FOXO1, FOXO3 and FOXO4 due to gene deletion, increased levels of reactive oxygen species (ROS) are detected. This correlates with altered expression of the detoxifying enzymes peroxiredoxin, glutathione peroxidase-1 and SESN3/sestrin-3. Since neuronal cells in particular depend on the thiol-redoxin system to defend themselves against ROS, regulation of these enzymes by FOXOs is critical for neuronal survival. FOXOs may therefore contribute to the self-renewal of neural stem cells by reducing ROS-accumulation, which is further supported by the observation that impaired self-renewal in the FOXO1/3/4 triple knock out neural stem cells can be rescued by the antioxidant N-acetyl cysteine (NAC) or the expression of SESN3 (Paik et al, 2009).

Genome wide microarray analysis from FOXO3$^{-/-}$ and FOXO3$^{+/+}$ neural stem cells from young adult mice revealed that FOXO3 regulates the neural stem cell pool by inducing genes that on one side promote quiescence and prevent premature differentiation and on the other side are involved in oxidative stress resistance and in control of glucose metabolism. When comparing the FOXO3-target genes with genes necessary during the process of aging in human and mouse brains, Renault et al observed a correlation between FOXO3-regulated genes and aging-regulated genes. This suggests that FOXO3 plays a critical role in the regulation of nerve stem cell homeostasis and may also be critical for brain-aging in mammals (Renault et al, 2009). The FOXO-dependent transcriptome of neural stem cells has little in common with the transcriptome of other cell types such as hematopoietic stem cells or endothelial cells. This indicates that FOXO transcription factors exert cell-type specific functions (Tothova et al, 2007a; Paik et al, 2007; Paik et al, 2009).

MicroRNAs have recently emerged as key regulators of embryonic and adult stem cells (Arnold et al, 2011). FOXO3 binds to a site in the first intron and thereby regulates the microRNA gene cluster miR-106b~25 consisting of miR-106b, miR-93 and miR-25 in primary cultures of neural stem/progenitor cells isolated from adult mice (Brett et al, 2011). Expression of this microRNA gene cluster promotes proliferation in self-renewal conditions and increased generation of new neurons in differentiation conditions. Therefore FOXO3 also regulates miRNAs which are necessary for the maintenance of adult stem cells and for the homeostasis of the neural stem cell pool during aging (Brett et al, 2011).

Similar to the hematopoietic system also during the development of the nerve system the effect of FOXO activation might completely differ between stem cells, progenitor cells and terminally differentiated cells. This has to be kept in mind when studying FOXO3 function in tumor cells that arise from different types of neuronal tumor stem cells, such as neuroblastoma. FOXO3 is expressed throughout the brain including hippocampal areas, cortex and cerebellum and may play a role during injuries that involve cerebral ischemia and oxidative stress (Chong et al, 2005). In primary cortical and cerebellar neurons NGF, NT-3 and -4, and IGF-1 mediate survival by inhibition of FOXO1 (Gan et al, 2005) and FOXO3 and its nuclear exclusion via the PI3K/PKB signaling pathway. Therefore during oxidative stress the inhibition of FOXO3 is necessary for the protective effect of trophic factors in neurons (Zheng et al, 2000; Zheng et al, 2002). High PKB-activity also accounts for neuroprotection in ischemic tolerance in hippocampal neurons (Yano et al, 2001) whereas a decreased PKB- and as a consequence thereof induced FOXO-activity mediates ischemia-induced cell death. Following ischemic brain injury FOXOs induce delayed neuronal apoptosis via induction of FASLG and the BH3-only protein Bim in hippocampal regions. Neurons can be rescued from this delayed apoptosis by sodium orthovanadate which increases PKB-activity and therefore inhibits FOXO-dependent death signals (Fukunaga et al, 2005). In neonatal mice FOXO3 expression is associated with the potential to promote cerebral hypoxic-ischemic injury (Pirianov et al, 2007) and the neuroprotective effects of estradiol during stroke are associated with inhibition of FOXO3 (Won et al, 2006). Stroke and reperfusion are associated with significant oxidative stress in neuronal cells and depending on the cell type, FOXO3 function may support survival or be detrimental. In neurons oxidative stress activates the tyrosine kinase c-Abl which in turn activates the protein kinase MST1 by phosphorylation at tyrosine-433. MST1 then phosphorylates serine-209 in the DNA-binding domain of FOXO3, which disrupts FOXO3 interaction with 14-3-3 proteins that are essential for the export of FOXO3 from the nucleus. This induces the nuclear accumulation and activation of FOXO3 even in presence of inhibitory PKB signals. Increased interaction of MST1 and FOXO3 activates the MST1-FOXO3 signaling pathway finally leading to cell death in both primary cultured neurons and rat hippocampal neurons (Xiao et al, 2011). Interestingly, in Drosophila the activation of the JNK/FOXO signaling pathway leads to neuronal resistance to oxidative stress via the expression of Jafrac1 the fly homologue of peroxiredoxin II. Neurons are susceptible to oxidative damage because of their high levels of ROS production and relatively low levels of antioxidant enzymes. Therefore JNK/FOXO suppresses oxidative stress-induced lethality and extends life span in Drosophila (Lee et al, 2009).

6. Are FOXOs tumor suppressor proteins or do they contribute to tumor development?

As FOXO transcription factors were discovered through the cloning of chromosomal breakpoints which were associated with cancer it was proposed that FOXOs act as tumor suppressors. Consistent with their putative role as tumor suppressors, overexpression of FOXOs in cell lines causes cell cycle arrest or cell death. However, depending on posttranslational modifications these transcription factors also regulate detoxification and stress resistance thereby protecting tumor cells from eradication during chemotherapy (Calnan and Brunet 2008). The dual role of FOXOs will be discussed in the following chapters.

6.1 Role of FOXO3 in cancer cell survival and in tumor stem cells

Although FOXOs were first described as tumor suppressor proteins, emerging data also suggest that FOXO transcription factors, in specific FOXO3, may have a "dark side": FOXO3 was shown to support cancer development by protecting tumor cells against oxidative stress by inducing the enzyme MnSOD and PTEN-induced putative kinase-1 (Pink1) (Kops et al, 2002a; Lee et al, 2009; Mei et al, 2009). Deletion of Pink1 sensitizes cells to growth factor withdrawal-induced cell death therefore demonstrating the important role of FOXO3 for protecting cells against growth factor depletion and oxidative stress mediated apoptosis (Mei et al, 2009). Furthermore FOXO3 induces via a negative feedback loop PKB survival signaling in chronic myelogenous leukemia cells. The acquisition of chemoresistance against doxorubicin correlates with activation of FOXO3 and an enhanced PI3K/PKB signaling via induction of PIK3CA, the PI3K catalytic subunit p110alpha (Hui et al, 2008b). In addition FOXO3 promotes multi-drug resistance in chronic myelogenous leukemia cells by inducing MDR1, a plasma membrane P-glycoprotein that functions as an efflux pump for different anticancer drugs. FOXO3 directly binds and activates the MDR1-promoter and increases the MDR1 drug efflux potential. In response to doxorubicin treatment FOXO3 induces in an early response cell cycle arrest and cell death but prolonged exposure promotes the development of cells that are drug resistant due to FOXO3-induced expression of MDR1

(Hui et al, 2008a). In such doxorubicin-resistant cells FOXO3 enhances PI3K/PKB signaling, but active PKB cannot induce the relocalization of FOXO3 from the nucleus to the cytoplasm suggesting that FOXO3 inactivation by PKB is hampered or that strong FOXO3 activating signals override inactivation by PKB. It is not clear, whether such cancer cells evolve by a selection process or whether a small, stem-cell like tumor cell population already exists which benefits from FOXO3 activation because of an already defined intrinsic "FOXO3-stemness longevity program". However, in such drug-resistant cancer cells active FOXO3 does not induce apoptosis or cell cycle arrest but leads to tumor progression and the development of an aggressive phenotype. Such a correlation between FOXO3 activation and adverse disease is not only observed in leukemic tumor cells but also in other types of cancer. For example in invasive ductal breast carcinoma nuclear localization of FOXO3 correlates with lymph node positivity and predicts poor survival (Chen et al, 2010). More recently it was discovered that FOXO3 supports tumor cell invasion via induction of matrix metalloproteinase (MMP)-9 and MMP-13, both of which induce invasion and metastasis of solid tumors (Storz et al, 2009). FOXO3 may not only protect cells against oxidative stress but also prevent the detrimental effects of transitory hypoxia. FOXO3 attenuates the pro-apoptotic response to hypoxia mediated by HIF1 in breast cancer cells by inducing the transcriptional cofactor CITED-2 which in turn controls HIF1 via a negative feedback loop (Bakker et al, 2007). These data clearly support the notion that the tumor suppressor and apoptosis-inducer FOXO3 may even promote cancer progression and metastasis depending on cell type and cellular differentiation stage.

Recently it was shown, that FOXO3 critically regulates tumor stem cell maintenance in chronic myeloid leukemia (CML) which is characterized by the Bcr-Abl genetic abnormality. Bcr-Abl induces the PI3K/PKB signaling pathway which represses the transcriptional activity of FOXO3 in these cancer cells. One of the major problems of CML treatment is the small population of leukemia initiating cells which promote recurrence of the disease. Naka et al. could demonstrate that in these leukemia-initiating cell population FOXO3 localizes to the nucleus and promotes their maintenance and stress resistance (Naka et al, 2010). FOXO3 seems to be the most important regulator of hematopoietic stem cells as FOXO3 is essential for the maintenance of the hematopoietic stem cell pool. Depletion of FOXO3 in hematopoietic stem cells leads to a reduced number of colony-forming cells in long-term co-cultures of bone marrow and stromal cells, an increase in ROS levels, a deficient repopulating capacity in serial transplantation assays, defective maintenance of quiescence and a higher sensitivity to cell cycle dependent myelotoxic agents such as 5-Fluorouracil (Miyamoto et al, 2007). These functions of FOXO3 in normal hematopoietic stem cells are apparently also important for the persistence of cancer stem cells in CML.

Neuroblastoma tumors are derived from embryonal neural stem cells in which FOXO3 may play an essential role in cell survival and replicative capacity similar to neural stem cells in the adult organism. Depending on the original cancer stem cell that gives rise to the tumor, FOXO3 regulation and function may differ explaining the phenomenon that some tumors respond well or even regress without chemotherapy, whereas others are highly resistant to high dose radiation and chemotherapy. Our own studies on neuroblastoma cells demonstrate that DNA-damaging chemotherapeutic drugs such as doxorubicin and etoposide which are also widely used for cancer therapy induce the accumulation of FOXO3 in the nucleus as determined via immunofluorescence analysis in SH-EP neuroblastoma cells expressing a wildtype FOXO3 allele (see Figure 2). FOXO3 induces programmed cell death in SH-EP/FOXO3 and NB15/FOXO3 cells (Obexer et al, 2007) but may also promote death resistance in neuroblastoma tumor cells after prolonged exposure of the cells to chemotherapeutic drugs (unpublished). In high stage neuroblastoma tumors it is frequently observed that almost no immune cells infiltrate the tumor tissue. The role of FOXO3 for immune-surveillance will be discussed in the next chapter.

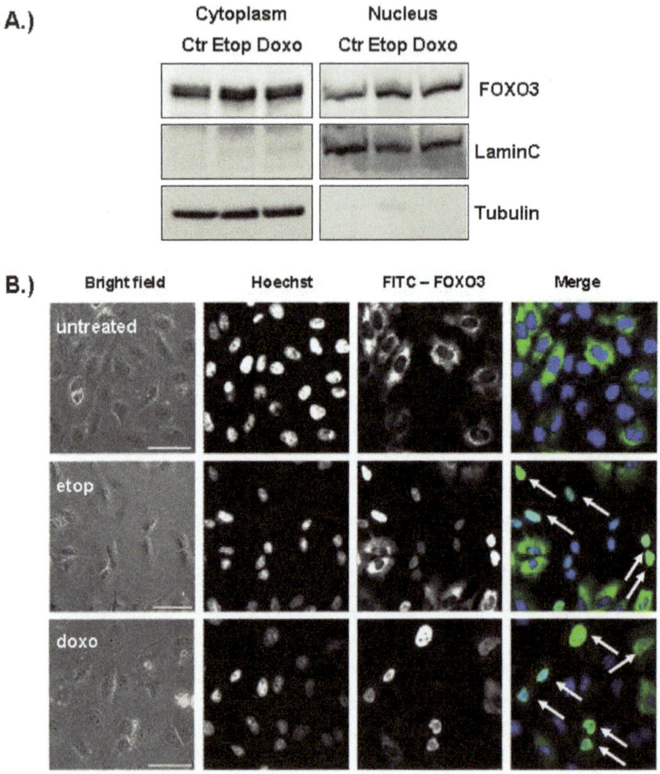

A) The localization of FOXO3 was demonstrated by immunoblot analysis of nuclear and cytoplasmic fractions of untreated, etoposide (20µg/ml) or doxorubicin-treated (0,25µg/ml, for 3 hours) SH-EP/FOXO3-wt cells expressing a wildtype FOXO3 allele. After etoposide and doxorubicin treatment FOXO3 accumulates in the nuclear fraction. Lamin A (nuclear protein) and Tubulin (cytoplasmic protein) were used as purification controls. B) Immunofluorescence analyses of SH-EP/FOXO3-wt cells reveal that in untreated cells FOXO3 localizes to the cytoplasm whereas in etoposide and doxorubicin-treated cells (for 3 hours) FOXO3-FITC is mainly present in the nucleus. Arrows mark nuclei with FOXO3-FITC staining.

Fig. 2. Localization of FOXO3 after treatment with the chemotherapeutic agents doxorubicin (doxo) and etoposide (etop).

6.2 FOXO3 represses immune function and immune surveillance

One aspect of cancer biology that is often neglected by those who focus on signal transduction in cancer cells is the essential role of the immune system in eliminating malignant and precancerous cells. FOXO3 is also involved in this aspect of cancer development as it coordinates immune responses by inducing apoptosis in T-cells thereby maintaining T-cell homeostasis and T-cell activity (Pandiyan et al, 2004; Dejean et al, 2009). Morever FOXO3 is involved in the persistence of $CD4^+$ memory T-cells (Riou et al, 2007). One hallmark of FOXO3 knockout mice is that they develop a multi-inflammatory disease involving the intestine and various other tissues (Lin et al, 2004). This is due to the fact that FOXO3 affects several different players of the immune system: FOXO3 is an essential transcriptional regulator of FoxP3 (Harada et al, 2010) and thereby controls the differentiation of naive T-cells into so-called regulatory T-cells (Treg). Tregs are important in confining the immune reaction and in preventing autoimmune disease. In cancer, however, these immunosuppressive T-cells also infiltrate tumors and repress the anti-cancer activity of cytotoxic T-cells. A deletion of Tregs during cancer therapy, e.g. by blocking FOXO3 could therefore boost the anti-tumor activity of the immune system. In addition it was shown that FOXO3 suppresses the expansion of antigen-specific effector T-cell populations (Wang et al, 2011) which might also hamper anti-cancer immunity. Also another branch of the immune system is significantly influenced by FOXO3: in stimulated dendritic cells, FOXO3 localizes to the nucleus and constrains the production of interleukin-6 and tumor necrosis factor (Dejean et al, 2009). Lack of FOXO3 in dendritic cells enhances T-cell viability and expansion thereby contributing to the pro-inflammatory phenotype. Importantly, in prostate cancer FOXO3 is highly expressed in tumor-associated dendritic cells and thereby induces a suppressive activity in the tumor-specific $CD8^+$ T-cell population. Repression of FOXO3 in dendritic cells using siRNAs upregulated the expression of co-stimulatory molecules and pro-inflammatory cytokines and enhanced the immune responses (Watkins et al, 2011). Silencing of FOXO3 in dendritic cells can be a strategy for the enhancement of anti-tumor immunity and also to overcome immune tolerance. It has not been investigated to date, whether FOXO3 is also involved in immune suppression in neuroblastoma. However, these recent publications imply that FOXO3 activity might rather support the progression of malignancies than preventing them due to its repressive function on the immune system.

6.3 FOXO3 regulates programmed cell death and death sensitivity in neuroblastoma cells

6.3.1 A brief overview on cell death regulation

Apoptosis plays a critical role in tumorigenesis and is a cellular process regulated either via membrane death receptors ("extrinsic pathway") or by the balance of pro- and anti-apoptotic proteins of the BCL2-family at the mitochondria ("intrinsic pathway", see figure 3) (Coultas and Strasser 2003). In the "extrinsic" apoptosis pathway death ligands such as TRAIL and FASLG bind to their cognate receptors thereby inducing the formation of the so called "death inducing signaling complex" (DISC) which consists of the adaptor protein Fas-associated death domain (FADD) and Procaspase-8. In this complex Caspase-8 is activated via autocleavage.

The "intrinsic pathway" is triggered by developmental cues and intracellular stresses such as DNA-damage, growth factor withdrawal and anoikis. It is regulated at the level of mitochondria by the balance of pro- and anti-apoptotic BCL2-proteins, which is also termed BCL2-rheostat (Cory and Adams 2002). The BCL2 protein family is divided into two subgroups: one is the so called "multidomain" family that consists of pro-apoptotic members such as BAX and BAK1/Bak and pro-survival proteins e.g. BCL2, Bcl-xL, BCL2L2/Bcl-w and MCL1. The other subgroup is the BH3-only family, a large group of apoptosis-inducers such as Noxa, BBC3/Puma, BID and Bim. The BH3-only proteins interact with the anti-apoptotic BCL2-proteins thereby antagonizing their pro-survival function (Coultas and Strasser 2003; Shibue and Taniguchi 2006). Two models have been proposed for apoptosis induction by BH3-only proteins: In the "direct activator/de-repressor model" (Kim et al, 2006) strong BH3-only proteins such as Bim, Puma and truncated BID act as direct activators of BAX, whereas in the "displacement model" (Labi et al, 2006; Willis et al, 2007) these three proteins are potent neutralizers of all five BCL2-like pro-survival proteins. Weak BH3-only proteins such as Noxa act as sensitizers by inactivating specific pro-survival BCL2-proteins. Oligomerization of BAX or Bak in the mitochondrial outer membrane causes release of Cytochrome-*c* from mitochondria. Cytochrome-*c* binds to APAF1 that recruits Procaspase-9 and activates the so-called "apoptosome". Once activated Caspase-8 and Caspase-9 cleave the downstream effector Caspases-3 and -7 which provoke cellular destruction, nuclear DNA fragmentation and apoptotic cell death. In some cells, the two pathways intersect since Caspase-8 can process the BCL2-family member BID into its active truncated form (Scaffidi et al, 1998) and thereby activate mitochondrial death signaling.

The activity of Caspases is counteracted by members of the inhibitor of apoptosis protein (IAP) family. In contrast to other IAPs (XIAP, c-IAP1, c-IAP2, NAIP) BIRC5/Survivin contains only a single baculovirus IAP repeat (BIR) and lacks the RING finger domain. Its apoptosis-protecting function therefore is still under debate: Survivin was shown to inhibit effector Caspases via its single BIR domain, but also to act upstream at the level of mitochondria (Shankar et al, 2001; Liu et al, 2004). Survivin is frequently expressed in various malignancies, among them neuroblastoma and leukemia (Adida et al, 1998; Adida et al, 2000; Granziero et al, 2001; Islam et al, 2000). In neuroblastoma the expression of Survivin has been reported to correlate with a reduced apoptotic index *in vivo,* with a shortened overall survival rate, an unfavorable prognosis and an increased relapse rate. We have shown that FOXO3 is an upstream regulator of Survivin in neuroblastoma and that Survivin is critical for sensitivity to chemotherapeutic agents (Obexer et al, 2009).

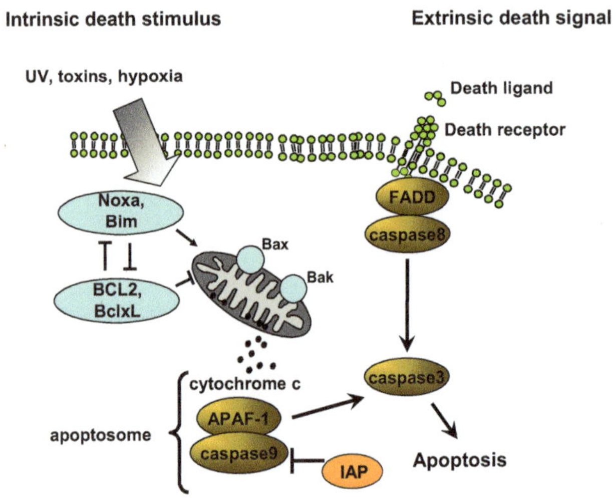

Fig. 3. Schematic presentation of "extrinsic" and "intrinsic" apoptosis signaling in mammalian cells.

6.3.2 FOXO3 in neuroblastoma cells

In neuroblastoma tumors the PI3K/PKB signaling pathway is frequently hyperactivated which leads to proliferation and therapy resistance of the tumor cells. PTEN mutations are rare (below 10%) in neuroblastoma but altered expression of PICT-1, a PTEN-stabilizing protein (Okahara et al, 2006) and aberrant neurotrophic factor signaling may be responsible for the hyperactivation of this signaling pathway. Hyperactivation of PKB was identified as a novel prognostic indicator for adverse clinical outcome and overall survival in neuroblastoma as it correlates with NMYC-amplification, 1p36 deletion, advanced disease stage, age at diagnosis and unfavorable histology (Opel et al, 2007). Several studies indicate that BDNF, by binding to its cognate receptor TrkB (BDNF and TrkB being markers for a poor 5-year survival outcome) increases neuroblastoma tumor cell survival (Feng et al, 2001; Matsumoto et al, 1995; Nakagawara et al, 1993), cell invasion (Matsumoto et al, 1995) and protects neuroblastoma cells from chemotherapy (Middlemas et al, 1999; Scala et al, 1996). BDNF promotes neurite extension (Nakagawara et al, 1993) and survival of sensory neurons (Acheson et al, 1995) under normal conditions. It was shown that the ability of BDNF to rescue neuroblastoma cells from chemotherapy-induced cell death was abrogated by the treatment with the tyrosine kinase inhibitor K252a or the PI3K-inhibitor Ly294002, indicating that both TrkB and PI3K activities are required for survival (Jaboin et al, 2002). In this context, the transcription factors FOXO1, FOXO3 and FOXO4 have been reported to be regulated downstream of Trk receptor signaling (Mai et al, 2002). They can induce apoptosis of cerebellar granule neurons (Brunet et al, 1999). In cortical neurons NGF, BDNF, NT-3 and NT-4 cause inactivation of FOXO3 by phosphorylation through PKB and SGK leading to neurotrophin-mediated cell survival of rat neurons. In concordance the PI3K inhibitor Ly294002 caused decreased phosphorylation of FOXO3 and induced cell death in these rat cells (Zheng et al, 2002). In SH-SY5Y neuroblastoma cells IGF-I signaling is associated with PKB-mediated phosphorylation of FOXO3 and its translocation into the cytoplasm. During growth factor withdrawal-induced apoptosis FOXO3 is imported into the nucleus in these cells (Schwab et al, 2005). Both, TrkB and BDNF may contribute to the chemoresistance of poor prognosis tumors and the suppression of PI3K activity or activation of further downstream targets of this pathway, such as FOXO3, could therefore significantly increase the effects of therapeutic agents on neuroblastoma tumors.

To analyze the connection between deregulated PI3K/PKB survival signaling and impaired apoptotic cell death in neuroblastoma, we determined the protein levels of PKB, FOXO3, phospho-PKB (serine-473) and phospho-FOXO3 (threonine-32) by immunoblot in different neuroblastoma cell lines and found that PKB and FOXO3 were phosphorylated, suggesting the inactivation of FOXO3. To study the function of FOXO3 we infected SH-EP and STA-NB15 neuroblastoma cells (Narath et al, 2007) with retroviruses coding for a 4OH-tamoxifen (4OHT)-regulated FOXO3(A3)ER^{tm} transgene. In the untreated condition this fusion protein is expressed in the cytoplasm. Upon addition of 4OHT it translocates into the nucleus and regulates FOXO3 target genes. Activation of FOXO3 in SH-EP/FOXO3 and NB15/FOXO3 cells promoted loss of mitochondrial activity, Cytochrome-*c*-release and Caspase-dependent apoptosis. FOXO3 induced TRAIL and the BH3-only proteins Noxa and Bim as measured by real time RT-PCR and immunoblot implicating both, extrinsic and intrinsic death pathways. However, expression of dominant negative FADD, which blocks the formation of the DISC and activation of Caspase-8, did not inhibit FOXO3-induced cell death, whereas transgenic expression of BCL2 protected against apoptosis. This excluded the death receptor pathway and suggested that cell death decision is regulated by BCL2-rheostat. Importantly, shRNA-knockdown of the pro-apoptotic BH3-only proteins Noxa or Bim decreased apoptosis, indicating that Noxa and Bim cooperate to mediate FOXO3-induced cell death. In this work we described for the first time that Noxa and Bim establish a connection between FOXO3 and mitochondria and that both BH3-only proteins are critically involved in FOXO3-induced apoptosis in neuroblastoma (Obexer et al, 2007). In a second paper we demonstrated for the first time that repression of the apoptosis inhibitor protein BIRC5/Survivin by FOXO3 sensitizes neuroblastoma cells to DNA-damage- and FOXO3-mediated apoptosis. The survivin gene is located at 17q25 an area that is frequently altered in neuroblastoma. Gain of chromosome 17q or the distal translocation of 17q is of prognostic relevance and correlates with aggressive tumors (Islam et al, 2000). Since activated PKB protects neuroblastoma cells from chemotherapy-induced apoptosis and both, active PKB and Survivin are predictive for an adverse clinical outcome we analyzed a possible connection between PKB and Survivin. We found that inhibition of the PI3K/PKB signaling pathway by the PI3K-inhibitor Ly294002 induces nuclear accumulation of FOXO3 and subsequently represses the pro-survival protein Survivin. Conditional FOXO3 activation repressed Survivin transcription and protein expression. Since the repression of Survivin by FOXO3 can be blocked by cycloheximide we found that in neuroblastoma FOXO3 rather indirectly downregulates the survivin promoter activity. Transgenic Survivin expression exerted a significant anti-apoptotic effect and prevented the accumulation of Bim and BAX at the mitochondria, the loss of mitochondrial membrane potential as well as the release of Cytochrome-*c* during FOXO3-activation and significantly delayed apoptosis. In concordance, Survivin knockdown by retroviral shRNA-technology accelerated FOXO3-induced apoptosis. In this paper we further demonstrated that low-level activation of FOXO3 sensitized neuroblastoma cells to the DNA-damaging agents doxorubicin and etoposide, whereas the overexpression of Survivin diminished FOXO3-sensitization to these drugs. These results suggest that repression of Survivin by FOXO3 facilitates FOXO3-induced apoptosis and sensitizes neuroblastoma cells to apoptosis induced by DNA-damaging agents, which supports the central role of PI3K-PKB-FOXO3 signaling in drug resistance of human neuroblastoma (Obexer et al, 2009).

As FOXO3 induction seems to be beneficial for the treatment in neuroblastoma, we searched for natural compounds that might activate FOXO3. The phytochemical indol-3-carbinol (I3C) which derives from cruciferous vegetables, has been shown to induce cell cycle arrest and apoptosis by targeting BCL2 and the cyclin-dependent kinase inhibitor $p27^{Kip1}$ in colon cancer cells (Aggarwal and Ichikawa 2005). In neuroblastoma cells I3C induces cell death in various cell lines, such as SH-EP, STA-NB1 and STA-NB15. I3C-mediated apoptosis can be blocked via the pan-Caspase-inhibitor zVAD and also via the Caspase-9 inhibitor LEHD demonstrating that I3C induces Caspases-dependent cell death (figure 4A). In SH-EP cells treatment with I3C induced the expression of the BH3-only proteins Noxa and Bim already 4 hours after I3C-treatment and reduced the expression of Survivin after 8 hours (figure 4C). As all three proteins are transcriptional targets of FOXO3 we hypothesized that I3C might induce the translocation and thereby activation of endogenous FOXO3 in neuroblastoma cells. To answer this question we generated SH-EP cells that express an enhanced cyan fluorescent protein (ECFP)-FOXO3 fusion protein which localizes to the cytoplasm in untreated cells. Already 30 minutes after I3C treatment FOXO3 shuttles into the nucleus and after 3 hours almost all cells show nuclear FOXO3 demonstrating that I3C leads to FOXO3-activation (Figure 4B).

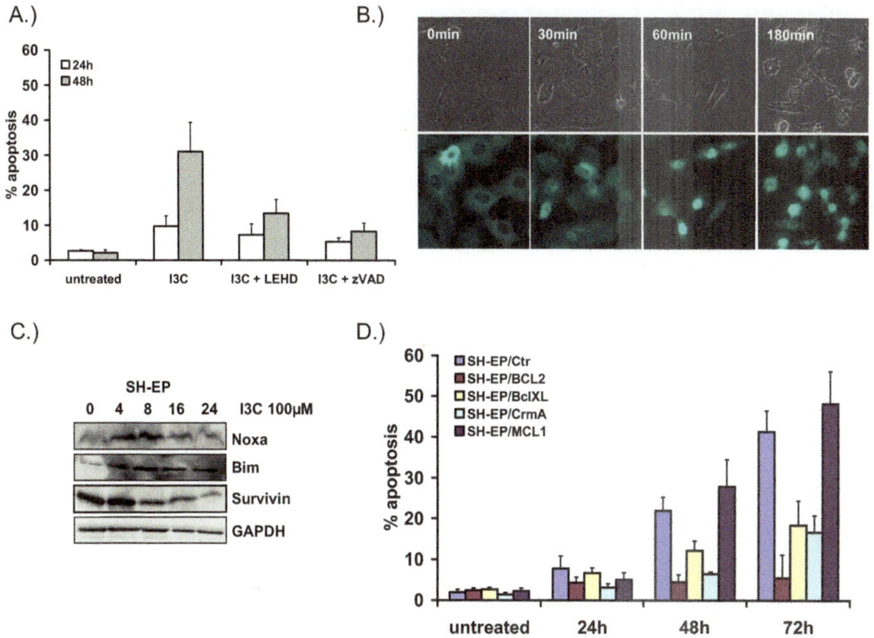

A) SH-EP cells were treated for 24 and 48 hours with I3C (100µM) alone or in combination with the Caspase-9 inhibitor LEHD, or the pan-Caspase-inhibitor zVAD. Apoptosis was determined by PI-FACS analysis. B) SH-EP cells were retrovirally infected with a plasmid coding for ECFP-FOXO3. Treatment of these SH-EP/ECFP-FOXO3 cells for 30, 60 and 180 minutes with 100µM I3C induced translocation of FOXO3 from the cytoplasm to the nucleus as analyzed by live cell fluorescence imaging in an Axiovert200M microscope (Zeiss). C) SH-EP cells were treated for 4, 8, 16 and 24 hours with 100µM I3C and the expression of Noxa, Bim and Survivin was determined by immunoblot. GAPDH was used as loading control. D) SH-EP cells were retrovirally infected with plasmids coding for BCL2, BclxL, CrmA and MCL1. These transgenic cell lines were treated for 24, 48 and 72 hours with 100µM I3C and apoptosis was analyzed by PI-FACS-analysis.

Fig. 4. I3C activates FOXO3 and induces apoptosis in neuroblastoma cells.

Similar to FOXO3-induced apoptosis also I3C-mediated cell death is inhibited by the prosurvival proteins BCL-2 and BclxL implicating that BCL2-rheostat is essential for the control of I3C-induced apoptosis (Obexer et al, 2007). In addition, ectopic expression of CrmA, a Caspase-8 inhibitor of the Cowpox virus, reduced I3C-induced apoptosis suggesting that active Caspase-3 might cleave Caspase-8 and thereby initiate a death-inducing feedback loop. This is also consistent with FOXO3-induced cell death in neuroblastoma cells. Ectopic expression of the pro-survival protein MCL1 had no effect on I3C-mediated apoptosis (figure 4D). The combined results implicate that I3C induces apoptosis at least in part via induction of FOXO3 which in turn activates the BH3-only proteins Bim and Noxa and represses the anti-apoptotic protein Survivin. As inactivation of FOXO3 in malignant neuroblastoma cells critically contributes to apoptosis resistance, strategies to activate FOXO3 in neuroblastoma despite aberrant PKB-signaling, for example by I3C and thereby to restore the function of a deregulated PKB-FOXO3 pathway, may improve the therapy of this malignant disease.

7. Conclusions: FOXO3 – a double-edged sword in therapeutic intervention

FOXO transcription factors were originally identified as tumor suppressor proteins that, when activated or overexpressed in tumor cells, trigger the expression of apoptosis-inducers of the BCL2-family or of the death ligand family. FOXOs integrate a plethora of different signals and translate them into complex, cell-type dependent gene expression patterns. Their transcriptional targets regulate cell cycle arrest and cell death, but may also promote stress resistance and longevity. Therefore the effects of FOXO3 activation might completely differ between different tumor types, but also between differentiation stages of cancer cells within one tumor. This is in particular of importance in human neuroblastoma, which frequently contain tumor cells of various differentiation states. Although in experimental systems with relatively homogenous cell populations FOXO3 is an efficient killer of neuroblastoma cells, the *in vivo* situation might completely differ and active FOXO3 may even support the survival of specific subpopulations of cancer-initiating cells during chemotherapy. The immune-suppressive function of FOXO3 adds an additional level of complexity in the role of FOXOs during cancer development and cancer surveillance. In particular in high-stage neuroblastoma, where immune infiltrations are almost absent, the activation of FOXO3 in immune cells, possibly as an unwanted side-effect of chemotherapy, may shut down tumor-specific cytotoxic immune responses. Therefore it has to be carefully investigated for which specific subtype of cancer FOXO3 is an attractive target and whether the inhibition of FOXO3 in immune cells may boost anti-cancer immune responses. So this double-edged sword has to be manipulated and handled with care otherwise it will cause detrimental damage.

8. References

Acheson, A., Conover J. C., Fandl J. P., DeChiara T. M., Russell M., Thadani A., Squinto S. P., Yancopoulos G. D. and Lindsay R. M. (1995). A BDNF autocrine loop in adult sensory neurons prevents cell death. *Nature* 374, 450-453.

Adida, C., Berrebi D., Peuchmaur M., Reyes-Mugica M. and Altieri D. C. (1998). Anti-apoptosis gene, survivin, and prognosis of neuroblastoma. *Lancet* 351, 882-883.

Adida, C., Recher C., Raffoux E., Daniel M. T., Taksin A. L., Rousselot P., Sigaux F., Degos L., Altieri D. C. and Dombret H. (2000). Expression and prognostic significance of survivin in de novo acute myeloid leukaemia. *Br. J. Haematol.* 111, 196-203.

Aggarwal, B. B. and Ichikawa H. (2005). Molecular targets and anticancer potential of indole-3-carbinol and its derivatives. *Cell Cycle* 4, 1201-1215.

Alvarez, B., Martinez A., Burgering B. M. and Carrera A. C. (2001). Forkhead transcription factors contribute to execution of the mitotic programme in mammals. *Nature* 413, 744-747.

Arden, K. C. (2008a). FOXO animal models reveal a variety of diverse roles for FOXO transcription factors. *Oncogene* 27, 2345-2350.

Arden, K. C. (2008b). FOXO animal models reveal a variety of diverse roles for FOXO transcription factors. *Oncogene* 27, 2345-2350.

Arnold, C. P., Tan R., Zhou B., Yue S. B., Schaffert S., Biggs J. R., Doyonnas R., Lo M. C., Perry J. M., Renault V. M. et al. (2011). MicroRNA programs in normal and aberrant stem and progenitor cells. *Genome Res.* 21, 798-810.

Bakker, W. J., Harris I. S. and Mak T. W. (2007). FOXO3a is activated in response to hypoxic stress and inhibits HIF1-induced apoptosis via regulation of CITED2. *Mol. Cell* 28, 941-953.

Biggs, W. H., Meisenhelder J., Hunter T., Cavenee W. K. and Arden K. C. (1999). Protein kinase B/Akt-mediated phosphorylation promotes nuclear exclusion of the winged helix transcription factor FKHR1. *Proc. Natl. Acad. Sci. U. S. A* 96, 7421-7426.

Bond, J., Roberts E., Mochida G. H., Hampshire D. J., Scott S., Askham J. M., Springell K., Mahadevan M., Crow Y. J., Markham A. F. et al. (2002). ASPM is a major determinant of cerebral cortical size. *Nat. Genet.* 32, 316-320.

Brett, J. O., Renault V. M., Rafalski V. A., Webb A. E. and Brunet A. (2011). The microRNA cluster miR-106b~25 regulates adult neural stem/progenitor cell proliferation and neuronal differentiation. *Aging* 3, 108-124.

Brunet, A., Bonni A., Zigmond M. J., Lin M. Z., Juo P., Hu L. S., Anderson M. J., Arden K. C., Blenis J. and Greenberg M. E. (1999). Akt promotes cell survival by phosphorylating and inhibiting a Forkhead transcription factor. *Cell* 96, 857-868.

Brunet, A., Sweeney L. B., Sturgill J. F., Chua K. F., Greer P. L., Lin Y., Tran H., Ross S. E., Mostoslavsky R., Cohen H. Y. et al. (2004). Stress-dependent regulation of FOXO transcription factors by the SIRT1 deacetylase. *Science* 303, 2011-2015.

Calnan, D. R. and Brunet A. (2008). The FoxO code. *Oncogene* 27, 2276-2288.

Carlsson, P. and Mahlapuu M. (2002). Forkhead transcription factors: key players in development and metabolism. *Dev. Biol.* 250, 1-23.

Castrillon, D. H., Miao L., Kollipara R., Horner J. W. and DePinho R. A. (2003). Suppression of ovarian follicle activation in mice by the transcription factor Foxo3a. *Science* 301, 215-218.

Chen, J., Gomes A. R., Monteiro L. J., Wong S. Y., Wu L. H., Ng T. T., Karadedou C. T., Millour J., Ip Y. C., Cheung Y. N. et al. (2010). Constitutively Nuclear FOXO3a Localization Predicts Poor Survival and Promotes Akt Phosphorylation in Breast Cancer. *Plos One* 5.

Chong, Z. Z., Li F. and Maiese K. (2005). Oxidative stress in the brain: novel cellular targets that govern survival during neurodegenerative disease. *Prog. Neurobiol.* 75, 207-246.

Coffer, P. J. and Burgering B. M. (2004). Forkhead-box transcription factors and their role in the immune system. *Nat. Rev. Immunol.* 4, 889-899.

Cory, S. and Adams J. M. (2002). The Bcl2 family: regulators of the cellular life-or-death switch. *Nat. Rev. Cancer* 2, 647-656.

Coultas, L. and Strasser A. (2003). The role of the Bcl-2 protein family in cancer. *Semin. Cancer Biol.* 13, 115-123.

Dejean, A. S., Beisner D. R., Ch'en I. L., Kerdiles Y. M., Babour A., Arden K. C., Castrillon D. H., DePinho R. A. and Hedrick S. M. (2009). Transcription factor Foxo3 controls the magnitude of T cell immune responses by modulating the function of dendritic cells. *Nat. Immunol.* 10, 504-513.

Dijkers, P. F., Medema R. H., Lammers J. W. J., Koenderman L. and Coffer P. J. (2000a). Expression of the pro-apoptotic Bcl-2 family member Bim is regulated by the forkhead transcription factor FKHR-L1. *Current Biology* 10, 1201-1204.

Dijkers, P. F., Medema R. H., Pals C., Banerji L., Thomas N. S., Lam E. W., Burgering B. M., Raaijmakers J. A., Lammers J. W., Koenderman L. et al. (2000b). Forkhead transcription factor FKHR-L1 modulates cytokine-dependent transcriptional regulation of p27(KIP1). *Mol. Cell Biol.* 20, 9138-9148.

Essers, M. A., Vries-Smits L. M., Barker N., Polderman P. E., Burgering B. M. and Korswagen H. C. (2005). Functional interaction between beta-catenin and FOXO in oxidative stress signaling. *Science* 308, 1181-1184.

Essers, M. A., Weijzen S., Vries-Smits A. M., Saarloos I., de Ruiter N. D., Bos J. L. and Burgering B. M. (2004). FOXO transcription factor activation by oxidative stress mediated by the small GTPase Ral and JNK. *EMBO J.* 23, 4802-4812.

Feng, X., Jiang H., Baik J. C., Edgar C. and Eide F. F. (2001). BDNF dependence in neuroblastoma. *J. Neurosci. Res.* 64, 355-363.

Fernandez, d. M., Essafi A., Soeiro I., Pietersen A. M., Birkenkamp K. U., Edwards C. S., Martino A., Nelson B. H., Francis J. M., Jones M. C. et al. (2004). FoxO3a and BCR-ABL regulate cyclin D2 transcription through a STAT5/BCL6-dependent mechanism. *Mol. Cell Biol.* 24, 10058-10071.

Fukunaga, K., Ishigami T. and Kawano T. (2005). Transcriptional regulation of neuronal genes and its effect on neural functions: expression and function of forkhead transcription factors in neurons. *J. Pharmacol. Sci.* 98, 205-211.

Furukawa-Hibi, Y., Yoshida-Araki K., Ohta T., Ikeda K. and Motoyama N. (2002). FOXO forkhead transcription factors induce G(2)-M checkpoint in response to oxidative stress. *J. Biol. Chem.* 277, 26729-26732.

Furuyama, T., Nakazawa T., Nakano I. and Mori N. (2000). Identification of the differential distribution patterns of mRNAs and consensus binding sequences for mouse DAF-16 homologues. *Biochem. J.* 349, 629-634.

Gan, L., Zheng W., Chabot J. G., Unterman T. G. and Quirion R. (2005). Nuclear/cytoplasmic shuttling of the transcription factor FoxO1 is regulated by neurotrophic factors. *J. Neurochem.* 93, 1209-1219.

Gilley, J., Coffer P. J. and Ham J. (2003). FOXO transcription factors directly activate bim gene expression and promote apoptosis in sympathetic neurons. *J. Cell Biol.* 162, 613-622.

Granziero, L., Ghia P., Circosta P., Gottardi D., Strola G., Geuna M., Montagna L., Piccoli P., Chilosi M. and Caligaris-Cappio F. (2001). Survivin is expressed on CD40 stimulation and interfaces proliferation and apoptosis in B-cell chronic lymphocytic leukemia. *Blood* 97, 2777-2783.

Harada, Y., Harada Y., Elly C., Ying G., Paik J. H., DePinho R. A. and Liu Y. C. (2010). Transcription factors Foxo3a and Foxo1 couple the E3 ligase Cbl-b to the induction of Foxp3 expression in induced regulatory T cells. *Journal of Experimental Medicine* 207, 1381-1391.

Hosaka, T., Biggs W. H., III, Tieu D., Boyer A. D., Varki N. M., Cavenee W. K. and Arden K. C. (2004). Disruption of forkhead transcription factor (FOXO) family members in mice reveals their functional diversification. *Proc. Natl. Acad. Sci. U. S. A* 101, 2975-2980.

Hu, M. C., Lee D. F., Xia W., Golfman L. S., Ou-Yang F., Yang J. Y., Zou Y., Bao S., Hanada N., Saso H. et al. (2004). IkappaB kinase promotes tumorigenesis through inhibition of forkhead FOXO3a. *Cell* 117, 225-237.

Hui, R. C., Francis R. E., Guest S. K., Costa J. R., Gomes A. R., Myatt S. S., Brosens J. J. and Lam E. W. (2008a). Doxorubicin activates FOXO3a to induce the expression of multidrug resistance gene ABCB1 (MDR1) in K562 leukemic cells. *Mol. Cancer Ther.* 7, 670-678.

Hui, R. C., Gomes A. R., Constantinidou D., Costa J. R., Karadedou C. T., Fernandez de M. S., Wymann M. P., Brosens J. J., Schulze A. and Lam E. W. (2008b). The forkhead transcription factor FOXO3a increases phosphoinositide-3 kinase/Akt activity in drug-resistant leukemic cells through induction of PIK3CA expression. *Mol. Cell Biol.* 28, 5886-5898.

Islam, A., Kageyama H., Takada N., Kawamoto T., Takayasu H., Isogai E., Ohira M., Hashizume K., Kobayashi H., Kaneko Y. et al. (2000). High expression of Survivin, mapped to 17q25, is significantly associated with poor prognostic factors and promotes cell survival in human neuroblastoma. *Oncogene* 19, 617-623.

Jaboin, J., Kim C. J., Kaplan D. R. and Thiele C. J. (2002). Brain-derived neurotrophic factor activation of TrkB protects neuroblastoma cells from chemotherapy-induced apoptosis via phosphatidylinositol 3'-kinase pathway. *Cancer Res.* 62, 6756-6763.

Katoh, M. and Katoh M. (2004). Human FOX gene family (Review). *Int. J. Oncol.* 25, 1495-1500.

Kim, H., Rafiuddin-Shah M., Tu H. C., Jeffers J. R., Zambetti G. P., Hsieh J. J. and Cheng E. H. (2006). Hierarchical regulation of mitochondrion-dependent apoptosis by BCL-2 subfamilies. *Nat. Cell Biol.* 8, 1348-1358.

Kops, G. J., Dansen T. B., Polderman P. E., Saarloos I., Wirtz K. W., Coffer P. J., Huang T. T., Bos J. L., Medema R. H. and Burgering B. M. (2002a). Forkhead transcription factor FOXO3a protects quiescent cells from oxidative stress. *Nature* 419, 316-321.

Kops, G. J. P. L., Medema R. H., Glassford J., Essers M. A. G., Dijkers P. F., Coffer P. J., Lam E. W. F. and Burgering B. M. T. (2002b). Control of cell cycle exit and entry by protein kinase B-regulated Forkhead transcription factors. *Molecular and Cellular Biology* 22, 2025-2036.

Labi, V., Erlacher M., Kiessling S. and Villunger A. (2006). BH3-only proteins in cell death initiation, malignant disease and anticancer therapy. *Cell Death. Differ.* 13, 1325-1338.

Lal, A. and Gorospe M. (2006). Egad, more forms of gene regulation: the gadd45a story. *Cell Cycle* 5, 1422-1425.

Lee, K. S., Iijima-Ando K., Iijima K., Lee W. J., Lee J. H., Yu K. and Lee D. S. (2009). JNK/FOXO-mediated neuronal expression of fly homologue of peroxiredoxin II reduces oxidative stress and extends life span. *J. Biol. Chem.* 284, 29454-29461.

Lehtinen, M. K., Yuan Z., Boag P. R., Yang Y., Villen J., Becker E. B., DiBacco S., de l., I, Gygi S., Blackwell T. K. et al. (2006). A conserved MST-FOXO signaling pathway mediates oxidative-stress responses and extends life span. *Cell* 125, 987-1001.

Leisser, C., Rosenberger G., Maier S., Fuhrmann G., Grusch M., Strasser S., Huettenbrenner S., Fassl S., Polgar D., Krieger S. et al. (2004). Subcellular localisation of Cdc25A determines cell fate. *Cell Death. Differ.* 11, 80-89.

Li, J., Yen C., Liaw D., Podsypanina K., Bose S., Wang S. I., Puc J., Miliaresis C., Rodgers L., McCombie R. et al. (1997). PTEN, a putative protein tyrosine phosphatase gene mutated in human brain, breast, and prostate cancer. *Science* 275, 1943-1947.

Lin, K., Dorman J. B., Rodan A. and Kenyon C. (1997). daf-16: An HNF-3/forkhead family member that can function to double the life-span of Caenorhabditis elegans. *Science* 278, 1319-1322.

Lin, L., Hron J. D. and Peng S. L. (2004). Regulation of NF-kappaB, Th activation, and autoinflammation by the forkhead transcription factor Foxo3a. *Immunity.* 21, 203-213.

Liu, T., Brouha B. and Grossman D. (2004). Rapid induction of mitochondrial events and caspase-independent apoptosis in Survivin-targeted melanoma cells. *Oncogene* 23, 39-48.

Mai, L., Jope R. S. and Li X. (2002). BDNF-mediated signal transduction is modulated by GSK3beta and mood stabilizing agents. *J. Neurochem.* 82, 75-83.

Matsumoto, K., Wada R. K., Yamashiro J. M., Kaplan D. R. and Thiele C. J. (1995). Expression of brain-derived neurotrophic factor and p145TrkB affects survival, differentiation, and invasiveness of human neuroblastoma cells. *Cancer Res.* 55, 1798-1806.

Mei, Y., Zhang Y., Yamamoto K., Xie W., Mak T. W. and You H. (2009). FOXO3a-dependent regulation of Pink1 (Park6) mediates survival signaling in response to cytokine deprivation. *Proc. Natl. Acad. Sci. U. S. A* 106, 5153-5158.

Middlemas, D. S., Kihl B. K., Zhou J. and Zhu X. (1999). Brain-derived neurotrophic factor promotes survival and chemoprotection of human neuroblastoma cells. *J. Biol. Chem.* 274, 16451-16460.

Miyaguchi, Y., Tsuchiya K. and Sakamoto K. (2009). P53 negatively regulates the transcriptional activity of FOXO3a under oxidative stress. *Cell Biol. Int.* 33, 853-860.

Miyamoto, K., Araki K. Y., Naka K., Arai F., Takubo K., Yamazaki S., Matsuoka S., Miyamoto T., Ito K., Ohmura M. et al. (2007). Foxo3a is essential for maintenance of the hematopoietic stem cell pool. *Cell Stem Cell* 1, 101-112.

Modur, V., Nagarajan R., Evers B. M. and Milbrandt J. (2002). FOXO proteins regulate tumor necrosis factor-related apoptosis inducing ligand expression. Implications for PTEN mutation in prostate cancer. *J. Biol. Chem.* 277, 47928-47937.

Naka, K., Hoshii T., Muraguchi T., Tadokoro Y., Ooshio T., Kondo Y., Nakao S., Motoyama N. and Hirao A. (2010). TGF-beta-FOXO signalling maintains leukaemia-initiating cells in chronic myeloid leukaemia. *Nature* 463, 676-680.

Nakagawara, A., Arima-Nakagawara M., Scavarda N. J., Azar C. G., Cantor A. B. and Brodeur G. M. (1993). Association between high levels of expression of the TRK gene and favorable outcome in human neuroblastoma. *N. Engl. J. Med.* 328, 847-854.

Narath, R., Ambros I. M., Kowalska A., Bozsaky E., Boukamp P. and Ambros P. F. (2007). Induction of senescence in MYCN amplified neuroblastoma cell lines by hydroxyurea. *Genes Chromosomes. Cancer* 46, 130-142.

Obexer, P., Geiger K., Ambros P. F., Meister B. and Ausserlechner M. J. (2007). FKHRL1-mediated expression of Noxa and Bim induces apoptosis via the mitochondria in neuroblastoma cells. *Cell Death. Differ.* 14, 534-547.

Obexer, P., Hagenbuchner J., Unterkircher T., Sachsenmaier N., Seifarth C., Bock G., Porto V., Geiger K. and Ausserlechner M. (2009). Repression of BIRC5/Survivin by FOXO3/FKHRL1 Sensitizes Human Neuroblastoma Cells to DNA-Damage-induced Apoptosis. *Mol. Biol. Cell.*

Obsil T and Obsilova V. Structural basis for DNA recognition by FOXO proteins. Biochim Biophys Acta 71(3), 946-954. 2010.

Okahara, F., Itoh K., Nakagawara A., Murakami M., Kanaho Y. and Maehama T. (2006). Critical role of PICT-1, a tumor suppressor candidate, in phosphatidylinositol 3,4,5-trisphosphate signals and tumorigenic transformation. *Mol. Biol. Cell* 17, 4888-4895.

Opel, D., Poremba C., Simon T., Debatin K. M. and Fulda S. (2007). Activation of Akt predicts poor outcome in neuroblastoma. *Cancer Res.* 67, 735-745.

Paik, J. H., Ding Z., Narurkar R., Ramkissoon S., Muller F., Kamoun W. S., Chae S. S., Zheng H., Ying H., Mahoney J. et al. (2009). FoxOs cooperatively regulate diverse pathways governing neural stem cell homeostasis. *Cell Stem Cell* 5, 540-553.

Paik, J. H., Kollipara R., Chu G., Ji H., Xiao Y., Ding Z., Miao L., Tothova Z., Horner J. W., Carrasco D. R. et al. (2007). FoxOs are lineage-restricted redundant tumor suppressors and regulate endothelial cell homeostasis. *Cell* 128, 309-323.

Pandiyan, P., Gartner D., Soezeri O., Radbruch A., Schulze-Osthoff K. and Brunner-Weinzierl M. C. (2004). CD152 (CTLA-4) determines the unequal resistance of Th1 and Th2 cells against activation-induced cell death by a mechanism requiring PI3 kinase function. *J. Exp. Med.* 199, 831-842.

Peltier, J., O'Neill A. and Schaffer D. V. (2007). PI3K/Akt and CREB regulate adult neural hippocampal progenitor proliferation and differentiation. *Dev. Neurobiol.* 67, 1348-1361.

Pirianov, G., Brywe K. G., Mallard C., Edwards A. D., Flavell R. A., Hagberg H. and Mehmet H. (2007). Deletion of the c-Jun N-terminal kinase 3 gene protects neonatal mice against cerebral hypoxic-ischaemic injury. *J. Cereb. Blood Flow Metab* 27, 1022-1032.

Ramaswamy, S., Nakamura N., Sansal I., Bergeron L. and Sellers W. R. (2002). A novel mechanism of gene regulation and tumor suppression by the transcription factor FKHR. *Cancer Cell* 2, 81-91.

Rena, G., Woods Y. L., Prescott A. R., Peggie M., Unterman T. G., Williams M. R. and Cohen P. (2002). Two novel phosphorylation sites on FKHR that are critical for its nuclear exclusion. *EMBO J.* 21, 2263-2271.

Renault, V. M., Rafalski V. A., Morgan A. A., Salih D. A., Brett J. O., Webb A. E., Villeda S. A., Thekkat P. U., Guillerey C., Denko N. C. et al. (2009). FoxO3 regulates neural stem cell homeostasis. *Cell Stem Cell* 5, 527-539.

Riou, C., Yassine-Diab B., Van grevenynghe J., Somogyi R., Greller L. D., Gagnon D., Gimmig S., Wilkinson P., Shi Y., Cameron M. J. et al. (2007). Convergence of TCR and cytokine signaling leads to FOXO3a phosphorylation and drives the survival of CD4+ central memory T cells. *J. Exp. Med.* 204, 79-91.

Sakai, A., Thieblemont C., Wellmann A., Jaffe E. S. and Raffeld M. (1998). PTEN gene alterations in lymphoid neoplasms. *Blood* 92, 3410-3415.

Scaffidi, C., Fulda S., Srinivasan A., Friesen C., Li F., Tomaselli K. J., Debatin K. M., Krammer P. H. and Peter M. E. (1998). Two CD95 (APO-1/Fas) signaling pathways. *EMBO J.* 17, 1675-1687.

Scala, S., Wosikowski K., Giannakakou P., Valle P., Biedler J. L., Spengler B. A., Lucarelli E., Bates S. E. and Thiele C. J. (1996). Brain-derived neurotrophic factor protects neuroblastoma cells from vinblastine toxicity. *Cancer Res.* 56, 3737-3742.

Schmidt, M., Fernandez d. M., van der H. A., Klompmaker R., Kops G. J., Lam E. W., Burgering B. M. and Medema R. H. (2002). Cell cycle inhibition by FoxO forkhead transcription factors involves downregulation of cyclin D. *Mol. Cell Biol.* 22, 7842-7852.

Schwab, T. S., Madison B. B., Grauman A. R. and Feldman E. L. (2005). Insulin-like growth factor-I induces the phosphorylation and nuclear exclusion of forkhead transcription factors in human neuroblastoma cells. *Apoptosis.* 10, 831-840.

Seoane, J., Le H. V., Shen L., Anderson S. A. and Massague J. (2004). Integration of Smad and forkhead pathways in the control of neuroepithelial and glioblastoma cell proliferation. *Cell* 117, 211-223.

Shankar, S. L., Mani S., O'Guin K. N., Kandimalla E. R., Agrawal S. and Shafit-Zagardo B. (2001). Survivin inhibition induces human neural tumor cell death through caspase-independent and -dependent pathways. *J. Neurochem.* 79, 426-436.

Shibue, T. and Taniguchi T. (2006). BH3-only proteins: Integrated control point of apoptosis. *Int. J. Cancer* 119, 2036-2043.

Siegrist,S.E., Hague,N.S., Chen,C.H., Hay,B.A. and Hariharan,I.K. (2010). Inactivation of Both foxo and reaper Promotes Long-Term Adult Neurogenesis in Drosophila. *Current Biology* 20, 643-648

Storz, P., Doppler H., Copland J. A., Simpson K. J. and Toker A. (2009). FOXO3a promotes tumor cell invasion through the induction of matrix metalloproteinases. *Mol. Cell Biol.* 29, 4906-4917.

Sunters, A., Madureira P. A., Pomeranz K. M., Aubert M., Brosens J. J., Cook S. J., Burgering B. M., Coombes R. C. and Lam E. W. (2006). Paclitaxel-induced nuclear translocation of FOXO3a in breast cancer cells is mediated by c-Jun NH2-terminal kinase and Akt. *Cancer Res.* 66, 212-220.

Tang, T. T., Dowbenko D., Jackson A., Toney L., Lewin D. A., Dent A. L. and Lasky L. A. (2002). The forkhead transcription factor AFX activates apoptosis by induction of the BCL-6 transcriptional repressor. *J. Biol. Chem.* 277, 14255-14265.

Tothova, Z., Kollipara R., Huntly B. J., Lee B. H., Castrillon D. H., Cullen D. E., McDowell E. P., Lazo-Kallanian S., Williams I. R., Sears C. et al. (2007b). FoxOs are critical mediators of hematopoietic stem cell resistance to physiologic oxidative stress. *Cell* 128, 325-339.

Tothova, Z., Kollipara R., Huntly B. J., Lee B. H., Castrillon D. H., Cullen D. E., McDowell E. P., Lazo-Kallanian S., Williams I. R., Sears C. et al. (2007a). FoxOs are critical mediators of hematopoietic stem cell resistance to physiologic oxidative stress. *Cell* 128, 325-339.

Tran, H., Brunet A., Grenier J. M., Datta S. R., Fornace A. J., Jr., DiStefano P. S., Chiang L. W. and Greenberg M. E. (2002). DNA repair pathway stimulated by the forkhead transcription factor FOXO3a through the Gadd45 protein. *Science* 296, 530-534.

van der Horst A., Vries-Smits A. M., Brenkman A. B., van Triest M. H., van den B. N., Colland F., Maurice M. M. and Burgering B. M. (2006). FOXO4 transcriptional activity is regulated by monoubiquitination and USP7/HAUSP. *Nat. Cell Biol.* 8, 1064-1073.

van der Vos, K. E. and Coffer P. J. (2008). FOXO-binding partners: it takes two to tango. *Oncogene* 27, 2289-2299.

Wang F, Chan CH, Chen K, Guan X, Lin HK and Tong Q. Deacetylation of FOXO3 by SIRT1 or SIRT2 leads to Skp2-mediated FOXO3 ubiquitination and degradation. Oncogene , 1-12. 2011.

Wang, S. T., Chang C. C., Yen M. C., Tu C. F., Chu C. L., Peng Y. T., Chen D. Y., Lan J. L. and Lin C. C. (2011). RNA interference-mediated silencing of Foxo3 in antigen-presenting cells as a strategy for the enhancement of DNA vaccine potency. *Gene Ther.* 18, 372-383.

Watkins, S. K., Zhu Z. Q., Riboldi E., Shafer-Weaver K. A., Stagliano K. E. R., Sklavos M. M., Ambs S., Yagita H. and Hurwitz A. A. (2011). FOXO3 programs tumor-associated DCs to become tolerogenic in human and murine prostate cancer. *Journal of Clinical Investigation* 121, 1361-1372.

Weigelt, J., Climent I., Dahlman-Wright K. and Wikstrom M. (2001). Solution structure of the DNA binding domain of the human forkhead transcription factor AFX (FOXO4). *Biochemistry* 40, 5861-5869.

Willis, S. N., Fletcher J. I., Kaufmann T., van Delft M. F., Chen L., Czabotar P. E., Ierino H., Lee E. F., Fairlie W. D., Bouillet P. et al. (2007). Apoptosis initiated when BH3 ligands engage multiple Bcl-2 homologs, not Bax or Bak. *Science* 315, 856-859.

Won, C. K., Ji H. H. and Koh P. O. (2006). Estradiol prevents the focal cerebral ischemic injury-induced decrease of forkhead transcription factors phosphorylation. *Neurosci. Lett.* 398, 39-43.

Woods, Y. L., Rena G., Morrice N., Barthel A., Becker W., Guo S., Unterman T. G. and Cohen P. (2001). The kinase DYRK1A phosphorylates the transcription factor FKHR at Ser329 in vitro, a novel in vivo phosphorylation site. *Biochem. J.* 355, 597-607.

Xiao, L., Chen D., Hu P., Wu J., Liu W., Zhao Y., Cao M., Fang Y., Bi W., Zheng Z. et al. (2011). The c-Abl-MST1 Signaling Pathway Mediates Oxidative Stress-Induced Neuronal Cell Death. *J. Neurosci.* 31, 9611-9619.

Xuan, Z. and Zhang M. Q. (2005). From worm to human: bioinformatics approaches to identify FOXO target genes. *Mech. Ageing Dev.* 126, 209-215.

Yamada, K. M. and Araki M. (2001). Tumor suppressor PTEN: modulator of cell signaling, growth, migration and apoptosis. *J. Cell Sci.* 114, 2375-2382.

Yano, S., Morioka M., Fukunaga K., Kawano T., Hara T., Kai Y., Hamada J., Miyamoto E. and Ushio Y. (2001). Activation of Akt/protein kinase B contributes to induction of ischemic tolerance in the CA1 subfield of gerbil hippocampus. *J. Cereb. Blood Flow Metab* 21, 351-360.

Zheng, W. H., Kar S. and Quirion R. (2000). Insulin-like growth factor-1-induced phosphorylation of the forkhead family transcription factor FKHRL1 is mediated by Akt kinase in PC12 cells. *J. Biol. Chem.* 275, 39152-39158.

Zheng, W. H., Kar S. and Quirion R. (2002). FKHRL1 and its homologs are new targets of nerve growth factor Trk receptor signaling. *J. Neurochem.* 80, 1049-1061.

17

Oncolytic Poliovirus Therapy in a Mouse Model of Neuroblastoma: Preclinical Data Analysis and Future Studies

Hidemi Toyoda, Eckard Wimmer and Jeronimo Cello
*Department of Molecular Genetics and Microbiology, Stony Brook University
Stony Brook, NewYork
USA*

1. Introduction

Neuroblastoma, a malignant embryonal tumor of the neural crest cells, is one of the most common solid extracranial tumors of early childhood (Brodeur et al., 2006). The prevalence of neuroblastoma in children is 7.5 cases /100, 000 infants (Brodeur et al., 2006; Gao et al, 1997; Gurney et al., 1997; Spix et al., 2006). Furthermore, the annual incidence of this tumor is nearly 1.0/100,000 children under the age of 15 years (Ries et al., 2005). Neuroblastoma comprises about 8-10% of all childhood cancers and for approximately 15% of cancer deaths in children (Gao et al., 1997; Ries et al., 2005). Neuroblastoma can arise anywhere along the sympathetic nervous system. Fifty percent of the tumors originate in the adrenal medulla. Additional sites of origin include the nerve tissue in the chest, neck, pelvis or abdomen (Ries et al., 2005). Clinical presentation of neuroblastoma is highly variable and is dependent on the site of the primary tumor, as well as on the disease extent and on the absence or presence of paraneoplastic syndromes (Maris & Matthay, 1999; Park et al., 2008). The three main clinical scenarios are: localized, metastatic and 4S (S for special).
In contrast to many other pediatric malignancies, progress in treatment of neuroblastoma (especially for advanced-stage tumors) has been relatively modest. Hence, at present, this tumor still poses a major challenge to the pediatric oncologist. Current treatment strategies include any or all of the following; watchfulwaiting, surgery, mild to aggressive chemotherapy, radiotherapy, and bone marrow transplants. Several new agents and combinations are in ongoing trials for relapsed neuroblastoma, including topoisomerase 1 inhibitors, radionuclides, histone deacetylase and tyrosine kinase inhibitors, monoclonal antibodies directed to disialoganglioside, and angiogenesis inhibitors (Maris & Matthay, 1999). As neuroblastoma is a disease that most often strikes young children, treating patients with aggressive therapy is a concern because of the potential for long-term health implications (from heart disease to second malignancies). Some children with neuroblastoma can be cured, and for these children, oncologists must try to give the minimum treatment possible while achieving cure. Although a fraction of the patients are cured with current treatments, approximately 40 per cent will die of this disease; for these patients improved treatment options are imperative (Matthay et al., 1999, 2009).

2. Virotherapy for cancer

Poor response to conventional treatment is not only observed in neuroblastoma but also in many prevalent tumors. In fact, despite aggressive radio-and chemotherapy, the long-term survival from common cancers such as prostate, breast, colorectal and lung has barely budged since the 1970s (Leaf, 2004). Therefore new cancer treatments with novel mechanisms of action are needed.

Such new treatments may be based on human non-pathogenic and pathogenic viruses (for review see Kirn et al., 2001; Parato et al., 2005; Vähä-Koskela et al., 2007). An oncolytic virus is a replicating agent that has either been naturally selected or engineered to single out and destroy tumor cells. For a long time, viruses have been under scrutiny for their potential antineoplastic effects (Sinkovics and Horvath, 1993). Historically, human trials were initiated with several potential oncolytic viruses during the 1950' and 1960's. Among the first viruses to be tested as oncolytic agents were rabies virus (DePace, 1912; Pack, 1950), several adenovirus serotypes (Huebner et al., 1956; Southam et al., 1952), mumps virus (Asada, 1974; Okuno et al., 1978), and West Nile virus (Southam & Moore, 1952). Moreover, 19 different viruses were evaluated in patients suffering from various types of cancer (Newman & Southam, 1954; Wheelock & Dingle, 1964). In general, the outcome of these treatments were tantalizing, but ultimately disappointing and the approach was temporarily abandoned. The onset of the gene therapy era in 1990s reinvigorated the field of viral therapy for cancer (virotherapy). Many of the basic principles of virus-mediated oncolysis apply equally to gene therapy vectors and oncolytic viruses. The main advantage of replication-competent oncolytic viruses over non-replicanting viral gene therapy is the ability to propagate and spread from the site of inoculation throughout tumor mass and beyond. Following the successful attempt to engineer a Herpes virus simplex-1 (HSV-1) mutant that selectively destroyed brain tumor cells (Martuza et al., 1991), the field of virotherapy has expanded considerably. There are now more 90 different DNA and RNA virus variants that have been tested for anti-tumor efficacy in animals and humans (for comprehensive list of oncolytic viruses see Kirn et al., 2001; Parato et al., 2005; Vähä-Koskela et al., 2007). Furthermore, more than 20 different oncolytic viruses have entered clinical trials (for review see Kirn et al., 2001; Parato et al., 2005; Vähä-Koskela et al., 2007).

Oncolytic viruses replicate preferentially in cancer cells because they are taking advantage of the same cellular defects that lead to tumor growth. Viruses that are not inherently selective for cancer cells can often be modified and engineered for tumor-selectivity. Generally, four main approaches have been described in the control of tumor progression through virotherapy: 1) the use of naturally occurring oncolytic viruses; e.g., Newcastle diseases virus (NDV) (Lorence et al., 1988); reovirus (Coffey et al., 1998), and vesicular stomatitis virus (VSV) (Stojdl et al., 2000); 2) engineered viruses with incorporate tissue-specific promoters that limit to tumor cells the expression of genes necessary for replication, e.g., HSV (Miyatake et al., 1997) and adenovirus (Hallenbeck et al., 1999); 3) modification of the viral coat to target uptake specifically to tumor cells, e.g., measles (Hammond et al, 2001); and 4) deletion of entire genes or functional gene regions that are necessary for efficient replication and/or toxicity but are nonessential in cancer cells, e.g., vaccinia virus (Mastrangelo et al.,) and adenovirus (Bischoff et al., 1996).

Oncolytic viruses are multimodality therapeutics that can be exploited as a treatment platform for cancer. One advantage of virotherapy is its use in combination with conventional chemo-, radio-or immunotherapy (Aghi & Martuzza, 2005; Kottke et al., 2008; Kumar et al., 2008;

Nandi et al., 2008). Another advantage of oncolytic viruses is the capacity to trigger tumor destruction by different mechanisms including stimulation of innate and adaptive immunity that have the potential anticancer activity (Bell et al., 2003). Despite the impressive improvements made in the field of virotherapy, the use of oncolytic viruses still face important hurdles in cancer therapy. Some of these problems are incomplete transduction, poor systemic distribution, immune response, intratumoral spread, and safety. These issues have to be resolved before oncolytic viral products became approved therapeutics.

3. Oncolytic poliovirus for treatment of neuroblastoma: Preclinical studies

Poliovirus (PV) has recently been added to the list of viruses that hold promise as possible agents in tumor therapy (Gromeier et al., 2000; Ochiai et al., 2004). A nonenveloped, plus-stranded enterovirus of the Picornaviridae family, poliovirus replicates in the gastrointestinal tract causing little, if any, clinical symptoms. Rarely (at a rate of 10^{-2} to 10^{-3}), the virus invades the central nervous system (CNS) where it targets predominantly motor neurons, thereby causing paralysis and even death (Mueller et al., 2005). Generally, poliovirus replicates efficiently in nearly all tumor cell lines tested, which has led to the suggestion that it may be suitable for the treatment of different cancers. However, the possibility that poliovirus can cause poliomyelitis calls for significant neuroattenuation to avoid collateral neurologic complications in cancer treatment. Therefore, the aim of our previous study was to develop highly attenuated polioviruses that may be suitable for the treatment of neuroblastoma in children (Toyoda et al., 2007). It was of concern, however, that the high coverage of antipolio vaccination in early childhood may interfere with the application of poliovirus in tumor therapy. Therefore, we also aimed to develop an immunocompetent animal model that would allow us to investigate the oncolytic capacity of neuroattenuated polioviruses for the treatment of neuroblastoma in the presence of high titers of poliovirus neutralizing antibodies (Toyoda et al., 2007). As shown by us and other investigators, pathogenesis of neurotropic viruses including poliovirus can be controlled by translation (Gromeier et al., 1996, 2000; Mohr, 2005). In poliovirus, an exchange of the internal ribosomal entry site (IRES) within the 5'-nontranslated region (NTR) with its counterpart from human rhinovirus type 2 (HRV2), another picornavirus, yielded viruses [called PV1(RIPO)] that are highly attenuated in mice transgenic for the human poliovirus receptor (PVR) CD155 (CD155 tg mice; Gromeier et al., 1996, 1999) yet replicate efficiently and lytically in cell lines derived from malignant glioma and breast cancer (Cello et al., 2008; Gromeier et al., 1996, 2000; Ochiai et al., 2004, 2006). However, PV1(RIPO) and PVS(RIPO), a derivative of PV1(RIPO) that is currently under investigation for the treatment of glioma, grow poorly in neuroblastoma cells (Cello et al., 2008; Gromeier et al., 1996, 2000;). This observation prompted us to search for other poliovirus derivatives with oncolytic properties against neuroblastoma. The whole genome synthesis of poliovirus (Cello et al., 2002) produced the surprising observation that a point mutation (A103G) in a "spacer region" between the cloverleaf and IRES in the 5'-NTR that was introduced as genetic marker attenuated poliovirus 10,000-fold (De Jesus et al., 2005). We found that the A103G variant of poliovirus replicates well in human neuroblastoma cell lines at 37°C (De Jesus et al., 2005). However, the attenuating mutation A103G in the spacer region was unstable on replication and direct revertant variants that had acquired the neurovirulent phenotype of wild-type (wt) poliovirus type 1 (Mahoney) [PV1(M)] (Fig. 1A) were readily scored (De Jesus et al., 2005). We reasoned that a stable attenuation phenotype could be generated if the spacer region would be interrupted by an essential RNA replication element that the virus cannot afford to delete. Such an element is the cre, a stem-loop structure mapping to the coding region of viral protein 2CATPase (Fig. 1B; Paul, 2002). Cre is absolutely required for poliovirus genome synthesis (Paul, 2002). Based on this concept, we have developed a stable attenuated poliovirus, replicating in neuroblastoma cells, by introducing the cre element into the spacer region between the cloverleaf and IRES in the 5'-NTR (mono-crePV) at the 104-nucleotide locus (Fig 1B) (Toyoda et al., 2007).

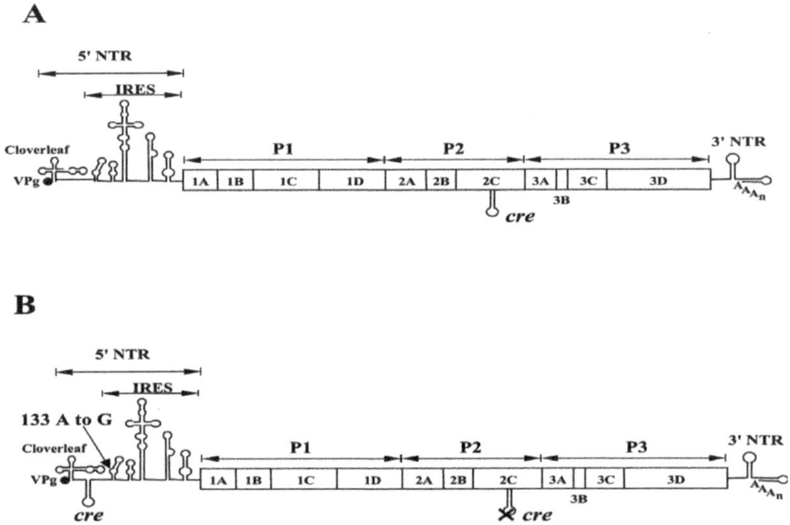

Fig. 1. Schematic diagram of full-length poliovirus genomes. (A) Genomic structure of PV1(M). The 5′ end is terminated with the genome-linked protein VPg and the 3′ end with polyadenylic acid. The 5′NTR, harboring the cloverleaf and the IRES, is followed by the single open reading frame (open box) encoding the viral polyprotein, and the 3′NTR. The cis replication element (*cre*) is indicated as an open stem-loop in the poliovirus polyprotein below polypeptide 2C. The polyprotein contains (Nterminus to C-terminus) structural (P1) and non-structural (P2 and P3) proteins that are released from the polypeptide chain by proteolytic processing. (B) Structure of A133G mono *cre* PV genomic RNA. The naïve *cre* in 2C was inactivated through three mutations G4462A C4465U A4472C of the poliovirus-*cre* loop. The cis replication element (*cre*) was inserted between cloverleaf and IRES. A point mutation was engineered at nt133 (A to G) of mono-*cre* PV.

To induce neuroblastoma in our animal model we used a mouse neuroblastoma cell line stably expressing CD155 ∝ (Neuro-2a^{CD155}). Neuro2a^{CD155} cell line was developed in our laboratory and is susceptible to poliovirus infection (Mueller & Wimmer, 2003). Using the nude mice model, we and others have shown previously that tumors of human origin can be successfully treated with neuroattenuated poliovirus strains, that is with PV(RIPO) derivatives (Groemeier et al., 2000), or with the Sabin vaccine strains (Toyoda et al., 2004). However, in the nude mice the lack of a possible immune response to the oncolytic agents mitigates the importance of the results. Therefore, we constructed fully immunocompetent mice (CD155 tg A/J mice) that express CD155 and accept Neuro-2a^{CD155} cells for the formation of lethal neuroblastoma (Toyoda et al., 2007). Using this animal model, we demonstrated that Neuro-2a^{CD155} subcutaneous tumors of Neuro-2a^{CD155} cells were eliminated by intratumoral administrations of a variant of mono-crePV (A_{133}Gmono-crePV) (Toyoda et al., 2007). Interestingly, we observed the complete regression of the established lethal subcutaneous Neuro-2a^{CD155} tumors without neurologic side effects despite the presence of high titers of anti-poliovirus antibodies (Toyoda et al., 2007). This result indicates that anti-polio response induced by immunization can exert protection against poliomyelitis without compromising the oncolytic capacity of poliovirus. Remarkably, the tumor-bearing mice, which were cured through treatment with A_{133}Gmono-crePV, resisted attempts to reestablish neuroblastoma with Neuro-2a^{CD155} cells. We hypothesized that destruction of tumor cells by A_{133}Gmono-crePV can increment the release of tumor antigens which may induce a more efficient antigen presentation and the development of a robust antitumor immunity (Toyoda et al., 2007).

Based on these results, we proposed to characterize the antitumor immune response evoked by the treatment of subcutaneous neuroblastoma by A_{133}Gmono-crePV. To evaluate the cellular anti-tumor immunity induced by oncolytic therapy with live attenuated poliovirus, we quantified the cytolytic anti-tumor activity of splenocytes collected from the neuroblastoma-implanted CD155 tg A/J mice cured by four intratumoral inoculations of A_{133}Gmono-crePV. Mock-treated mice received equivalent intratumoral injections of PBS. These animals were killed after the tumor had reached a volume of ~500 mm^3 and their splenocytes were used as a control in cytotoxic assays. The development of tumor specific cytotoxicity was assessed by standard lactate dehydrogenase-release assays (Decker & Lohmann-Matthes, 1988). Splenocytes isolated from mice cured from neuroblastoma exhibited significantly higher lytic activity against both target cells tested (Neuro-2a^{CD155} and Neuro-2a) than did those from splenocytes derived from control mice (16.0% vs 1.5 %, $P< 0.001$). Thus, this result confirmed that treatment with a neuroattenuated oncolytic PV strain induces antitumor immunity against neuroblastoma (Toyoda et al., 2011).

To determine which cell subpopulations are responsible for the cell-mediated antitumor immune responses, splenocytes from the cured mice were depleted in vitro of NK, CD4+ or CD8+ cells respectively, prior to cytotoxic assay. As shown in Fig. 2, incubation of splenocytes with neutralizing antibody NK1.1 or anti-CD4 had little or no effect on their ability to kill Neuro-2a^{CD155} cells. In contrast, depletion of CD8+ cells abrogated the cytolytic activity of splenocytes from cured mice by about 70% compared to non-depleted splenocytes (Fig. 2). These data indicate that cytotoxic CD8+ T cells are the principal mediators of antineuroblastoma immunity elicited by A_{133}Gmono-crePV virotherapy (Toyoda et al., 2011)

Any firm conclusion about the capacity of A_{133}Gmono-crePV induced antitumor immunity requires direct demonstration of that ability. We thus adoptively transferred the splenocytes harvested from mice cured of neuroblastoma by four A_{133}Gmono-crePV inoculations into mice that had developed subcutaneous Neuro-2a^{CD155} tumor. Splenocytes from naïve mice served as a negative control. Splenocytes from cured or naïve mice were adoptively transferred by tail vein injection ($2x10^7$ splenocytes in 100 μl of PBS) to neuroblastoma implanted mice when their subcutaneous tumor volumes were ~ 170mm^3. After the splenocyte transfer, tumor sizes were measured and tumor volumes calculated every day. Our results showed that adoptive transfer of splenocytes from A_{133}GmonocrePV-treated mice produced a significant inhibition of tumor growth by comparison with the negative control (average tumor volume: 583 mm^3 vs. 2183 mm^3, $p < 0.01$ at day 10 post splenocytes transfer) (Toyoda et al., 2011). This result confirms that oncolytic therapy for neuroblastoma with attenuated poliovirus induces tumor-specific immune response.

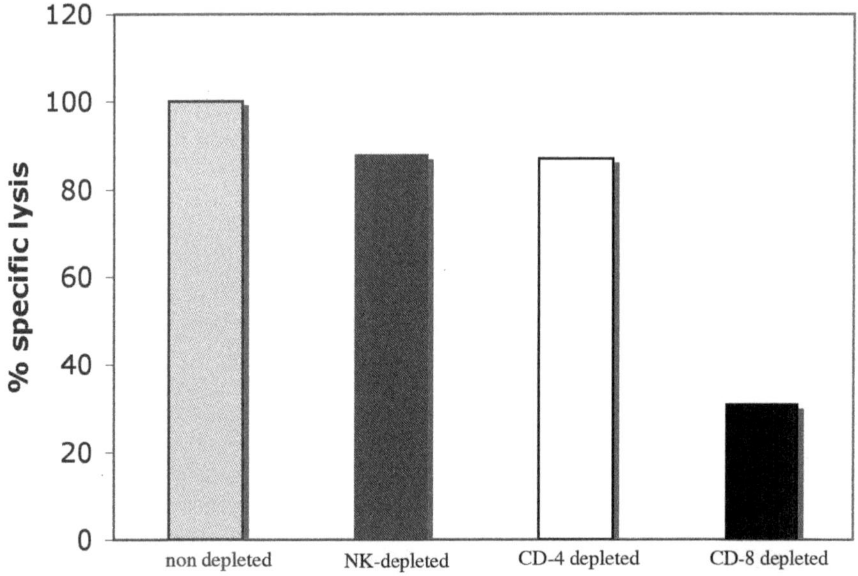

Fig. 2. Characterization of effector cytotoxic cells. Mice were sacrificed 2 months after tumor rechallenge. Splenocytes purified from the mice were incubated with neutralizing antibody against CD4, CD8, NK or PBS (as control) and then tested for cytotoxicity against Neuro-2aCD155 cells.

In line with our findings, previous investigations in mice and humans have also shown that treatment with oncolytic viruses can result in the enhancement of antitumor immune response (Diaz et al., 2007; Greiner et al., 2006; Moehler et al., 2005; Liu et al., 2007a, 2007b; Qiao et al., 2008; Toda et al., 1999).

Tumor destruction by an oncolytic virus can release a wide range of tumor specific antigens that will be taken up by infiltrating antigen-presenting cells for cross-presentation to T cells for priming of antigen-specific immune response (O'Shea, 2005). Moreover, different stimuli can promote an immunogenic cell death of tumor cells. Immunogenic cell death implies that dying tumor cells release several cellular signals that will facilitate immune recognition and elimination of tumor cells (Obeid et al., 2007a, 2007b). Noteworthy, it has been speculated that virus infection of tumor cells may induce an immunogenic cell death (Blachere et al., 2005). Based on these premises, we reasoned that immunization with in vitro PV-infected neuroblastoma cells should be able to prime an effective immune response against tumor cells and subsequently hinder neuroblastoma growth. To this end, 3 freeze-thaw cycles followed by 10 strokes of dounce homogenizer were performed for preparation of noninfected and PV-infected Neuro-2a^{CD155} lysates. The poliovirus titer in the PV-infected Neuro-2a^{CD155} lysate was 5x 10^8 pfu/ml. For the tumor rejection assays, polio Neuro-2a^{CD155} immunized CD155 tgA/J mice were injected intraperitoneally with PV-infected lysate, or noninfected Neuro-2aCD155 lysate, or a mixture of noninfected Neuro-2aCD155 lysate plus poliovirus (poliovirus titer in the mixture was 5x 108 pfu/ml) or PBS thrice at 1-week interval. All mice were injected intravenously with 2 x 10^6 Neuro-2aCD155 cells 21 days after last vaccination. Survival of the mice was monitored.

Examination of dead mice showed multiple liver and perirenal tumors. Analysis of Kaplan-Meier curves using the log-rank test showed no difference in the survival kinetics among mice immunized with PBS, noninfected Neuro2aCD155 lysate and the mixture of noninfected Neuro-2aCD155 lysate and poliovirus ($p > 0.05$, Fig 3). All mice from these groups died before 90 days of tumor challenge. In contrast, 70% of mice immunized with PV-infected Neuro-2aCD155 lysate, survived beyond 100 days after tumor challenge. Furthermore, statistical analyses showed that immunization with PV-infected Neuro-2aCD155 lysate was superior to each immunization with other lysate or PBS ($p < 0.01$, Fig 3).

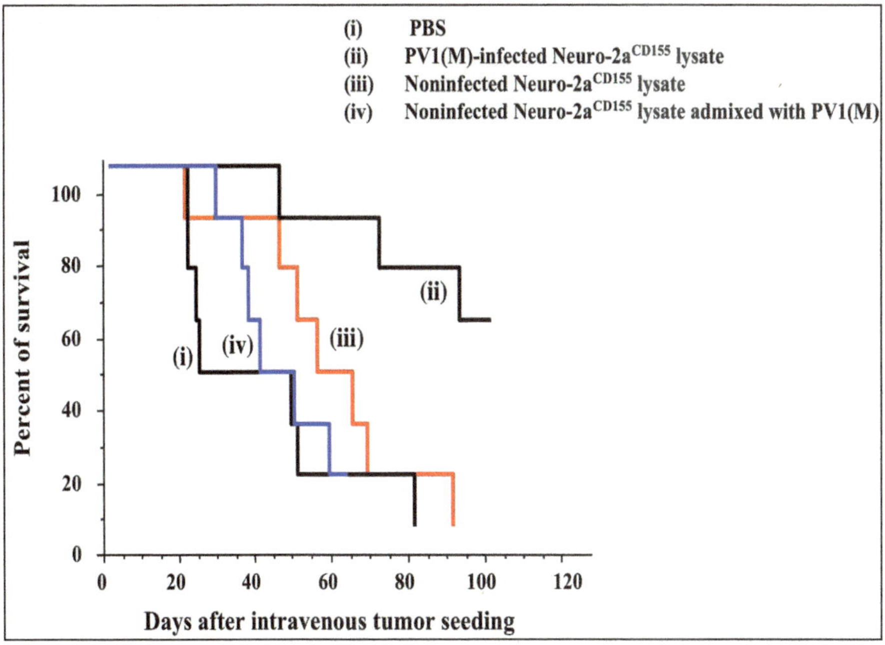

Fig. 3. Survival of mice inoculated withNeuro-2aCD155. Before challenge, mice were vaccinated with different lysates or PBS. Mice were observed every day and survival was plotted using a Kaplan-Meier survival curve.

We ruled out the possibility that protection effect seen in mice immunized with PV-infected Neuro-2aCD155 lysate is due to a cytolitic effect by an ongoing poliovirus infection after lysate injection. Our assertion is based in the following facts: i) no poliovirus were isolated from the lung, liver, spleen, brain and spinal cord of mice at the time of tumor challenge, i.e., 21 days after vaccination with homogenates prepared from PV1(M)-infected Neuro-2aCD155 cells or noninfectedNeuro-2aCD155 admixed with poliovirus, ii) No protection was induced by noninfected Neuro-2aCD155 admixed with poliovirus, and iii) all mice are vaccinated with different lysates or previously immunized against poliovirus. Altogether, our results clearly suggest that in vitro infection of neuroblastoma cells turn these cells into a potent tumor immunogen.

It has long been assumed that most therapeutic agents kill tumor cells through apoptosis. Notably, apoptosis has been considered to be a non-immunogenic or even a tolerogenic cell death mechanism as opposed to necrosis (an immunogenic cell death). However, depending on the cell death inducer, tumor cells can become highly immunogenic and induce a potent antitumor response in vivo (Zitvogel et al., 2006). Furthermore, there is now persuasive evidence that cell death can trigger an immune response only if the dying cells emit 'eat-me', 'danger' and 'killing' signals that mediate their efficient phagocytosis by dendritic cells (DC's) and the maturation of DCs (Blachere et al., 2005; Casares et al., 2005; Kepp et al., 2009; Melcher et al., 1998; Sauter et al., 2000).

DCs are the most important professional antigen-presenting cells and play a central role in initiating innate and adaptive immune response against tumor associate antigens (TAA). Antigen presentation by immature DCs (iDCs), associated with a lack of costimulation, induces tolerance. A number of molecules released from dying cells have been identified to elicit immune signaling during immunogenic cell death.

These include, among others, high mobility group box 1 (HMGB1, also known as amphoterin), purine metabolites (uric acid), calreticulin (CRT), and heat shock proteins (HSP) (Freedman et al., 1988; Obeid et al., 2007a; Shi et al., 2003; Udono & Srivastava, 1994). Induction of HSP is one of the earliest indications of cellular stress following infection with both RNA and DNA viruses (Asea, 2007; Liu et al., 2008). HSPs have been found to play key roles in the stimulation of the immune system when located on the plasma membrane or in the extracellular space (Udono & Srivastava, 1994). These proteins can promote tumor antigen cross-priming by binding to DC (Schild et al., 1999; Srivastava et al., 1998). Moreover, HSP 70 and 90 expressions act as "eat me" signals and enhance phagocytosis and maturation of DC (Binder & Srivastava, 2004; Lehner et al., 2004). CRT, another 'eat me' signal, is located in the lumen of the endoplasmic reticulum (ER) (Obeid et al., 2007a). Upon stress, CRT is translocated and exposed on the outer leaflet of cells during the early phase of cell death (Obeid et al., 2007a, 2007b). The exposure of CRT dictates the immunogenicity of tumor cells death because exposed CRT help the engulfment of dying tumor cells by DC (Obeid et al., 2007a). Investigators have previously identified uric acid as a novel endogenous danger signal capable of alerting the immune system (Shi et al., 2003). Injury cells rapidly degrade their DNA and RNA and release uric acid that activates DCs. Another signal molecule is HMGB1, which is loosely bound to chromatin and is referred to as 'danger signal' or alarmin (27). Dying cells release this molecule massively in the extracellular environment (Scaffidi et al., 2002). Extracellular HGMB1 induces functional maturation of DCs and acts as immune adjuvant for soluble and particulate antigens (Dumitriu et al., 2005; Rovere-Querini et al., 2004).

Until now, most of the identified inducers of immunogenic cell death of tumors cells are chemotherapheutics (Ulrich et al., 2008). The potent antitumor response elicited by virotherapy, observed by us and other investigators, clearly suggests that viruses are in vivo inducers of immunogenic death of tumor cells. Moreover, our finding that inoculation of PV-infected neuroblastoma lysate protects against live tumor challenge indicates that poliovirus is also an in vitro inducer of immunogenic death. Interestingly, necrosis by freeze-thawing is also considered as an immunological cell death (Ulrich et al., 2008). However, we observed that immunization with freeze-thawed noninfected neuroblastoma lysate, as opposed to the PV-infected lysate, did not protect against live tumor challenge. This result underscores the capacity of poliovirus to trigger the release of danger signals from tumor cells, which in turn it could induce an antitumor response.

Significantly, cells infected with encephalomyocarditis virus, a picornavirus as polio, have been shown to be effective at presenting nonviral antigens for cross-priming of DCs in vivo (Schulz et al., 2005). Viral lysates (called oncolysate) have been used in the past to vaccinate human against cancer (Sinkovics & Horvth, 2006). Those few trials have shown some degrees of success, but results have been ambiguous (Cassel & Murray, 1992; Freedman et al., 1988; Murray et al., 1977).

Remarkably, treatment with viral oncolysates showed better overall survival than radio-and chemo-therapy, probably because of the harmful effects of conventional therapies has on the immune system (White et al., 2002). On the other hand, using live viruses in humans for the treatment of cancer comes with some drawbacks. Inoculation of a virus, mainly a high dose, could elicit an unwanted inflammatory reaction, or cause an opportunistic infection or an unexpected complication (Bell et al., 2003; Kirn et al., 2001). Furthermore, the majority of human population is immune to several of the potential therapy viruses (Bell et al., 2003). Therefore, innate and pre-existing immunity may inactive the oncolytic virus which limits its use in systemic virotherapy (Ikeda et al., 1999; Kirn et al., 2001). Tumor vaccine therapy using virus lysate may overcome some of these hurdles. Viral oncolysate can be prepared with nonpathogenic virus without losing its tumor immunogenicity. Hypothetically, inactivation of the live virus present in the viral oncolysate should not affect the antitumor response induced by viral oncolysate. Finally, immunotherapy with viral oncolysate can be more effective than tumor virotherapy in controlling minimal residual and metastatic diseases states, thereby preventing or prolonging the time of recurrence.

4. Hypothesis and future studies

We hypothesize that in vitro poliovirus infection of neuroblastoma cells induces an immunogenic tumor cell death through a massive upregulation of endogenus alarm signals. We entertain the idea that the main alarm signals induced by poliovirus infection of tumor cells are CRT, HSP 70 and 90, uric acid and HMGB1, which in turn mediate DC activation. Therefore, we also hypothesize that PV-infected neuroblastoma lysate induces an effective DC maturation and tumor antigen cross-presentation. Finally, we postulate that immunization with PV-infected neuroblastoma lysate generates a systemic and potent anti tumor response that will eradicate established tumors and will confer a long-lasting tumor immunity.

Overall, there is enough information to expect that the immunization with polio lysate might represent a new treatment for neuroblastoma. However, the antitumor response induced by polio oncolysate remains largely uncharacterized. Therefore, a detailed knowledge of the immune response and therapeutic protection elicited by polio-infected neuroblastoma lysates is needed. Specifically, future studies should aim to determine:

- Aim I. If poliovirus infection of neuroblastoma cells induces upregulation, translocation and release of endogenous danger signals.
- Aim II. If polio-infected neuroblastoma lysates can induce DC maturation and presentation of tumor-derived antigens
- Aim III. Whether immunization with polio-infected neuroblastoma lysates can induce a systemic immune response capable of eradicating established cancer and stimulating a long-lasting anti-tumor immunity

Aim I

Rationale

Tumors evoke mechanism to induce immune tolerance. In this context, tumor cells are nonimmunogenic and their death will not stimulate an antitumor response. On the other hand, tumor cells can be stressed by multiple stimuli and may promote membrane expression or release of endogenous danger signals. The upregulation of these signals will turn nonimmunogenic tumor cells into immunogenic tumor cells, and facilitate immune recognition and final elimination of the stressed tumor cells. It has been shown that chemotherapeutic agents activates pro-apoptotic promoter BAX, which in turn induce translocation and exposure of two potent danger signals, CRT and HMGB1 (Kepp et al., 2009; Krynetskaia et al., 2008). Interestingly, poliovirus infection activates BAX in neuroblastoma cells (Autret et al., 2007). It is tempting to speculate that different inducers of immunogenic cell death activate common pathways to upregulate, translocate and release endogenous warning molecules. Thus, we postulate that poliovirus infection of neuroblastoma cells induce the upregulation and translocation of CRT, uric acid, HSP 70 and 90, and HMGB1. We also hypothesize that signal-inducing capacity of poliovirus depends on virus strain and infectious dose.

Approach.

Neuroblastoma cells will be infected with different poliovirus strains at different multiplicity of infection (MOI). At different time points after infection, the presence of CRT, uric acid, HSP 70 and 90, and HMGB1 in virus-infected cells and/or their supernatants will be determined. It also important to determine apoptosis/death of infected cells by Annexin V/PI test.

Expected results and alternatives.

Based in our previous results (see above in point 3), we think that poliovirus is a potent inducer of immunogenic cell death. Therefore, it is expected that infection of neuroblastoma cells will lead to surface exposure of CRTL, translocation of HMGB1 from nucleus to cytoplasm of infected cells followed by release into cell culture medium. We also anticipate a rapid increase in the expression of inducible HSP70 and HSP 90 and in the concentration of uric acid within cells and in supernatant of polio-infected cells.

With this approach, we should be able to determine the kinetic of different danger signal expressions induced by poliovirus before overt CPE is developed. We should also be capable of correlating the kinetic of danger signals and apoptotic or necrotic profile of the virus-infected tumor cells. Finally, we speculate that there are differences between different poliovirus strains in their capacity to induce upregulation of danger signals, and with our experimental approach we should be able to determine these differences. It is possible that the endogenous danger signals that we are going to analyze are poorly or not at all induced by poliovirus. In this case, we will look for other potential immunogenic determinants of dying tumor cells such as NKG2D ligands, RNA, HSP27, DNA, PTX3, IL-1β. Alternatively, proteomic analyses can be done to identify new putative "alarming" signals induced by poliovirus infection.

The way in which exogenous insults kill a tumor cell is likely to be a key determinant of the interaction of dying cells with the immune system and whether this interaction will lead to an immune response. Here we will define if poliovirus infection of neuroblastoma cells induces an immunogenic cell death through upregulation and translocation of endogenous danger signals. cell death through upregulation and translocation of endogenous danger signals.

Aim II

Rationale

In response to various cell death associated stimuli, Dcs have been shown to play a central role in the recognition of apoptotic cell death and in the initiation of an immune response,. Only when danger signals are correctly emitted by dying cells, in response to a stimulus, and perceived by DC, an immune response is elicited.

On the other hand, pathogen induced cell death can be immunogenic and hence stimulate an immune response against antigens that derive from dying cells and are presented by dendritic cells (DCs). Here we postulate that poliovirus infection of neuroblastoma cells induces an immunogenic death of these tumor cells. Therefore, lysate from these cells contain several immunogenic (danger) signals and tumor associated antigens that will induce DC maturation and tumor antigen-presentation.

Approach

Initially, mouse DC will be treated with polio oncolysates to determine whether these oncolysate could stimulate DC maturation. To assess DC activation by different viral lysates, phenotypic DC maturation and production of cytokines will be measured. To address whether the DC response to viral lysate could impact on downstream pathways of anti-tumor immune response, we will test stimulation of splenocytes from neuroblastoma-challenged mice via presentation by viral lysate-actived DC. As markers of splenocytes activation, IL 2, 4, 10 and IFN-γ release and cytotoxic activity will be determined.

Expected results and alternatives. As mentioned in Aim 1, poliovirus infection of neuroblastoma cells provokes an immunogenic cell death. Therefore, we expect that the interaction between polio-infected neuroblastoma lysate and iDCs will result in DC maturation, allowing the DCs to activate relevant cell mediated immunity against tumor cells. Our experimental approach will allow us to determine the ability of viral oncolysate pulsed DC to present tumor and viral antigens to primed T cells. Moreover, we expect that oncolysate-pulsed DCs will be able to prime naïve splenocytes against tumor antigens. In line with our theory, we speculate that wild type poliovirus is a stronger inducer of immunogenic cell death than the other strains used in this study. Thus, PV1(M)-oncolysate will induce a stronger activation of DC than those stimulated by the polio replicon or the neuroattenuated polio oncolysate. However, we think that DCs will mature and acquire the ability of presenting tumor antigens upon stimulation with polio replicon oncolysate or the neuroattenuated polio oncolysate.

It might be possible that the activation signals provided by oncolysate induce a poor maturation of DCs. To solve this problem, we can concentrate the oncolysates and test their capacity to induce DC maturation. Alternatively, we can mix oncolysate with small amounts of LPS (10-50 pg) to boost DC maturation. It is expected that polio oncolysate has a high concentration of poliovirus proteins. Therefore, DCs may preferentially present poliovirus antigens. In this case, oncolysate-pulsed DC will induce a poor antitumor response. We propose to increase the amount of tumor antigens presented to DCs. For this purpose, we will use cell membrane isolated from neuroblastoma cells as source of tumor antigens. After concentration, cell membranes will be mixed with oncolysate and the mixture will be used to pulse DCs.

Aim III

Rationale

Unfortunately, the prognosis for many children diagnosed with neuroblastoma is poor despite aggressive surgical resection and simultaneous radiochemotherapy regimens. Moreover, the frequency of relapse and the subsequent failure of further treatment have created the need to develop non-toxic and more effective treatments. Immunotherapy has the theoretical appeal that tumor-reactive lymphocyte may seek and eliminate tumor cells with greater accuracy than conventional therapy. A limiting impediment to successful immunotherapeutic treatment is the stimulation of adequate tumor antigen-specific effector cells. To attain this, tumor-associated antigens should be processed by antigen presenting cells (APCs), and presented to T cells along with enough costimulatory signals to avoid tolerance. Our previous results showed that polio oncolysate is able to prime an anti-neuroblastoma response. This result indicate that viral oncolysate contain tumor associated antigens and immunoadjuvant molecules which activate the immune system to elicit a prophylatic tumor response. Based on this finding, we propose to continue our studies and determine if immunization with polio-infected neuroblastoma oncolysate could evoke a tumor-specific immunity capable of eradicating established neuroblastoma as well as maintaining immunological memory. On the other hand, viral oncolysate contain infectious virus. Therefore, inoculation of viral oncolysate may cause severe complications. To circumvent this problem, we also propose to obtain viral oncolysate from neuroblastoma cells infected with polio replicon. These RNA-based vectors are generated by providing the capsid proteins in trans, they can undergo only a single round of replication in the infected cell and they are genetically incapable of producing infectious virus.

Therefore, we will also determine the capacity of noninfectious poliovirus replicon-infected lysate to induce a therapeutic effect against established tumor.

Approach.

We will establish hepatic and subcutaneous Neuro-2aCD155 tumors in polio-immunized CD155 tg A/J. Ten days after tumor cell inoculation, animals will be vaccinated intraperitonally (i.p) or intramuscuraly (i.m) with neuroblastoma lysates prepared from tumor cells infected with wild type PV1 (M), neuroattenuated A133GmonocrePV or propagation-defective poliovirus (poliovirus replicon). Control mice will be inoculated with noninfected neuroblastoma lysates or PBS. To determine long-lasting anti tumor immunity evoked by oncolysate vaccination, mice previously cured with any experimental treatment described above or 6 months after immunization with different lysates will be challenged i.v. or s.c with neuroblastoma cells. Protection response to each experimental therapy will be measured by survival rates and tumor growth. Splenocytes and sera from each experimental group will be obtained to test tumor-and virus specific immunity.

Expected results and alternatives. First, we expect to obtain a comprehensive characterization of tumor-specific and virus-specific induced by in vivo vaccination with poliovirus oncolysate. We think that in vivo administration of polio oncolysates will mediate a strong therapeutic benefit and eliminate or slow significantly tumor growth, preferentially on established liver metastases. Based on our previous results, we anticipate that in vivo vaccination with polio oncolysate will induce a robust memory response. Since tumor immunogenicity of polio oncolysates might be different depending on poliovirus strain used for their preparation, we expect to see differences in the therapeutic effect induced by each of the oncolysate tested. There is concern that immunity induced by repetitive inoculation of viral oncolysate will be biased towards a viral immune response. Our experimental approach will allow us to determine the tumor-specific and virus-specific and therapeutic effect induce by in vivo immunization with oncolysate. Correlation of these data should identify whether the biased response affects the effectiveness of immunotherapeutic treatment.

It is possible, although unlikely, that in vivo vaccination with oncolysate will induce a poor anti-tumor response. If we detect that the reason of this poor anti-tumor response is due to oncolysate vaccination bias the immune response to virus, we will increase the tumor antigens in the oncolysate as described in Aim 2. Another possibility for a poor antit-tumor response is a low adjuvanticity of viral oncolysate in vivo. In this case, we propose to mix viral oncolysate with CpG oligodeoxynucleotides. CpG has been successful used as an adjuvant in other mouse models of immunotherapy for treatment of several tumors. Alternatively, we may improve the immune response against the tumor by combining frequency, timing, dose and route of administration of viral oncolysate.

5. Conclusion

In the current state of the art, it is likely that virotherapy using attenuated poliovirus will be capable of eradicating neuroblastoma when used in combination with other therapies. Moreover, immunotherapy with PV oncolysate alone or in combination with virotherapy can be effective in controlling minimal residual and metastatic diseases states, thereby preventing recurrence or prolonging the time of recurrence in patient suffering from neuroblastoma. Therefore, we think that our data and the directions of future studies presented here will lead to practical applications of attenuated poliovirus and polio oncolysate for the treatment of neuroblastoma

6. References

Aghi, M., & Martuza, R. (2005). Oncolytic viral therapies: the clinical experience. *Oncogene,* 24, pp. 7802–7816

Asada, T. Treatment of human cancer with mumps virus. (1974). *Cancer,* 34, pp. 1907–1928

Asea A. Mechanisms of HSP72 release. (2007). *J Biosci,* 32, pp. 579-84

Autret, A., Martin-Latil, S., Mousson, L., Wirotius, A., Petit, F, Arnoult, D., Colbère-Garapin, F., Estaquier, J., & Blondel, B. (2007). Poliovirus induces Bax-dependent cell death mediated by c-Jun NH2-terminal kinase. *J Virol,* 81, pp. 7504-7516

Bell, C., Lichty, B., & Stojdl, D. Getting oncolytic virus therapies off the ground. (2003). *Cancer Cell,*4, pp. 7-11

Binder, R., & Srivastava, P. (2004). Essential role of CD91 in re-presentation of gp96-chaperoned peptides. Proc Natl Acad Sci USA, 101, pp. 6128–6133

Bischoff, J., Kirn, D., Williams, A., Heise, C., Horn, S., Muna, M., Ng, L., Nye, J., Sampson-Johannes, A., Fattaey, A., & McCormick, F. (1996). An adenovirus mutant that replicates selectively in p53-deficient human tumor cells. *Science,* 274, pp. 373–376

Blachère, N., Darnell, R., & Albert M. (2005). Apoptotic cells deliver processed antigen to dendritic cells for cross-presentation PLoS Biol 3:e185.

Brodeur, G., & Maris, J. (2006). Neuroblastoma. In: Pizzo PA, Poplack DG (eds) *Principles and practice of pediatric oncology.* 5th edn. Lippincott Williams and Wilkins, Philadelphia, pp 933–970

Casares, N., Pequignot, M., Tesniere, A., Ghiringhelli, F., Roux, S., Chaput, N., Schmitt, E., Hamai, A., Hervas-Stubbs, S., Obeid, M., Coutant, F., Métivier, D., Pichard, E., Aucouturier, P., Pierron, G., Garrido C., Zitvogel, L., & Kroemer, G. (2005). Caspase dependent immunogenicity of doxorubicin- induced tumor cell death. *J Exp Med,* 202, pp. 1691–1701

Cassel, W., & Murray, D. (1992). A ten-year follow-up on stage II malignant melanoma patients treated postsurgically with Newcastle disease virus oncolysate. *Med Oncol Tumor Pharmacother,* 9, pp. 169–171.

Cello, J., Paul, A., & Wimmer, E.. (2002). Chemical synthesis of poliovirus cDNA: generation of infectious virus in the absence of natural template. *Science,* 297, pp. 1016–1018

Cello, J., Toyoda, H., Dejesus, N., Dobrikova, E., Gromeier, M., & Wimmer, E. (2008). Growth phenotypes and biosafety profiles in poliovirus-receptor transgenic mice of recombinant oncolytic polio/human rhinoviruses. J Med Virol, 80, pp. 352-359

Coffey, M., Strong, J., Forsyth, P., & Lee, P. (1998). Reovirus therapy of tumors with activated ras pathway, *Science,* 282, pp. 1332–1334.

DePace, N. (1912). Rabies virus treatment of cervical cancer. *Ginecologia,* 9, pp. 82

Decker, T., & Lohmann-Matthes, M. (1988). A quick and simple method for the quantitation of lactate dehydrogenase release in measurements of cellular cytotoxicity and tumor necrosis factor (TNF) activity. *J Immunol Methods,* 115, pp. 61-69

De Jesus, N., Franco, D., Paul, A., Wimmer, E., & Cello, J. (2005). Mutation of a single conserved nucleotide between the cloverleaf and internal ribosome entry site attenuates poliovirus neurovirulence. J Virol 79, pp. 14235–14243

Diaz, R., Galivo, F., Kottke, T., Wongthida, P., Qiao, J., Thompson, J., Valdes, M., Barber, G., & Vile, R. (2007). Oncolytic immunovirotherapy for melanoma using vesicular stomatitis virus. *Cancer Res,* 67, pp. 2840-2848

Dumitriu, I., Baruah, P., Manfredi A., Bianchi, M., & Rovere-Querini, P. (2005). HMGB1: guiding immunity from within. *Trends Immunol,* 26, pp. 381-387

Freedman, R., Edwards, C., Bowen, J., Lotzova, E., Katz, R., Lewis, E., Atkinson, N., & Carsetti, R. (1988). Viral oncolysates in patients with advanced ovarian cancer. *Gynecol Oncol,* 29, pp. 337–347

Gao, R.N., I. G. Levy, W. G. Woods, B. A. Coombs, L. A. Gaudette, and G. B. Hill. 1997. Incidence and mortality of neuroblastoma in Canada compared with other childhood cancers. *Cancer Causes and Control,* 8, pp. 745–754

Greiner, S., Humrich, J., Thuman, P., Sauter, B., Schuler, G., & Jenne, L. (2006). The highly attenuated vaccinia virus strain modified virus Ankara induces apoptosis in melanoma cells and allows bystander dendritic cells to generate apotent anti-tumoral immunity. *Clin Exp Immunol,* 146, pp. 344-353

Gromeier, M., Alexander, L., & Wimmer, E. (1996). Internal ribosomal entry site substitution eliminatesneurovirulence in intergeneric poliovirus recombinants. *Proc Natl Acad Sci U S A,* 93, pp. 2370-2375

Gromeier, M., Bossert, B., Arita, M., Nomoto, A., & Wimmer, E. (1999). Dual stem loops within the poliovirus internal ribosomal entry site control neurovirulence. *J Virol,* 73, pp. 958–964

Gromeier, M., Lachmann, S., Rosenfeld, M., Gutin, P., & Wimmer, E. (2000). Intergeneric poliovirus recombinants for the treatment of malignant glioma. *Proc Natl Acad Sci U S A,* 97, pp. 6803–6808

Gurney, J., Ross, J., Wall, D., Bleyer, W., Severson, R., & Robison, L. (1997). Infant cancer in the U.S.: histology-specific incidence and trends, 1973 to 1992. *J PediatricHematology/Oncology*, 19, pp. 428–432

Hammond, A., Plemper, R., Zhang, J., Schneider, U., Russell, S., & Cattaneo, R. (2001). Single-chain antibody displayed on a recombinant measles virus confers entry through the tumor-associated carcinoembryonic antigen. *J Virol*, 75, pp. 2087–2096

Hallenbeck, P., Chang, Y., Hay, C., Golightly, D., Stewart, D., Lin, J., Phipps, S., & Chiang, Y. (1999). A novel tumor-specific replication-restricted adenoviral vector for gene therapy of hepatocellular carcinoma. *Hum Gene Ther*, 10, pp. 1721–1733

Huebner, R., Rowe, W., Schatten, W., Smith. R., & Thomas, L. (1956). Studies on the use of viruses in the treatment of carcinoma of the cervix. *Cancer*, 9, pp. 1211–1218

Ikeda, K., Ichikawa, T., Wakimoto, H., Silver, J., Deisboeck, T., Finkelstein, D., Harsh G., Louis, D., Bartus, R., Hochberg F., & Chiocca, E. (1999). Oncolytic virus therapy of multiple tumors in the brain requires suppression of innate and elicited antiviral responses. *Nat Med*, 5, pp. 881-887

Kepp, O., Senovilla, L., Galluzzi, L., Panaretakis, T., Tesniere, A., Schlemmer, F., Madeo, F., Zitvogel, L., & Kroemer, G.. (2009). Viral subversion of immunogenic cell death. *Cell Cycle*, 8, pp. 860-869

Kirn, D., Martuza, R., & Zwiebel, J. (2001). Replication-selective virotherapy for cancer: Biological principles, risk management and future directions. *Nat Med*, 7, pp. 781-787

Kottke, T., Diaz, R., Kaluza, K., Pulido, J., Galivo, F., Wongthida, P., Thompson, J., Willmon, C., Barber, G., Chester, J., Selby, P., Strome, S., Harrington, K., Melcher, A., & Vile, R. (2008). Use of biological therapy to enhance both virotherapy and adoptive T-cell therapy for cancer. *Mol Ther*, 16, pp. 1910-1918

Krynetskaia, N., Xie, H., Vucetic, S., Obradovic, Z., & Krynetskiy, E. (2008). High mobility group protein B1 is an activator of apoptotic response to antimetabolite drugs. *Mol Pharmacol*, 73, pp. 260-269

Kumar, S., Gao, L., Yeagy, B., & Reid, T. (2008). Virus combinations and chemotherapy for the treatment of human cancers. *Curr Opin Mol Ther*, 10, pp. 371-379

Maris, J., & Matthay, K. (1999). Molecular biology of neuroblastoma, *J Clin Oncol*, 17, pp. 2264–2279

Martuza, R., Malick, A., Markert, J., Ruffner, K., & Coen, D. (1991). Experimental therapy of human glioma by means of a genetically engineered virus mutant. *Science*, 252, pp. 854-856

Mastrangelo, M., Eisenlohr, L., Gomella, L., & Lattime, E. (2000). Poxvirus vectors: Orphaned and underappreciated. *J Clin Invest*, 105, pp. 1031–1034

Matthay, K., Villablanca, J., Seeger, R., Stram, D., Harris R., Ramsay N., Swift, P., Shimada, H., Black, C., Brodeur, G., Gerbing, R., & Reynolds, C. (1999). Treatment of high-risk neuroblastoma with intensive chemotherapy, radiotherapy, autologous bone marrow transplantation, and 13-*cis*-retinoic acid: a Children's Cancer Group study. *N Engl J Med*, 341, pp. 1165–1173

Matthay, K., Reynolds, C., Seeger, R., Shimada, H., Adkins, E., Haas-Kogan, D., Gerbing, R., London, W., & Villablanca, J. (2009). Long-term results for children with high-risk neuroblastoma treated on a randomized trial of myeloablative therapy followed by 13-*cis*-retinoic acid: a Children's Oncology Group study. *J Clin Oncol*, 27, pp. 1007-1013

Melcher, A., Todryk, S., Hardwick, N., Ford, M., Jacobson, M., & Vile, R. (1998). Tumor immunogenicity is determined by the mechanism of cell death via induction of heat shock protein expression. *Nat Med*, 4, pp. 581–587

Miyatake, S., Iyer, A., Martuza, R., & Rabkin, S. (1997). Transcriptional targeting of herpes simplex virus for cell-specific replication. J Virol, 71, pp. 5124–1532

Moehler, M., Zeidler, M., Wilsberg, V., Cornelis, J., Woelfel, T., Rommelaere J., Galle P., & Heike, M. (2005). Parvovirus H-1-induced tumor cell death enhances human immune response in vitro via increased phagocytosis, maturation, and cross-presentation by dendritic cells. *Hum Gene Ther*, 16, pp. 996- 1005

Mohr, I. (2005). To replicate or not to replicate: achieving selective oncolytic virus replication in cancer cells through translational control. *Oncogene*, 24, pp. 7697–709

Mueller, S., & Wimmer, E. (2003). Recruitment of nectin-3 to cell-cell junctions through transheterophilic interaction with CD155, a vitronectin and poliovirus receptor that localizes to {alpha}(v)ß3 integrin-containing membrane microdomains. *J Biol Chem*, 278, pp. 31251–31260

Mueller, S., Wimmer, E., & Cello, J. (2005). Poliovirus and poliomyelitis: a tale of guts, brains, and an accidental event. *Virus Res*, 111, pp. 175–193

Murray, D., Cassel, W., Torbin, A., Olkowski, Z., & Moore, M. (1977). Viral oncolysate in the management of malignant melanoma. II. Clinical studies. *Cancer*, 40, pp. 680–686

Nandi, S., Ulasov, I., Tyler, M., Sugihara, A., Molinero, L., Han, Y., Zhu, Z., & Lesniak, M. (2008). Low-dose radiation enhances survivin-mediated virotherapy against malignant glioma stem cells. *Cancer Res*, 68, pp. 5778-5784

Newman, W., & Southam, C. (1954). Virus treatment in advanced cancer; a pathological study of fifty- seven cases. Cancer, 7, pp. 106–118

Leaf, C. (2004). Why we're losing the war on cancer and how to win it. *Fortune*, pp. 76–92

Lehner, T., Wang, Y., Whittall, T., McGowan, E., Kelly, C., & Singh, M. (2004). Functional domains of HSP70 stimulate generation of cytokines and chemokines, maturation of dendritic cells and adjuvanticity. *Biochem Soc Trans*, 32, pp. 629–632

Li, H., Dutuor, A., Fu, X., & Zhang, X. (2007a). Induction of strong antitumor immunity by an HSV-2-based oncolytic virus in a murine mammary tumor model. *J Gene Med*, 9, pp. 161-169

Li, H., Dutuor, A, Tao, L., Fu, X., & Zhang, X. (2007b). Virotherapy with a type 2 herpes simplex virus derived oncolytic virus induces potent antitumor immunity against neuroblastoma. *Clin Cancer Res*, 13, pp. 316-322

Liu, C., Erlichman, C., McDonald, C., Ingle, J., Zollman, P., Iankov, I., Russell, S., & Galanis, E. (2008). Heat shock protein inhibitors increase the efficacy of measles virotherapy. *Gene Ther*, 15, pp. 1024-1034

Lorence, R., Rood, P., & Kelley, K. (1988). Newcastle disease virus as an antineoplastic agent: Induction of tumor necrosis factor-alpha and augmentation of its cytotoxicity. *J Natl Cancer Inst*, 80, pp. 1305–1312

Obeid, M., Tesniere, A., Ghiringhelli, F., Fimia, G., Apetoh, L., Perfettini, J., Castedo, M., Mignot, G., Panaretakis, T., Casares, N., Métivier , D., Larochette, N., van Endert, P., Ciccosanti, F., Piacentini, M., Zitvogel, L., & G. Kroemer. (2007a). Calreticulin exposure dictates the immunogenicity of cancer cell death. *Nat Med*, 13, pp. 54-61

Obeid, M., Panaretakis, T., Joza, N., Tufi, R., Tesniere, A., van Endert, P., Zitvogel, L., & Kroemer, G. (2007b). Calreticulin exposure is required for the immunogenicity of gamma-irradiation and UVC light induced apoptosis. *Cell Death Differ*, 14, pp. 1848-1850

Ochiai, H., Moore, S., Archer, G., Okamura, T., Chewning, T., Marks, J., Sampson, J., & Gromeier, M. (2004). Treatment of intracerebral neoplasia and neoplastic meningitis with regional delivery of oncolytic recombinant poliovirus. *Clin Cancer Res*, 10, pp. 4831–4838

Ochiai, H., Campbell, S., Archer, G., Chewning, T., Dragunsky, E., Ivanov, A., Gromeier, M., & Sampson, J. (2006). Targeted therapy for glioblastoma multiforme neoplastic meningitis with intrathecal delivery of an oncolytic recombinant poliovirus. *Clin Cancer Res*, 12, pp. 1349–1354

Okuno, Y., Asada, T., Yamanishi, K., Otsuka, T., Takahashi, M., Tanioka, T., Aoyama, H., Fukui, O., Matsumoto, K., Uemura, F., & Wada, A. (1978). Studies on the use of mumps virus for treatment of human cancer. *Biken J*, 21, pp. 37–49

O'Shea, C. (2005). Viruses- seeking and destroying the tumor program. *Oncogene*, 24, pp. 7640-7655

Pack, G. (1950). Note on the experimental use of rabies vaccine for melanomatosis. *AMA Arch Derm Syphilol*, 62, pp. 694–695

Parato, K. A., D. Senger, P. A. Forsyth, and J. C. Bell. (2005). Recent progress in the battle between oncolytic viruses and tumours. *Nat Rev Cancer*, 5, pp. 965–976

Park, J., Eggert, A., & Caron, H. (2008). Neuroblastoma: Biology, Prognosis and Treatment. *Pediatr Clin North Am*, 55, pp. 97-120

Paul, A. (2002). Possible unifying mechanism of picornavirus genome replication. In: Semler BL, Wimmer E, editors. Molecular biology of picornaviruses. Washington (DC): *ASM Press*, p. 227–246

Qiao, J., Kottke, T., Willmon, C., Galivo, F., Wongthida, P., Diaz, R., Thompson, J., Ryno, P., Barber, G., Chester, J., Selby, P., Harrington, K., Melcher, A., & Vile, R. (2008). Purging metastases in lymphoid organs using a combination of antigen non-specific adoptive T cell therapy, oncolytic virotherapy and immunotherapy. *Nat Med*, 14, pp. 37-44

Ries, L., Eisner, M., Kosary, C., Hankey, B., Miller, B., & Clegg, L. (2005). SEER Cancer Statistics Review, 1975–2002. Bethesda, MD: National Cancer Institute

Rovere-Querini, P., Capobianco, A., Scaffidi, P., Valentinis, B., Catalanotti, F., Giazzon, M., Dumitriu, I., Muller, S., Iannacone, M., Traversari, C., Bianchi, M., & A. Manfredi, A. (2004). HMGB1 is an endogenous immune adjuvant released by necrotic cells. *EMBO Rep*, 5, pp. 825–830

Sauter, B., Albert, M., Francisco, L., Larsson, M., Somersan, S., & Bhardwaj, N. (2000). Consequences of cell death: exposure to necrotic tumor cells, but not primary tissue cells or apoptotic cells, induces the maturation of immunostimulatory dendritic cells. *J Exp Med*, 191, pp. 423–434

Scaffidi, P., Misteli, T., & Bianchi, M. (2002). Release of chromatin protein HMGB1 by necrotic cells triggers inflammation. *Nature*, 418, pp. 191–195

Schild, H., Arnold-Schild, D., Lammert, E., & Rammensee, H. (1999). Stress proteins and immunity mediated by cytotoxic T lymphocytes. *Curr Opin Immunol*, 11, pp. 109–113

Schulz, O., Diebold, S., Chen, M., Näslund, T., Nolte, M., Alexopoulou, L., Azuma, Y., Flavell, R., Liljeström, P., & Reis e Sousa, C. (2005). Toll-like receptor 3 promotes cross-priming to virus infected cells. *Nature*, 433, pp. 887-892

Shi, Y., Evans, J., & Rock, K. (2003). Molecular identification of a danger signal that alerts the immune system to dying cells. *Nature*, 425, pp. 516–521

Sinkovics, J., & Horvath, J. (1993). New developments in the virus therapy of cancer: a historical review. *Intervirology*, 36, pp. 193–214

Sinkovics, J., & Horvath, J. (2006). Evidence accumulating in support of cancer vaccines combined with chemotherapy: a pragmatic review of past and present efforts. *Int J Oncol*, 29, pp. 765–777

Spix, C., Pastore, G., Sankila, R., Stiller, C., & Steliarova-Foucher, E. (2006). Neuroblastoma incidence and survival in European children (1978–1997): report from the Automated Childhood Cancer Information System project. *European J Cancer*, 42, pp. 2081–2091

Southam, C., & Moore, A. (1952). Clinical studies of viruses as antineoplastic agents with particular reference to Egypt 101 virus. *Cancer*, 5, pp. 1025–1034

Southam, C., Hilleman, M., & Werner, J. (1956). Pathogenicity and oncolytic capacity of RI virus strain RI-67 in man. *J. Lab. Clin. Med.*, 47, pp. 573–582

Srivastava, P., Menoret, A., Basu, S., Binder, R., & McQuade, K. (1998). Heat shock proteins come of age: primitive functions acquire new roles in an adaptive world. *Immunity*, 8, pp. 657–665

Stojdl, D., Lichty, B., Knowles, S., Marius, R., Atkins, H., Sonenberg, N., & Bell, J. (2000). Exploiting tumor-specific defects in the interferon pathway with a previously unknown oncolytic virus. *Nature Med*, 6, pp. 821–825

Toda, M., Rabkin, S., Kojima, H., & L. Martuza, R. (1999). Herpes simplex virus as an in situ cancer vaccine for the induction of specific anti-tumor immunity. *Hum Gene Ther*, 10, pp. 385-393

Toyoda, H., Ido, M., Hayashi, T., Gabazza, E., Suzuki, K., Kisenge, R., Kang, J., Hori, H., & Komada, Y. (2004). Experimental treatment of human neuroblastoma using live-attenuated poliovirus. *Int J Oncol*, 24, pp. 49–58.

Toyoda, H., Yin, J., Mueller, S., Wimmer, E., & Cello, J. (2007). Oncolytic treatment and cure of neuroblastoma by a novel attenuated poliovirus in a novel poliovirus-susceptible animal model. Cancer Res, 67, pp. 2857-2864

Toyoda, H., Wimmer, E., & Cello, J. (2011). Oncolytic polio therapy and immunization with poliovirus-infected cell lysate induces potent antitumor immunity against neuroblastoma *in vivo*. *Int J Oncology*, 38, pp. 81-87

Udono, H., & Srivastava, P. (1994). Comparison of tumor-specific immunogenicities of stress induced proteins gp96, hsp90, and hsp70. *J Immunol*, 152, pp. 5398–5403

Ullrich, E., Bonmort, M., Mignot, G., Kroemer, G., & Zitvogel, L. (2008). Tumor stress, cell death and the ensuing immune response. *Cell Death Differ*, 15, pp. 21-28

Vähä-Koskela, M., Heikkilä, J., & Hinkkanen, A. (2007). Oncolytic viruses in cancer therapy. *Cancer Lett*, 254, pp. 178-216

Wheelock, E., & Dingle, J. (1964). Observations on the repeated administration of viruses to a patient with acute leukemia: A preliminary report. *N Engl J Med*, 271, pp. 645–651

White, R., Stanley, W., Johnson, J., Tyler, D., & Seigler, H. (2002). Long-term survival in 2505 patients with melanoma with regional lymph node metastasis. *Ann Surg*, 235, pp. 879–887

Zitvogel, L., Tesniere, A., & Kroemer, G. (2006). Cancer despite immunosurveillance: immunoselection and immunosubversion. Nat Rev Immunol, 6, pp. 715-727

Permissions

The contributors of this book come from diverse backgrounds, making this book a truly international effort. This book will bring forth new frontiers with its revolutionizing research information and detailed analysis of the nascent developments around the world.

We would like to thank Hiroyuki Shimada, for lending his expertise to make the book truly unique. He has played a crucial role in the development of this book. Without his invaluable contribution this book wouldn't have been possible. He has made vital efforts to compile up to date information on the varied aspects of this subject to make this book a valuable addition to the collection of many professionals and students.

This book was conceptualized with the vision of imparting up-to-date information and advanced data in this field. To ensure the same, a matchless editorial board was set up. Every individual on the board went through rigorous rounds of assessment to prove their worth. After which they invested a large part of their time researching and compiling the most relevant data for our readers. Conferences and sessions were held from time to time between the editorial board and the contributing authors to present the data in the most comprehensible form. The editorial team has worked tirelessly to provide valuable and valid information to help people across the globe.

Every chapter published in this book has been scrutinized by our experts. Their significance has been extensively debated. The topics covered herein carry significant findings which will fuel the growth of the discipline. They may even be implemented as practical applications or may be referred to as a beginning point for another development.

The editorial board has been involved in producing this book since its inception. They have spent rigorous hours researching and exploring the diverse topics which have resulted in the successful publishing of this book. They have passed on their knowledge of decades through this book. To expedite this challenging task, the publisher supported the team at every step. A small team of assistant editors was also appointed to further simplify the editing procedure and attain best results for the readers.

Our editorial team has been hand-picked from every corner of the world. Their multi-ethnicity adds dynamic inputs to the discussions which result in innovative outcomes. These outcomes are then further discussed with the researchers and contributors who give their valuable feedback and opinion regarding the same. The feedback is then collaborated with the researches and they are edited in a comprehensive manner to aid the understanding of the subject.

Apart from the editorial board, the designing team has also invested a significant amount of their time in understanding the subject and creating the most relevant covers. They scrutinized every image to scout for the most suitable representation of the subject and create an appropriate cover for the book.

The publishing team has been involved in this book since its early stages. They were actively engaged in every process, be it collecting the data, connecting with the contributors or procuring relevant information. The team has been an ardent support to the editorial, designing and production team. Their endless efforts to recruit the best for this project, has resulted in the accomplishment of this book. They are a veteran in the field of academics and their pool of knowledge is as vast as their experience in printing. Their expertise and guidance has proved useful at every step. Their uncompromising quality standards have made this book an exceptional effort. Their encouragement from time to time has been an inspiration for everyone.

The publisher and the editorial board hope that this book will prove to be a valuable piece of knowledge for researchers, students, practitioners and scholars across the globe.

List of Contributors

Loretta M.S. Lau
The Children's Hospital at Westmead and University of Sydney, Australia

Wendy B. London
Dana-Farber Harvard Cancer Center and Children's Hospital Boston; Children's Oncology Group Statistics and Data Center, USA

Diana T. Lau and Lesley J. Ashton
Children's Cancer Institute Australia for Medical Research, Lowy Cancer Research Centre, UNSW, Australia

John B. Denny
Department of Ophthalmology, University of Texas Health Science Center, San Antonio, Texas, USA

Andrew Tee, Pei Y. Liu, Glenn M. Marshall and Tao Liu
Children's Cancer Institute Australia for Medical Research, Australia

Antonietta R. Farina, Lucia Cappabianca, Pierdomenico Ruggeri, Natalia Di Ianni, Marzia Ragone, Stefania Merolle and Andrew R. Mackay
Department of Experimental Medicine, University of L'Aquila, L'Aquila, Italy

Alberto Gulino
Department of Experimental Medicine and Pathology, University of Rome "La Sapienza", Rome, Italy

George Leondaritis, Xenia Koliou, Shalini Johnson, Chengjun Li, Andreas Florakis and Dimitra Mangoura
Neurosciences, Biomedical Research Foundation of the Academy of Athens (BRFAA) Athens, Greece

Konstantinos Dimas and Nikos Sakellaridis
Department of Pharmacology, Medical School, University of Thessaly, Larissa, Greece

Mehrdad Rahmaniyan, Amr Qudeimat and Jacqueline M. Kraveka
Division of Pediatric Hematology Oncology, Hollings Cancer Center and Darby Children's Research Institute, Medical University of South Carolina, USA

Vanessa Andries, Karl Vandepoele and Frans van Roy
Department for Molecular Biomedical Research, VIB, Belgium
Department of Biomedical Molecular Biology, Ghent University, Belgium

Magdalena Czarnecka, Jason Tilan and Joanna Kitlinska
Georgetown University, USA

Pietro Luigi Poliani
Department of Pathology, University of Brescia, Brescia, Italy

Domenico Ribatti
Department of Human Anatomy, University of Bari, Bari, Italy

Victoria R. Chu and Inhan Lee
miRcore, U.S.A.

Juan M. Escamilla, Christine Bäuerl, Carlos M. R. López, Satu P. Pekkala, and Domingo Barettino
Instituto de Biomedicina de Valencia, Consejo Superior de Investigaciones Científicas, Valencia,

Samuel Navarro
Dept. of Pathology, School of Medicine, University of Valencia, Valencia, Spain

Irena Horwacik and Hanna Rokita
The Jagiellonian University, Faculty of Biochemistry, Biophysics and Biotechnology, Laboratory of Molecular Genetics and Virology, Poland

Chengyuan Xue, Michelle Haber and Murray D. Norris
Children's Cancer Institute Australia for Medical Research, Lowy Cancer Research Centre, UNSW, Sydney, Australia

Andrei Gudkov
Roswell Park Cancer Institute, Buffalo, New York, USA

Yung-Feng Liao
Institute of Cellular and Organismic Biology, Academia Sinica, Taipei, Taiwan

Wen-Ming Hsu
Departments of Surgery, National Taiwan University Hospital and National Taiwan University, College of Medicine, Taipei, Taiwan

Hsiu-Hao Chang
Departments of Pediatrics, National Taiwan University Hospital and National Taiwan University, College of Medicine, Taipei, Taiwan

Yeou-Guang Tsay
Institute of Biochemistry and Molecular Biology and Proteomics Research Center, National Yang-Ming University, Taipei, Taiwan

Min-Chuan Huang
Graduate Institute of Anatomy and Cell Biology, National Taiwan University College of Medicine, Taipei, Taiwan

Ming-Kuan Hu
School of Pharmacy, National Defense Medical Center, Taipei, Taiwan

Hsinyu Lee
Department of Life Science and Institutes of Zoology, National Taiwan University, Taipei, Taiwan

Hsueh-Fen Juan
Department of Life Science and Institutes of Molecular and Cellular Biology, National Taiwan University, Taipei, Taiwan

Bo-Jeng Wang and Yu-Yin Shih
Institutes of Zoology, National Taiwan University, Taipei, Taiwan
Institute of Cellular and Organismic Biology, Academia Sinica, Taipei, Taiwan

Michael J. Ausserlechner
Medical University Innsbruck, Department of Pediatrics II, Tyrolean Cancer Research Institute, Austria

Stefan Fuchs and Kathrin Geiger
Medical University Innsbruck, Tyrolean Cancer Research Institute, Austria

Judith Hagenbuchner and Petra Obexer
Medical University Innsbruck, Department of Pediatrics IV, Tyrolean Cancer Research Institute, Austria

Hidemi Toyoda, Eckard Wimmer and Jeronimo Cello
Department of Molecular Genetics and Microbiology, Stony Brook University, Stony Brook, New York, USA